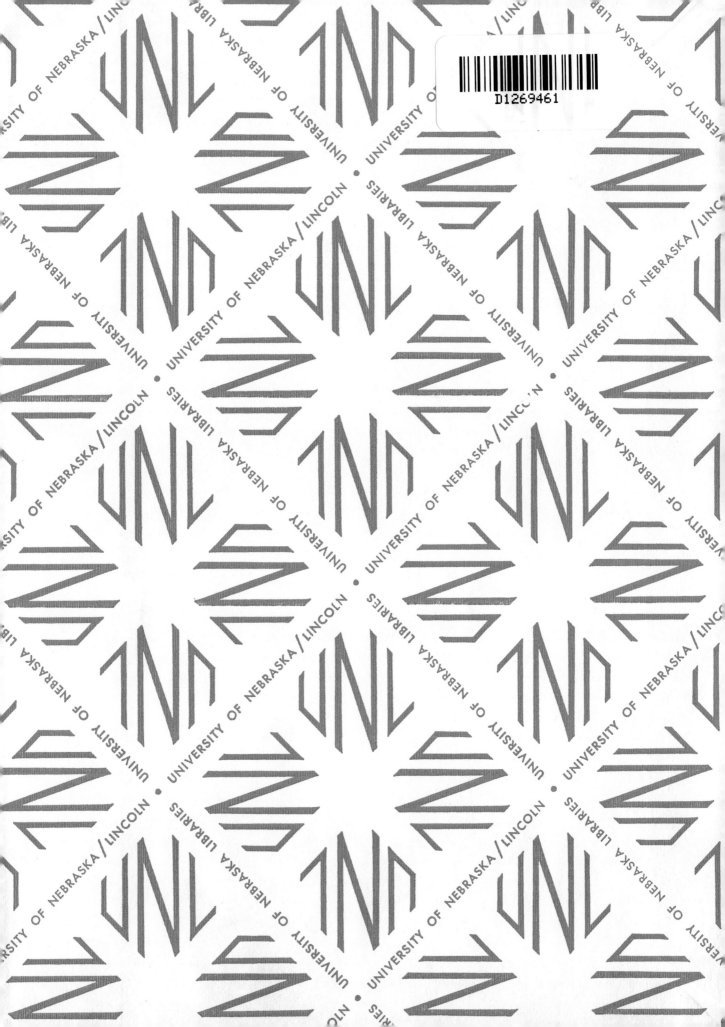
D1269461

ESTHETIC DENTISTRY

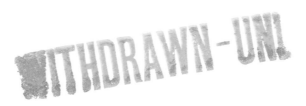
WITHDRAWN-UNI

BARRY G. DALE, D.M.D., F.A.C.D.

Assistant Clinical Professor, Department of Dentistry
Mount Sinai School of Medicine of the City University of New York
Assistant Attending Dentist, The Mount Sinai Hospital
New York, New York
Private Practice
Englewood, New Jersey

KENNETH W. ASCHHEIM, D.D.S., F.A.C.D.

Assistant Clinical Professor, Department of Dentistry
Mount Sinai School of Medicine of the City University of New York
Assistant Attending Dentist, The Mount Sinai Hospital
Private Practice
New York, New York

ESTHETIC DENTISTRY

A Clinical Approach to Techniques and Materials

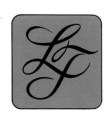

LEA & FEBIGER, Philadelphia, London 1993

Lea & Febiger
200 Chester Field Parkway
Box 3024
Malvern, Pennsylvania 19355-9725
U.S.A.
(215) 251-2230

Library of Congress Cataloging-in-Publication Data
Esthetic Dentistry : a clinical approach to techniques and materials /
   [edited by] Barry G. Dale, Kenneth W. Aschheim.
      p.   cm.
   Includes index.
   ISBN 0-8121-1467-1
   1. Dentistry—Aesthetics.   I. Dale, Barry G.   II. Aschheim,
Kenneth W.
   [DNLM: 1. Dental Materials.   2. Dental Restoration, Permanent.
3. Esthetics, Dental.   WU 100 E79]
RK54.E88 1992
617.9′676—dc20
DNLM/DLC   91-37519
for Library of Congress   CIP

Reprints of chapters may be purchased from Lea & Febiger in quantities of 100 or more. Contact Sally Grande in the Sales Department.

Copyright © 1993 by Lea & Febiger. Copyright under the International Copyright Union. All Rights Reserved. This book is protected by copyright. *No part of it may be reproduced in any manner or by any means without written permission from the publisher.*

PRINTED IN THE UNITED STATES OF AMERICA

Print number: 5 4 3 2 1

To my parents, Jack and Frances Dale, who built a strong foundation and to my wife, Ellen, my son, Adam and our child-to-be, who assure me the stars.

In memory of my parents, David and Edith Aschheim; together they pointed me in the right direction. And to my wife, Susan and children, Sara and Joshua, without whom I could not continue to find the way.

FOREWORD

Esthetic dentistry has become a reality. It is among the most stimulating and active areas in all of clinical dentistry. Most patients want to look better and feel better about themselves. This evolution from nothing to a major part of dentistry has happened in just a few years. As a result of the rapid changes that have occurred, it has been impossible for dentists to have state-of-the-art knowledge when graduating from dental school. Additionally, concepts and techniques have changed so fast that it is difficult for practitioners to keep their knowledge current.

Dental schools are responding as quickly as possible to the presence of procedures in esthetic dentistry, but changes in curricula come slowly. There are many dental continuing education courses in esthetic dentistry, but to this time there has not been a comprehensive textbook on the subject.

There are numerous subtopics in esthetic dentistry, because it spans nearly all of the clinical disciplines in dentistry as well as some in other parts of medicine. This book provides comprehensive consideration of this very broad subject of esthetic dentistry. This text provides authoritative, thorough, practical, and up-to-date information for those practitioners interested in knowing more about esthetic dentistry.

Gordon J. Christensen D.D.S., Ph.D.

PREFACE

Dental restorations exhibiting exquisite esthetics and physiologic function are well within the province of today's dentist. For the majority of practitioners, however, most of the information in the vast area of esthetic dentistry has changed dramatically or was simply unavailable during their formal dental training. The myriad choices of techniques and materials available may initially appear overwhelming. In reality, when properly organized, this body of knowledge is easily managed. This, then, was the challenge in preparing this book: to create a definitive, all encompassing, single source of information presented in a clinically relevant, "user-friendly" manner.

Resolution of a cosmetic dental problem requires the practitioner to determine a diagnosis, formulate a treatment plan, and select the appropriate instruments and materials. Treatment must then be performed in an orderly fashion with an understanding of proper clinical technique and specific material manipulations.

The confident clinician approaches any cosmetic dilemma in the above manner. We, therefore, organized this text to duplicate this sequence of thought processes and clinical operations.

A problem-oriented "trouble-shooting" section quickly guides the practitioner to appropriate information. It permits diagnosis and treatment planning at a glance followed by appropriate cross-referencing to more detailed discussions of material selection and clinical technique.

A materials-oriented section aids in selecting the correct materials for a specific clinical situation. The concise discussion of basic material science enables the clinician to fully understand the ramifications of differences in currently available materials. This further serves as a basis of comparison, enabling an effective evaluation of new materials as they are introduced. Detailed step-by-step clinical techniques delineate appropriate armamentarium and include specific procedural nuances and numerous highlighted "clinical tips." This facilitates a sound clinical approach. Also included is a comprehensive discussion of special considerations, indications, and contraindications for each technique and material presented, as well as numerous case presentations.

A specialty-oriented section presented by eminent practitioners addresses dental photography, color science, marketing, jurisprudence, orthodontics, periodontics, oral surgery, plastic surgery, dermatology, cosmetology, and psychology. The clinical relevance to the esthetic dentist is stressed through the use of case studies, sample laboratory prescriptions, office forms, and clinical techniques. Advanced techniques and criteria are presented to aid the dentist in determining when to refer a patient for specialty care.

As our profession enters the twenty-first century, esthetic dentistry offers a new era of doctor and patient satisfaction and excitement. We hope we have shared our own enthusiasm in the pages of this text.

Barry G. Dale, D.M.D., F.A.C.D.
Kenneth W. Aschheim, D.D.S., F.A.C.D.

ACKNOWLEDGMENTS

A textbook of this magnitude is not the undertaking of a few individuals; it is the culmination of the combined efforts of many. We owe an enormous debt not only to those pioneers of esthetics who have preceded us, but also to the gifted clinicians of today who seek to expand the envelope of knowledge. These people are our contributors. Their willingness and ability to surpass all expectations and to share in the common goal of creating a "state-of-the-art" text made this book possible. We wish to thank Dr. Rella Christensen for graciously providing the resource list. We also would like to extend a special thank you to Dr. Gordon Christensen for his contribution of the foreword.

We are greatly indebted to Ray Kersey and the executives at Lea & Febiger for having confidence in us during the book's gestation and early infancy. We also want to thank Tanya Lazar and Lisa Stead who guided us through the formative years and aided us in the editing of the text and to Mike DeNardo, our production manager, for his creativity and diligence. A particular debt of gratitude goes to Darlene Cooke, our executive editor, who, with her seasoned professional skills guided us through the intricacies of publishing and made certain that we did not lose sight of the forest for the trees. In addition, we wish to thank everyone else at both Lea & Febiger and Waverly Press, from marketing to production, from the art department to the editorial department, without whose efforts this book could not have been a success.

We also wish to thank all the laboratory technicians and manufacturers' representatives who supplied us with much of the necessary technical information. We must extend a special thank you to Adrian Jurim at McAndrews-Northern Laboratories and both Jack Karp and Arthur Saltzman at Jack Karp Laboratories, our reservoirs of information for some of the laboratory aspects of dental esthetics. An additional thank you goes to Barry Mermelstein of Healthco, Inc. for supplying us with information about many of the products in this textbook.

We also would like to thank Bonnie Young and Inez Felliciano for help in preparing the text. A special note of gratitude goes to Debbie Baer, Catherine Hill, Darlene Butko, and Millie Errante, as well as former and present dental assistants who helped "mind the store" while we worked on the book as well as aided us in compiling many of the clinical cases necessary for this text. We also owe particular gratitude to Dr. Jack Hirsch who, despite seeing his office overrun with "bookwork," was always there to provide much appreciated insight and guidance. An additional thank you to Eric Zaidins, Esq. for his advice and counsel.

We owe much to our colleagues at the Department of Dentistry of The Mount Sinai Medical Center for their continued support and guidance, especially Dr. Jack Klatell, Dr. Andrew Kaplan, and Dr. Daniel Buchbinder. We also must acknowledge the invaluable help provided by Dr. Brian Pollack, whose encyclopedic knowledge of dental materials helped ensure the accuracy of much of the material in this text. Also, a special thank you to Dr. Alfred Carin whose thoughtful insight from his many years in clinical practice was a welcome and necessary balance to much of the technical information presented.

A note of appreciation must be extended to our medical illustrator Caroline Meinstein. She never complained when asked to redraw an illustration a second and even a third time so as to ensure accuracy and clarity. Her good spirits, combined with her excellent technical skills, were an integral part of conveying many of the techniques illustrated in the book.

Finally, we wish to thank our families. For four years they have been textbook widows and orphans, often going to sleep as we continued to work late into the night only to awaken to see us back at work. Their unwavering love, encouragement and moral support not only made our lives easier but was ultimately the most important force ensuring a successful conclusion.

This is not merely a book of our experiences with dental esthetics, but a work of the combined experiences of all of the above people as well as many others whom we do not have the space to acknowledge separately. Through their efforts, we have been able to define and describe the state of esthetic dentistry today and lay the basic framework for the esthetic dentist of tomorrow.

Barry G. Dale, D.M.D., F.A.C.D.
Kenneth W. Aschheim, D.D.S., F.A.C.D.

CONTRIBUTOR LIST

FRED B. ABBOTT, D.D.S., M.D.S., F.A.C.D.
Practice Limited to Prosthodontics
Salisbury, Maryland
Former Associate Professor, School of Dentistry
Northwestern University
Chicago, Illinois

NELLIE ABBOTT, Ph.D., R.N.
Business Manager, Former Associate Administrator
Nursing Hospital of the University of Pennsylvania
Former Associate Dean, Nursing Practice
School of Nursing, University of Pennsylvania
Philadelphia, Pennsylvania

MILTON B. ASBELL, D.D.S., M.Sc., M.A.
Clinical Associate Professor, Department of Community
    Dentistry
Temple University School of Dentistry
Staff, Department of Dental Medicine Einstein Medical Center
Philadelphia, Pennsylvania

KENNETH W. ASCHHEIM, D.D.S., F.A.C.D.
Assistant Clinical Professor, Department of Dentistry
Mount Sinai School of Medicine of the City University of
    New York
Assistant Attending Dentist, The Mount Sinai Hospital
Private Practice
New York, New York

DAVID E. BELLER, D.M.D.
Diplomate, American Board of Oral and Maxillofacial Surgery
Fellow, American Association of Oral and Maxillofacial
    Surgeons
Assistant Clinical Professor of Oral and Maxillofacial Surgery,
New York University School of Dentistry
Private Practice
New York, New York

JERRY B. BLACK, D.M.D., M.S., F.A.C.D.
Private Practice
Birmingham, Alabama

PHILLIP BONNER, D.D.S.
President, Spectrum Healthcare Group, Inc.
Atlanta, Georgia

VINCENT CELENZA, D.M.D., F.A.C.P.
Diplomate, American Board of Prosthodontics
Clinical Assistant Professor, Department of Graduate Fixed
    Prosthodontics
New York University School of Dentistry
New York, New York
Private Practice
Scarsdale, New York

CHARLES I. CITRON, D.D.S., M.S.D.
Diplomate, American Academy of Pediatric Dentistry
Director of Pediatric Dentistry
Booth Memorial Medical Center
Flushing, New York

BARRY G. DALE, D.M.D., F.A.C.D.
Assistant Clinical Professor, Department of Dentistry
Mount Sinai School of Medicine of the City University of New
    York
Assistant Attending Dentist, The Mount Sinai Hospital
New York, New York
Private Practice
Englewood, New Jersey

DAVID R. FEDERICK, D.M.D., M.Sc.D.
Biomaterials Researcher, UCLA School of Dentistry
Los Angeles, California
Private Practice
Marina Del Rey, California

SAUL HOFFMAN, M.D., F.A.C.S.
Clinical Professor of Surgery, Mount Sinai School of Medicine of
    the City University of New York
Attending Surgeon, The Mount Sinai Hospital
Attending Surgeon, Beth Israel Hospital
Chief of Plastic Surgery, Doctors Hospital
New York, New York

PETER R. HUNT, B.D.S, M.Sc., L.D.S.R.C.S. Eng.
Clinical Associate Professor of Periodontics
University of Pennsylvania, School of Dental Medicine
Philadelphia, Pennsylvania

MARK JENSEN, MS, DDS, PhD., F.A.C.D., F.A.D.M.
Minnesota Dental Research Associates
Former Associate Professor, College of Dentistry
The University of Iowa
Private Practice
Iowa City, Iowa

MARK P. KING, D.D.S., M.S.
Assistant Professor
University of Texas, Dental Branch
Houston, Texas

AL KLIGMAN, M.D., Ph.D.
Professor of Dermatology, Center for Human Appearance
University of Pennsylvania Medical Center
Philadelphia, Pennsylvania

RICHARD LAZZARA, D.M.D., M.Sc.D
Clinical Assistant Professor, Advanced Education
Prosthodontics, USC School of Dentistry
Los Angeles, California
President, Implant Innovations
West Palm Beach, Flordia

MARK LEES, Ph.D, M.S.
CIDESCO Diplomate
Immediate Past Chairman
Esthetics Division, National Cosmetology Association
Private Practice
Pensacola, Florida

MARC R. LEFFLER, D.D.S.
Diplomate, American Board of Oral and Maxillofacial Surgery
Fellow, American Association of Oral and Maxillofacial
    Surgeons
Lecturer, Mount Sinai School of Medicine
Assistant, Department of Dentistry, Beth Israel Medical Center
New York, New York

CHARLES A. LENNON, D.M.D.
Assistant Attending Dentist (Prosthodontist)
New York Hospital Dental Center
Private Practice
New York, New York

RICHARD D. MILLER, D.D.S.
Clinical Associate Professor, Division of Restorative and
    Prosthodontic Sciences
New York University College of Dentistry
Private Practice
New York, New York

EDWARD C. MCNULTY, D.M.D., M.D.S., F.A.C.D., F.I.C.D.
Co-Chief, Orthodontic Division
Lenox Hill Hospital
Private Practice
New York, New York
Staff, Dental Clinic, Greenwich Hospital
Greenwich, Connecticut

ROSS W. NASH, D.D.S.
Clinical Instructor, Department of Restorative Dentistry
Medical College of Georgia
Augusta, Georgia
Private Practice
Charlotte, North Carolina

FRANCIS V. PANNO, B.S., D.D.S., F.A.C.P.
Diplomate, American Board of Prosthodontics
Professor and Chairman, Division of Restorative and
    Prosthodontics Sciences
New York University College of Dentistry
Private Practice
New York, New York

HERBERT M. PARKER, M.A., D.D.S.
Clinical Professor, Division of Restorative and Prosthodontic
    Sciences
New York University College of Dentistry
New York, New York

MICHAEL PERTSCHUK, M.D.
Clinical Associate Professor of Psychiatry
University of Pennsylvania Medical Center
Chairman, Department of Psychiatry
Graduate Hospital
Philadelphia, Pennsylvania

MITCHELL S. PINES, D.D.S.
Clinical Professor, Department of Restorative and Prosthodontic
    Sciences (Dental Materials)
New York University College of Dentistry
New York, New York
Private Practice
Rosyln Heights, New York

BURTON R. POLLACK, D.D.S., M.P.H., J.D.
Professor, School of Dental Medicine
State University of New York at Stony Brook
Stony Brook, New York

BRIAN POLLACK, D.D.S., F.A.C.D., F.I.C.D., M.A.G.D.
Associate Clinical Professor
Director of Dental Materials Research
Section Chief, General Dentistry
Mount Sinai Medical Center
Private Practice
New York, New York

EDWIN S. ROSENBERG, B.D.S., H.D.D., D.M.D., F.I.C.D., F.A.C.D., F.C.R
Professor and Chairman, Department of Periodontics
Director and Chairman, Dental Implantology
Temple University School of Dentistry
Clinical Professor, Department of Periodontics
University of Pennsylvania, School of Dental Medicine
Clinical Professor of Dental Medicine
Medical College of Pennsylvania
Philadelphia, Pennsylvania

SIDNEY I. SILVERMAN, D.D.S.
Diplomate, American Board of Prosthodontics and Occlusion
Research Professor, Division of Restorative and Prosthodontic
  Services
Attending Dentist, Department of Oral Surgery, University
  Hospital
New York University College of Dentistry
Clinical Professor, Department of Clinical Neurology
New York University School of Medicine
New York, New York

BRUCE A. SINGER, B.S., D.D.S.
Clinical Assistant Professor, Department of General Restorative
  Dentistry
University of Pennsylvania School of Dental Medicine
Philadelphia, Pennsylvania
Director of Scientific Photography, Dental Division
Albert Einstein Medical Center, North Division
Jenkintown, Pennsylvania

VAN P. THOMPSON, D.D.S, Ph.D.
Director of Biomaterials and Clinical Research Unit
Professor of General Dentistry
University of Maryland School of Dentistry
Baltimore, Maryland

JAMES TOROSIAN, D.M.D.
Assistant Clinical Professor Department of Dental Hygiene
Thomas Jefferson University Hospital
Philadelphia, Pennsylvania

MORTON WOOD, D.D.S., M.Ed.
Assistant Professor of Restorative Dentistry
University of Maryland School of Dentistry
Baltimore, Maryland

IRA D. ZINNER, D.D.S., M.S.D., F.A.C.P.
Diplomate, American Board of Prosthodontics
Clinical Professor, Division of Restorative and Prosthodontics
  Sciences
New York University College of Dentistry
Private Practice
New York, New York

CONTENTS

CHAPTER 4. COLOR MODIFIERS AND OPAQUERS

Jerry B. Black

CHAPTER 5. COMPOSITE RESIN—FUNDAMENTALS AND DIRECT TECHNIQUE RESTORATIONS

Brian Pollack

CHAPTER 6. COMPOSITE RESIN — INDIRECT TECHNIQUE RESTORATIONS

Ross W. Nash

CHAPTER 7. GLASS IONOMER CEMENTS

Peter R. Hunt

CHAPTER 8. CERAMOMETAL — FULL COVERAGE RESTORATIONS

Ira D. Zinner
Francis V. Panno
Richard D. Miller
Herbert M. Parker
Mitchell S. Pines

CHAPTER 11. PORCELAIN—LAMINATE VENEERS AND OTHER PARTIAL COVERAGE RESTORATIONS

Kenneth W. Aschheim
Barry G. Dale

CHAPTER 12. ADHESIVE RESIN BONDED CAST RESTORATIONS

Morton Wood
Van Thompson

CHAPTER 13. ACRYLIC AND OTHER RESINS— PROVISIONAL RESTORATIONS

David Federick

CHAPTER 14. ACRYLIC AND OTHER RESINS— REMOVABLE PROSTHESES

Sidney I. Silverman

CHAPTER 15. BLEACHING AND RELATED AGENTS

Barry G. Dale

CHAPTER 16. ESTHETICS AND PSYCHOLOGY

Fred B. Abbott
Nellie Abbott

CHAPTER 17. ESTHETICS AND ORAL PHOTOGRAPHY

Mark King

CHAPTER 20. ESTHETICS AND PEDODONTICS

Charles I. Citron

CHAPTER 21. ESTHETICS AND PERIODONTICS

Edwin S. Rosenberg
James Torosian

CHAPTER 22. ESTHETICS AND ORTHODONTICS
Edward McNulty

CHAPTER 23. ESTHETICS AND ORAL SURGERY
David Beller
Marc R. Leffler

CHAPTER 24. ESTHETICS AND PLASTIC SURGERY

Saul Hoffman

CHAPTER 25. ESTHETICS AND DERMATOLOGY

Michael J. Pertschuk
Albert M. Kligman

CHAPTER 26. ESTHETICS AND COSMETOLOGY

Mark Lees

CHAPTER 27. ESTHETICS AND DENTAL MARKETING   **Phillip Bonner**

CHAPTER 28. ESTHETICS AND DENTAL JURISPRUDENCE   **Burton R. Pollack**

CHAPTER 29. ESTHETICS AND ADVANCED TECHNOLOGY   Kenneth W. Aschheim

APPENDIX A—CUSTOM STAINING   Kenneth W. Aschheim
Barry G. Dale

APPENDIX B. NINETY-SECOND RUBBER DAM PLACEMENT

Barry G. Dale

APPENDIX C. SMILE ANALYSIS

Barry G. Dale
Kenneth W. Aschheim

APPENDIX D. SAMPLE LEGAL FORMS

APPENDIX E. LIST OF MANUFACTURERS

INDEX

TROUBLESHOOTING GUIDE

This problem-oriented troubleshooting guide serves as an efficient treatment planning aid. Each esthetic problem is cross referenced to the appropriate chapter or chapters which provide more detailed technique and material information. Clinical conditions that are common to more than one category are appropriately repeated.

The guide is divided into the following categories:

Clinical conditions which are common to more than one category are appropriately repeated.

TOOTH RELATED PROBLEMS

Size And Shape Problems

Problem	Solution	Chapter	Title
Abrasion	Direct composite resin restoration	CHAPTER 4	Color Modifiers and Opaquers
		CHAPTER 5	Composite Resin — Fundamentals and Direct Technique Restorations
	Indirect composite resin restoration	CHAPTER 6	Composite Resin — Indirect Technique Restorations
	Glass ionomer restoration (non-stress bearing areas only)	CHAPTER 7	Glass Ionomer Cements
	Ceramometal restoration	CHAPTER 8	Ceramometal — Full Coverage Restorations
	Cast glass restoration	CHAPTER 9	Cast Glass Ceramic — Full Coverage Restorations
	All-porcelain restoration	CHAPTER 10	Porcelain — Full Coverage Restorations
	Porcelain laminate veneer or partial coverage restoration	CHAPTER 11	Porcelain — Laminate Veneer and Other Partial Coverage Restorations
Aged Teeth — Worn	Direct composite resin veneers	CHAPTER 4	Color Modifiers and Opaquers
		CHAPTER 5	Composite Resin — Fundamentals and Direct Technique Restorations
	Indirect composite resin veneers	CHAPTER 6	Composite Resin — Indirect Technique Restorations
	Ceramometal — full coverage restorations	CHAPTER 8	Ceramometal — Full Coverage Restorations
	Cast glass restorations	CHAPTER 9	Cast Glass Ceramic — Full Coverage Restorations
	All-porcelain restorations	CHAPTER 10	Porcelain — Full Coverage Restorations
	Porcelain laminate veneers or partial coverage restorations	CHAPTER 11	Porcelain — Laminate Veneer and Other Partial Coverage Restorations
Anterior Tooth — Chipped or Fractured	Cosmetic recontouring	CHAPTER 2	Fundamentals of Esthetics
	Direct composite resin veneer	CHAPTER 4	Color Modifiers and Opaquers
		CHAPTER 5	Composite Resin — Fundamentals and Direct Technique Restorations

Problem	Solution	Chapter	Title
Anterior Tooth — Chipped or Fractured (continued)	Indirect composite resin veneer	CHAPTER 6	Composite Resin — Indirect Technique Restorations
	Glass ionomer restoration (non-stress bearing areas only)	CHAPTER 7	Glass Ionomer Cements
	Ceramometal restoration	CHAPTER 8	Ceramometal — Full Coverage Restorations
	Cast glass restoration	CHAPTER 9	Cast Glass Ceramic — Full Coverage Restorations
	All-porcelain restoration	CHAPTER 10	Porcelain — Full Coverage Restorations
	Porcelain laminate veneer	CHAPTER 11	Porcelain — Laminate Veneer and Other Partial Coverage Restorations
Attrition	Direct composite resin veneer (in selected cases)	CHAPTER 4	Color Modifiers and Opaquers
		CHAPTER 5	Composite Resin — Fundamentals and Direct Technique Restorations
	Indirect composite resin restoration (in selected cases)	CHAPTER 6	Composite Resin — Indirect Technique Restorations
	Ceramometal restoration	CHAPTER 8	Ceramometal — Full Coverage Restorations
	Cast glass restoration (in selected cases)	CHAPTER 9	Cast Glass Ceramic — Full Coverage Restorations
	All-porcelain restoration (in selected cases)	CHAPTER 10	Porcelain — Full Coverage Restorations
	Porcelain laminate veneer or partial coverage restoration (in selected cases)	CHAPTER 11	Porcelain — Laminate Veneer and Other Partial Coverage Restorations
Chipped Tooth	Cosmetic recontouring	CHAPTER 2	Fundamentals of Esthetics
	Direct composite resin restoration	CHAPTER 4	Color Modifiers and Opaquers
		CHAPTER 5	Composite Resin — Fundamentals and Direct Technique Restorations
	Indirect composite resin restoration	CHAPTER 6	Composite Resin — Indirect Technique Restorations
	Glass ionomer restoration (non-stress bearing areas only)	CHAPTER 7	Glass Ionomer Cements
	Ceramometal restoration	CHAPTER 8	Ceramometal — Full Coverage Restorations
	Cast glass restoration	CHAPTER 9	Cast Glass Ceramic — Full Coverage Restorations

Problem	Solution	Chapter	Title
Chipped Tooth (continued)	All-porcelain restoration	CHAPTER 10	Porcelain — Full Coverage Restorations
	Porcelain laminate veneer or partial coverage restoration	CHAPTER 11	Porcelain — Laminate Veneer and Other Partial Coverage Restorations
	Direct composite resin restoration	CHAPTER 4	Color Modifiers and Opaquers
		CHAPTER 5	Composite Resin — Fundamentals and Direct Technique Restorations
	Indirect composite resin restoration	CHAPTER 6	Composite Resin — Indirect Technique Restorations
Erosion	Glass ionomer restoration (non-stress bearing areas only)	CHAPTER 7	Glass Ionomer Cements
	Ceramometal restoration	CHAPTER 8	Ceramometal — Full Coverage Restorations
	Cast glass restoration	CHAPTER 9	Cast Glass Ceramic — Full Coverage Restorations
	All-porcelain restoration	CHAPTER 10	Porcelain — Full Coverage Restorations
	Porcelain laminate veneer or partial coverage restoration	CHAPTER 11	Porcelain — Laminate Veneer and Other Partial Coverage Restorations
	Cosmetic recontouring	CHAPTER 2	Fundamentals of Esthetics
	Ceramometal restoration (possibly combined with endodontic and periodontal therapy)	CHAPTER 8	Ceramometal — Full Coverage Restorations
	Cast glass restoration (possibly combined with endodontic and periodontal therapy)	CHAPTER 9	Cast Glass Ceramic — Full Coverage Restorations
	All-porcelain restoration (possibly combined with endodontic and periodontal therapy)	CHAPTER 10	Porcelain — Full Coverage Restorations
Extruded Tooth	Porcelain laminate veneer or partial coverage restoration (possibly combined with endodontic and periodontal therapy)(sufficient tooth structure must be present)	CHAPTER 11	Porcelain — Laminate Veneer and Other Partial Coverage Restorations
	Gingival recontouring — electrosurgery (if necessary)	CHAPTER 18	Esthetics and Electrosurgery
	Gingival grafting (if accompanied by recession)	CHAPTER 21	Esthetics and Periodontics
	Artificial gingiva (if accompanied by recession)	CHAPTER 21	Esthetics and Periodontics

Problem	Solution	Chapter	Title
Extruded Tooth (continued)	Gingival recontouring (if necessary)	CHAPTER 21	Esthetics and Periodontics
	Orthodontic therapy	CHAPTER 22	Esthetics and Orthodontics
	Orthognathic surgery	CHAPTER 23	Esthetics and Oral Surgery
Feminine Teeth — Exaggerated	Cosmetic recontouring	CHAPTER 2	Fundamentals of Esthetics
	Cosmetic recontouring	CHAPTER 2	Fundamentals of Esthetics
		CHAPTER 4	Color Modifiers and Opaquers
	Direct composite resin restoration	CHAPTER 5	Composite Resin — Fundamentals and Direct Technique Restorations
	Indirect composite resin restoration	CHAPTER 6	Composite Resin — Indirect Technique Restorations
Fractured Tooth	Glass ionomer restoration (non-stress bearing areas only)	CHAPTER 7	Glass Ionomer Cements
	Ceramometal restoration	CHAPTER 8	Ceramometal — Full Coverage Restorations
	Cast glass restoration	CHAPTER 9	Cast Glass Ceramic — Full Coverage Restorations
	All-porcelain restoration	CHAPTER 10	Porcelain — Full Coverage Restorations
	Porcelain laminate veneer or partial coverage restoration	CHAPTER 11	Porcelain — Laminate Veneer and Other Partial Coverage Restorations
High Smile Line	Cosmetic recontouring	CHAPTER 2	Fundamentals of Esthetics
	Gingival recontouring — electrosurgery (with restoration — see Long Tooth)	CHAPTER 18	Esthetics and Electrosurgery
	Gingival recontouring (with restoration — see Long Tooth)	CHAPTER 21	Esthetics and Periodontics
	Oral surgery (with restoration — see Long Tooth)	CHAPTER 23	Esthetics and Oral Surgery
Large Tooth	Cosmetic recontouring	CHAPTER 2	Fundamentals of Esthetics

Problem	Solution	Chapter	Title
Large Tooth (continued)	Direct composite resin restoration	CHAPTER 4	Color Modifiers and Opaquers
		CHAPTER 5	Composite Resin — Fundamentals and Direct Technique Restorations
	Indirect composite resin restoration	CHAPTER 6	Composite Resin — Indirect Technique Restorations
	Ceramometal restoration	CHAPTER 8	Ceramometal — Full Coverage Restorations
	Cast glass restoration	CHAPTER 9	Cast Glass Ceramic — Full Coverage Restorations
	All-porcelain restoration	CHAPTER 10	Porcelain — Full Coverage Restorations
	Porcelain laminate veneer or partial coverage restoration	CHAPTER 11	Porcelain — Laminate Veneer and Other Partial Coverage Restorations
Long Tooth	Cosmetic recontouring	CHAPTER 2	Fundamentals of Esthetics
	Direct composite resin restoration	CHAPTER 4	Color Modifiers and Opaquers
		CHAPTER 5	Composite Resin — Fundamentals and Direct Technique Restorations
	Indirect composite resin restoration	CHAPTER 6	Composite Resin — Indirect Technique Restorations
	Ceramometal restoration (possibly combined with endodontic and periodontal therapy)	CHAPTER 8	Ceramometal — Full Coverage Restorations
	Cast glass restoration (possibly combined with endodontic and periodontal therapy)	CHAPTER 9	Cast Glass Ceramic — Full Coverage Restorations
	All-porcelain restoration (possibly combined with endodontic and periodontal therapy)	CHAPTER 10	Porcelain — Full Coverage Restorations
	Porcelain laminate veneer or partial coverage restoration (possibly combined with endodontic and periodontal therapy)(sufficient tooth structure must be present)	CHAPTER 11	Porcelain — Laminate Veneer and Other Partial Coverage Restorations
	Gingival grafting (if accompanied by recession)	CHAPTER 21	Esthetics and Periodontics
	Artificial gingiva	CHAPTER 21	Esthetics and Periodontics
	Orthodontic therapy	CHAPTER 22	Esthetics and Orthodontics
	Orthognathic surgery	CHAPTER 23	Esthetics and Oral Surgery

Problem	Solution	Chapter	Title
Malformed Teeth — Mild	Cosmetic recontouring	CHAPTER 2	Fundamentals of Esthetics
	Direct composite resin restorations	CHAPTER 4	Color Modifiers and Opaquers
		CHAPTER 5	Composite Resin — Fundamentals and Direct Technique Restorations
	Indirect composite resin restorations	CHAPTER 6	Composite Resin — Indirect Technique Restorations
	Ceramometal — full coverage restorations	CHAPTER 8	Ceramometal — Full Coverage Restorations
	Cast glass restorations	CHAPTER 9	Cast Glass Ceramic — Full Coverage Restorations
	All-porcelain restorations	CHAPTER 10	Porcelain — Full Coverage Restorations
	Porcelain laminate veneers or partial coverage restorations	CHAPTER 11	Porcelain — Laminate Veneer and Other Partial Coverage Restorations
Malformed Teeth — Severe	Direct composite resin restorations	CHAPTER 4	Color Modifiers and Opaquers
		CHAPTER 5	Composite Resin — Fundamentals and Direct Technique Restorations
	Indirect composite resin restorations	CHAPTER 6	Composite Resin — Indirect Technique Restorations
	Ceramometal — full coverage restorations	CHAPTER 8	Ceramometal — Full Coverage Restorations
	Cast glass restorations	CHAPTER 9	Cast Glass Ceramic — Full Coverage Restorations
	All-porcelain restorations	CHAPTER 10	Porcelain — Full Coverage Restorations
	Porcelain laminate veneers or partial coverage restorations	CHAPTER 11	Porcelain — Laminate Veneer and Other Partial Coverage Restorations
Masculine Teeth — Exaggerated	Cosmetic recontouring	CHAPTER 2	Fundamentals of Esthetics
Narrow Tooth	Cosmetic recontouring	CHAPTER 2	Fundamentals of Esthetics
	Direct composite resin restoration	CHAPTER 4	Color Modifiers and Opaquers
		CHAPTER 5	Composite Resin — Fundamentals and Direct Technique Restorations

Problem	Solution	Chapter	Title
Narrow Tooth (continued)	Indirect composite resin restoration	CHAPTER 6	Composite Resin — Indirect Technique Restorations
	Glass ionomer restoration (non-stress bearing areas only)	CHAPTER 7	Glass Ionomer Cements
	Ceramometal restoration	CHAPTER 8	Ceramometal — Full Coverage Restorations
	Cast glass restoration	CHAPTER 9	Cast Glass Ceramic — Full Coverage Restorations
	All-porcelain restoration	CHAPTER 10	Porcelain — Full Coverage Restorations
	Porcelain laminate veneer or partial coverage restoration	CHAPTER 11	Porcelain — Laminate Veneer and Other Partial Coverage Restorations
Peg Lateral Incisor	Direct composite resin restoration	CHAPTER 4	Color Modifiers and Opaquers
		CHAPTER 5	Composite Resin — Fundamentals and Direct Technique Restorations
	Indirect composite resin restoration	CHAPTER 6	Composite Resin — Indirect Technique Restorations
	Ceramometal restoration	CHAPTER 8	Ceramometal — Full Coverage Restorations
	Cast glass restoration	CHAPTER 9	Cast Glass Ceramic — Full Coverage Restorations
	All-porcelain restoration	CHAPTER 10	Porcelain — Full Coverage Restorations
	Porcelain laminate veneer or partial coverage restoration	CHAPTER 11	Porcelain — Laminate Veneer and Other Partial Coverage Restorations
Short Tooth	Cosmetic recontouring	CHAPTER 2	Fundamentals of Esthetics
	Direct composite resin restoration	CHAPTER 4	Color Modifiers and Opaquers
		CHAPTER 5	Composite Resin — Fundamentals and Direct Technique Restorations
	Indirect composite resin restoration	CHAPTER 6	Composite Resin — Indirect Technique Restorations
	Ceramometal restoration	CHAPTER 8	Ceramometal — Full Coverage Restorations
	Cast glass restoration	CHAPTER 9	Cast Glass Ceramic — Full Coverage Restorations
	All-porcelain restoration	CHAPTER 10	Porcelain — Full Coverage Restorations

Problem	Solution	Chapter	Title
Short Tooth (continued)	Porcelain laminate veneer or partial coverage restoration	CHAPTER 11	Porcelain — Laminate Veneer and Other Partial Coverage Restorations
	Gingival recontouring — electrosurgery	CHAPTER 18	Esthetics and Electrosurgery
	Gingival recontouring	CHAPTER 21	Esthetics and Periodontics
	Cosmetic recontouring	CHAPTER 2	Fundamentals of Esthetics
		CHAPTER 4	Color Modifiers and Opaquers
	Direct composite resin restoration	CHAPTER 5	Composite Resin — Fundamentals and Direct Technique Restorations
	Indirect composite resin restoration	CHAPTER 6	Composite Resin — Indirect Technique Restorations
Small Tooth	Glass ionomer restoration (non-stress bearing areas only)	CHAPTER 7	Glass Ionomer Cements
	Ceramometal restoration	CHAPTER 8	Ceramometal — Full Coverage Restorations
	Cast glass restoration	CHAPTER 9	Cast Glass Ceramic — Full Coverage Restorations
	All-porcelain restoration	CHAPTER 10	Porcelain — Full Coverage Restorations
	Porcelain laminate veneer or partial coverage restoration	CHAPTER 11	Porcelain — Laminate Veneer and Other Partial Coverage Restorations
	Gingival recontouring — electrosurgery	CHAPTER 18	Esthetics and Electrosurgery
	Gingival recontouring	CHAPTER 21	Esthetics and Periodontics
Wide Tooth	Cosmetic recontouring	CHAPTER 2	Fundamentals of Esthetics
		CHAPTER 4	Color Modifiers and Opaquers
	Direct composite resin restoration	CHAPTER 5	Composite Resin — Fundamentals and Direct Technique Restorations
	Indirect composite resin restoration	CHAPTER 6	Composite Resin — Indirect Technique Restorations
	Ceramometal restoration	CHAPTER 8	Ceramometal — Full Coverage Restorations
	Cast glass restoration	CHAPTER 9	Cast Glass Ceramic — Full Coverage Restorations
	All-porcelain restoration	CHAPTER 10	Porcelain — Full Coverage Restorations

Problem	Solution	Chapter	Title
Wide Tooth (continued)	Porcelain laminate veneer or partial coverage restoration	CHAPTER 11	Porcelain — Laminate Veneer and Other Partial Coverage Restorations
Position Problems			
Anterior Flared Teeth — Major	Orthodontic therapy	CHAPTER 22	Esthetics and Orthodontics
	Direct composite resin restorations	CHAPTER 4	Color Modifiers and Opaquers
		CHAPTER 5	Composite Resin — Fundamentals and Direct Technique Restorations
	Indirect composite resin restorations	CHAPTER 6	Composite Resin — Indirect Technique Restorations
	Ceramometal — full coverage restorations	CHAPTER 8	Ceramometal — Full Coverage Restorations
	Cast glass restorations	CHAPTER 9	Cast Glass Ceramic — Full Coverage Restorations
	All-porcelain restorations	CHAPTER 10	Porcelain — Full Coverage Restorations
Anterior Flared Teeth — Minor	Porcelain laminate veneers or partial coverage restorations	CHAPTER 11	Porcelain — Laminate Veneer and Other Partial Coverage Restorations
	Orthodontic therapy	CHAPTER 22	Esthetics and Orthodontics
	Cosmetic recontouring	CHAPTER 2	Fundamentals of Esthetics
	Direct composite resin restorations	CHAPTER 4	Color Modifiers and Opaquers
		CHAPTER 5	Composite Resin — Fundamentals and Direct Technique Restorations
	Indirect composite resin restorations	CHAPTER 6	Composite Resin — Indirect Technique Restorations
Crowding	Glass ionomer restorations (non-stress bearing areas only)	CHAPTER 7	Glass Ionomer Cements
	Ceramometal — full coverage restorations	CHAPTER 8	Ceramometal — Full Coverage Restorations
	Cast glass restorations	CHAPTER 9	Cast Glass Ceramic — Full Coverage Restorations
	All-porcelain restorations	CHAPTER 10	Porcelain — Full Coverage Restorations

Problem	Solution	Chapter	Title
Crowding (continued)	Porcelain laminate veneers or partial coverage restorations	CHAPTER 11	Porcelain — Laminate Veneer and Other Partial Coverage Restorations
	Orthodontic therapy	CHAPTER 22	Esthetics and Orthodontics
Diastemata	Direct composite resin restorations	CHAPTER 4	Color Modifiers and Opaquers
		CHAPTER 5	Composite Resin — Fundamentals and Direct Technique Restorations
	Indirect composite resin restorations	CHAPTER 6	Composite Resin — Indirect Technique Restorations
	Ceramometal — full coverage restorations	CHAPTER 8	Ceramometal — Full Coverage Restorations
	Cast glass restorations	CHAPTER 9	Cast Glass Ceramic — Full Coverage Restorations
	All-porcelain restorations	CHAPTER 10	Porcelain — Full Coverage Restorations
	Porcelain laminate veneers or partial coverage restorations	CHAPTER 11	Porcelain — Laminate Veneer and Other Partial Coverage Restorations
	Orthodontic therapy	CHAPTER 22	Esthetics and Orthodontics
Excessive Spacing	Direct composite resin veneers	CHAPTER 4	Color Modifiers and Opaquers
		CHAPTER 5	Composite Resin — Fundamentals and Direct Technique Restorations
	Indirect composite resin veneers	CHAPTER 6	Composite Resin — Indirect Technique Restorations
	Ceramometal — full coverage restorations	CHAPTER 8	Ceramometal — Full Coverage Restorations
	Cast glass restorations	CHAPTER 9	Cast Glass Ceramic — Full Coverage Restorations
	All-porcelain restorations	CHAPTER 10	Porcelain — Full Coverage Restorations
	Porcelain laminate veneers	CHAPTER 11	Porcelain — Laminate Veneer and Other Partial Coverage Restorations
	Orthodontic therapy	CHAPTER 22	Esthetics and Orthodontics
Extruded Tooth	Cosmetic recontouring	CHAPTER 2	Fundamentals of Esthetics
	Ceramometal restoration (possibly combined with endodontic and periodontal therapy)	CHAPTER 8	Ceramometal — Full Coverage Restorations

Problem	Solution	Chapter	Title
Extruded Tooth (continued)	Cast glass restoration (possibly combined with endodontic and periodontal therapy)	CHAPTER 9	Cast Glass Ceramic — Full Coverage Restorations
	All-porcelain restoration (possibly combined with endodontic and periodontal therapy)	CHAPTER 10	Porcelain — Full Coverage Restorations
	Porcelain laminate veneer or partial coverage restoration (possibly combined with endodontic and periodontal therapy)(sufficient tooth structure must be present)	CHAPTER 11	Porcelain — Laminate Veneer and Other Partial Coverage Restorations
	Gingival recontouring — electrosurgery (if necessary)	CHAPTER 18	Esthetics and Electrosurgery
	Gingival grafting (if accompanied by recession)	CHAPTER 21	Esthetics and Periodontics
	Artificial gingiva (if accompanied by recession)	CHAPTER 21	Esthetics and Periodontics
	Gingival recontouring — electrosurgery (if necessary)	CHAPTER 21	Esthetics and Periodontics
	Orthodontic therapy	CHAPTER 22	Esthetics and Orthodontics
	Orthognathic surgery	CHAPTER 23	Esthetics and Oral Surgery
Generalized Spacing	Direct composite resin veneers	CHAPTER 4	Color Modifiers and Opaquers
		CHAPTER 5	Composite Resin — Fundamentals and Direct Technique Restorations
	Indirect composite resin veneers	CHAPTER 6	Composite Resin — Indirect Technique Restorations
	Ceramometal — full coverage restorations	CHAPTER 8	Ceramometal — Full Coverage Restorations
	Cast glass restorations	CHAPTER 9	Cast Glass Ceramic — Full Coverage Restorations
	All-porcelain restorations	CHAPTER 10	Porcelain — Full Coverage Restorations
	Porcelain laminate veneers	CHAPTER 11	Porcelain — Laminate Veneer and Other Partial Coverage Restorations
	Orthodontic therapy	CHAPTER 22	Esthetics and Orthodontics
High Smile Line	Cosmetic recontouring	CHAPTER 2	Fundamentals of Esthetics
	Gingival recontouring — electrosurgery (with restoration — see Long Tooth)	CHAPTER 18	Esthetics and Electrosurgery

Problem	Solution	Chapter	Title
High Smile Line (continued)	Gingival recontouring (with restoration — see Long Tooth)	CHAPTER 21	Esthetics and Periodontics
	Oral surgery (with restoration — see Long Tooth)	CHAPTER 23	Esthetics and Oral Surgery
	Cosmetic recontouring	CHAPTER 2	Fundamentals of Esthetics
	Direct composite resin restoration	CHAPTER 4	Color Modifiers and Opaquers
		CHAPTER 5	Composite Resin — Fundamentals and Direct Technique Restorations
	Indirect composite resin restoration	CHAPTER 6	Composite Resin — Indirect Technique Restorations
	Ceramometal restoration (possibly combined with endodontic and periodontal therapy)	CHAPTER 8	Ceramometal — Full Coverage Restorations
	Cast glass restoration (possibly combined with endodontic and periodontal therapy)	CHAPTER 9	Cast Glass Ceramic — Full Coverage Restorations
	All-porcelain restoration (possibly combined with endodontic and periodontal therapy)	CHAPTER 10	Porcelain — Full Coverage Restorations
Long Tooth	Porcelain laminate veneer or partial coverage restoration (possibly combined with endodontic and periodontal therapy)(sufficient tooth structure must be present)	CHAPTER 11	Porcelain — Laminate Veneer and Other Partial Coverage Restorations
	Gingival recontouring — electrosurgery (if necessary)	CHAPTER 18	Esthetics and Electrosurgery
	Gingival grafting (if accompanied by recession)	CHAPTER 21	Esthetics and Periodontics
	Artificial gingiva (if accompanied by recession)	CHAPTER 21	Esthetics and Periodontics
	Gingival recontouring — electrosurgery (if necessary)	CHAPTER 21	Esthetics and Periodontics
	Orthodontic therapy	CHAPTER 22	Esthetics and Orthodontics
	Orthognathic surgery	CHAPTER 23	Esthetics and Oral Surgery
Midline Disharmony	Cosmetic recontouring	CHAPTER 2	Fundamentals of Esthetics

Problem	Solution	Chapter	Title
Midline Disharmony (continued)	Ceramometal — full coverage restorations	CHAPTER 8	Ceramometal — Full Coverage Restorations
	Cast glass restorations	CHAPTER 9	Cast Glass Ceramic — Full Coverage Restorations
	All-porcelain restorations	CHAPTER 10	Porcelain — Full Coverage Restorations
	Porcelain laminate veneer	CHAPTER 11	Porcelain — Laminate Veneer and Other Partial Coverage Restorations
	Orthodontic therapy	CHAPTER 22	Esthetics and Orthodontics
Migrated Teeth	Orthodontic therapy	CHAPTER 22	Esthetics and Orthodontics
Multiple Diastemata	Direct composite resin veneers	CHAPTER 4	Color Modifiers and Opaquers
		CHAPTER 5	Composite Resin — Fundamentals and Direct Technique Restorations
	Indirect composite resin veneers	CHAPTER 6	Composite Resin — Indirect Technique Restorations
	Ceramometal — full coverage restorations	CHAPTER 8	Ceramometal — Full Coverage Restorations
	Cast glass restorations	CHAPTER 9	Cast Glass Ceramic — Full Coverage Restorations
	All-porcelain restorations	CHAPTER 10	Porcelain — Full Coverage Restorations
	Porcelain laminate veneers	CHAPTER 11	Porcelain — Laminate Veneer and Other Partial Coverage Restorations
Open Bite — Mild	Direct composite resin veneers	CHAPTER 4	Color Modifiers and Opaquers
		CHAPTER 5	Composite Resin — Fundamentals and Direct Technique Restorations
	Indirect composite resin veneers	CHAPTER 6	Composite Resin — Indirect Technique Restorations
	Ceramometal — full coverage restorations	CHAPTER 8	Ceramometal — Full Coverage Restorations
	Cast glass restorations	CHAPTER 9	Cast Glass Ceramic — Full Coverage Restorations
	All-porcelain restorations	CHAPTER 10	Porcelain — Full Coverage Restorations
	Porcelain laminate veneers	CHAPTER 11	Porcelain — Laminate Veneer and Other Partial Coverage Restorations
	Orthodontic therapy	CHAPTER 22	Esthetics and Orthodontics
	Orthognathic surgery	CHAPTER 23	Esthetics and Oral Surgery

Problem	Solution	Chapter	Title
Open Bite — Severe	Orthodontic therapy	CHAPTER 22	Esthetics and Orthodontics
	Orthognathic surgery	CHAPTER 23	Esthetics and Oral Surgery
Overbite/ Overjet	Orthodontic therapy	CHAPTER 22	Esthetics and Orthodontics
	Orthognathic surgery	CHAPTER 23	Esthetics and Oral Surgery
Spacing	Direct composite resin veneers	CHAPTER 4	Color Modifiers and Opaquers
		CHAPTER 5	Composite Resin — Fundamentals and Direct Technique Restorations
	Indirect composite resin veneers	CHAPTER 6	Composite Resin — Indirect Technique Restorations
	Ceramometal — full coverage restorations	CHAPTER 8	Ceramometal — Full Coverage Restorations
	Cast glass restorations	CHAPTER 9	Cast Glass Ceramic — Full Coverage Restorations
	All-porcelain restorations	CHAPTER 10	Porcelain — Full Coverage Restorations
	Porcelain laminate veneers	CHAPTER 11	Porcelain — Laminate Veneer and Other Partial Coverage Restorations
Traumatic Injury — Luxation	Temporary splinting	CHAPTER 20	Esthetics and Pedodontics
Color Problems			
Aged (Dark) Teeth	Direct composite resin veneers	CHAPTER 4	Color Modifiers and Opaquers
		CHAPTER 5	Composite Resin — Fundamentals and Direct Technique Restorations
	Indirect composite resin veneers	CHAPTER 6	Composite Resin — Indirect Technique Restorations
	Ceramometal — full coverage restorations	CHAPTER 8	Ceramometal — Full Coverage Restorations
	Cast glass restorations	CHAPTER 9	Cast Glass Ceramic — Full Coverage Restorations
	All-porcelain restorations	CHAPTER 10	Porcelain — Full Coverage Restorations

Problem	Solution	Chapter	Title
Aged (Dark) Teeth (continued)	Porcelain laminate veneers	CHAPTER 11	Porcelain — Laminate Veneer and Other Partial Coverage Restorations
	Bleaching — vital/non-vital	CHAPTER 15	Bleaching and Related Agents
	Cosmetics (adjusting skin color to alter contrast)	CHAPTER 26	Esthetics and Cosmetology
Coloration	Direct composite resin veneers	CHAPTER 4	Color Modifiers and Opaquers
		CHAPTER 5	Composite Resin — Fundamentals and Direct Technique Restorations
	Indirect composite resin veneers	CHAPTER 6	Composite Resin — Indirect Technique Restorations
	Ceramometal — full coverage restorations	CHAPTER 8	Ceramometal — Full Coverage Restorations
	Cast glass restorations	CHAPTER 9	Cast Glass Ceramic — Full Coverage Restorations
	All-porcelain restorations	CHAPTER 10	Porcelain — Full Coverage Restorations
	Porcelain laminate veneers	CHAPTER 11	Porcelain — Laminate Veneer and Other Partial Coverage Restorations
	Bleaching — vital/non-vital	CHAPTER 15	Bleaching and Related Agents
	Prophylaxis (extrinsic stains)	CHAPTER 15	Bleaching and Related Agents
	Cosmetics (adjusting skin color to alter contrast)	CHAPTER 26	Esthetics and Cosmetology
Congenital Discoloration	Direct composite resin veneer	CHAPTER 4	Color Modifiers and Opaquers
		CHAPTER 5	Composite Resin — Fundamentals and Direct Technique Restorations
	Indirect composite resin veneer	CHAPTER 6	Composite Resin — Indirect Technique Restorations
	Ceramometal restoration	CHAPTER 8	Ceramometal — Full Coverage Restorations
	Cast glass restoration	CHAPTER 9	Cast Glass Ceramic — Full Coverage Restorations
	All-porcelain restoration	CHAPTER 10	Porcelain — Full Coverage Restorations
	Porcelain laminate veneer	CHAPTER 11	Porcelain — Laminate Veneer and Other Partial Coverage Restorations
	Bleaching — vital/non-vital	CHAPTER 15	Bleaching and Related Agents

Problem	Solution	Chapter	Title
Endodontic Discoloration	Direct composite resin veneers	CHAPTER 4	Color Modifiers and Opaquers
		CHAPTER 5	Composite Resin — Fundamentals and Direct Technique Restorations
	Indirect composite resin veneers	CHAPTER 6	Composite Resin — Indirect Technique Restorations
	Ceramometal — full coverage restorations	CHAPTER 8	Ceramometal — Full Coverage Restorations
	Cast glass restorations	CHAPTER 9	Cast Glass Ceramic — Full Coverage Restorations
	All-porcelain restorations	CHAPTER 10	Porcelain — Full Coverage Restorations
	Porcelain laminate veneers	CHAPTER 11	Porcelain — Laminate Veneer and Other Partial Coverage Restorations
	Bleaching — vital/non-vital	CHAPTER 15	Bleaching and Related Agents
	Cosmetics (adjusting skin color to alter contrast)	CHAPTER 26	Esthetics and Cosmetology
Fluorosis	Direct composite resin veneer	CHAPTER 4	Color Modifiers and Opaquers
		CHAPTER 5	Composite Resin — Fundamentals and Direct Technique Restorations
	Indirect composite resin veneer	CHAPTER 6	Composite Resin — Indirect Technique Restorations
	Ceramometal restoration	CHAPTER 8	Ceramometal — Full Coverage Restorations
	Cast glass restoration	CHAPTER 9	Cast Glass Ceramic — Full Coverage Restorations
	All-porcelain restoration	CHAPTER 10	Porcelain — Full Coverage Restorations
	Porcelain laminate veneer	CHAPTER 11	Porcelain — Laminate Veneer and Other Partial Coverage Restorations
	Bleaching — vital/non-vital	CHAPTER 15	Bleaching and Related Agents
	Cosmetics (adjusting skin color to alter contrast)	CHAPTER 26	Esthetics and Cosmetology
Post-Endodontic Discoloration	Direct composite resin veneer	CHAPTER 4	Color Modifiers and Opaquers
		CHAPTER 5	Composite Resin — Fundamentals and Direct Technique Restorations
	Indirect composite resin veneer	CHAPTER 6	Composite Resin — Indirect Technique Restorations

Problem	Solution	Chapter	Title
Post-Endodontic Discoloration (continued)	Ceramometal restoration	CHAPTER 8	Ceramometal — Full Coverage Restorations
	Cast glass restoration	CHAPTER 9	Cast Glass Ceramic — Full Coverage Restorations
	All-porcelain restoration	CHAPTER 10	Porcelain — Full Coverage Restorations
	Porcelain laminate veneer	CHAPTER 11	Porcelain — Laminate Veneer and Other Partial Coverage Restorations
	Bleaching — vital/non-vital	CHAPTER 15	Bleaching and Related Agents
	Cosmetics (adjusting skin color to alter contrast)	CHAPTER 26	Esthetics and Cosmetology
Staining	Direct composite resin veneer	CHAPTER 4	Color Modifiers and Opaquers
		CHAPTER 5	Composite Resin — Fundamentals and Direct Technique Restorations
	Indirect composite resin veneer	CHAPTER 6	Composite Resin — Indirect Technique Restorations
	Ceramometal restoration	CHAPTER 8	Ceramometal — Full Coverage Restorations
	Cast glass restoration	CHAPTER 9	Cast Glass Ceramic — Full Coverage Restorations
	All-porcelain restoration	CHAPTER 10	Porcelain — Full Coverage Restorations
	Porcelain laminate veneer	CHAPTER 11	Porcelain — Laminate Veneer and Other Partial Coverage Restorations
	Bleaching — vital/non-vital	CHAPTER 15	Bleaching and Related Agents
	Prophylaxis (extrinsic stains)	CHAPTER 15	Bleaching and Related Agents
	Cosmetics (adjusting skin color to alter contrast)	CHAPTER 26	Esthetics and Cosmetology
Tetracycline Discoloration	Direct composite resin veneer	CHAPTER 4	Color Modifiers and Opaquers
		CHAPTER 5	Composite Resin — Fundamentals and Direct Technique Restorations
	Indirect composite resin veneer	CHAPTER 6	Composite Resin — Indirect Technique Restorations
	Ceramometal restoration	CHAPTER 8	Ceramometal — Full Coverage Restorations
	Cast glass restoration	CHAPTER 9	Cast Glass Ceramic — Full Coverage Restorations
	All-porcelain restoration	CHAPTER 10	Porcelain — Full Coverage Restorations

Problem	Solution	Chapter	Title
Tetracycline Discoloration (continued)	Porcelain laminate veneer	CHAPTER 11	Porcelain — Laminate Veneer and Other Partial Coverage Restorations
	Bleaching — vital/non-vital	CHAPTER 15	Bleaching and Related Agents
	Cosmetics (adjusting skin color to alter contrast)	CHAPTER 26	Esthetics and Cosmetology
Tooth Color — Too Dark	Direct composite resin veneer	CHAPTER 4	Color Modifiers and Opaquers
		CHAPTER 5	Composite Resin — Fundamentals and Direct Technique Restorations
	Indirect composite resin veneer	CHAPTER 6	Composite Resin — Indirect Technique Restorations
	Ceramometal restoration	CHAPTER 8	Ceramometal — Full Coverage Restorations
	Cast glass restoration	CHAPTER 9	Cast Glass Ceramic — Full Coverage Restorations
	All-porcelain restoration	CHAPTER 10	Porcelain — Full Coverage Restorations
	Porcelain laminate veneer	CHAPTER 11	Porcelain — Laminate Veneer and Other Partial Coverage Restorations
	Bleaching — vital/non-vital	CHAPTER 15	Bleaching and Related Agents
	Prophylaxis (extrinsic stains)	CHAPTER 15	Bleaching and Related Agents
	Cosmetics (darkening of skin to reduce color contrast)	CHAPTER 26	Esthetics and Cosmetology
Tooth Color — Too Light	Direct composite resin veneer	CHAPTER 4	Color Modifiers and Opaquers
		CHAPTER 5	Composite Resin — Fundamentals and Direct Technique Restorations
	Indirect composite resin veneer	CHAPTER 6	Composite Resin — Indirect Technique Restorations
	Ceramometal restoration	CHAPTER 8	Ceramometal — Full Coverage Restorations
	Cast glass restoration	CHAPTER 9	Cast Glass Ceramic — Full Coverage Restorations
	All-porcelain restoration	CHAPTER 10	Porcelain — Full Coverage Restorations
	Porcelain laminate veneer	CHAPTER 11	Porcelain — Laminate Veneer and Other Partial Coverage Restorations
	Bleaching — vital/non-vital (white spot lesions)	CHAPTER 15	Bleaching and Related Agents

Problem	Solution	Chapter	Title
Tooth Color — Too Light (continued)	Prophylaxis (extrinsic stains)	CHAPTER 15	Bleaching and Related Agents
	Cosmetics (lightening of skin to reduce color contrast)	CHAPTER 26	Esthetics and Cosmetology
	Direct composite resin veneer	CHAPTER 4	Color Modifiers and Opaquers
		CHAPTER 5	Composite Resin — Fundamentals and Direct Technique Restorations
	Indirect composite resin veneer	CHAPTER 6	Composite Resin — Indirect Technique Restorations
	Ceramometal restoration	CHAPTER 8	Ceramometal — Full Coverage Restorations
	Cast glass restoration	CHAPTER 9	Cast Glass Ceramic — Full Coverage Restorations
	All-porcelain restoration	CHAPTER 10	Porcelain — Full Coverage Restorations
	Porcelain laminate veneer	CHAPTER 11	Porcelain — Laminate Veneer and Other Partial Coverage Restorations
	Bleaching — vital/non-vital	CHAPTER 15	Bleaching and Related Agents
	Cosmetics (adjusting skin color to alter contrast)	CHAPTER 26	Esthetics and Cosmetology
Traumatic Discoloration	Direct composite resin veneer	CHAPTER 4	Color Modifiers and Opaquers
		CHAPTER 5	Composite Resin — Fundamentals and Direct Technique Restorations
	Indirect composite resin veneer	CHAPTER 6	Composite Resin — Indirect Technique Restorations
	Ceramometal restoration	CHAPTER 8	Ceramometal — Full Coverage Restorations
	Cast glass restoration	CHAPTER 9	Cast Glass Ceramic — Full Coverage Restorations
	All-porcelain restoration	CHAPTER 10	Porcelain — Full Coverage Restorations
	Porcelain laminate veneer	CHAPTER 11	Porcelain — Laminate Veneer and Other Partial Coverage Restorations
White Spots	Bleaching — vital/non-vital	CHAPTER 15	Bleaching and Related Agents
	Prophylaxis (extrinsic stains)	CHAPTER 15	Bleaching and Related Agents
	Cosmetics (adjusting skin color to alter contrast)	CHAPTER 26	Esthetics and Cosmetology

Missing Teeth Problems

Problem	Solution	Chapter	Title
Migrated Teeth — Multiple	Ceramometal — full coverage restorations	CHAPTER 8	Ceramometal — Full Coverage Restorations
	All-porcelain restorations (experimental)	CHAPTER 10	Porcelain — Full Coverage Restorations
	Cast glass restorations (experimental)	CHAPTER 9	Cast Glass Ceramic — Full Coverage Restorations
	Acid etched retained ceramometal restoration	CHAPTER 12	Adhesive Resin Bonded Cast Restorations
	Removable prosthesis	CHAPTER 14	Acrylic and Other Resins — Removable Prostheses
	Orthodontic therapy	CHAPTER 22	Esthetics and Orthodontics
Migrated Tooth — Single	Direct composite resin veneer	CHAPTER 4	Color Modifiers and Opaquers
		CHAPTER 5	Composite Resin — Fundamentals and Direct Technique Restorations
	Indirect composite resin veneer	CHAPTER 6	Composite Resin — Indirect Technique Restorations
	Ceramometal — full coverage restorations	CHAPTER 8	Ceramometal — Full Coverage Restorations
	Cast glass restorations (experimental)	CHAPTER 9	Cast Glass Ceramic — Full Coverage Restorations
	All-porcelain restorations (experimental)	CHAPTER 10	Porcelain — Full Coverage Restorations
	Acid etched retained ceramometal restorations	CHAPTER 12	Adhesive Resin Bonded Cast Restorations
	Removable prosthesis	CHAPTER 14	Acrylic and Other Resins — Removable Prostheses
	Orthodontic therapy	CHAPTER 22	Esthetics and Orthodontics
Missing Teeth — Multiple	Ceramometal — full coverage restorations	CHAPTER 8	Ceramometal — Full Coverage Restorations
	Cast glass restorations (experimental)	CHAPTER 9	Cast Glass Ceramic — Full Coverage Restorations
	All-porcelain restorations (experimental)	CHAPTER 10	Porcelain — Full Coverage Restorations
	Acid etched retained ceramometal restorations	CHAPTER 12	Adhesive Resin Bonded Cast Restorations
	Removable prosthesis	CHAPTER 14	Acrylic and Other Resins — Removable Prostheses
	Implant retained restorations	CHAPTER 19	Esthetics and Implant Prosthetics

Problem	Solution	Chapter	Title
Missing Tooth — Single	Ceramometal restoration	CHAPTER 8	Ceramometal — Full Coverage Restorations
	Cast glass restoration (experimental)	CHAPTER 9	Cast Glass Ceramic — Full Coverage Restorations
	All-porcelain restoration (experimental)	CHAPTER 10	Porcelain — Full Coverage Restorations
	Acid etched retained ceramometal restoration	CHAPTER 12	Adhesive Resin Bonded Cast Restorations
	Removable prosthesis	CHAPTER 14	Acrylic and Other Resins — Removable Prostheses
	Implant retained restoration	CHAPTER 19	Esthetics and Implant Prosthetics
Traumatic Injury — Avulsion	Temporary splinting	CHAPTER 20	Esthetics and Pedodontics
Caries			
Carious Restoration Margins	See Repairs		
	Direct composite resin restoration	CHAPTER 4	Color Modifiers and Opaquers
		CHAPTER 5	Composite Resin — Fundamentals and Direct Technique Restorations
	Indirect composite resin restoration	CHAPTER 6	Composite Resin — Indirect Technique Restorations
	Glass ionomer restoration (non-stress bearing areas only)	CHAPTER 7	Glass Ionomer Cements
Carious Tooth	Ceramometal restoration	CHAPTER 8	Ceramometal — Full Coverage Restorations
	Cast glass restoration	CHAPTER 9	Cast Glass Ceramic — Full Coverage Restorations
	All-porcelain restoration	CHAPTER 10	Porcelain — Full Coverage Restorations
	Porcelain laminate veneer or partial coverage restoration	CHAPTER 11	Porcelain — Laminate Veneer and Other Partial Coverage Restorations

Repairs

Problem	Solution	Chapter	Title
Acrylic Veneer Facing — Dislodgement	Acrylic veneer repair	CHAPTER 4	Color Modifiers and Opaquers
Carious Restoration Margins	Porcelain bonding agents	CHAPTER 4	Color Modifiers and Opaquers
Porcelain Fractures — Ceramometal Restorations	Porcelain bonding agents	CHAPTER 4	Color Modifiers and Opaquers

NON-TOOTH RELATED PROBLEMS

Periodontal Problems

Problem	Solution	Chapter	Title
Gingival Asymmetry	Gingival recontouring — electrosurgery	CHAPTER 18	Esthetics and Electrosurgery
	Artificial gingiva	CHAPTER 21	Esthetics and Periodontics
	Gingival grafting (if caused by recession)	CHAPTER 21	Esthetics and Periodontics
	Gingival recontouring	CHAPTER 21	Esthetics and Periodontics
Gingival Hypertrophy	Gingival recontouring — electrosurgery	CHAPTER 18	Esthetics and Electrosurgery
	Gingival recontouring	CHAPTER 21	Esthetics and Periodontics
Gingival Inflammation	Evaluate restoration margins and contours	CHAPTER 5	Composite Resin — Fundamentals and Direct Technique Restorations
	Evaluate restoration margins and contours	CHAPTER 6	Composite Resin — Indirect Technique Restorations
	Evaluate restoration margins and contours	CHAPTER 7	Glass Ionomer Cements
	Evaluate restoration margins and contours	CHAPTER 8	Ceramometal — Full Coverage Restorations
	Evaluate restoration margins and contours	CHAPTER 9	Cast Glass Ceramic — Full Coverage Restorations
	Evaluate restoration margins and contours	CHAPTER 10	Porcelain — Full Coverage Restorations
	Evaluate restoration margins and contours	CHAPTER 11	Porcelain — Laminate Veneer and Other Partial Coverage Restorations
	Evaluate restoration margins and contours	CHAPTER 13	Acrylic and Other Resins — Provisional Restorations
	Periodontal therapy	CHAPTER 21	Esthetics and Periodontics
	Evaluate medical status		
Gingival Recession	Gingival graft	CHAPTER 21	Esthetics and Periodontics
	Artificial gingiva	CHAPTER 21	Esthetics and Periodontics

Problem	Solution	Chapter	Title
High Frenum Attachment with or without Diastema	Frenectomy	CHAPTER 22	Esthetics and Orthodontics
High Smile Line	Gingival recontouring — electrosurgery (possibly with restoration — see Long Tooth)	CHAPTER 18	Esthetics and Electrosurgery
	Gingival recontouring (possibly with restoration — see Long Tooth)	CHAPTER 21	Esthetics and Periodontics
	Oral surgery (possibly with restoration — see Long Tooth)	CHAPTER 23	Esthetics and Oral Surgery
Mobile Teeth	Ceramometal — full coverage restorations	CHAPTER 8	Ceramometal — Full Coverage Restorations
	Splinting	CHAPTER 21	Esthetics and Periodontics

Dermatologic Problems

Problem	Solution	Chapter	Title
Aging	Restore lip support — direct composite resin restorations	CHAPTER 4	Color Modifiers and Opaquers
		CHAPTER 5	Composite Resin — Fundamentals and Direct Technique Restorations
	Restore lip support — indirect composite resin restorations	CHAPTER 6	Composite Resin — Indirect Technique Restorations
	Restore lip support — ceramometal restorations	CHAPTER 8	Ceramometal — Full Coverage Restorations
	Restore lip support — cast glass restorations	CHAPTER 9	Cast Glass Ceramic — Full Coverage Restorations
	Restore lip support — all-porcelain restorations	CHAPTER 10	Porcelain — Full Coverage Restorations
	Restore lip support — porcelain laminate veneers	CHAPTER 11	Porcelain — Laminate Veneer and Other Partial Coverage Restorations
	Restore lip support — removable prostheses	CHAPTER 14	Acrylic and Other Resins — Removable Prostheses
	Plastic surgery	CHAPTER 24	Esthetics and Plastic Surgery
	Dermatologic therapy	CHAPTER 25	Esthetics and Dermatology
	Cosmetic cover-up	CHAPTER 26	Esthetics and Cosmetology

Problem	Solution	Chapter	Title
Bruising	Plastic surgery	CHAPTER 24	Esthetics and Plastic Surgery
	Dermatologic therapy	CHAPTER 25	Esthetics and Dermatology
	Cosmetic cover-up	CHAPTER 26	Esthetics and Cosmetology
Scars	Plastic surgery	CHAPTER 24	Esthetics and Plastic Surgery
	Dermatologic therapy	CHAPTER 25	Esthetics and Dermatology
	Cosmetic cover-up	CHAPTER 26	Esthetics and Cosmetology
Wrinkles	Restore lip support — direct composite resin restorations	CHAPTER 5	Composite Resin — Fundamentals and Direct Technique Restorations
	Restore lip support — indirect composite resin restorations	CHAPTER 6	Composite Resin — Indirect Technique Restorations
	Restore lip support — ceramometal restorations	CHAPTER 8	Ceramometal — Full Coverage Restorations
	Restore lip support — cast glass restorations	CHAPTER 9	Cast Glass Ceramic — Full Coverage Restorations
	Restore lip support — all-porcelain restorations	CHAPTER 10	Porcelain — Full Coverage Restorations
	Restore lip support — porcelain laminate veneers	CHAPTER 11	Porcelain — Laminate Veneer and Other Partial Coverage Restorations
	Restore lip support — removable prostheses	CHAPTER 14	Acrylic and Other Resins — Removable Prostheses
	Plastic surgery	CHAPTER 24	Esthetics and Plastic Surgery
	Dermatologic therapy	CHAPTER 25	Esthetics and Dermatology
	Cosmetic cover-up	CHAPTER 26	Esthetics and Cosmetology
Facial Contours and Skeletal Problems			
Asymmetry	Orthognathic surgery	CHAPTER 23	Esthetics and Oral Surgery
	Plastic surgery	CHAPTER 24	Esthetics and Plastic Surgery
	Cosmetic cover-up	CHAPTER 26	Esthetics and Cosmetology
Bimaxillary Prognathism/ Protrusion	Orthodontic therapy	CHAPTER 22	Esthetics and Orthodontics
	Orthognathic surgery	CHAPTER 23	Esthetics and Oral Surgery
	Plastic surgery	CHAPTER 24	Esthetics and Plastic Surgery
	Cosmetic cover-up	CHAPTER 26	Esthetics and Cosmetology

Problem	Solution	Chapter	Title
Excessive Lip Support	Orthodontic therapy	CHAPTER 22	Esthetics and Orthodontics
	Orthognathic surgery	CHAPTER 23	Esthetics and Oral Surgery
	Plastic surgery (severe)	CHAPTER 24	Esthetics and Plastic Surgery
	Cosmetic cover-up	CHAPTER 26	Esthetics and Cosmetology
Facial Asymmetry	Orthognathic surgery	CHAPTER 23	Esthetics and Oral Surgery
	Plastic surgery	CHAPTER 24	Esthetics and Plastic Surgery
	Cosmetic cover-up	CHAPTER 26	Esthetics and Cosmetology
Hypogenia	Orthognathic surgery	CHAPTER 23	Esthetics and Oral Surgery
	Plastic surgery	CHAPTER 24	Esthetics and Plastic Surgery
	Dermatologic therapy	CHAPTER 25	Esthetics and Dermatology
	Cosmetic cover-up	CHAPTER 26	Esthetics and Cosmetology
Insufficient Lip Support	Restore lip support — direct composite resin restorations	CHAPTER 4	Color Modifiers and Opaquers
		CHAPTER 5	Composite Resin — Fundamentals and Direct Technique Restorations
	Restore lip support — indirect composite resin restorations	CHAPTER 6	Composite Resin — Indirect Technique Restorations
	Restore lip support — ceramometal restorations	CHAPTER 8	Ceramometal — Full Coverage Restorations
	Restore lip support — cast glass restorations	CHAPTER 9	Cast Glass Ceramic — Full Coverage Restorations
	Restore lip support — all-porcelain restorations	CHAPTER 10	Porcelain — Full Coverage Restorations
	Restore lip support — porcelain laminate veneers	CHAPTER 11	Porcelain — Laminate Veneer and Other Partial Coverage Restorations
	Restore lip support — removable prostheses	CHAPTER 14	Acrylic and Other Resins — Removable Prostheses
	Orthodontic therapy	CHAPTER 22	Esthetics and Orthodontics
	Orthognathic surgery (severe)	CHAPTER 23	Esthetics and Oral Surgery
	Plastic surgery (severe)	CHAPTER 24	Esthetics and Plastic Surgery
	Cosmetic cover-up	CHAPTER 26	Esthetics and Cosmetology
Macrogenia	Orthognathic surgery	CHAPTER 23	Esthetics and Oral Surgery
	Plastic surgery	CHAPTER 24	Esthetics and Plastic Surgery

Problem	Solution	Chapter	Title
Macrogenia (continued)	Cosmetic cover-up	CHAPTER 26	Esthetics and Cosmetology
Mandibular Prognathism/ Protrusion	Orthodontic therapy	CHAPTER 22	Esthetics and Orthodontics
	Orthognathic surgery	CHAPTER 23	Esthetics and Oral Surgery
	Plastic surgery	CHAPTER 24	Esthetics and Plastic Surgery
	Cosmetic cover-up	CHAPTER 26	Esthetics and Cosmetology
Mandibular Retrognathism/ Retrusion	Orthodontic therapy	CHAPTER 22	Esthetics and Orthodontics
	Orthognathic surgery	CHAPTER 23	Esthetics and Oral Surgery
	Plastic surgery	CHAPTER 24	Esthetics and Plastic Surgery
	Cosmetic cover-up	CHAPTER 26	Esthetics and Cosmetology
Maxillary Prognathism/ Protrusion	Orthodontic therapy	CHAPTER 22	Esthetics and Orthodontics
	Orthognathic surgery	CHAPTER 23	Esthetics and Oral Surgery
	Plastic surgery	CHAPTER 24	Esthetics and Plastic Surgery
	Cosmetic cover-up	CHAPTER 26	Esthetics and Cosmetology
Maxillary Retrognathism/ Retrusion	Orthodontic therapy	CHAPTER 22	Esthetics and Orthodontics
	Orthognathic surgery	CHAPTER 23	Esthetics and Oral Surgery
	Plastic surgery	CHAPTER 24	Esthetics and Plastic Surgery
	Cosmetic cover-up	CHAPTER 26	Esthetics and Cosmetology
Open Bite — Mild	Direct composite resin veneers	CHAPTER 4	Color Modifiers and Opaquers
		CHAPTER 5	Composite Resin — Fundamentals and Direct Technique Restorations
	Indirect composite resin veneers	CHAPTER 6	Composite Resin — Indirect Technique Restorations
	Ceramometal — full coverage restorations	CHAPTER 8	Ceramometal — Full Coverage Restorations
	Cast glass restorations	CHAPTER 9	Cast Glass Ceramic — Full Coverage Restorations
	All-porcelain restorations	CHAPTER 10	Porcelain — Full Coverage Restorations

Problem	Solution	Chapter	Title
Open Bite — Mild (continued)	Porcelain laminate veneers	CHAPTER 11	Porcelain — Laminate Veneer and Other Partial Coverage Restorations
	Orthodontic therapy	CHAPTER 22	Esthetics and Orthodontics
	Orthognathic surgery	CHAPTER 23	Esthetics and Oral Surgery
Open Bite — Severe	Orthodontic therapy	CHAPTER 22	Esthetics and Orthodontics
	Orthognathic surgery	CHAPTER 23	Esthetics and Oral Surgery
Prognathism	Orthodontic therapy	CHAPTER 22	Esthetics and Orthodontics
	Orthognathic surgery	CHAPTER 23	Esthetics and Oral Surgery
	Plastic surgery	CHAPTER 24	Esthetics and Plastic Surgery
	Cosmetic cover-up	CHAPTER 26	Esthetics and Cosmetology
Protrusion	Orthodontic therapy	CHAPTER 22	Esthetics and Orthodontics
	Orthognathic surgery	CHAPTER 23	Esthetics and Oral Surgery
	Plastic surgery	CHAPTER 24	Esthetics and Plastic Surgery
	Cosmetic cover-up	CHAPTER 26	Esthetics and Cosmetology
Retrognathism	Orthodontic therapy	CHAPTER 22	Esthetics and Orthodontics
	Orthognathic surgery	CHAPTER 23	Esthetics and Oral Surgery
	Plastic surgery	CHAPTER 24	Esthetics and Plastic Surgery
	Cosmetic cover-up	CHAPTER 26	Esthetics and Cosmetology
Retrusion	Orthodontic therapy	CHAPTER 22	Esthetics and Orthodontics
	Orthognathic surgery	CHAPTER 23	Esthetics and Oral Surgery
	Plastic surgery	CHAPTER 24	Esthetics and Plastic Surgery
	Cosmetic cover-up	CHAPTER 26	Esthetics and Cosmetology

Milton B. Asbell, D.D.S., M.Sc., M.A.

INTRODUCTION TO ESTHETICS

The search for beauty can be traced to the earliest civilizations. Dental art has been part of this quest to enhance the esthetics of the teeth and mouth. Assyrio-Babylonian cuneiform tablets dating from the dawn of recorded history advise the following:

"If a man's teeth become yellow . . . thou shalt bray together "salt of Akkad," ammi, lolium, pine-turpine with these, with thy fingers shalt bur his teeth."

One recalls the chant of the Psalmist (Song of Songs 4:2 c. 900 B.C.):

"Thy teeth are like a flock of well-selected sheep, which are come up from the washing, all of which bear twins, and there is not one among them that is deprived of her young."

Both the Phoenicians (c. 800 B.C.) and Etruscans (c. 900 B.C.) carefully carved animal tusks to simulate the shape, form, and hue of natural teeth for use as pontics (Fig. 1–1). The American Mayas (c. 1000 A.D.) "beautified" themselves by filing incisal edges of anterior teeth into various shapes and designs (Figs. 1–2, 1–3). They also placed plugs of iron pyrites, obsidian or jade into the labial surfaces of the maxillary anterior teeth (Fig. 1–4). This practice was common among both sexes and tooth mutilation is still practiced in some societies (Figs. 1–5, 1–6).

During the Roman Empire, dental cosmetic treatment was available only to the affluent classes. Oral hygiene was practiced primarily by women for reasons of beauty rather than dental health. Mouthwashes, dentifrices, and toothpicks were prominent in the boudoirs, and when teeth were lost, they were replaced with substitutes of bone or ivory carved to the likeness of the missing ones.

Interest in dental esthetics was virtually absent during the Middle Ages. It was not until the eighteenth century that dentistry was established as a separate discipline and its various branches established. The leader of this movement was Pierre Fauchard (1678–1761) of France. He, together with several colleagues, advocated such esthetic practices as proper oral hygiene and the use of gold shell crowns with enamel "veneers." They introduced a technique for the manufacture of mineral "incorruptible" teeth to replace those of ivory and bone in the fabrication of dentures. In England, *The British Journal* carried the following advertisement (1724):

"The incomparable powder for cleaning the teeth which has given great satisfaction to most of the nobility and gentry for above these twenty years . . . it, at one using, makes the teeth as white as ivory, and never black or yellow."

ESTHETICS IN THE UNITED STATES

In the colonial United States, primitive conditions existed for almost a century (c. 1670–1770) until the arrival of European-trained "operators for the teeth." They brought with them not only medications for toothache, but prescriptions for "toothpowder to make teeth white," to "attend to your teeth and preserve your health and beauty," and which "prepares and fixes real enameled teeth, the best contrivance yet to substitute the loss of natural ones" (Figs. 1–7, 1–8). Transplantation of teeth between patients was practiced: "any person that will dispense of the front teeth, five guineas for each" (Fig. 1–9).

Cosmetic dentistry was not met with universal acceptance, however. The following is an official edict published by His Britannic Majesty at Perth Amboy, New Jersey:

"All women of whatever age, rank, profession or degree, whether virgins, maids, or widow, who after this Act shall impose upon, seduce and betray unto matrimony any of His Majesty's subjects by virtue of cosmetics, scents, washes, paints, artificial teeth, false hair or high-heeled shoes, shall incur the penalty of the law in force against witchcraft and like misdemeanors."

The early years of the nineteenth century found competent practitioners in the leading cities of the country. After the introduction of mineral teeth (1817), the manufacture of porcelain teeth was established. Dentures were made with a gingival component made of carved ivory or animal bone designed to be adapted to ivory or bone bases (Fig. 1–10). These denture bases were common until the 1850s when various alternative materials were introduced to afford more esthetic results. A technique was patented of mounting artificial teeth on gold or platinum fused with a continuous pink gingival body made of porcelain. "Auroplasty," colored gutta percha; "parkesine," a celluloid-like material; "cheoplasty," an alloy of tin, silver, and bismuth; "rose pearl," collodion, pink colored hecolite, and even tortoise shells were used. Vulcanite was the first universally acceptable denture material. Patented by Nelson Goodear in 1851, it was made by heating caoutchouc (Indian rubber) with sulphur, resulting in a firm, yet flexible material. Vulcanite, which was relatively inexpensive and simple to make, propelled the use of dentures out of the luxury category by allowing for relatively inexpensive and simple fabrication. Synthetic materials, such as vinyl acrylic resins, copolymer acrylic resins, and styrene acrylic resins were introduced about 1934.

In the late nineteenth century, various techniques of esthetic fixed prosthodontics were introduced. The open faced crown (c. 1880), the interchangeable porcelain facing (a ridged facing that fitted into a grooved pontic) (c. 1880s), and the venerable porcelain jacket crown (c. 1900s) came into vogue. The three-quarter crown was introduced in 1907.

In operative dentistry, the search was on for more esthetic material than the gold, lead, tin, and platinum then in use. One option was "Hill's Stopping," a mixture of bleached gutta-percha, carbonates of lime and quartz, plastic, bone, and fused glass. Porcelain as a restorative material was another. By 1897, a relatively modern composition of silicate cement was developed. It consisted of powdered aluminum and zinc oxide mixed with phosphoric and hydrofluoric acid. Abandoned because it was difficult to manage and ultimately became brittle, it resurfaced in modified form in 1904 and revolutionized operative dentistry. The inventive combination of acid-soluble glasses blended with a liquid containing phosphoric acid produced dentistry's first truly translucent restorative material. Further modifications continued until the American Dental Association, in 1938, created definitive specifications of acceptability known as "A.D.A. Specification No. 9." This was the first cosmetic dental material to be accepted by the American Dental Association. However, newer and more exciting innovations were about to arrive.

In the 1930s, chemically activated acrylic resins were developed. In the 1940s, the acrylic veneer facings came into widespread use. Thirty years later, composite resin virtually replaced acrylic resins and silicate cements as "permanent" restorations. Refinements of this basic formula of resin matrix and glass filler are currently in use.

Acid etching, often called "bonding," radically changed cavity design, with an emphasis on conservation of tooth structure. It also allowed for the numerous veneering techniques first introduced in the 1970s. Variations include direct resin veneers, commercially produced acrylic "shells," and laboratory processed veneers of resin and porcelain.

Research continues. Study groups, societies, journals, and continuing education courses dedicated to the discipline of cosmetic dentistry have proliferated. Undoubtedly, the persistent drive for the evasive ultimate restoration will continue to unveil new vistas in the art and science of cosmetic dentistry.

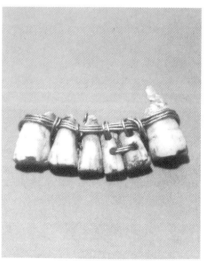

FIG. 1–1

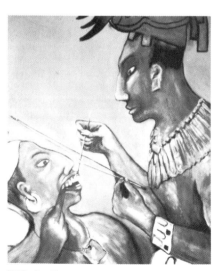

FIG. 1–2

FIG. 1–1. Ancient Phonecian "bridge." Pontics are extracted central and lateral incisors that were attached to the remaining canines with wires. (From Ring ME: Dentistry. An Illustrated History. New York, Harry N. Abrams, 1985.)

FIG. 1–2. Ancient painting depicting a probable method of preparing teeth used by the Mayas about 1000 A.D. (From Ring ME: Dentistry. An Illustrated History. New York, Harry N. Abrams, 1985.)

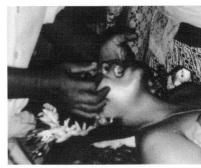

FIG. 1—3. Various forms of tooth mutilation that were considered a beautification technique. (From Weinberger BW: An Introduction to the History of Dentistry, Vol. 1. St. Louis, Mosby, 1948.)

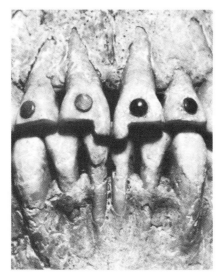

FIG. 1—4. Specimen showing multiple inlays and turquoise restorations by Mayas circa 1000 A.D. (From Ring ME: Dentistry. An Illustrated History. New York, Harry N. Abrams, 1985.)

FIG. 1—5. Filing of maxillary anterior teeth to beautify brides-to-be (Polynesia, 1987).

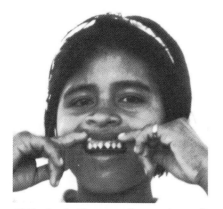

FIG. 1—6. Ticuana tribe tooth mutilation. (From Ring ME: Dentistry. An Illustrated History. New York, Harry N. Abrams, 1985.)

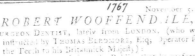

FIG. 1—7. Colonial United States advertisement that appeared in the *Pennsylvania Chronicle and Universal Advocate* on November 5, 1767, sells "artificial teeth, so as to escape discernment."

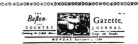

FIG. 1—8. Paul Revere's advertisement for his services as a dentist (dated September 5, 1768). (From Ring ME: Dentistry. An Illustrated History. New York, Harry N. Abrams, 1985.)

FIG. 1—9. Eighteenth century Thomas Rowlanson etching depicting the transplantation of a tooth from a maid to her mistress. (From Ring ME: Dentistry. An Illustrated History. New York, Harry N. Abrams, 1985.)

FIG. 1—10. George Washington's denture. (From the National Museum of American History, Smithsonian Institution, Washington, D.C.)

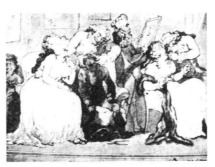

FIG. 1—9

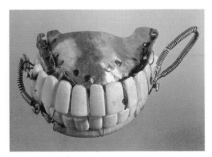

FIG. 1—10

BIBLIOGRAPHY

Asbell, M.B.: A Bibliography of Dentistry in America: 1790–1840. Cherry Hill, NJ, Sussex House, 1973.

Asbell, M.B.: Dentistry: A Historical Perspective. Pittsburgh, Dorrance & Co., 1988.

Bremmer, M.D.K.: The Story of Dentistry. New York, Dental Items of Interest, 1954.

Foley, G.P.H.: Foley's Footnotes: A Treasury of Dentistry. Wallingford, PA, Washington Square East Publishing Co., 1972.

Guerini, V.: A History of Dentistry from the Most Ancient Times until the End of the Eighteenth Century. Philadelphia, Lea & Febiger, 1969.

Herschfeld, J.: The Progress of Esthetics Restorations in Dentistry. Unpublished paper.

Kanner, L.: Folklore of the Tooth. New York, Macmillin, 1934.

Prinz, H.: Dental Chronology. A Record of More Important Historic Events in the Evolution Of Dentistry. Philadelphia, Lea & Febiger, 1945.

Ring, M.E.: Dentistry: An Illustrated History. New York, Harry N. Abrams, Inc., 1985.

Weinberger, B.W.: An Introduction to the History of Dentistry, 2 Vol. St. Louis, C.V. Mosby, 1948.

Bruce A. Singer, B.S., D.D.S.

FUNDAMENTALS OF ESTHETICS

2

The development of new materials and techniques in dentistry has created a responsibility for the enlightened practitioner to develop new artistic skills. Manipulation of light, color, illusion, shape, and form to create a more esthetic situation than existed originally is the responsibility of the restorative dentist. Expertise in these areas differentiates the technically proficient dentist from one practicing a higher level of care, that of being an artist.

LIGHT AND SHADOW

Objects cannot be distinguished without light. When lit, the most fundamental objects (Fig. 2–1) exhibit two dimensions—length and width. True natural light, however, is multidirectional; it reveals texture and throws shadows, which adds the lifelike third dimension of depth (Fig. 2–2). Therefore, *the communication of form is by shadow.* By comparing Figures 2–1 and 2–2 this concept becomes apparent. Dental restorations can *mimic* the shadows of adjacent teeth to create a shape that blends with the surrounding tooth forms. Shadow manipulation can make poorly shaped teeth esthetically pleasing.

THE PRINCIPLES OF COLOR

In 1666, Sir Isaac Newton observed that white light passing through a prism divided into an orderly pattern of colors now termed the spectrum. He also discovered that these colors would reproduce white light when passed back through the prism proving that all spectral colors were in the original beam.[1]

Color, as the eye interprets it, is either a result of absorption or reflection. In absorption, a white light is passed through a filter. The colors that pass through the filter and reach the eye are perceived as the color of the filter. In reflection, as with solid objects, the color that we see is the portion of the spectrum that is reflected back to the eye.

Light entering the eye stimulates the photoreceptor rods and cones in the retina. The energy is converted through a photochemical reaction into nerve impulses and carried through the optic nerve into the occipital lobe of the cerebral cortex. The rod cells are responsible for interpreting brightness differences and value. The cone cells function in hue and chroma interpretation. If the light source contains all of the colors of the spectrum, a true reading will occur. But if the original light is deficient in a certain color, then we will perceive that object as having an untrue color (see the section on Metamerism later in this chapter). Precisely describing these colors and organizing their inter-relationships, however, required another 249 years after Newton's work. Robert Louis Stevenson, one of the most concise writers in the English language, demonstrated the prob-

FIG. 2–1. Unidirectional unnatural lighting throws no shadows. Only length and width are represented.

FIG. 2–2. Natural lighting is multidirectional. It throws shadows and, therefore, promotes a feeling of depth—a three dimensional effect.

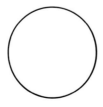

FIG. 2–1

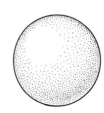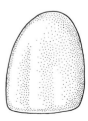

FIG. 2–2

lems of describing color: "red—it's not Turkish and it's not Roman and it's not Indian, but it seems to partake of the two last."[2] In 1915, Albert Henry Munsell created an orderly numeric system of color description, which is still the standard today. In this system color is divided into three parameters—hue, chroma, and value.[3]

Hue

Hue (Fig. 2–3) is the name of the color. Roy G. Biv (*Red, Orange, Yellow, Green, Blue, Indigo, Violet*) is an acronym for the hues of the spectrum. In a younger permanent dentition, hue tends to be similar throughout the mouth. With aging, variations in hue often occur because of intrinsic and extrinsic staining from restorative materials, foods, beverages, smoking, and other influences.

Chroma

Chroma (Fig. 2–4) is the saturation or intensity of hue and, therefore, chroma can only be present with hue. For example, to increase the chroma of a porcelain restoration more of that hue is added. Chroma is the quality of hue that is most amenable to decrease by bleaching. Almost all hues are amenable to chroma reduction in vital and nonvital bleaching.[4] In general, the chroma of teeth increases with age.

Value

Value (Fig. 2–5) is the relative whiteness or blackness of a color. A light tooth has a high value; a dark tooth has a low value. It is not the *quantity* of the "color" gray, but rather the *quality* of brightness, on a gray scale.[5] That is, does the shade of color (hue + chroma)

seem light and bright or dark and dim? It is helpful to regard value in this way because the use of value in restorative dentistry does not involve adding gray but rather manipulating colors to increase or decrease amounts of grayness.

CLINICAL TIP. *Value is the most important factor in shade matching. If the value blends, small variations in hue and chroma will not be noticeable.*[5]

COLOR (HUE) RELATIONSHIP
The Color Wheel

Hues, as used in dentistry, have a relationship to one another that can be demonstrated in a color wheel. The relationships of primary, secondary, and complementary hues are graphically explained by the color wheel (Fig. 2–6).

Primary Hues

The primary hues—red, yellow, and blue—form the basis of the dental color system. In dentistry, the metal oxide pigments used in coloring porcelains are limited in forming certain reds, therefore, pink is substituted. The primary hues have a relationship to one another and form the basic structure of the color wheel.

Secondary Hues

Any two primary hues, when mixed, form a secondary hue. When red and blue are mixed they create violet, blue and yellow create green, and yellow and red create orange. Altering the proportions of the primary hues in a mixture will vary the hue of the secondary hue produced. Primary and secondary hues can be graphically related in a circular fashion with secondary hues positioned between primary hues.

Complementary Hues

Colors directly opposite each other on the color wheel are termed complementary hues. A peculiarity of this system is that a primary hue is always opposite a secondary hue and vice versa. When a primary hue is mixed with a complementary secondary hue, the effect is to "cancel" out both colors and produce gray. *This is the most important relationship in dental color manipulation.*

CLINICAL TIP. *To change hue or lessen chroma or lower value, place the complementary hue over the color to be modified.*

When a portion of a crown is too yellow, lightly washing with violet (the complementary hue of yellow) will produce an area that is no longer yellow. The yellow color is canceled out and the area will have an increased grayness (a lower value). This is especially useful if the body color of a crown has been brought too far incisally and more of an incisal color is desired toward the cervical area. If a cervical area is too yellow,

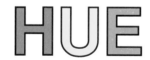

FIG. 2–3. Hue is the name of the color.

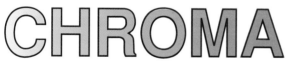

FIG. 2–4. Chroma is the saturation or amount of hue.

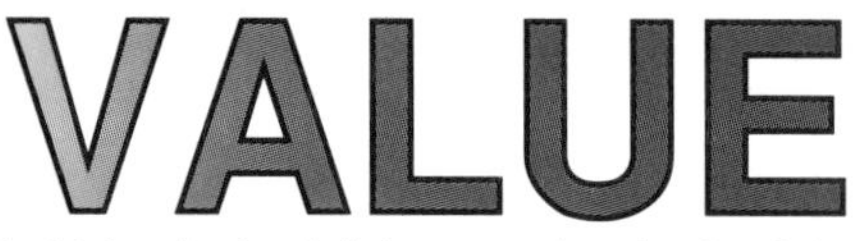

VALUE

FIG. 2–5. Value is the brightness of a shade. A low value is darker than a high value.

and a brown color is desired, washing the area with violet will cancel the yellow. This is followed by the application of the desired color, in this case brown.

Complementary hues also exhibit the useful phenomenon of intensification. When complementary hues are placed next to one another, they each intensify the other and appear to have a higher chroma. A light orange line on the incisal edge will intensify the blue nature of an incisal color.

Hue Sensitivity

After 5 seconds of staring at a tooth or shade guide, the eye accommodates and becomes biased. If one stares at any color for longer than 5 seconds and then stares away at a white surface, or closes one's eyes, the image appears, but in the complementary hue. This phenomenon, known as hue sensitivity, adversely effects shade selection.

CLINICAL TIP. After 5 seconds, look away or stare briefly at a blue surface (such as a patient napkin), which will readapt vision to the orange-yellow portion of the spectrum. This is the portion that is most involved in color matching.

Metamerism

Basic Theory. Metamerism can cause two color samples to appear as the same hue under one light source, but as unmatched hues under a different light source.

There is more than one way to produce a color. It can either be pure, or a mixture of two other colors (i.e., pure green versus a mix of blue and yellow). A pure green color will reflect light in the green band, but the green mixture color will reflect light in the blue and yellow bands simultaneously. If both colors are exposed to a light with a full color spectrum they will appear similar. If, however, they are exposed to a light source that does not contain light in the blue band, the two colors will appear dissimilar. True green will still appear green, however, the mixture will appear yellow because without a source of light in the blue band the blue component of the mix will not be visible to the eye. A spectral curve is a measure of the wavelength of light reflected from a surface and reveals the actual component colors reflected from an object (Fig. 2–7).[5]

Clinical Relevance. Metamerism complicates the color matching of restorations. A shade button may match under incandescent lighting from the dental operatory lamp but not under fluorescent lighting in the patient's workplace.

CLINICAL TIP. The best approach to color matching is to use three light sources.

A color selection that works well under a variety of lights is preferred to a match that is exact under one source of light but completely wrong under others.[6] Usually, three sources of light are available in the dental operatory.

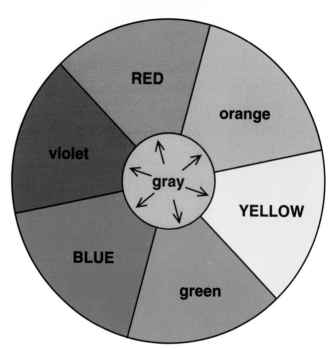

FIG. 2–6. The color wheel. The primary colors, red, yellow, and blue, when mixed two at a time produce the secondary colors, orange, green, and violet. Opposite colors on the color wheel, when mixed together, cancel each other out and produce gray.

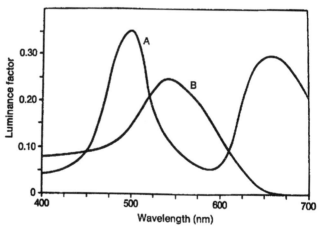

FIG. 2–7. The spectral curves of two metameric green surfaces that appear identical but exhibit different reflection properties. Surface B reflects light in the green wavelengths and, thus, appears green. Surface A, on the other hand, reflects both cyan and yellow light, which also results in the perception of a green surface. As long as all the required wavelengths of light are present these two metameric pairs will look identical. If, however, the incident light is deficient in either the yellow or cyan, Surface A will not appear green and the colors will not match (Adapted from Preston, J.D., and Bergen, S.F.: Color Science and Dental Art—A Self Teaching Program. St. Louis, CV Mosby, 1980.)

1. Outside daylight through a window.
2. Incandescent lighting from the dental operatory lamp.
3. A cool white fluorescent overhead light.

Color-corrected fluorescent lamps more closely approximate natural daylight and some practitioners prefer them as the standard in dental operatories. If the entire office is illuminated by color-corrected fluorescent lamp, one room should have cool white fluorescent lighting for comparative shade matching. The color match that holds up the best in these three lights is the best choice.

CLINICAL TIP. *If the patient spends a great deal of time in one lighting situation, then this light source should take precedence during shade selection.*

Opacity

Basic Theory. An opaque material does not permit any light to pass through. It reflects all of the light that is shined upon it.

Clinical Relevance. A porcelain-fused-to-metal restoration must have a layer of opaque porcelain applied to the metal substructure to prevent the color of the metal from appearing through the translucent body and incisal porcelains. Improper tooth reduction results in two unacceptable results:

1. An ideally contoured restoration with minimal porcelain thickness and too much opaque porcelain, resulting in a "chalky" appearance.
2. A bulky, poorly contoured restoration with ideal porcelain thickness.

Tooth reduction must be sufficient to allow enough room for an adequate bulk of body and incisal porcelains (Fig. 2–8).

CLINICAL TIP. *The usual areas of underpreparation are in the cervical one-third and, if a second plane of reduction is not placed, in the incisofacial aspect of the preparation.*

Translucency

Translucent materials allow some light to pass through them. Only some of the light is absorbed. Translucency provides realism to an artificial dental restoration.

Depth

Basic Theory. In restorative dentistry, depth is a spacial concept of color blending combining the concepts of opacity and translucency. In the natural dentition, light passes through the translucent enamel and is reflected out from the depths of the relatively opaque dentin.

Clinical Relevance. White porcelain colorants used in color modification are opaque. Gray porcelain colorants are a mixture of black and white. A tooth restoration with a white opaque colorant on the surface appears artificial because it lacks the quality of depth that would be seen if the opaque layer was placed *beneath* a translucent layer of porcelain. Similarly, a bright restoration (high value) in need of graying (a decrease in value) would appear falsely opaque if simply painted gray. Adding a complementary hue, however, both decreases the value and adds to the translucency. If characterization needs to be added to porcelain to represent white hypoplastic spots or gray amalgam stains, white or gray colorant can be used, but with the knowledge that translucency will be reduced in these areas.

Depth may be problematic when translucent composite resins are used to restore class III or class IV cavities that extend completely from facial to lingual surfaces. The restoration may appear gray or overly translucent. However, if a more opaque composite resin is placed on the lingual portion of the restoration, and then overlaid with a translucent resin, a natural illusion of depth results.

THE PRINCIPLES OF FORM
Perception

As we look at a tooth in an environment of other teeth we perceive unconsciously many qualities of that tooth. Perceptions about color, size, shape, age, and sex are based upon certain natural biases that are indigenous to an individual's cultural background. Perceptual biases can be divided into two types: cultural and artistic.

Cultural Biases

Cultural biases are naturally occurring environmental observations about the world around us. We perceive (and believe) that darker, heavily worn, highly stained, longer teeth belong to a person of an older age because we know that teeth naturally darken, wear, and stain in grooves and along the cervical area with age, and that they lengthen because of gingival recession. We perceive (and believe) rounded, smooth flowing forms are feminine, whereas harsher, more angular forms are masculine.

Masculine and Feminine. Culturally defined masculine qualities may enhance the appearance of a female (many feminine fashions include a modification of a shirt and a tie, or a black bowler hat). But usually these masculine nuances look best on a very attractive female, and not a woman who has many other masculine characteristics. Square, angular anterior teeth, therefore, may be desirable for a more "feminine" female, but on a large, masculine-looking woman this tooth shape would only accentuate her "un-femininity." In our culture, contrast evokes a certain allure. With no contrast, the allure is gone.

The Golden Proportion. Western civilization has drawn the conclusion that for objects to be proportional to one another the ratio of 1:1.618 is esthetically pleasing. Much has been hypothesized in this area, from the mathematical relationship of the chambers of the multichambered nautilus shell to facial proportions. As a general rule, if the *apparent* (see the section on The Law of the Face later in this chapter) size of each tooth, as observed from the frontal view, is 60% of the size of the tooth anterior to it, the relationship is considered to be artistically pleasing. That is, if the *apparent* width of the central incisor is 1.608, the lateral incisor and canine should be 1.0 and .608 respectively.[7]

Artistic Biases

Artistic biases are inherent subconsciously in our perception of form. The most important of these is the perception that light approaches and dark recedes; this is the *principle of illumination*.[8] Those areas in Figure 2–2 that are light appear to come forward, whereas the darker areas appear to recede. This produces the illusion of a third dimension (depth) despite the two dimensional nature (length and width) of the printed page. This bias applies equally to clothes, makeup, or teeth. The purpose of make-up is to give contour to the face (Fig. 2–9).

The second artistic bias of great importance in dentistry is the use of horizontal and vertical lines. A horizontal line will make an object *appear* wider, whereas a vertical line will make an object *appear* longer (Fig. 2–10). This can be termed the *principle of line*.

These cultural and artistic biases are so entrenched in our subconscious thought that they are unavoidable and automatic. Manipulation of these biases allows the cosmetic dentist to artistically fool the eye of the observer when fabricating artificial esthetic restorations.

Illusion

Illusion is the art of changing perception to cause an object to appear different than it actually is. Teeth can be made to appear wider, narrower, smaller, larger, shorter, longer, older, younger, masculine, or feminine. However, an understanding of the basic principles of perception must precede the utilization of these principles to control illusion.

USING THE PRINCIPLES OF PERCEPTION TO CONTROL ILLUSION

Principle of Illumination

The basic artistic bias exhibited in the principle of illumination can be manipulated to change the size and shape of a tooth through illusion. This bias is the key to *The Law of the Face*.

The Law of the Face

The law of the face is the most important single concept in shaping dental restorations. Understanding this concept and its interplay with the preceding concept of light and dark will enable the esthetic dentist to correctly shape all esthetic restorations.

The *face* of a tooth is that area on the facial surface, on both anterior and posterior teeth, that is bounded by the transitional line angles as viewed from the facial (buccal) aspect (Fig. 2–11). The transitional line angles mark the transition from the facial surface to the mesial, cervical, distal, and incisal surfaces. The tooth surface slopes lingually toward the mesial and distal approximating surfaces and toward the cervical root surface from these line angles. Often, no transitional line angle appears on the incisal portion of the facial surface; in this case, the face is bounded by the incisal edge or the occlusal tip. Shadows created as light strikes the labial surface of the tooth begin at the transitional line angles. *These shadows delineate the boundaries of the face.*

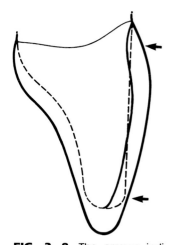

FIG. 2–8. The arrows indicate underprepared areas in a typical full crown or veneer preparation. Underpreparation results in opaque areas in the finished restoration. The correct preparation is illustrated by the solid line.

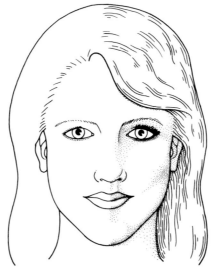

FIG. 2–9. The principle of illumination: Light approaches and dark recedes. The illusion of contour is produced as makeup is applied to the face or shadows are drawn on a drawing.

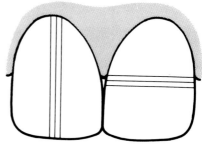

FIG. 2–10. The principle of line: Horizontal lines created by cervical staining, texturing, white hypoplastic lines, and straight incisal edges create the illusion of width; vertical lines created by narrowing the face of the tooth, carving the incisal edges to slope cervically, and deepening the incisal embrasures create the illusion of length.

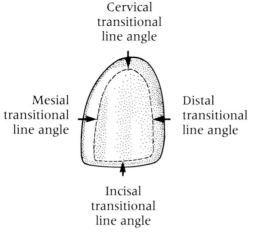

FIG. 2–11. The face of the tooth is bound by the transitional line angles.

The apparent face is that portion of the face that is visible to the viewer from any single view. The perimeter of the apparent face is dictated by the position of the viewer relative to the tooth. For example, from the front view, the entire incisor faces are visible, but usually only the mesial half of the faces of the maxillary canines (Fig. 2–12).

The *law of the face* states that to make dissimilar teeth appear similar, make the apparent faces equal (Figs. 2–13, 2–14). Creating equal apparent faces in two dissimilar adjacent teeth will produce dissimilar areas outside the transitional line angles (outside the faces). These dissimilarities are esthetically acceptable because they are essentially not visible; the similar faces of the teeth catch the light and appear to protrude while the dissimilar areas are in shadow and appear to recede (see Fig. 2–13). Through cultural biases we are conditioned to expect the faces of contralateral teeth to be equal even though exposed roots may be unequal in length. The six teeth in Figure 2–13 are dissimilar. Shaping the maxillary right central incisior, lateral incisor, and canine so that their faces equal that of the maxillary left central incisor, lateral incisor, and canine produces the illusion that these teeth are equal.

CLINICAL TIP. Equal faces can be most effectively created by shaping the labial surface to reposition the transitional line angles. This promotes a natural shadow.

When the transitional line angle cannot be repositioned on a ceramic restoration the artistic principle of illumination can be employed. A portion of the tooth can be stained darker to create the illusion that the transitional line angle has been moved and that the portion of the tooth is receding. In reality, the tooth contour remains unchanged (Fig. 2–15). *Only the "apparent face" should be manipulated, not the actual face.* This becomes particularly significant in posterior regions where the apparent face significantly differs from the actual face (see the section on Canines and The Law of The Face later in this chapter).

Alteration of the Face—Incisors

For clarity, the tooth to be mimicked is referred to as the "guide" tooth and the tooth to be altered as the "related" tooth.

Armamentarium

- Pencil
- Greenstones (porcelain)
- Multifluted carbides or finishing diamonds (tooth structure, composite resin)
- Aluminum oxide disks in varying coarseness, 4 grits are preferred (e.g., Sof-Flex, 3M Inc.) (tooth structure, acrylic, composite resin)
- Diamond disks (porcelain modification)
- Porcelain stains

Clinical Technique

1. Outline the face of the guide tooth with a pencil.
2. Examine the related tooth from the incisal angle to determine the buccolingual dimensions.
3. Using greenstones, multifluted carbides, finishing diamonds, or coarse disks, flatten the labial surface to the same level of protrusion as the guide tooth provided sufficient tooth structure (or restorative material) is available.
4. Using a pencil, draw a mirror image of the face of the guide tooth onto the related tooth.
5. Carve back toward the proximal surfaces from the boundaries of the face first using greenstones, multifluted carbides, finishing diamonds, and coarse disks followed by diamond disks and successively finer aluminum oxide disks. If this is not possible, shade the restorative material a darker color in the areas lateral to the face (pencil lines). In the case of porcelain, surface staining can be employed. In the case of

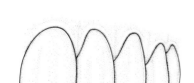

FIG. 2–12. From a frontal view, the canine displays only the mesial portion of the tooth, up to and including the midlabial ridge.

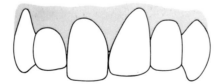

FIG. 2–13. Teeth with numerous, disharmonious esthetic problems.

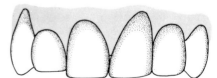

FIG. 2–14. Selective grinding of the incisal edges, moving the labial prominence of the left canine mesially, and altering the transitional line angles to make the apparent faces equal, creates an esthetic illusion of harmony.

composite resin, use a resin with a lower value or increased chroma.

Canines and the Law of the Face

The concept of the apparent face becomes more important when dealing with teeth posterior to the incisor teeth. From a frontal view, only a portion of the canine and posterior teeth are visible (see Figure 2–12). In the frontal view, the canine face is bounded by the mesial transitional line angle, the cervical transitional line angle, and the midlabial ridge. Usually the distal half of the tooth is not visible from a frontal view. The left and right side views cannot be seen simultaneously and are of secondary importance. Therefore, to blend a poorly shaped canine into a smile, four steps are needed.

Alteration of the Face—Canines

For clarity, the tooth to be mimicked is referred to as the "guide" tooth and the tooth to be altered as the "related" tooth.

Armamentarium. Same setup as above.

Clinical Technique

1. Using the frontal view, outline the apparent face of the guide tooth (the contralateral canine) with a pencil (Fig. 2–16A).
2. Again looking from the front, draw a mirror image of the apparent face of the guide tooth onto the related canine with a pencil.
3. Using these lines, move the midlabial ridge of the related tooth either mesially or distally to approximate the amount of tooth structure shown on the guide canine. Because only the area mesial to this ridge is seen from the frontal view, the viewer extrapolates the full size of the tooth as twice that size (Fig 2-16B).
4. From the side view, if the mesial half of the related tooth has been made smaller by moving the midla-

bial ridge toward the mesial, make the distal half of the face equal by locating the distal transitional line angle in a symmetric position to the mesial transitional line angle. Do this by carving the tooth structure back toward the lingual area from the distal transitional line angle (Fig. 2–16C).

Principle of Line

Horizontal lines, in the form of cervical staining, texturing, white hypoplastic lines, or long, straight incisal edges create the illusion of width. Widening the face will also produce that illusion (Fig. 2–17).

Vertical lines in the form of accentuated developmental grooves, hypoplastic lines, and vertical texturing accentuate height. Incisal edges of anterior teeth carved to slope cervically toward the distal area with larger incisal embrasures and a narrower (mesio-distally) incisal edge aid in creating an illusion of increased height. Narrowing the face will also create this illusion (see Fig. 2–17).

These same concepts apply for clothing and makeup. Individuals wearing clothing with vertical lines appear thinner. Conversely, horizontal stripes accentuate width and should be avoided by short overweight people. To "lengthen" and "slim" the nose with makeup, a light highlighter is placed in a vertical line down the center bridge of the nose. Then a darker contour shade of makeup is applied on each side of the nose to make that area recede.[9]

Age

The cultural bias of age is a sensitive issue for patients seeking esthetic care and must be considered.

Older Teeth. Older teeth (Fig. 2–18)

1. Are smoother
2. Are darker (i.e., not as bright, lower value)
3. Have a higher saturation (higher chroma)
4. Are shorter incisally (less tooth shows when the patient is smiling)

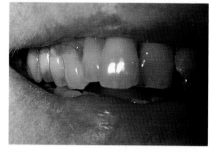

FIG. 2–15. The porcelain-fused-to-metal crown restoring the maxillary right second premolar has been darkened at the gingival third to create the illusion of a discolored restoration. The root surface appears to recede because it has a lower (darker) value.

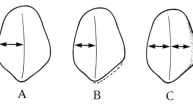

FIG. 2–16. From a frontal view the canine appears too wide. These steps are required to create the illusion of a narrower tooth. A. Preoperative view of the canine with the width delineated by an arrow. B. The midlabial ridge is moved mesially, creating the illusion of a narrower tooth. The incisal tip is also moved mesially by removing tooth structure from the distal aspect of the incisal edge. C. The distal transitional line angle is moved mesially, until the distal face is equal to the mesial face. The canine now appears narrower from both the frontal and side views.

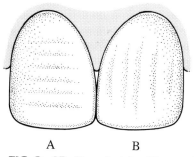

FIG. 2–17. The principle of line can be used to create the illusion of a longer or shorter tooth. Stain lines, texturing, and modifying the face and incisal edge all contribute to the illusion.

5. Are longer gingivally (although they may be shorter incisally)
6. Have worn, even incisal edges with little incisal embrasures
7. Have wider more open gingival embrasures
8. Are more characterized.

The lower incisors exhibit flat broad incisal edges, which show a dentin core.

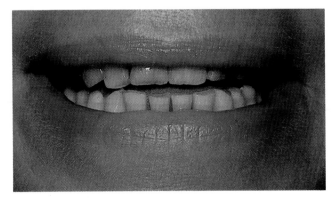

FIG. 2–18. Older teeth are smoother, darker, shorter, have worn incisal edges, and are more characterized.

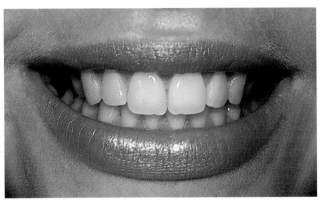

FIG. 2–19. Younger teeth are more textured, brighter, have lower chroma, and have gingival margins at the cemento-enamel junction (CEJ). They have pronounced incisal embrasures, small gingival embrasures, and are only lightly characterized. Lateral incisors are shorter than the central incisors and the canines. These feminine-looking teeth are more rounded at the transitional line angles with pronounced incisal embrasures.

Younger Teeth. Younger teeth (Fig. 2–19):

1. Are more textured
2. Are lighter (i.e., brighter, higher value)
3. Have a lower saturation (lower chroma)
4. Have a gingival margin at approximately the cementoenamel junction
5. Have incisal edges that make the laterals appear shorter than the incisors or canines
6. Have significant incisal embrasures
7. Have small gingival embrasures
8. Have light characterization, often with white hypoplastic lines or spots.

Clinically, the ultimate esthetic goal is to make artificial prostheses appear natural. (This should elicit a third party response of: "What beautiful teeth you have," rather than an observer noticing an artificial substitution.) Beautiful natural teeth or artificial substitutes should be harmonious with the patient's personality, age, and sex.

Sex

Lombardi[8] described a theory of anterior esthetics in which he proposed that the age, sex, and personality of a person was reflected in the shape and form of the teeth. Factually, the concept of sexual dimorphism is difficult to prove or disprove. Alternately, this concept should be considered in the light of a cultural bias.

Feminine. Feminine teeth are more rounded, both on the incisal edges and at the transitional line angles. The incisal embrasures, therefore are more pronounced. The incisal edges are more translucent and white hypoplastic striations may be used to give the illusion of delicacy (see Figure 2–20). The translucency on the incisal edges appears as a gray line in the incisal one-eighth of the facial surface paralleling the incisal edge with a white hypoplastic rim on the edge.

Masculine. Masculine teeth are more angular and rugged. In older men, chroma is greater and body color often extends to the incisal edges. The incisal embrasures are more squared and not as pronounced as in teeth appearing more flowing and feminine. Characterization is often stronger, incorporating darker craze lines (Fig. 2–21).

Cultural and artistic biases are central to understand-

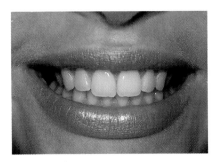

FIG. 2–20

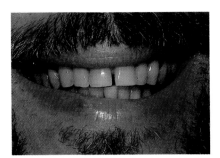

FIG. 2–21

FIG. 2–20. Feminine-looking teeth are more rounded and translucent, giving an appearance of delicacy.

FIG. 2–21. Masculine-looking teeth are more angular, have a higher chroma, square incisal edges, and have darker craze lines.

ing dental esthetics. They must be thoroughly understood so that the dentist, as an artist, can use these biases to create illusions to satisfy the esthetic demands of the patient. Only then can the technically proficient dentist rise to the level of an artist, thus, providing a higher level of care.

LABORATORY COMMUNICATIONS

There are many practical ways to enhance communication with the dental laboratory. Shape and texture can be communicated by intraoral photographs, either in the form of slides or prints. Desired form may also be conveyed via video imaging technology (see Chapter 29—Esthetics and Advanced Technology). Shape, though, is perhaps best communicated three dimensionally. Preoperative study models, wax-ups on these models for development of the provisional phase, and models of the provisional restorations are helpful. Models of the seated bisque bake allow the technician to see the relation of tooth shape to the soft tissue.

Color communication can be accomplished by demonstration or prescription. Demonstration is by far the most accurate method. Custom colored shade tabs sent to the laboratory as a three-dimensional prescription are most effective. They can be shaded with the same materials used in chairside dental porcelain staining with the only modification being the use of a product such as Ceramco Stain Set (Ceramco, Dentsply) as a liquid media (see Appendix A, Custom Staining). The same technique can be used to communicate final coloring when the case is at the bisque bake stage.

REFERENCES

1. Waltke, R.: Color in the Human Dentition. New Rochelle, Jelenko, 1977.
2. Clark, E.B.: Tooth color selection. JADA, June:1065, 1933.
3. Munsell, A.H.: A Grammar of Color. New York, Van Nostrand Reinhold Co., 1969.
4. Feinman, R.A., Goldstein, R.E., Garber, D.A.: Bleaching Teeth. Chicago, Quintessence Publishing Co., Inc., 1987.
5. Preston, J.D., Bergen, S.F.: Color Science and Dental Art, A Self-Teaching Program. St. Louis, C.V. Mosby Co., 1980.
6. Sproull, R.C.: Color matching in dentistry. Part III. Color control. J Prosthet Dent 31:146, 1974.
7. Feigenbaum, N., Mopper, K.W.: A Complete Guide to Dental Bonding. East Windsor, Johnson and Johnson, 1984.
8. Lombardi, R.E.: Visual perception and denture esthetics. J Prosthet Dent 29:363, 1973.
9. Jackson, C.: Color Me Beautiful Makeup Book. New York, Ballantine Books, 1988.

BIBLIOGRAPHY

Adams, A.: Artificial-Light Photography. Hastings-on-Hudson, Morgan and Morgan, Inc., 1968.
Agoston, G.A.: Color Theory and its Application in Art and Design. New York, Springer-Verlag. 1979.
Appleby, D.S., Craig, C.: Subtleties of contour: a system for recognition and correction. Compend Contin Ed 7:109, 1986.
Beder, O.E.: Esthetics—an enigma. J Prosthet Dent 25:588, 1971.
Bergen, S.F., McCasland, J.: Dental operatory lighting and tooth color discrimination. JADA, 94:130, 1977.

Culpepper, W.D.: A comparative study of shade-matching procedures. J Prosthet Dent 24:166, 1970.
Culpepper, W.D.: Esthetic factors in anterior tooth restoration. J Prosthet Dent 30:576, 1973.
Ceramco Stain System Manual. East Windsor, Johnson and Johnson, 1977.
De Van, M.: Methods of procedure in a diagnostic service to the edentulous patient. JADA 29:1981, 1942.
Edwards, B.: Drawing on the right side of the brain: a course in enhancing creativity and artistic confidence. New York, St. Martin's Press, 1979.
Edwards, B.: Drawing on the artist within: a guide to innovation, invention, imagination, and creativity. New York, Simon and Schuster, 1986.
Edwards, B.: Drawing on the artist within: an inspirational and practical guide to increasing your creative powers. New York, Simon and Schuster, 1986.
Feigenbaum, N., Mopper, K.W.: A Complete Guide to Dental Bonding. East Windsor, Johnson and Johnson, 1984.
Friedman, M.: Staining and shade control of dental ceramics. Part I. Trends and Techniques, April, 1987.
Friedman, M.: Staining and shade control of dental ceramics. Part II. Trends and Techniques. May:24, 1987.
Frush, J.P., Fisher, R.D.: Introduction to dentogenic restorations. J Prosthet Dent 5:586, 1955.
Frush, J.P., Fisher, R.D.: How dentogenic restorations interpret the sex factor. J Prosthet Dent 6:160, 1956.
Frush, J.P., Fisher, R.D.: How dentogenics interprets the personality factor. J Prosthet Dent 6:441, 1956.
Frush, J.P., Fisher, R.D.: The age factor in dentogenics. J Prosthet Dent 7:5, 1957.
Frush, J.P., Fisher, R.D.: The dysesthetic interpretation of the dentogenic concept. J Prosthet Dent 8:558, 1958.
Frush, J.P., Fisher, R.D.: Dentogenics: its practical application. J Prosthet Dent 9:914, 1959.
Garber, D.A., Goldstein, R.E., Feinman, R.A.: Porcelain Laminate Veneers. Chicago, Quintessence Publishing Co., Inc., 1988.
Goldstein, R.E.: Esthetics in Dentistry. Philadelphia, J.B. Lippincott Co., 1976.
Goldstein, R.E.: Change Your Smile. Chicago, Quintessence Publishing Co., Inc., 1987.
Held, R.: Readings from Scientific American, Image, Object, and Illusion. San Francisco, W.H. Freeman Co., 1974.
Jackson, C.: Color Me Beautiful. New York, Ballantine Books, 1985.
Light and Film. New York, Time-Life Books, 1970.
Pincus, C.L.: Cosmetics—the psychologic fourth dimension in full mouth rehabilitation. Dent Clin North Am, March, 1967.
Rickets, R.M.: The Golden Divider. J Clin Ortho 15:752, 1981.
Rogers, L.R.: Sculpture. Toronto, Oxford University Press, 1969.
Sorensen, J.A., Torres, T.J.: Improved color matching of metal-ceramic restorations. Part I. A systematic method for shade determination. J Prosthet Dent 58:133, 1987.
Sorensen, J.A., Torres, T.J.: Improved color matching of metal-ceramic restorations. Part II. Procedures for visual communication. J Prosthet Dent 58:669, 1987.
Sorensen, J.A., Torres, T.J.: Improved color matching of metal-ceramic restorations. Part III. Innovations in porcelain application. J Prosthet Dent 59:1, 1988.
Sproull, R.C.: Color matching in dentistry. Part I. The three-dimensional nature of color. J Prosthet Dent 29:416, 1973.
Sproull, R.C.: Color matching in dentistry. Part II. Practical applications of the organization of color. J Prosthet Dent 29:556, 1973.
Swedlund, C.: Photography. New York, Holt, Rinehart and Winston, Inc., 1974.
Torlakson, J., Gordon, J.: Deepening the third dimension. The Artist's Magazine, 6:50, 1989.

Mark Jensen, M.S., D.D.S., Ph.D.

DENTIN BONDING AGENTS

3

Significant advances in adhesive dentistry have occurred over the past three decades. The bonding of bis-GMA resin to etched enamel[1] introduced esthetic restorations without the need for mechanical retention within the cavity preparation. Many cavity preparations, however, have significant amounts of exposed dentin, and many have cavosurface margins of cementum or dentin. An obvious goal was to develop an adhesive material that would bond to dentin with at least a strength equal to that of resin bonded to etched enamel. Creating this type of dentin bonding is extremely difficult because of the composition of this vital tissue. The composition of dentin is only about 50% inorganic by volume as compared to approximately 98% for enamel. The remaining volume is primarily water and collagen. In addition, a surface or a physically altered layer is created by instrumentation during operative procedures. This layer is a mechanically altered surface that is relatively homogenous and covers the instrumented dentin, occluding open tubules. This layer is most commonly referred to as a smear layer and has a distinctive scanning electron microscopic appearance (Fig. 3–1). These factors have made the goals of dentin bonding difficult to achieve.

HISTORIC PERSPECTIVE

Dentin bonding has evolved through essentially three generations of materials. The first generation materials were developed in the late 1950s and early 1960s and included polyurethanes, cyanoacrylates, glycerophosphoric acid dimethacrylate, and NPG-GMA (N-phenyl glycine and glycidylmethacrylate). All of these approaches proved to be clinically unsuccessful. Bond strengths to dentin surfaces, when tested on a "shear-like" model, were only approximately 10 to 20 kg/cm^2.[2]

Second generation dentin bonding agents were introduced nearly 2 decades later. These materials include the commercial products Scotchbond, Dentin Bonding Agent, Creation Bonding Agent, Dentin-Adhesit, Bondlite, and Prisma Universal Bond. Most of these agents were halophosphorus esters of bis-GMA that attempted to bond to the mineral portion of dentin as a phosphate-calcium bond. The bond, however, was hydrolyzed over time in the oral environment. This factor may help account for their clinical failure. A wide range of in vitro bond strengths of approximately 30 to 90 kg/cm^2, which is well below that of etched enamel bonding, has been reported with these materials.[3] Clinical success, however, was not satisfactory.[3,4,5,6,7]

Within the last decade, a third generation of dentin bonding materials has flooded the commercial dental market beginning with the oxalate dentin bonding system introduced by Bowen in 1982.[8] Originally, this system was very cumbersome and often unpredictable, but it exhibited improved bond strengths of approximately 100 to 150 kg/cm^2. The acidified ferric oxalate in this system is believed to be a source of marginal discoloration and the complicated series of reagents made the system clinically difficult to use. However, in vitro bond strength for improved versions of these agents has been reported to reach 200 to 220 kg/cm^2, approximately the strength of resin bonded to etched enamel.

IDEAL CHARACTERISTICS OF DENTIN BONDING AGENTS

The ideal characteristics of a dentin bonding agent include:

1. Bond strength to dentin that is equivalent to or higher than that of the etched enamel-resin bond.
2. Rapid attainment of maximal bond strength.
3. Biocompatible with and nonirritating to the pulp.
4. Elimination of microleakage.
5. Long range stability within the oral environment.
6. Ease of application with little technique sensitivity.

Third-generation agents have undergone testing[9] over a 3-year period, and show significant promise. These studies have focused upon performance of the materials in nonretentive cervical abrasion lesions without etching enamel. However, results concerning bond strengths vary considerably. Uniform research protocol and testing standardization is lacking.[10] In addition, a direct extrapolation from in vitro tests to the oral environment is not possible.[11]

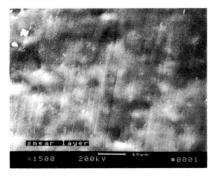

FIG. 3—1. Scanning electron micrograph (SEM) of "smear layer" on the dentin surface (uncoated specimen).

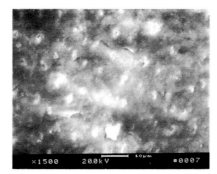

FIG. 3—2. Different types of instrumentation produce variations in the smear layer and it is generally thicker when a rotary instrument is used without a water coolant.

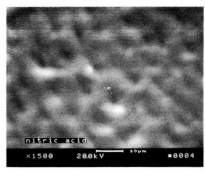

FIG. 3—3. Modification of the smear layer following treatment with a solution of phenylglycine in a 2.5% nitric acid. The dentinal tubules are not completely opened but can be readily seen beneath the altered smear layer.

INDICATIONS

A dentin bonding agent is indicated under composite resin restorations when cavity preparation exposes dentin or when any cavosurface margin involves cementum or dentin. It helps reduce marginal leakage, even if it is not totally eliminated, thus lessening pulpal irritation and sensitivity, marginal discoloration, and recurrent caries.

Clinical data is insufficient to allow the practitioner to rely solely on dentin bonding for retention, even in Class V low stress-bearing areas. Until further clinical data is obtained, even third-generation dentin bonding agents should be used in conjunction with cavity preparations that include mechanical retention form. Hopefully, this can be eliminated as dentin bonding improves.

Although third-generation dentin bonding materials may not be ideal, they certainly offer much more promise than before for clinical success. Sufficient data exists to warrant the clinical application of these agents in a very conservative manner. Appropriate case selection should involve informed consent on the patient's behalf. When used in this way, the third-generation dentin bonding agents become an adjunct to current esthetic restorative techniques and help to improve dentistry for the patient. If case selection is improper or if correct techniques are not adhered to strictly, failure is almost certain. The future of dentin bonding appears bright and, hopefully, the ideal bonding agent for dentin will be developed and incorporated into the practice of clinical dentistry in the coming years.

CHEMISTRY

Most third-generation dentin bonding agents incorporate either smear layer removal during the treatment sequence or a substantial modification, usually with an acidic liquid. Previous generations of dentin bonding agents simply adhered to the unaltered smear layer. Failure apparently occurred at the dentin to smear layer interface or within the smear layer itself. Variations in this layer occur with different types of instrumentation and this layer is generally thicker when a water coolant is not used with the rotary instrument (Fig. 3—2). After removal or conditioning of the smear layer, a bonding resin is applied, which creates the adhesion to dentin as well as a coupled bond to the restorative material.

Total Etch Technique

A controversial modality, the total etch technique involves the application of acid-etch to the entire external and internal aspect of the preparation. Besides etching both the enamel and dentin, it serves to totally remove the smear layer, leaving the dentinal tubules completely open. The sequela of etching dentin has yet to be determined. In addition, because a true bond to the organic portion of the dentin has not been adequately demonstrated, this technique deserves more scientific investigation before its widespread clinical application.

Oxalate Systems (e.g., Tenure, Mirage Bond II)

The iron of the original Bowen formulation was replaced with aluminum and the system evolved into a clinically applicable product. A solution of phenylglycine in a 2.5% nitric acid solution is used to alter the smear layer (Fig. 3—3). The dentin surface is then treated with an oxalate solution and PMDM and acetone. The crystalline structure is believed to create the bond to the dentin surface (Fig. 3—4).

Glutaraldehyde/HEMA (e.g., Gluma)

This third-generation dentin bonding agent was introduced initially in Europe.[12] The manufacturer claimed the material bonds to collagen in the dentin in addition to the mechanical bond to dentin structure. Although this has not been substantiated with physicochemical evidence, the dentin adhesive has been extensively investigated in both the laboratory and clinical setting and results are promising. A 0.5M EDTA solution is used to remove the smear layer (Fig. 3—5) by chelation at a pH of 7.4. The glutaraldehyde/HEMA solution is then applied to create a bond. A layer of unfiltered bis-GMA is

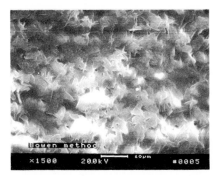

FIG. 3–4. Following phenylglycine/nitric acid treatment an oxalate, PMDM, and acetone solution is applied. The resultant crystalline structure is believed to create the bond to the dentin surface.

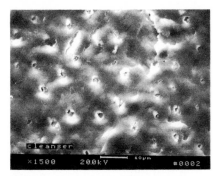

FIG. 3–5. A 0.5M EDTA solution or "cleanser" is used to remove the smear layer. The dentinal tubules are evident but not fully opened.

FIG. 3–7. Phosphonated dimethacrylate and a camphorquinone photoinitiator are applied to the dentin surface, and then photocured.

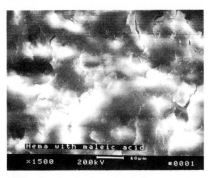

FIG. 3–6. A hydrophobic monomer (HEMA) and a bis-GMA system are applied to the dentin surface.

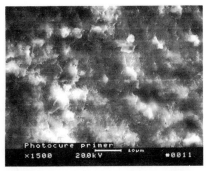

FIG. 3–7

placed over the bonded surface and photocured prior to application of the restorative composite resin.

Hydrophobic Monomer/Bis-GMA (e.g., Scotchbond 2)

A hydrophobic monomer (HEMA) and bis-GMA system was also recently introduced as a third-generation dentin adhesive. This approach consists of a two-component system comprised of a primer and a photocuring adhesive. The primer is an aqueous solution of hydrophilic methacrylate monomers (hydroxyethyl methacrylate or HEMA) acidified with maleic acid. The acidic nature of the primer acts to modify the smear layer while incorporating the HEMA onto the surface in a controlled manner. The HEMA contains a hydroxyl group and is, therefore, considered to be hydrophilic or "water loving." This allows the product to more easily coat or wet the surface of the dentin, which is relatively high in water content.

The Scotchbond 2 primer is incorporated into the modified smear layer although often most tubules are observed to be almost entirely patent (Fig. 3–6). The dentin surface is treated with this acidified HEMA primer. Note the material has altered the smear layer and covered the entire surface even over the area of the tubules. The adhesive consists of photoactive initiators for light-curing, as well as both HEMA and the hydrophobic monomer bis-GMA. The surface of this adhesive layer is oxygen-inhibited, which allows the bonding resin to bond to the dentin adhesive. Composite resin is then placed over the bonded surface to act as a restorative material.

Polyhexanide Methacrylate Resin (e.g., Tripton)

The primer for this system consists of a 0.1% weight by volume aqueous solution of polyhexanide of polyhex-

anethylene biguanide hydrochloride. This acts to condition the smear layer and modify the surface energy of the dentin so it can be better wet by the bonding resin. The bonding resin consists of a mixture of MPDM (methacryl propane diol monophosphate), TEGDM, (triethylene glycol dimethacrylate), urethane dionethacrylate, and camphorquinine as a photocuring catalyst. The bonding resin is photocured and then composite resin is placed over the "bonded" dentin as a restorative material.

Phosphonated Dimethacrylate/ Phosponated Bis-GMA (e.g., XR-Primer)

The conditioning agent in this system is a photocuring primer consisting of phosponated dimethacrylate and a camphorquinone photo-initiator or catalyst. The primer solution is brushed onto the prepared dentin surface and then air-dried. The material is then photocured for 10 seconds (Fig. 3–7). A phosphorated bis-GMA resin is then placed over the cured point and photocured for 20 seconds. The preparation is then restored with composite resin.

Citric Acid-Ferric Chloride/4 Meta (e.g., Superbond, Metadent, Phenyl-P)

These systems substantially remove the smear layer during priming through the use of acid. Superbond uses a 10% citric acid with 3% ferric chloride; Phenyl-P uses phosphoric acid in glycerin. The bonding agent in Superbond is 4 META (methacryloxyethyl trimellitic anhydride) and PMMA (poly-methyl-methacrylate) with RTBB-O (partially oxidized tri-n-butyl ketone). The 4 META/PMMA-TBB enhances wetting of the cleaned dentin and creates a graft polymerization onto the collagen, which is initiated by the TBB. Photocuring composite resin is used as a restorative material over the bonded dentin.

GENERAL CONSIDERATIONS

Cavity preparation, basing, and placement of composite restoration materials are generally the same for all dentin bonding systems. It is extremely important that the tooth surfaces are not contaminated in any way during the procedure. Therefore, adequate isolation is absolutely essential. Should contamination occur at any step, the entire process must be repeated beginning with thorough surface cleansing achieved by mechanically cleaning the tooth surface with a prophylaxis brush or cup and nonfluoridated pumice. The cleaned tooth surface should be rinsed with a water/air or water spray for 15 seconds and dried with an oil-free stream of air from the triple syringe.

Dentin adhesive materials are sensitive to variations in clinical techniques. The agents are often operator-dependent and success is most often found with strict adherence to manufacturers instructions. If a clear understanding of each step and why it is performed is not obtained, the practitioner may deviate from the ideal and meet with failure. For example, rinsing after placement of the Scotchbond 2 primer, Scotchprep, in the same manner as is done after the Gluma II cleanser would most likely remove the HEMA or contaminate it with moisture and result in failure.

CLINICAL PROCEDURES

In order to gain a clinical appreciation for various third-generation dentin bonding agents, the clinical procedures for four representative systems are listed and discussed. The clinical procedures for one—Polyhexanide (Tripton)—are illustrated with clinical photographs and schematic diagrams.

Polyhexanide/Methacrylate (e.g., Tripton)
Armamentarium

- Standard dental setup
  Explorer
  Mouth mirror
  Periodontal probe
  Suitable anesthesia
  Rubber dam setup
  High-speed handpiece
  Low-speed handpiece
  No. 2 Round Bur
- Calcium hydroxide (e.g., Dycal)
- Orthophosphoric acid etch gel
- Tripton

Clinical Technique

1. Administer local anesthesia if necessary.
2. Isolate the lesion with a rubber dam.

3. Cleanse the tooth with a nonfluoridated pumice (Figs. 3–8, 3–9).
4. Prepare the cavity in a conventional manner (Fig. 3–10).
5. Using a round bur and slow-speed handpiece, place mechanical retention slots, grooves, or points. (Fig. 3–11).

CLINICAL TIP. In preparations without mechanical retention, such as cervical abrasion, the enamel should be beveled.

---

6. In deep cavities, (within approximately 0.5 mm of the pulp) place an acid-resistant calcium hydroxide base over the deep areas. This area should be kept to a minimum in order to leave an adequate amount of exposed dentin (Fig. 3–12).
7. Place orthophosphoric acid gel on the enamel margins for 15 seconds (Fig. 3–13).
8. Wash the preparation for 20 seconds with a water spray.
9. Dry the area with a stream of oil-free air (Fig. 3–14).
10. If the enamel does not appear etched (frosty white) reapply orthophosphoric acid gel (15 seconds), rinse with water (20 seconds), dry, and re-evaluate. The enamel must be properly etched in order to obtain an adequate bond.
11. Apply the primer to all exposed dentin surfaces for 30 seconds (Fig. 3–15).

CLINICAL TIP. Inadvertent placement of primer on etched enamel will *not* effect subsequent enamel bond strength.

CLINICAL TIP. The surface must be kept wet with primer for the entire 30 second period in order to obtain an optimal bond.

---

12. *Gently* air-dry the preparation. *Do not rinse the primer off with water.*
13. Apply a thin layer of bonding resin to all primed dentin and etched enamel surfaces (Fig. 3–16).

CLINICAL TIP. Avoid excess puddling of resin by gently blowing it with oil-free air or absorbing it with a dry endodontic paper point.

---

14. Photocure the dentin bonding resin for 30 seconds (Fig. 3–17). If the curing surface of the lamp is inadequate to cure the entire restoration at one time, the tip should be repositioned and the polymerization process repeated until all the resin is cured.
15. Restore the cavity with an appropriate composite resin system. (See Chapter 5—Composite Resin—Fundamentals and Direct Technique Restorations).
16. Following the finishing of the restoration, a final glaze of the Tripton resin may be applied over the completed restoration to help seal any marginal microgaps that may have been created by the finishing process (Fig. 3–18).

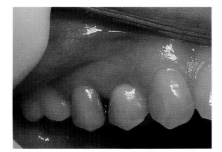

FIG. 3–8. Preoperative class V lesion.

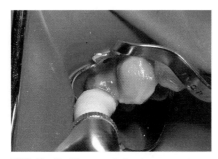

FIG. 3–9. The tooth is cleaned with a nonfluoridated flour of pumice.

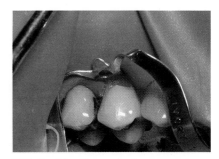

FIG. 3–10. The cavity is prepared.

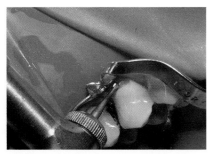

FIG. 3–11. Mechanical retention slots, grooves, or points are placed using a round bur in a slow-speed handpiece.

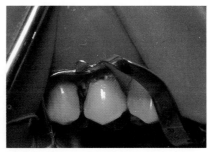

FIG. 3–12. An acid-resistant calcium hydroxide liner is placed in deep areas of the preparation.

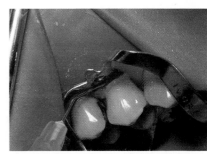

FIG. 3–13. The orthophosphoric acid gel is placed on the enamel margins for 15 seconds.

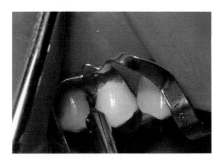

FIG. 3–14. The preparation is washed for 20 seconds with a water spray and dried with a stream of oil-free air.

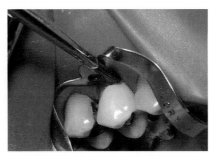

FIG. 3–15. The primer is applied to all exposed dentin surfaces for 30 seconds.

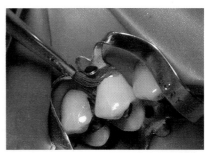

FIG. 3–16. A thin layer of bonding resin is applied to all primed dentin and etched enamel surfaces.

FIG. 3–17. The dentin bonding resin is photocured for 30 seconds.

FIG. 3–18. A final glaze of the resin may be applied over the completed restoration to help seal any marginal microgaps that may have been created by the finishing process.

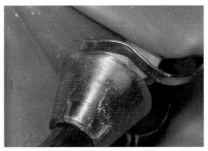

FIG. 3–17

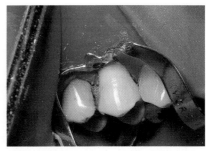

FIG. 3–18

Glutaraldehyde/HEMA—(e.g., Gluma)

Armamentarium. Identical to polyhexanide/methacrylate (e.g., Tripton) armamentarium listed previously except:

■ Gluma kit

Clinical Technique

1. Administer local anesthesia.
2. Isolate the lesion with a rubber dam (Fig. 3–19).
3. Cleanse the tooth with a nonfluoridated pumice.
4. Prepare the cavity in a conventional manner.
5. Using a round bur and slow-speed handpiece, place mechanical retention slots, grooves, or points.

CLINICAL TIP. In preparations without mechanical retention, such as cervical abrasion, the enamel should be beveled.

---

6. In deep cavities, (within approximately 0.5 mm of the pulp) place an acid-resistant calcium hydroxide base over the deep areas. This area should be kept to a minimum in order to leave an adequate amount of exposed dentin (Fig. 3–20).
7. Place orthophosphoric acid gel (Gluma I) on the enamel margins for 15 seconds (Fig. 3–21).
8. Wash the preparation for 20 seconds with a water spray (Fig. 3–22).
9. Dry the area with a stream of oil-free air.
10. If the enamel does not appear etched (frosty white) reapply orthophosphoric acid gel (15 seconds), rinse with water (20 seconds), dry, and re-evaluate. The enamel must be properly etched in order to obtain an adequate bond.
11. Remove the smear layer by rubbing neutralized aqueous EDTA (Gluma II) to the dentin with a cotton pledget. Leave the solution on for 30 seconds.

CLINICAL TIP. Inadvertent placement of cleanser (Gluma II) primer on etched enamel will *not* effect subsequent enamel bond strength.

CLINICAL TIP. The surface must be kept wet with cleanser (Gluma II) for the entire 30 second period in order to obtain an optimal bond.

---

12. *Rinse the Gluma II off with water* for 30 seconds in order to completely remove the smear layer.
13. Dry the dentin with a gentle stream of oil-free air.
14. Apply glutaraldehyde and HEMA (Gluma III) to the dentin with a cotton pledget or brush. Leave the solution on for 30 seconds (Fig. 3–23).

CLINICAL TIP. Inadvertent placement of primer (Gluma III) on etched enamel will *not* effect subsequent enamel bond strength.

CLINICAL TIP. The surface must be kept wet with primer (Gluma III) for the entire 30 second period in order to obtain an optimal bond.

---

15. Gently air-dry the preparation. *Do not rinse the primer off with water* (Fig. 3-24).
16. Apply a thin layer of bonding resin (Gluma IV) to all primed dentin and etched enamel surfaces (Fig. 3-25).

CLINICAL TIP. Avoid excess puddling of resin by gently blowing it with oil-free air or absorbing it with a dry endodontic paper point.

---

17. Photocure the dentin bonding resin for 30 seconds. If the curing surface of the lamp is inadequate, the tip should be repositioned and the polymerization process repeated until all resin is cured (Fig. 3–26).
18. Restore the cavity with an appropriate composite resin system (Fig. 3–27). (See Chapter 5—Composite Resin—Fundamentals and Direct Technique Restorations).

Although the manufacturer claims that the Gluma IV layer does not have to be photocured prior to placement of the resin, if the preparation is being restored directly with composite resin recent data indicates photocuring the Gluma IV is necessary.[13] When used with indirect restorations that require low film thickness of luting agents, this step is not indicated because the thickness of the material can prevent full setting of the restoration. In addition, the air-inhibited layer will not be a factor in this case.

Oxalate Systems (e.g., Tenure)

This dentin adhesive system has changed dramatically since it was first introduced. The application procedure only includes acid etching the enamel as an optional step. Den-Mat contends that the nitric acid in the conditioner is adequate to etch the enamel. Oxalate systems (e.g., Tenure) are solutions of 2.5% nitric acid, malic acid, and oxalate mordant. Although promising, their clinical application to dentin and enamel has not been tested adequately. Until further research is conducted, orthophosphoric acid-etching of enamel and mechanical retention are still highly recommended in order to avoid clinical failures.

Armamentarium. Identical to polyhexanide/methacrylate (e.g., TRIPTON) armamentarium listed previously except:

■ Tenure kit

Clinical Technique

1. Administer local anesthesia.
2. Isolate the lesion with a rubber dam.
3. Cleanse the tooth with a nonfluoridated flour of pumice.
4. Prepare the cavity in a conventional manner.
5. Using a round bur and slow-speed handpiece, place mechanical retention slots, grooves, or points.

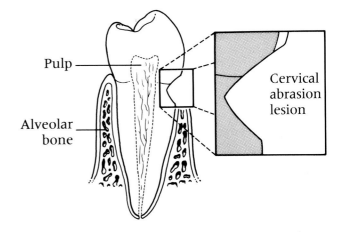

FIG. 3–19. Initial cervical abrasion. (Rubber dam not shown for clarity.)

Pulp

Alveolar bone

Cervical abrasion lesion

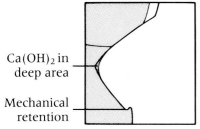

Ca(OH)₂ in deep area

Mechanical retention

FIG. 3–20. An acid-resistant calcium hydroxide base is placed in deep cavities. Note mechanical retention.

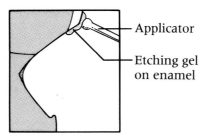

Applicator

Etching gel on enamel

FIG. 3–21. Orthophosphoric acid gel is placed on the enamel margins for 15 seconds.

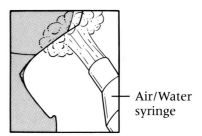

Air/Water syringe

FIG. 3–22. The preparation is washed for 20 seconds with a water spray and dried with a stream of oil-free air.

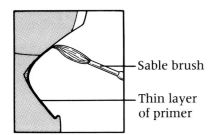

Sable brush

Thin layer of primer

FIG. 3–23. A thin layer of primer is applied to all exposed dentin surfaces following the removal of the smear layer.

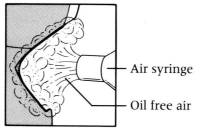

Air syringe

Oil free air

FIG. 3–24. The tooth is dried with oil-free air.

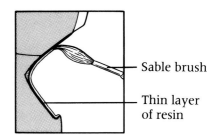

Sable brush

Thin layer of resin

FIG. 3–25. A thin layer of bonding resin is applied to all primed dentin and etched enamel surfaces.

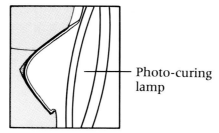

Photo-curing lamp

FIG. 3–26. The dentin bonding resin is photocured for 30 seconds.

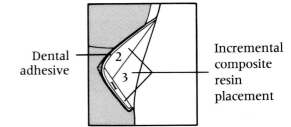

Dental adhesive

Incremental composite resin placement

FIG. 3–27. The cavity is restored with incremental layers of composite resin.

6. In deep cavities, (approximately 0.5 mm of the pulp) an acid-resistant calcium hydroxide base should be placed over the deep areas. This area should be kept to a minimum in order to leave an adequate amount of exposed dentin.
7. Place orthophosphoric acid gel on the enamel margins for 15 seconds (see note above).
8. Wash the preparation for 20 seconds with a water spray.
9. Dry the area with a stream of oil-free air.
10. If the enamel does not appear etched (frosty white), reapply orthophosphoric acid gel (15 seconds), rinse with water (20 seconds), dry, and re-evaluate. Enamel must be properly etched in order to obtain an adequate bond.
11. Condition the enamel and dentin with 2.5% nitric acid, maleic acid, and oxalate mordant (Den-Mat conditioner) for 30 to 60 seconds (see note above).
12. *Rinse the conditioner off with water* for 30 seconds.
13. Dry the dentin with a gentle stream of oil-free air.
14. Mix the Tenure A and Tenure B (NTG-GMA and PDM, respectively) bonding agents for 10 to 20 seconds with a brush and immediately apply it to the cavity preparation.
15. Dry with a stream of oil-free air.
16. Reapply the solution.
17. Once again, dry thoroughly with a stream of oil-free air.
18. Apply an unfilled bis-GMA resin (Visor Seal) to all primed dentin and etched enamel surfaces.

CLINICAL TIP. Avoid excess puddling of resin by gently blowing it with oil-free air or absorbing it with a dry endodontic paper point.

19. Apply a thin layer of bonding resin.
20. Photocure the dentin bonding resin for 30 seconds. If the curing surface of the lamp is inadequate, the tip should be repositioned and the polymerization process repeated until all resin is cured.
21. Restore the cavity with an appropriate composite resin system. (see Chapter 5, Composite Resins—Fundamentals and Direct Technique Restorations).

Hydrophobic Monomer/Bis-GMA—(e.g., Scotchbond 2)

Armamentarium. Identical to polyhexanide/methacrylate (e.g., Tripton) armamentarium listed previously except:

■ Scotchbond II Kit

Clinical Technique

1. Administer local anesthesia.
2. Isolate the lesion with a rubber dam.
3. Cleanse the tooth with a nonfluoridated flour of pumice.

4. Prepare the cavity in a conventional manner.
5. Using a round bur and slow-speed handpiece, place mechanical retention slots, grooves or points.

CLINICAL TIP. In preparations without mechanical retention, such as cervical abrasion, the enamel should be beveled.

6. In deep cavities (within approximately 0.5 mm of the pulp), an acid-resistant calcium hydroxide base should be placed over the deep areas. This area should be kept to a minimum in order to leave an adequate amount of exposed dentin.
7. Place orthophosphoric acid gel on the enamel margins for 15 seconds.
8. Wash the preparation for 20 seconds with a water spray.
9. Dry the area with a stream of oil-free air.
10. If the enamel does not appear etched (frosty white) reapply orthophosphoric acid gel (15 seconds), rinse with water (20 seconds), dry, and re-evaluate. Enamel must be properly etched in order to obtain an adequate bond.
11. Condition the teeth with aqueous solution of HEMA and maleic acid (Scotchprep), which mixes with and solubilizes the smear-layer.
12. Gently air dry the preparation. *Do not rinse the primer off with water.*
13. With a sable brush, apply the dentin adhesive resin (Scotchbond 2) to the primed dentin and etched enamel.

CLINICAL TIP. A layer of 75 to 100 microns is desired. Because the resin pools readily in line and point angles of the cavity preparation, careful attention and practice are required. Although thinning with an air stream has been advocated, this is not advisable. The excess resin should be removed with a dry sable brush or with an endodontic paper point.

14. Photocure the dentin bonding resin for 20 seconds. If the curing surface of the lamp is inadequate to cure the entire restoration at one time, the tip should be repositioned and the polymerization process repeated until all the resin is cured.
15. Restore the cavity with an appropriate composite resin system. (See Chapter 5—Composite Resin—Fundamentals and Direct Technique Restorations).

Since Scotchbond 2 is not radiopaque, a radiolucent line may appear on radiographs, especially if the liquid is allowed to pool. Another drawback with this resin is that the 100-micron thick layer of resin may be visible in some cases, especially if the margins are on etched enamel. This system is contraindicated for indirect restorations unless dentin bonding is carried out prior to taking the impression.

CONCLUSION

Wider applications of dentin bonding have been in the developmental stages for some time. Laboratory and clinical studies have been conducted or are underway to evaluate the use of dentin bonding agents for all kinds of resin-bonded ceramics, for root desensitization, and even for caries prevention as possible root surface sealants.

REFERENCES

1. Buonocore, M.G., Wileman, W., and Brudevold, F.: Simple methods of increasing adhesion of acrylic filling materials to enamel surfaces. J Dent Res 34:849, 1955.
2. Asmussen, E.: Clinical relevance of physical, chemical and bonding properties of composite resins. Oper Dent 10:61, 1985.
3. Fan, P.L.: Dentin bonding systems. An update. J Am Dent Assoc 114:91, 1987.
4. Doering, J.V. and Jensen, M.E. Clinical evaluation of dentin bonding materials on cervical "abrasion" lesions. J Dent Res 65:173, 1986.
5. Tyas, M.J., Beech, D.R.: Clinical performance of three restorative materials for nonundercut cervical abrasion lesions. Aust Dent J 30:260, 1985.
6. Dennison, J.B., Ziemiecki, T.L., and Charbeneau, G.T.: Retention of unprepared cervical restorations utilizing a dentin bonding agent. Two year report. J Dent Res 65:173, 1986.
7. Ziemiecki, T.L., Dennison, J.B., and Charbeneau, G.T.: Clinical evaluation of cervical composite resin restorations placed without retention. Oper Dent 12:27, 1987.
8. Bowen, R.L., Cobb, E.N., and Rapson, J.E.: Adhesive bonding of various materials to hard tooth tissues. Improvement in bond strength to dentin. J Dent Res 61:1070, 1982.
9. Horsted-Blindslev, P., Knudsen, J., and Baelum, V.: Dentin adhesive materials for restoration of cervical erosions. Two and three-year clinical observations. Am J Dent 195, 1988.
10. Finger, W.J.: Dentin bonding agents. Relevance of in vitro investigations. Am J Dent 1:184, 1988.
11. Retief, H.D., O'Brien, J.A., Smith, L.A., and Marchman, J.L.: In vitro investigation and evaluation of dentin bonding agents. Am J Dent 1:176, 1988.
12. Asmussen, E. and Munksgaard, E.C.: Adhesion of restorative resins to dentinal tissues. *In* Vanherle G. and Smith D.C.: Posterior composite resin dental restorative materials. Utrecht, Peter Szulc Publishing Co., 1985.
13. Hanson, S.E. and Swift, E.J. Jr.: Microleakage with gluma: effects of unfilled resin polymerization and storage time. Am J Dent 2:266, 1989.

Jerry B. Black, D.M.D., M.S.

COLOR MODIFIERS AND OPAQUERS

4

The introduction of the acid-etch technique in 1955[1] and the bis-GMA resin by Bowen in 1962[2] set the stage for a new era in dentistry. As the chairside or direct bonding technique gained impetus, many dentists found themselves lacking in a basic knowledge of dental anatomy, a subject that had traditionally been relegated to the laboratory technician. In addition to external anatomic features, dentists began to appreciate internal anatomy and the individual roles that enamel and dentin play in the determination of tooth color. The facial enamel could be visualized as a translucent window through which light could pass and reflect off the dentin background. The direct bonded veneer became, in a sense, the anatomic equivalent of the facial enamel. The challenge to reproduce normal shades stimulated interest in the components of color: hue, chroma, and value.

Enamel reduction and the desire for reversibility was a subject of debate in the early days of direct enamel bonding. In order to prevent overcontouring, it became obvious that enamel reduction was often necessary to provide space for color modifiers, opaquers, and the veneer resin. At least one study showed that even minimal enamel reduction resulted in a significant increase in the shear bond strength between etched enamel and composite resin.[3]

In cases involving intrinsically stained teeth, efforts were concentrated on opaquing or masking the dark background. In 1982, a definitive technique was described which included enamel reduction and masking of severe tetracycline stain in the fabrication of direct bonded composite resin veneers.[4] Color modifiers and opaquers helped create highly esthetic and realistic restorations.

HISTORY

The first color modifiers (Estilux Color, Kulzer, Inc., USA,) were introduced in 1982. These low chroma tooth colored tints expanded the possibilities for shade matching, characterization, and opaquing. Two years later, high chroma color modifiers were introduced by Kulzer, Inc., USA, (Durafill Color) and Den-Mat Corp. (Rembrandt). When diluted with low viscosity bonding resins these color modifiers allowed unlimited variation of chroma and provided the dentist more flexibility.

In 1984, Cosmedent, Inc., introduced its Creative Color and Renamel opaquing system. The opaques, available in five colors, have a putty-like consistency and are mixed with a clear, low viscosity resin to produce the desired thickness or opacity. The opaquers create the desired natural tooth appearance before the final resin layer is applied.

In 1987, Kulzer, Inc., USA, introduced Durafill Color VS, a series of highly pigmented Vita opaque shades, which when coordinated with corresponding Vita composite resin, provide a high degree of color predictability in the composite resin veneer.

The need for intense metal opaquers prompted the introduction of many products, including Heliocolor Opaque (Vivadent USA, Inc.) Prisma Metal Opaque (Caulk/Dentsply), Panavia (J. Morita USA, Inc.) and Cover Up (Parkell).

CHEMISTRY

Most of the visible light-cured color modifiers contain metal oxide pigments suspended in a low viscosity bis-GMA resin or a mixture of bis-GMA and urethane dimethylacrylate resins. Moderate opaquers, such as Durafill Color VS (Kulzer, Inc., USA), contain 20 to 30% microfilled pigmented bis-GMA resin by weight. Helio-color Opaque (Vivadent USA, Inc.) is supplied in solid opaque tablets, which are used with diethyl ketone solvent for complete opaquing of metal and for intensely stained teeth. The opaquing tablets contain titanium dioxide, iron oxide, and polymethyl methacrylate.

Recently introduced metal opaques, such as Cover Up II (Parkel), are reported to chemically bond resin opaquers to nickel-chromium alloys and to amalgam. The bond is mediated through a 4 META component. Panavia contains a modified ester of bis-GMA, which provides chemical adhesion to nonprecious alloys, tin-plated noble alloys, porcelain, tooth enamel, and un-etched dentin. Because the long-term strength of these adhesive formulations is unknown, wherever possible, mechanical retention should be used in addition to chemical adhesion.

GENERAL CONSIDERATIONS

Color modifiers can be mixed with composite resins to change their shades; however, this procedure can result in:

1. Incorporation of air, which may result in surface porosity
2. Decreased filler loading
3. Increased curing times because of the pigments in the modifiers.

The introduction of composite resins in an extended range of shades, including Vita shades, makes the admixing of color modifiers with composite resins seldom necessary.

The color characteristic of a natural tooth is the result of the subtle interplay of light reflected from the underlying dentin through the relatively translucent enamel. This phenomenon is simulated through the creative use of opaquers and color modifiers that are subsequently overlaid with a relatively translucent composite resin.

TABLE 4–1. VISUAL EFFECTS OF COLOR MODIFIERS

COLOR	INDICATIONS
Yellow-Orange	Creates illusion of narrowness
	Simulates craze lines
Yellow-Brown	Masks blue tetracycline stains
Blue, Gray, Violet	Simulates translucency
	Decreases value or brightness
White	Increases the brightness of any color modifier
	Simulates craze lines
	Simulates enamel hypocalcifications; white spots
	Masks yellow spots
Red, Pink	Simulates gingival tones
	Enhances vitality
	Masks blue tetracycline stains

CLINICAL TIP. The rough enamel surface created by diamond burs should be smoothed with fine diamond burs or flexible disks prior to placing an opaquer. This allows the opaquer to flow evenly over the prepared surface and results in a uniform background

CLINICAL TIP. Always mask out in very thin layers and be certain to observe the required curing time for each layer. Thicker layers result in incomplete curing and uneven layers caused by pooling of the material.

INDICATIONS FOR COLOR MODIFIERS

The most frequently used color modifiers are white, gray, yellow, yellow-brown, blue, and red (Table 4–1).

CLINICAL TIP. Because most color modifiers have high chromas, they must be diluted with a low viscosity resin prior to use.

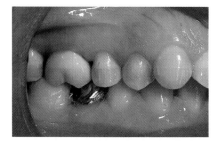

FIG. 4–1. Preparation of the maxillary right first and second premolars for direct bonded veneers.

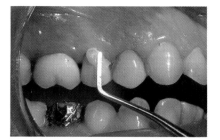

FIG. 4–2. The color of the cervical one-third of the veneers must harmonize with the adjacent teeth. A diluted yellow-brown color modifier (Durafill Color) was placed on the cervical one-third and overlaid with Durafill VS A-30.

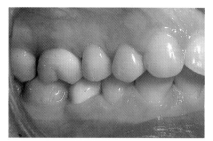

FIG. 4–3. Color harmony from the maxillary right first molar to the maxillary right canine has been established.

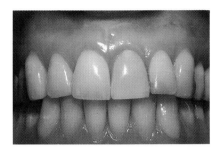

FIG. 4–4. Intrinsic yellow discoloration of maxillary left central incisor.

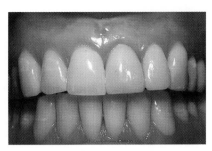

FIG. 4–5. White color modifier was used to mask the yellow background and blue color modifier was added to the incisal to simulate translucency.

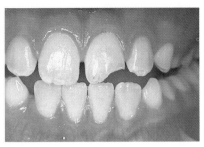

FIG. 4–6. Fractured distoincisal angle. Adjacent teeth exhibit white hypoplastic enamel areas. (Courtesy of Dr. William Mopper.)

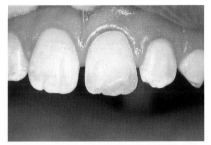

FIG. 4–7. A layer of Multifill VS (Kulzer, Inc.) is placed on the lingual wall and cured. (Courtesy of Dr. William Mopper.)

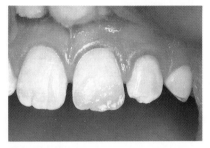

FIG. 4–8. Creative Color white is added to simulate the hypoplastic areas. (Courtesy of Dr. William Mopper.)

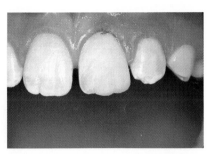

FIG. 4–9. The completed restoration. (Courtesy of Dr. William Mopper.)

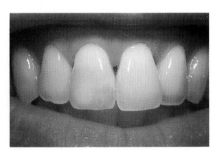

FIG. 4–10. A maxillary right central incisor with intrinsic yellow discoloration.

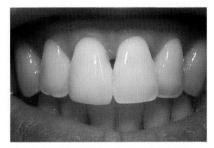

FIG. 4–11. White color modifier is used to mask the yellow background.

1. **Yellow and yellow-brown.** These shades are most often used in the cervical one-third of the crown (Figs. 4–1 to 4–3). Sometimes they are used along proximal surfaces to create the illusion of narrowness. (See Chapter 2—Fundamentals of Esthetics.) They can also be used to simulate craze lines. Because yellow is the complementary color of violet, it is effective in neutralizing and masking blue-gray tetracycline stains. (See Chapter 2—Fundamentals of Esthetics.) Yellow can also be used in combination with white to mask brown tetracycline stains.
2. **Blue, Gray, or Violet.** These shades are used on the incisal one-third of the tooth to simulate translucency (Figs. 4–4, 4–5). They can also be used to reduce value (brightness).
3. **White.** White is used to increase the value (brightness) of any color modifier. It can also be effectively used to simulate craze lines and enamel hypocalcifications (Figs. 4–6 to 4–9). White can be effectively used to mask yellow stains (Figs. 4–10, 4–11).
4. **Red or pink.** Red or pink simulates gingival tones, enhances vitality, and can neutralize blue tetracycline stains. (See Chapter 2—Fundamentals of Esthetics.)

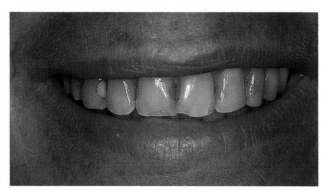

FIG. 4–12. Preoperative view of discolored Class III composite resin restorations. (Courtesy of Dr. William Mopper.)

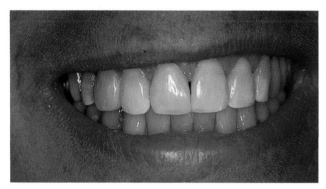

FIG. 4–13. Postoperative view of "invisible restoration." (Courtesy of Dr. William Mopper.)

CLASS III AND CLASS IV RESTORATIONS

Truly "invisible" Class III and Class IV restorations are possible only through proper cavity preparation in conjunction with proper color matching (Figs. 4–12, 4–13).[5] Blending the color of the restorative resin into the color of the tooth is essential. Color modifiers are indispensable in fine tuning the final color.

In Class III or Class IV cavity preparations involving a "through and through" loss of both the labial and lingual enamel, the final restoration can exhibit undesirable "shine-through" (Fig. 4–14). This shine-through occurs because the missing lingual tooth structure is replaced by a composite resin that is more translucent than the original dentin. The result is a visible outline of the restoration. Shine-through can be prevented by careful cavity preparation, the judicious use of color modifiers and opaquers, and a "sandwich" of various types of composite resins.

Armamentarium

- Standard dental setup
  rubber dam
  cotton rolls
  explorer
  high-speed handpiece
  low-speed handpiece
  mouth mirror
  periodontal probe
  2 × 2 Gauze
- Mylar matrix strips
- Wooden or plastic wedge (optional)
- Assorted round carbide dental burs
- Flame-shaped, tapered, and ovoid coarse diamonds for cavity preparations.
- Oil-free pumice
- Rubber prophy cup
- Cavity liner (optional)
  light-cured glass ionomer: (e.g., Vitrabond 3M, Inc; XR Ionomer, Kerr; LC Zionomer, Den-Mat Corp.) or light-cured resin liners: (e.g., Timeline, Caulk/Dentsply; Fluorolite, George Taub Products, Universal Dentinal Sealant, Ultradent Products, Inc.; Dentin Protector, Vivadent USA, Inc.)
- Acid etchant
- Bonding agent of choice (See Chapter 3—Dentin Bonding Agents.)
- Composite resin placement instruments (e.g., 8A, Hu-Friedy, American Dental, Brasseler USA; 1PC-1, Premier Dental Products, Inc.; Goldstein Series 1-4 and mini 1 and 3, GC International Corp.)
- Hybrid composite resin of choice (See Chapter 5—Composite Resin—Fundamentals and Direct Technique Restorations.)
- Microfilled composite resin of choice (See Chapter 5—Composite Resin—Fundamentals and Direct Technique Restorations.)
- Diamond finishing burs
  For microfilled composite resins low-speed water-cooled diamond burs are best for trimming and finishing. For small particle hybrid composite resins, high-speed tungsten carbide burs and low-speed water-cooled diamond burs are recommended.
- 12-fluted finishing burs (e.g., 7901—Premier OR ET-9 and ET-OSI ovoid; Brasseler USA)
- Finishing and polishing disks (e.g., Sof-Lex, 3M; Super Snaps, Shofu; or Flexi-Discs, Cosmedent, Inc.)
- Finishing and polishing strips
  Metal backed (e.g., Compo Strips, Premier Dental Products Co.) or
  Plastic backed (e.g., Sof-Lex, 3M or Flexi Strips, Cosmedent, Inc.)
- Rubber wheels, cups, and points containing abrasives
  Medium grit rubber wheels for prepolishing (e.g., Burlew, J.F. Jelenko & Company), or complete systems (e.g., Shofu Dental Corp., Vivadent USA, Inc., Brasseler USA, Kulzer Inc., USA, or Cosmedent, Inc., Enhance, L.D. Caulk Co.)
- Composite resin polishing paste (containing aluminum oxide)
- Dry felt wheel
- Padded discs (e.g., Cosmedent, Inc.)
- Color modifiers and opaquers
  Color modifiers: yellow, yellow-brown, white, blue, gray, violet. (e.g., Durafill Color, Kulzer, Inc. USA; Creative Color, Cosmedent Inc.; Porcelite Color Modifiers, Kerr Manufacturing Co.; Prisma Enhancers, Caulk/Dentsply)

Clinical Technique

1. Administer local anesthesia (optional).
2. Cleanse the tooth and neighboring teeth with pumice.
3. Determine the appropriate shade while the teeth are wet with saliva.
4. Isolate the lesion with a rubber dam.
5. Prepare the cavity in a conventional manner (Fig. 4–15).
6. Round the cavosurface angle and place a long bevel in order to create an invisible transition from resin to tooth (Fig 4–16).

CLINICAL TIP. If the enamel is very translucent, create a longer and deeper bevel. If the tooth is more opaque, the bevel can be shorter and less pronounced.

---

7. Place a light-cured glass ionomer cavity liner (e.g., Vitrabond 3M; XR Ionomer, Kerr Manufacturing Co.; LC Zionomer, Den-Mat Corp.), if necessary.

CLINICAL TIP. Avoid the use of opaque lining materials beneath very translucent enamel. They interfere with the transmission of light through the enamel into the underlying tooth structure or composite resin.

---

8. To prevent "shine-through," place a more opaque hybrid composite resin in the lingual portion of the preparation.
9. Build up the resin to the level of the original dento-enamel junction.
10. If necessary, place custom tinting resins over this layer and blend the background color of the resin with the color of the tooth (Fig 4–17).

CLINICAL TIP. Always apply color modifiers in very thin layers and be certain to observe the required curing time for each layer. Thicker layers result in incomplete curing and uneven layers caused by pooling of the material.

CLINICAL TIP. Chroma (intensity) must be appropriately diluted with a bonding resin to create a tooth-colored hue.

CLINICAL TIP. Place custom tints, such as gray, blue, or violet, to simulate incisal translucency in Class IV restorations. Place yellow or yellow-brown custom tints for fine tuning the background color. Place white for increasing value. (Figs 4–18, 4–19).

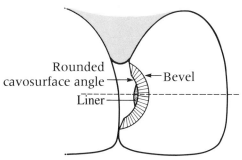

FIG. 4–14. Typical Class III preparation with a "through and through" loss of both the labial and lingual enamel. The line denotes the cross-section area of subsequent drawings.

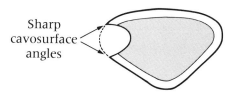

FIG. 4–15. The cavity is prepared in a conventional manner.

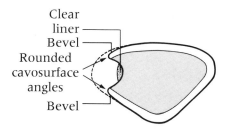

FIG. 4–16. The cavosurface angle is rounded and a long bevel is placed in order to facilitate an invisible transition from resin to tooth.

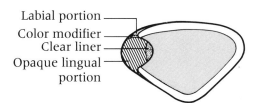

FIG. 4–17. An opaque composite resin is placed on the lingual portion of the restoration. This is followed by color modifiers or opaquers (if necessary) and completed with a labial veneer of a microfilled composite resin.

FIG. 4–18. Maxillary central incisors in open bite relationship.

FIG. 4–19. A lingual wall of Multifill VS was first created. Durafill Color VS (white) was then used to simulate white hypoplastic enamel areas. A Multifill VS (incisal) overlay on the labial surface completed the restoration.

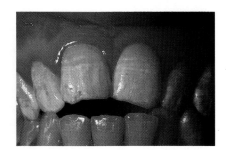

FIG. 4–18

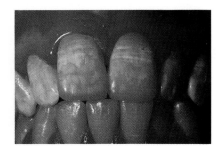

FIG. 4–19

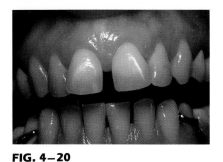

FIG. 4–20

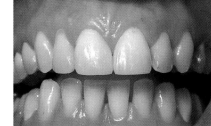

FIG. 4–21

FIG. 4–20. Malposed maxillary right and left central incisors with a 2-mm diastema.

FIG. 4–21. The distal surface was re-contoured and a mesial partial composite resin veneer (Durafill Color VS) was placed. Usually a matching composite resin shade can be blended into the tooth without the need for color modifiers.

11. To complete the restoration, fill the remaining labial portion with a translucent microfilled composite resin.
12. Contour the restoration.
13. Prepolish the restoration with rubber wheels or cups.
14. Smooth with a microfine diamond at low speed with water cooling.
15. Polish with disks or strips.

CLINICAL TIP. An excellent final high gloss can be obtained by using a dry felt wheel or padded disk without paste on the dry composite resin surface.

DIASTEMA CLOSURES

A microfilled composite resin is the material of choice for diastema closure because of its excellent polishability and enamel-like luster (Figs. 4–20, 4–21). If the diastema is very large, the lingual surface of the composite resin could be subjected to high functional stress in patients with heavy centric contacts. In these cases, the dentist may elect to use a hybrid composite resin for the entire restoration or a hybrid on the lingual portion overlaid on the labial surface with a microfilled composite resin. Shine-through is usually not a problem in diastema closure because of the labiolingual thickness of the add-on composite resin in the body area of the clinical crown. In many cases, some translucency is desirable because the composite resin thins out at the incisal edge. If shine-through is a problem, follow the procedure described for the Class III and Class IV restorations.

DIRECT LABIAL VENEERS

Direct composite resin veneers can be divided into two types; those that require incisal lengthening and those that do not. If tooth length is to be maintained, place an opaque or color modifying layer underneath a microfilled layer (Fig. 4–22). If incisal lengthening is required, materials are used in the following order, from lingual to labial (Fig. 4–23).

1. hybrid or small particle composite resin
2. opaquer
3. color modifiers
4. microfilled composite resins

The shades and distribution of color modifiers are related to the three zones of the clinical crown. Each of the three zones may require a different combination of colors based on the individual requirements of the tooth to be restored (Fig. 4–24). A color modifier with a high value (usually white), can make teeth appear larger and more prominent in the arch (Fig. 4–25). A gray tint lowers value, which creates a less prominent appearance (Fig. 4–26).

In addition, teeth can be made to appear narrow by staining the interproximal surfaces yellow-brown or orange. This results in the central aspect appearing relatively lighter, i.e., a higher value (Fig. 4–27). (See Chapter 2—Fundamentals of Esthetics.) By staining the central vertical axis of the crown, the lateral aspects appear lighter and, therefore, the entire crown appears wider (Fig. 4–28).

Armamentarium. Same dental setup as used for Class III and Class IV composite resin restorations except:

- Assorted diamond burs for the preparation, such as 850-014, 6850-016, 8392-016, 8392-016EF, and Nixon II Kit (Brasseler USA).
- Retraction cord
    Ultrapak No. 0 (Ultradent Products, Inc.)
    Gingibraid No. 0 (Van R Products, Inc.)
- Mylar strips (optional)
- Wooden or clear plastic wedges (optional)
- Opaquers or color modifiers, as dictated by the individual case. Opaquers for tetracycline and other severe intrinsic stains include: Durafill Color and Durafill Color VS (Kulzer, Inc, USA), Creative Color (Cosmedent, Inc.), Tetrapaque (Den-Mat Corp.), Prisma Enhancers (Caulk/Dentsply), Command Opaque (Kerr Manufacturing Co.), Heliomolar Opaque (Vivadent USA, Inc.), and Masking Agens (3M, Inc.).
- Artist's brushes.

Clinical Technique

1. Administer local anesthesia (optional).
2. Cleanse the tooth and neighboring teeth with pumice.
3. Determine the appropriate shade while the teeth are wet with saliva.
4. Isolate the area to maintain a dry field.

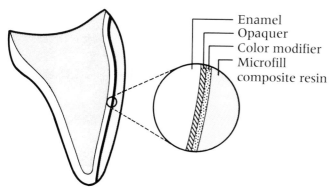

Enamel
Opaquer
Color modifier
Microfill
composite resin

FIG. 4—22. Cross-sectional view of a direct labial veneer when incisal lengthening was not required.

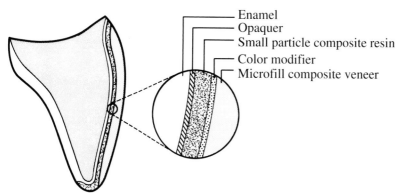

Enamel
Opaquer
Small particle composite resin
Color modifier
Microfill composite veneer

FIG. 4—23. Cross-sectional view of a direct labial veneer when incisal lengthening was required.

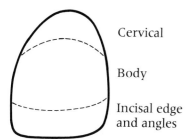

Cervical

Body

Incisal edge and angles

FIG. 4—24. The three zones of the clinical crown.

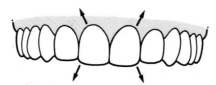

FIG. 4—25. Using a color modifier with a high value (usually white), teeth can be made to appear larger and more prominent in the arch.

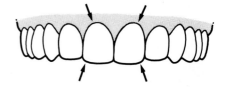

FIG. 4—26. Using a color modifier with a low value (usually gray), teeth can be made to look less prominent in the arch.

FIG. 4—27. Teeth can be made to appear narrow by staining the interproximal surfaces yellow-brown or orange.

FIG. 4—28. Teeth can be made to appear wider by staining the central vertical axis yellow-brown or orange.

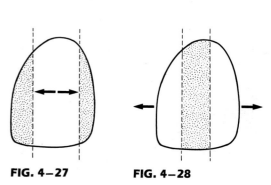

FIG. 4—27   **FIG. 4—28**

CLINICAL TIP. A rubber dam is not recommended for direct labial veneers because the creative (artistic) nature of the work requires an unobstructed view of the patient in order to harmonize tooth color and form with the patient's face. Moisture can usually be controlled with cotton rolls, cheek retractors, and retraction cord.

5. Prepare the teeth (Fig. 4–29). The need for enamel reduction depends upon the reason for veenering.
   1. If the reason for veneering is to close diastemata and change the length of teeth with a blending shade of composite resin, minimal or no enamel reduction is necessary.
   2. If the reason for veneering is to affect a color change, enamel reduction is usually necessary to create space for color modifiers and veneer resins. In most cases, reduce the enamel by 0.3 mm in the gingival one-third, and by 0.5 mm in the body area. Depth cutting diamonds (Nixon II Kit, Brasseler USA) can be used to establish appropriate levels of enamel reduction. (If the intrinsic discoloration is severe, as in the case of tetracycline stain, reduce the enamel by 0.5 mm in the gingival one-third and by 1.0 mm in the body.) The gingival margin must be subgingival for major color changes. In all other cases the gingival margin should be supragingival if possible.
6. Place the opaquers and color modifiers (Figs. 4–30, 4–31).
7. Finish and polish (See the section on Class III and Class IV restorations)

CLINICAL TIP. It is usually better to complete one veneer at a time, including final polishing (Fig. 4–32). This allows for precise evaluation of the final color and prevents bonding through the contact area. Uncured resin from the adjacent veneer will not bond readily to the highly polished resin surface of the finished veneer.

8. In order to minimize the possibility of chipping, eliminate all premature centric contacts and all interferences in labial excursive movements. Provide for cuspid guidance whenever possible.

REPAIR OF ACRYLIC VENEER CROWNS

Partial or total separation of the acrylic veneer from an otherwise serviceable crown or bridge is common. Composite resin can be used to restore the veneer, however, an adequate layer of opaquer is necessary to conceal the metal (Fig. 4–33). Both mechanical and chemical retention assist in preventing dislodgement of the restorative material.

Armamentarium. Same dental setup as used for Class III and Class IV composite resin restorations except:

- Small round or inverted cone high-speed tungsten carbide burs for providing mechanical retention (e.g., No. 1 round or 33½ inverted cone bur)
- Metal coupling agent (e.g., Cover-Up II, Parkell, or Goldlink, DenMat)
- Bonding resin of choice
- Composite resin of choice
- Composite resin instruments (same as those listed under the section on Direct Labial Veneers)
- Composite resin color opaquer of choice
- Composite resin color modifiers of choice

Clinical Technique

1. Cleanse the tooth and neighboring teeth with pumice.
2. Determine the appropriate shade while the teeth are wet with saliva.
3. Using a water-cooled high-speed small round or inverted cone bur, remove any remaining acrylic.

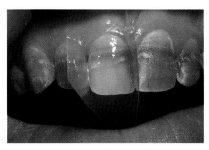

FIG. 4–29

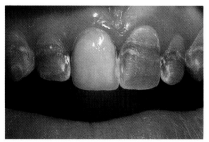

FIG. 4–30

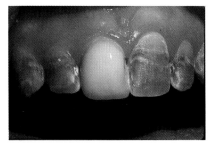

FIG. 4–31

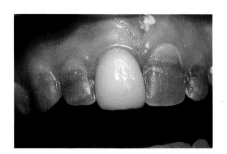

FIG. 4–32

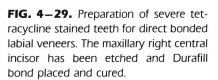

FIG. 4–29. Preparation of severe tetracycline stained teeth for direct bonded labial veneers. The maxillary right central incisor has been etched and Durafill bond placed and cured.

FIG. 4–30. To neutralize the blue-gray tetracycline stain, a complementary color (Durafill Color yellow) was placed.

FIG. 4–31. Estilux Color (white) was placed over the yellow to create a normal dentin background color.

FIG. 4–32. Durafill VS A-10 was used to complete the veneer.

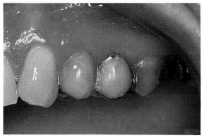
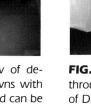

FIG. 4–33. Preoperative view of defective acrylic veneer gold crowns with an inadequate opaquer. The gold can be seen through the composite resin. (Courtesy of Dr. William Mopper.)

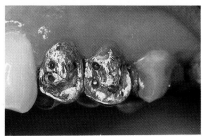

FIG. 4–34. Retention holes are placed through the metal into dentin. (Courtesy of Dr. William Mopper.)

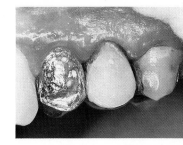

FIG. 4–35. After treatment with a metal bonding agent, a layer of opaquer is placed. (Courtesy of Dr. William Mopper.)

FIG. 4–36. Color modifiers are placed over the opaque resin. (Courtesy of Dr. William Mopper.)

FIG. 4–37. Incremental layers of composite resin are added. (Courtesy of Dr. William Mopper.)

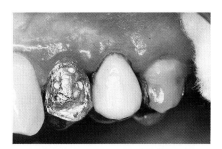

FIG. 4–36

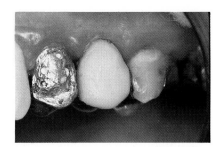

FIG. 4–37

FIG. 4–38. Postoperative view of the repair. (Courtesy of Dr. William Mopper.)

FIG. 4–39. Postoperative view of the repair of the adjacent tooth. (Courtesy of Dr. William Mopper.)

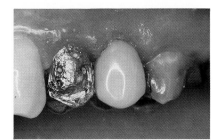

FIG. 4–38

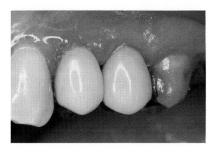

FIG. 4–39

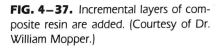
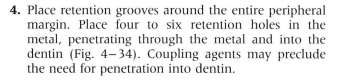

4. Place retention grooves around the entire peripheral margin. Place four to six retention holes in the metal, penetrating through the metal and into the dentin (Fig. 4–34). Coupling agents may preclude the need for penetration into dentin.

CLINICAL TIP. It is important to seal the entire labial or buccal surface with composite resin to assure an adequate seal and prevent marginal leakage through the retention holes.

5. For all remaining steps, maintain a dry operating field.

CLINICAL TIP. It is often difficult to match shades when a rubber dam is used. However, it is vital to maintain a dry field to assure maximum bond strength.

6. Treat and coat the exposed metal surface with a 4 META coupling agent and opaquer, according to the manufacturer's recommendation (e.g., Cover-Up II) (Fig 4–35).
7. Place a color modifier (if necessary) to adjust the background color (Fig. 4–36).

CLINICAL TIP. Always apply color modifiers in very thin layers and be certain to observe the required curing time for each layer. Thicker layers result in incomplete curing and uneven layers caused by pooling of the material.

8. Apply the composite resin in increments (Fig. 4–37).
9. Finish and polish (Figs. 4–38, 4–39).

PORCELAIN REPAIRS

Repair of Fractured Porcelain With No Exposed Metal

Recent advances in silane coupling agents and opaques and color modifiers have allowed for the repair of porcelain fractures of ceramometal restorations.

Armamentarium. Same dental setup as used for Class III and Class IV composite resin restorations except:

■ Microetcher (Danville Engineering) (optional)
■ Hydrofluoric acid etching gel
■ Silane

- Bonding resin of choice
- Composite resin of choice
- Composite resin instruments (same as those listed under the section on Direct Labial Veneers)
- Color modifiers of choice

Clinical Technique

1. Cleanse the tooth and neighboring teeth with pumice. Determine the appropriate shade while the teeth are wet with saliva.
2. Using water-cooled high-speed coarse diamonds, remove any loose porcelain and place a broad 2-mm bevel in the porcelain around the fracture site. Featheredge the porcelain peripheral to the bevel.

CLINICAL TIP. Featheredging beyond the beveled porcelain will facilitate the blending of the resin into the porcelain.

---

3. For all of the remaining steps maintain a dry operating field.
4. Sandblast or etch the prepared porcelain with hydrofluoric acid gel for 3 to 6 minutes, according to the manufacturer's instructions.

CLINICAL TIP. Although hydrofluoric acid for dental use is buffered, it should be handled with care. When applying it to teeth, take precautions to avoid contact with skin and mucosal surfaces. (e.g., use a rubber dam or protective gel).

---

5. Apply silane to the prepared porcelain.
6. Let dry for 2 minutes.
7. Apply bonding resin; gently remove excess with an air syringe and cure.
8. Apply the composite resin in increments.
9. Apply color modifiers (if necessary).

CLINICAL TIP. Always apply color modifiers in very thin layers and be certain to observe the required curing time for each layer. Thicker layers result in incomplete curing and uneven layers caused by pooling of the material.

---

10. Complete the application of composite resin.
11. Finish and polish.

Repair of Fractured Porcelain With Exposed Metal

The use of metal bonding agents (Table 4–2) has

TABLE 4–2. METAL BONDING AGENTS

PRODUCT	MANUFACTURER
Cover-Up II	Parkell
Metabond	Parkell
Panavia OP (nonprecious only)	J. Morita USA, Inc.
Gold Link	Den-Mat Corp.

greatly enhanced the ability to repair porcelain that has fractured and exposed metal (Figs. 4–40, 4–41).

Armamentarium. Same dental setup as used for Class III and Class IV composite resin restorations and:

- Small round or inverted cone high-speed tungsten burs for providing mechanical retention
- Metal opaquer of choice

Clinical Technique

1. Cleanse the tooth and neighboring teeth with pumice.
2. Determine the appropriate shade while the teeth are wet with saliva.
3. Using water-cooled high-speed diamonds remove any loose porcelain and place a broad 2-mm bevel in the porcelain around the fracture site. Featheredge the porcelain peripheral to the bevel.

CLINICAL TIP. Featheredging beyond the bevel porcelain will facilitate the blending of the resin into the porcelain.

---

4. Retention can be accomplished in two ways.
   A. Place retentive holes through the metal or
   B. Use a coarse diamond or a microetcher to roughen the metal surface and remove the oxide layer.

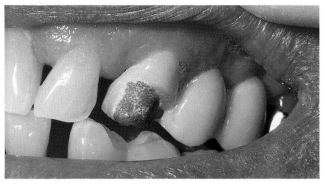

FIG. 4–40. Fractured porcelain veneers with exposed metal. The metal was roughened with a coarse diamond. The porcelain was beveled, feather edged, etched, and silanated.

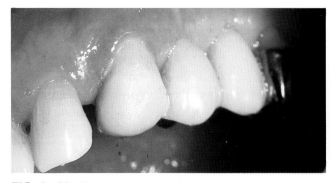

FIG. 4–41. The completed repair.

5. For all remaining steps maintain a dry operating field.
6. Sandblast or etch the prepared porcelain with hydrofluoric acid gel for 3 to 6 minutes, according to the manufacturer's instructions.

CLINICAL TIP. *Although hydrofluoric acid for dental use is buffered, it should be handled with care. When applying it to teeth, take precautions to avoid contact with skin and mucosal surfaces (e.g., use a rubber dam or protective gel).*

7. Apply silane to the prepared porcelain.
8. Let dry for 2 minutes.
9. Apply a thin layer of the metal opaquer of choice.

CLINICAL TIP. *Panavia OP will not set in the presence of oxygen. Cover the Panavia with Oxyguard for 2 to 3 minutes, then rinse off the Oxyguard and dry.*

CLINICAL TIP. *It is not necessary to apply a bonding resin between the metal opaquer and the composite resin.*

10. Incrementally apply the composite resin of choice.
11. Apply color modifiers (if necessary).

CLINICAL TIP. *Always apply color modifiers in very thin layers and be certain to observe the required curing time for each layer. Thicker layers result in incomplete curing and uneven layers caused by pooling of the material.*

12. Complete the application of the composite resin.
13. Finish and polish.

REPAIR OF CERAMOMETAL MARGINS

Cervical Addition to Exposed Metal Crown Margins or Restorations of Recurrent Caries Around Ceramometal Margins

Restorations of ceramometal margins are especially complex because of the necessity for bonding to cementum, dentin, metal, and porcelain (Fig. 4–42). The clinician should be aware of the importance of following the proper sequence in the use of the material because the materials have specific chemistries or formulations for specific functions.

Armamentarium. Use the armamentarium listed under the sections on Repair of Acrylic Veneer Crowns, Porcelain Repairs, and Repair of Fractured Porcelain with Exposed Metal, plus:

- Dentin bonding agent (see Chapter 3—Dentin Bonding Agents)
- Metal opaquer of choice
- Polyacrylic acid: (e.g., Dentin Conditioner, GC International Corp.; Polyacrylic Conditioner, Ultradent Products, Inc.; Durelon Liquid, ESPE Premier Sales Corp.)

Clinical Technique

CLINICAL TIP. *It is often difficult to place a rubber dam on these types of restorations (Fig. 4–43). Take extra care to maintain a dry field and avoid contact with skin and mucosal surfaces.*

1. Cleanse the tooth and neighboring teeth with pumice.
2. Determine the appropriate shade while the teeth are wet with saliva.
3. Prepare the tooth. Remove the metal collar to greatly simplify the restoration. Hold a coarse diamond at an angle to the crown and tooth and create a long bevel on the adjacent portion of the porcelain and remove the metal collar. The crown margin should be located at a more cervical level (Fig. 4–44). Featheredge the occlusal porcelain and bevel the gingival margin (Fig. 4–45). A retention groove can be optionally placed in the gingival wall (Fig. 4–46).

CLINICAL TIP. *Featheredging beyond the bevel porcelain will facilitate the blending of the resin into the porcelain.*

4. For all remaining steps maintain a dry operating field.
5. Sandblast or etch the prepared porcelain with hydrofluoric acid gel for 3 to 6 minutes, according to the manufacturer's instructions.

CLINICAL TIP. *Although hydrofluoric acid for dental use is buffered, it should be handled with care. When applying it to teeth, take precautions to avoid contact with skin and mucosal surfaces (e.g., use a rubber dam or protective gel).*

6. Rinse and dry thoroughly.
7. Apply silane to the prepared porcelain (Fig. 4–47).
8. Let dry for 2 minutes.
9. If significant metal is exposed, apply the metal opaquer of choice in thin layers.

CLINICAL TIP. *Panavia OP will not set in the presence of oxygen. Cover the Panavia with Oxyguard for 2 to 3 minutes, then rinse off the Oxyguard and dry.*

10. If exposed dentin remains, apply a dentin bonding agent to the exposed dentin and enamel only (Fig. 4–48).
11. Incrementally apply the composite resin of choice (Fig. 4–49).

CLINICAL TIP. *In general, more opaque composite resins are needed in the cervical area (e.g., Cervical Opaque Composite Shade BO [brown] or YO [yellow], Kulzer, Inc. USA).*

12. Apply color modifiers (if necessary).

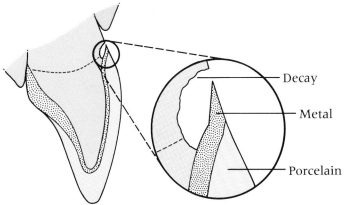

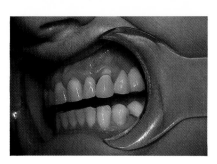

FIG. 4–43. Exposed ceramometal crown margin with class V caries.

FIG. 4–42. Recurrent caries around ceramo-metal margins.

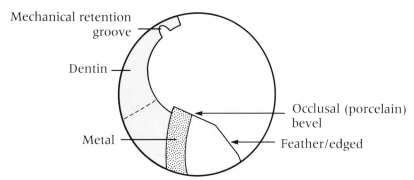

FIG. 4–44. The prepared tooth following removal of the metal collar and placement of a long bevel and featheredge on the porcelain. A retention groove can be optionally placed in the gingival floor.

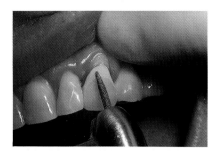

FIG. 4–45. A bevel and featheredge was placed on porcelain.

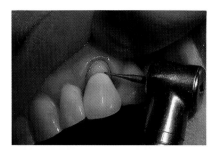

FIG. 4–46. Class V preparation and caries removal. Note retraction cord in place.

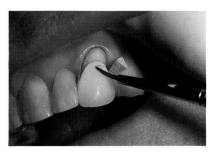

FIG. 4–47. The etched porcelain was silanted.

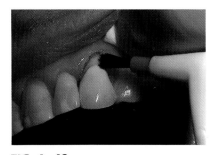

FIG. 4–48

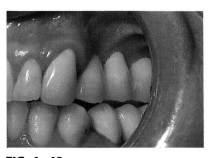

FIG. 4–49

FIG. 4–48. Application of Durafill bonding resin.

FIG. 4–49. The completed restoration with Durafill Color VS A-30.

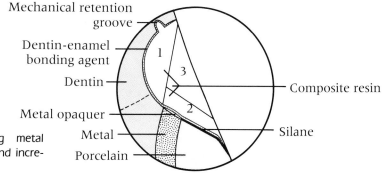

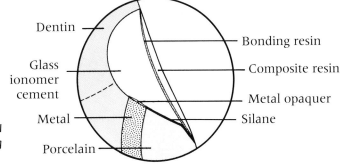

FIG. 4–50. The completed restoration showing metal opaquer, silanated porcelain, dentin bonding agent, and incremental placement of composite resin.

FIG. 4–51. The completed restoration showing metal opaquer, silanated porcelain, glass ionomer base, bonding agent, and single layer of composite resin.

13. Complete the application of composite resin.
14. Finish and polish (Fig. 4–50).

CLINICAL TIP. *Always apply color modifiers in very thin layers and be certain to observe the required curing time for each layer. Thicker layers result in incomplete curing and uneven layers caused by pooling of the material.*

Alternative Use of Glass Ionomer Cement for the Repair of Exposed Metal Crown Margins or Restorations of Recurrent Caries Around Ceramometal Margins

Armamentarium. In addition to the armamentarium listed in the section on Cervical Addition to Exposed Metal Crown Margins or Restorations of Recurrent Caries:

- Dentinal bonding agent (see Chapter 3—Dentin Bonding Agents)
- Metal opaquer of choice
- Polyacrylic acid (e.g., Dentin Conditioner, GC International Corp.; Polyacrylic Conditioner, Ultradent Products, Inc., Durelon Liquid, ESPE Premier Sales Corp.)
- Glass ionomer cement of choice (see Chapter 7—Glass Ionomer Cements)

Clinical Technique

1. Cleanse the tooth and neighboring teeth with pumice.
2. Determine an appropriate shade while the teeth are wet with saliva.

3. Using a low-speed round carbide bur, excavate all recurrent decay within the dentin and around the margins and metal substructure.
4. Place pulp protection if necessary.
5. Place a long bevel on the most occlusal portion of the porcelain and featheredge the porcelain below the bevel.
6. For all remaining steps maintain a dry operating field.

CLINICAL TIP. *It is often difficult to place a rubber dam on these types of restorations. Take extra care to maintain a dry field and avoid contact with skin and mucosal surfaces.*

CLINICAL TIP. *Although hydrofluoric acid for dental use is buffered, it should be handled with care. When applying it to teeth, take precautions to avoid contact with skin and mucosal surfaces (e.g., use a rubber dam or protective gel).*

---

9. Rinse and dry thoroughly.
10. Place glass ionomer restoration of choice. Use a light-cured resin to protect the surface while setting.
11. Apply silane to the prepared porcelain.
12. Let dry for 2 minutes.
13. If significant metal is exposed, apply a thin layer of primer followed by a thin layer of metal opaquer.
14. Apply a dentin bonding agent to any remaining exposed dentin.

CLINICAL TIP. *Panavia OP will not set in the presence of oxygen. Cover the Panavia with Oxyguard for 2 to 3 minutes, then rinse off the Oxyguard and dry.*

---

15. Incrementally apply the composite resin of choice.

CLINICAL TIP. In general, more opaque composite resins are needed in the cervical area (e.g., Cervical Opaque Composite Shade BO [brown] or YO [yellow] Kulzer, Inc. USA).

16. Apply color modifiers (if necessary).

CLINICAL TIP. If needed, use color modifiers to fine tune the background color or for custom tinting prior to the application of the last (surface) layer of composite resin.

17. Complete the application of composite resin.
18. Finish and polish (Fig. 4–51).

CONCLUSION

Composite resins have vastly increased the range of options available to the dentist. The use of color modifiers and opaquers, along with agents capable of bonding to porcelain or metal, have allowed the dentist to not only create an "invisible filling," but also to greatly improve the esthetics of the patient's existing dentition.

REFERENCES

1. Buonocore, M.G.: A simple method of increasing the adhesion of acrylic filling materials to enamel surfaces. J Dent Res 34:849, 1955.
2. Bowen, R.L.: Dental filling material comprising vinyl silane treated fused silica and a binder consisting of the reaction product of bisphenol and glycidyl acrylate. US Patent 3,006,112, 1962.
3. Schneider, R.M., Messer, L.B., and Douglas, W.H.: The effect of enamel surface reduction in vitro on the bonding of composite resin to permanent human enamel. J Dent Res 60(5):895, 1981.
4. Black, J.B.: Esthetic restoration of tetracycline stained teeth. J Am Dent Assoc 104:846, 1982.
5. Belvedere, P.C.: Universal material, wide shade range make for invisible anterior restorations. Restor Dent 3:4, 1989.

Brian Pollack, D.D.S.

COMPOSITE RESIN— FUNDAMENTALS AND DIRECT TECHNIQUE RESTORATIONS

5

In 1955, Michael Buonocore introduced the concept of bonding acrylic to teeth. It evoked little excitement in the dental profession initially. Today, the marriage of bonding and composite resins is the basis for a new era of restorative adhesive dentistry. Bis-GMA, polyurethane, and tricyclodecane dimethacrylates resins were formulated in an effort to overcome the shortcomings of acrylic.

HISTORY

Buonocore's original paper showed that the bond between acrylic and enamel could be tremendously strengthened if the enamel was first etched with phosphoric acid. In 1962, Raphael Bowen introduced a new resin, the reaction product of bisphenol A and a glycidyl methacrylate, which has been abbreviated as bis-GMA. This formulation was originally marketed in a powder-liquid or paste-paste system, i.e., a chemically cured resin. In 1972, ultraviolet-cured resins were formulated. This resulted in controlled working and setting times and improved physical properties. More recently, visible light-cured systems have been introduced.

The filler particles used in resin systems have been improved. Loading was increased for better physical properties and particle size was reduced for better polishability.

Originally, composite resins and bonding agents were conceived as anterior filling materials. Later, uses were expanded to include esthetics. Today, it is possible to bond to:

1. enamel
2. dentin and cementum
3. existing composite resins
4. porcelain
5. etched and unetched metals

Furthermore, application of indirect system technology has allowed fabrication of resins using tremendous heat, light, and pressure, and in one case, using a nitrogen atmosphere. This treatment of resin, which cannot be performed intraorally, results in plastics with more optimal physical properties. Marginal adaptation of the resin restorations to the dies, and ultimately to the tooth, surpasses that of porcelain and wear of the opposing dentition is decreased. The future of resin chemistry appears very promising.

BASIC CHEMISTRY

Composite resins consist of three phases: the matrix phase, the dispersed phase, and the coupling phase. The matrix phase consists of the resin: bisphenol A glycidyl methacrylate and urethane or tricyclodecane dimethacrylates (similar to bis-GMA chemically but not in physical geometry, i.e., sterically; it is more saturated, hence has lower water absorption). Most resins contain mixtures of the first two polymers in various proportions. Additional resins are added to control viscosity and to alter the affinity of the resin for water. Initiators and accelerators are added to produce the free radicals needed for polymerization. Resins can be hardened with heat, which splits benzoyl peroxide into free radicals. A chemically activated system uses benzoyl peroxide, which reacts with a tertiary aromatic amine to produce the free radicals. In the ultraviolet systems, a 365 nm light source can split benzoin methyl ether into free radicals (no amine is necessary). Most visible light-cured systems utilize a 460 to 480 nm light source to cause camphoroquinone (or another diketone) to react with an aliphatic amine to initiate free radical production. This amine is more color stable than the aromatic amine used in chemically cured formulations, hence the improved color stability of light-cured resin systems. Inhibitors may be added to increase shelf life of the chemically cured systems.

The dispersed phase contains filler particles to provide stability and to improve physical properties, i.e., reduce water sorption, polymerization contraction, and the coefficient of thermal expansion, and increase the hardness of the resin matrix. Common filler particles include quartz, lithium aluminum silicate, borosilicate, barium, and other glasses. Particle sizes in modern formulations range from approximately one-half to 10 microns, and constitute about 75 to 85% of the resin by weight. A special filler of silicon dioxide, with particle sizes between 0.007 and 0.04 microns, can be loaded into the resin to constitute about 35 to 70% by weight. This results in a composite resin capable of receiving an ultra smooth finish, but that has somewhat reduced physical properties because of reduced loading. This composite resin is frequently termed a microfilled resin. (See the section on Particle Size below.)

The final phase is the coupling phase. Filler particles are coated with a silane agent (1 to 6% of the weight of the filler). Resin and filler particles have very different chemistries; the silane can function as a "glue" to bind these two phases together. It probably does this by lowering the surface energy of the filler (wetting), allowing better adaptation of the resin to the filler.

Chemically cured and light-cured composite resins may contain ultraviolet-absorbing compounds, which act as color stabilizers. These compounds are not found in ultraviolet-cured composite resins because they would inhibit polymerization.

PARTICLE SIZE

First-generation composite resins contained particles as large as 90 microns. These were frequently referred to as *macrofilled resins.* Clinically, they produced a rough surface but were strong and serviceable. Examples of such materials were the original Adaptic and Concise, and ultraviolet-cured Nuvafill.

Over the years, manufacturers have been able to reduce particle size dramatically first to about 30 microns and later to about 1 to 5 microns. This resulted in composite resins with smoother surfaces, but which still are not totally polishable. These resins are frequently referred to as *small particle composite resins.* Examples include Prisma, Estilux, Aurafill, and Command.

Microfilled resins present an ultrasmooth surface, but fracture resistance is the lowest in the group. Examples include chemically cured Silar, Estic Microfill, and Isopast, and visible light-cured varieties such as Durafill, Silux, Heliomolar, Paste Laminate, Prisma Microfine, Renamel, and Comp Plus (a glaze).

Hybrid resins are a most exciting evolution of composite resin chemistry. As the name indicates, they combine particles of different sizes. A typical example combines particles ranging from 0.04 micron to less than 5 microns. These resins can receive a high polish, which often rivals a microfilled resin, but may not be as lasting. Furthermore, they appear to be as strong as the macrofilled and small particle composite resins, and can be used for posterior restorations. Chemically cured examples include Conclude, Miradapt, Finesse and P-10. Visible light-cured hybrid resins include Brilliant Lux, Command Ultrafine, Herculite XR, APH, Multifil VS, Bis Fil M, Occlusion, Visarfill, Ultrabond, P-30, and P-50.

Dental composite resins must be both strong and polishable. Hybrids appear to have the strength of macrofilled or small particle resins. Furthermore, they can be

polished to almost the luster of a microfilled resin. Newest formulations of hybrids, such as Herculite XR and APH, are available in a wide range of shades for both anterior and posterior use. Hybrids are a good choice for the practitioner who wishes to stock only one composite resin. The introduction of hybrid resins may make macrofilled and small particle composite resins obsolete.

Radiopacity is desirable for Class II and Class III restorations. This can, however, be detrimental when veneering the labial area of a tooth because radiographic contrast is reduced, making caries detection more difficult.

Different composite resins have different degrees of fill and radiopacity, and different numbers of shades. (Table 5-1). There are advantages and disadvantages to composite resin versus microfilled resin placement. Composite resin is less technique-sensitive than microfilled resin and shrinks less on polymerization. This would indicate less microleakage at the gingival margin of Class II or Class V restorations if shrinkage and strength of the dentin bonding agent were the only considerations. Paradoxically, several in vitro studies have shown that microfilled resins can produce a better seal than composite resins.[1,2] In addition, resins with a low Young's modulus (rigidity), such as Silux, produce a better seal than many composite resins.[3,4,5]

GENERAL CONSIDERATIONS
Acid Etch Considerations

Etching selectively dissolves away calcified portions of enamel, leaving small microporosites. Composite resin can enter these microporosites, resulting in a strong mechanical bond to enamel, which reduces or eliminates microleakage. Important clinical tips follow.

1. Liquid acid etchants should be continuously applied to the tooth to prevent drying. A gel etch need only be left in place for the required time, as stated by the manufacturer.
2. Prior to etching, remove the top layer of fluoriderich enamel with a diamond bur, and by prophylaxis, remove all plaque on the treated tooth and on the area immediately adjacent to it. Contrary to most instructions, a commercial fluoride prophylaxis paste can be used, provided the paste vehicle is completely water soluble. Fluoridated water may be used for rinsing.[6,7,8]
3. Because moisture or gingival fluid contamination inhibits bonding, adequate precautions, such as placing a rubber dam, are advisable.
4. Etch for 15 seconds. If this does not produce a frosted appearance on the enamel after washing and drying, re-etch in 15 second increments until the frosted surface is obtained. Recent studies have shown that shorter etching times produce the same or greater adhesive strength than the original 60 second recommendations.[9] Etching for over 120 seconds creates an insoluble calcium precipitate, which decreases bond strength.
5. Some evidence suggests that agitation with a soft brush of either liquid or gel agents produces superior

TABLE 5–1. COMPOSITE RESINS

NAME	MANUFACTURER	RADIOPAQUE	SHADES	% FILLER
MICROFILLED 0.04 MICRONS				
Durafill VS	Kulzer	N	12	50
Heliomolar	Vivadent	Y	8	79
Helioprogress	Vivadent	N	14	75
Perfection	Den-Mat	N	42	51
Prisma Microfine	Caulk/Dentsply	N	7	47
Renamel	Cosmedent	N	16	60
Silux Plus	3M	N	14	52
Visio Dispers	ESPE/Premier	N	6	66
SMALL PARTICLE 1–5 MICRONS				
Estilux	Kulzer	N	4	84
Estilux C	Kulzer	N	3	84
Healthco VLC	Healthco	Y	7	76
Paste Laminate	Den-Mat	Y	6	84
Prisma Fill	Caulk/Dentsply	Y	7	78
Valux	3M	N	9	78
Visiofil	ESPE/Priemer	N	6	80
HYBRID 0.04 + 5 MICRONS				
A.P.H	Caulk/Dentsply	Y	16	78
Bisfil M	Bisco	N	11	73
Bisfil P	Bisco	Y	6	86
Brilliant Lux	Coltene	Y	15	78
Command Ultrafine	Kerr	Y	6	76
Conquest	Jeneric/Pentron	Y	25	77
Herculite	Kerr	Y	18	78
Lite-fil A	Shofu	Y	8	84
Lite-fil P	Shofu	Y	2	85
Multi-fil	Kulzer	N	11	78
Occlusion	COE/GC	Y	6	85.9
P-50	3M	Y	4	87.5
Pentra-fil II	Jeneric/Pentron	Y	6	78.7
Pertac Hybrid	ESPE/Premier	Y	15	80
Post Com II	Jeneric/Pentron	Y	3	79.2
Photo Clearfill	J. Morita	N	7	86
Status	Healthco	Y	8	79
Ultrabond	Den-Mat	Y	21	75–82
Visarfil	Den-Mat	Y	8	84
Visiomolar	ESPE/Premier	Y	4	86

scanning electron microscope (SEM) etch patterns and possibly better retention.[10] Agitation places "new" acid in contact with the enamel and displaces the neutralized acid.

6. Shiny etched areas can indicate plaque or incomplete removal of old composite resin. These can be removed with a diamond bur and re-etched so that a uniformly etched enamel surface is obtained.

7. Throughly wash to remove the reaction products from the etch solution. Wash times using water or water/air spray should exceed 10 seconds (25 ml) for gel etchants, but need not exceed 20 seconds.[11,12]

CLINICAL TIP. Spraying for more than 60 seconds may damage the etched enamel surface, resulting in decreased bond strength.[11,12]

---

8. Studies of bovine enamel exposed to 35% hydrogen peroxide for 1 hour (as might be used in successive 30 minute bleaching sessions) suggest that similar treatment of human enamel might be contraindi-

cated prior to placing composite resin or porcelain veneers because of reduced enamel bond strength.[13] More research is needed in this area.

9. Nitric acid (e.g., Mirage Bond, Chameleon Dental Products, Inc.) etchant may require constant rubbing of enamel to achieve an etched surface.

Enamel and Enamel-Dentin Bonding Considerations

1. Enamel bonding agents are unfilled or lightly filled fluid composite resins. Application of a bonding agent reduces microleakage. Dentin-enamel bonding agents are more hydrophilic and can strengthen the bond between composite resin and dentin.

2. Because the bond between the composite resin and cervical enamel is much weaker than the bond between the composite resin and occlusal enamel, increased microleakage occurs in cervical areas.[14,15]

3. Brushing to distribute a thin layer of bonding agent may be better than air drying, which can incorporate

air into the composite resin and inhibit curing. Air drying from a "triple" syringe can incorporate moisture into the preparation.

CLINICAL TIP. Dry with a syringe that is not connected to a water line or with a hair dryer to avoid moisture contamination.

---

4. See Chapter 3 for a complete discussion of dentin bonding agents and total etch (enamel and dentin) technique.
5. See Chapter 7 for a complete discussion of glass ionomer cements.

Polymerization Shrinkage

Upon curing, composite resin shrinks about 3% linearly and about 1.5% volumetrically. This can have adverse consequences on the quality of the final restoration. Bonding to enamel is instantaneous and very strong. Bonding to dentin, particularly with older dentin bonding adhesives, is less reliable, much slower, and in almost all cases, weaker than the enamel bond. This can result in the composite resin pulling away from the dentin while it is curing.

Polymerization contraction can also cause problems when bonding resin to cervical enamel. Contraction is strong enough to tear enamel rods from cervical enamel. Polymerization contraction is partially compensated for by water sorption, which causes composite resin expansion, but this process takes time. In addition, leakage may have occurred and the dentin bond may have been destroyed.

Dentin Bonding and Polymerization Shrinkage

Class V preparations may contain margins which are totally surrounded by enamel, surrounded by both enamel and root structure, or are completely contained within root structure. These three situations typically demonstrate the devastating effects of polymerization shrinkage in Class V restorations.[2]

Polymerization contraction causes stresses. If the lesion is completely surrounded by enamel (Fig. 5–1), these stresses are relieved by detachment of composite resin from the dentin. However, marginal integrity in enamel is maintained.

Dentin bonding agents that are as strong as enamel bonding agents do not solve the problem of the detrimental effect that polymerization contraction has on marginal integrity.[2] Paradoxically, a dentin bonding agent with a bond strength equal to or exceeding the bond of composite resin to enamel would not be desirable in terms of polymerization shrinkage. If a strong bond exists between the dentin and the composite resin, no gap could be formed between the composite resin and the dentin to relieve the stresses caused by polymerization contraction. In this situation only the labial composite resin surface is free to move. However, because of its proximity to the curing light, the labial surface is also the first area of the composite resin that would be hardened. If the composite resin-to-dentin bond held, contraction would pull the composite resin

away from enamel either by breaking the bond or by actually pulling the enamel rods out of the tooth, resulting in leakage at this critical area. In the unlikely event that the enamel bond held, and the enamel rods did not break off from the tooth, the tooth and the composite resin would be under tremendous stress from the contraction shrinkage.

If the lesion is completely contained within the root surface (Fig. 5–2) and polymerization shrinkage forces exceed the instantaneous strength of the dentin bonding agent, the restoration may leak and most likely will dislodge.

The most common occurrence is when the restoration is bonded to enamel incisally and to root structure at the gingival margin (Fig. 5–3). If the dentin bond is not instantaneous and not stronger than the composite resin shrinkage, a contraction gap forms at the gingival margin and the restoration will probably leak there.

Because even the new dentin bonding agents do not always produce reliable, instantaneous, high-strength bonds, gingival groove placement for mechanical retention is recommended. (Refer to the discussion of Class III restorations for a technique of compensating for gingival gaps with additional bonding resin). Some reports state that even thin layers of composite resin, such as those produced under porcelain inlays, can produce shrinkage stresses which challenge the dentin bond.[16]

Liner and Base Considerations

Calcium hydroxide in its various forms has a long, safe clinical track record when used in close proximity to the pulp or as a pulp capping material. Unfortunately, calcium hydroxide tends to disappear under composite resins and even under amalgams.[17] This can leave gaps that can fill with tissue fluid and become secondarily infected under leaking restorations. Therefore, it is prudent to use calcium hydroxide in small amounts and only when preparations are in close proximity to the pulp. Glass ionomer cements are a preferred liner and base (see Chapter 7—Glass Ionomer Cements).

Marginal Bevel Considerations

1. Bevels are extremely useful in gaining a gradual optical transition from composite resin to enamel in Class III, IV, and V restorations. If performed correctly, they can help create an almost invisible restoration.
2. Occlusal bevels in Class I and Class II situations should be avoided. Composite resins wear faster than enamel; therefore, occlusal enamel should not be sacrificed for a bevel. Furthermore, thin composite resin bevels are vulnerable to fracture.
3. Preparations ending near the cementoenamel junction should not be beveled to avoid inadvertent removal of this thin area of enamel. Although bonds to gingival enamel exhibit more microleakage than bonds to occlusal enamel, it is preferable to terminate the preparation on any enamel rather than on dentin or cementum.[14,15]
4. The choice of rotary instrument type for beveling is equivocal. Rough surfaces provided by coarse diamonds increase available enamel surface area result-

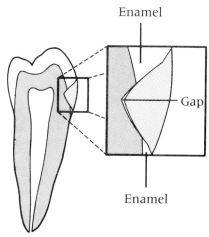

Enamel

Enamel

FIG. 5–1. In a restoration completely surrounded by enamel, polymerization contraction causes the detachment of the composite resin from the dentin. Although a gap may form under the restoration, the marginal integrity in the enamel is maintained. In the unlikely event that a dentin bonding agent could be formulated as strong as an enamel bonding agent this could cause the composite resin to break away from the enamel or cause a pulling out of the enamel rods or, if both the enamel and dentin bonds hold, place the tooth and the resin under tremendous stresses.

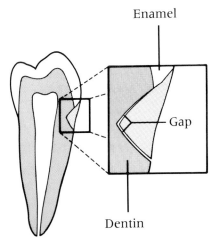

Enamel

Gap

Dentin

FIG. 5–3. The most common clinical situation is a restoration bonded to enamel incisally and to root at the gingival margin. If the dentin bond is not instantaneous and stronger than the composite resin shrinkage, a contraction gap forms at the gingival margin. Microleakage may occur at the gingival margin, resulting in restoration failure. (Adapted from Davidson CL, Kemp-Shulte CM: Shortcomings of Composite Resins in Class V Restorations. J Esthetic Dent 1:1, 1986.)

ing in a stronger bond. However, this added surface area may be unnecessary, and the irregular surface that is produced has a greater chance of trapping air bubbles. A bubble presents the possibilities of inner oxygen inhibition or porosities, which may lead to future discoloration.[18]

Finishing Considerations

All etched surfaces must be covered with bonding agent. Etched enamel that is not covered with resin

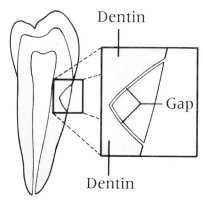

Dentin

Gap

Dentin

FIG. 5–2. If the restoration is completely contained within the root surface and polymerization shrinkage forces exceed the instantaneous strength of the dentin bonding agent, a gap may form around the entire restoration. This may lead to leakage and restoration failure.

may take as long as 2 to 3 months to remineralize,[18] leaving the tooth surface vulnerable to discoloration. Therefore, the bonding agent should extend beyond the area that was etched. When the bonding agent is placed, the tooth returns to its original color and it is difficult to tell the original area of etched enamel. This results in a layer of bonding agent lying invisibly against, but not bonded to, enamel, which could be a source of future discoloration and caries. To remedy this, use rotary instruments to reduce the restoration to its proper topography and completely align it with the remaining enamel. Then, run a composite resin carving knife, a No. 12 Bard Parker blade, or a gold foil finishing instrument from the enamel to the composite resin to remove all unattached bonding agent. (These instruments are also excellent for removing small proximal overhangs in Class II restorations prior to finishing with aluminum oxide strips [see Figure 5–17].) This will leave a small step, which can be finished flush with the enamel with composite resin finishing diamonds, burs, or discs.

Polishing Considerations

Optimal polish can be obtained with microfilled composite resins; however, because of low filler content, optimal polish is obtained at the expense of physical properties, such as increased water sorption, polymerization shrinkage, coefficient of thermal expansion, and brittleness. The gap between the stronger, more filled composite resins and the microfilled composite resins is narrowing with microfilled resin loading approaching 50 to 70% (versus 75 to 85% for composite resins) and the development of the new hybrid composite resins loaded in excess of 75% and containing some submicron particles. Polish may not be retained on a hybrid and periodic polishing may, therefore, be necessary.

One study shows that eliminating conventional finishing procedures accomplished with burs on the occlusal surface of posterior composite resins, resulted in a substantial reduction in wear of the composite resin in Class II restorations.[19] Because it is usually necessary to shape and adjust the occlusal area of composite resins, micron diamond burs should be used, as described by Lutz and others.[20] (See also Chapter 4—Color Modifiers and Opaquers—Class III and Class IV Restorations.)

TECHNIQUES AND MATERIALS

Class I Composite Resin Restorations

Armamentarium

- Standard dental setup
  explorer
  mouth mirror
  anesthesia (if necessary)
  rubber dam setup
  high-speed handpiece
  burs
  30 to 50% phosphoric acid, liquid or gel
  flat contrangle placement instrument
  suitable liner (if necessary)
  suitable base (if necessary)
- Articulating paper or wax
- A radiopaque composite or microfilled resin designed for posterior use (e.g., APH, Caulk/Dentsply; P-50, 3M, Inc.; Herculite XR, Kerr, Inc.; Heliomolar, Vivadent, Inc.)
- Oil-free pumice
- Composite resin placement syringe (e.g., Centrix Syringe, Centrix, Inc.)
- Composite resin polishing paste

Clinical Technique

1. Cleanse the tooth with pumice.
2. Determine the appropriate shade of the tooth while it is wet with saliva.
3. Prior to cavity preparation, use articulating paper to ensure that the cavity design avoids including occlusal contacts, if possible.
4. Administer local anesthesia if necessary.
5. Place a rubber dam.
6. The preparation may be entirely based in enamel because extension to dentin for retention is not necessary.
7. Place appropriate liner and base if necessary. (See the section on Liner and Base Considerations.)
8. Etch the enamel for 15 seconds. (See the section on Acid Etch Considerations.)
9. Wash with water or a water/air spray for a minimum of 10 seconds (25 ml) for gel etchants, but not longer than 20 seconds. (See the Clinical Tip in the section on Acid Etch Considerations.)
10. Air-dry the preparation. (See the Clinical Tip in the section on Acid Etch Considerations.)
11. Repeat if a frosted white appearance is not present.
12. Place the appropriate bonding agent. (See the section on Enamel and Enamel-Dentin Bonding Considerations.)
13. Use three pie-shaped wedges of composite resin to fill the restoration. Place the first layer on the buccal wall and extend it diagonally to the pulpal floor. Cure through the buccal enamel for at least

60 seconds with a 13-mm curved light tip and then cure for 60 seconds from the occlusal direction. Because polymerization shrinkage occurs toward the light source, curing from the buccal direction first provides buccal adaptation of the restoration.

CLINICAL TIP. Bonding agent is a better lubricant than alcohol for preventing composite resin from sticking to the plastic instrument. Alcohol could weaken the composite resin. This consideration is particularly important for Class II restorations, which are subjected to heavy occlusal stress.

CLINICAL TIP. A preferred method of composite resin placement is to use a Centrix-type syringe. Placing the material with a syringe lessens the chance of bubble formation and eliminates composite resin "pull back" that occurs when the material is placed with hand instruments.

14. Repeat this procedure on the lingual wall. Cure through the lingual enamel for at least 60 seconds with a 13-mm curved light tip and then cure for 60 seconds from the occlusal direction.
15. Place composite resin in the mid portion of the tooth and cure from the occlusal direction for 60 seconds.
16. Adjust the occlusion; contour and finish the restoration. (See the section on Finishing Considerations.)
17. Polish the restoration. (See the section on Polishing Considerations.)

CLINICAL TIP. The composite resin that is closest to the light tip is often the most polymerized and, thus, the hardest part of the restoration. Because this layer will be removed with occlusal adjustment and polishing, cure occlusally for an additional 60 seconds following polishing.

Class II Composite Resin Restorations

The chief problems with Class II restorations appear to be occlusal wear, poor proximal contact, and postoperative sensitivity.

Occlusal Wear. Manufacturers have been designing more wear-resistant resins. In addition to wear resistance, these composite resins are radiopaque making detection of proximal overhangs and recurrent caries easier.

Postoperative Sensitivity. Postoperative sensitivity reportedly occurs in 10 to 50% of cases.[21] This has been attributed to inadvertent acid etching of the dentin. In many non-Class II situations acid inadvertently contacts the dentin (especially when placed in liquid rather than gel form). However, sensitivity in other restorations is rare and, therefore, little reported in the literature. (See Chapter 3—Dentin Bonding Agents—Total Etch Technique.)

Light-cured composite resins are generally used for posterior restorations because they are better resistant to occlusal wear. Unlike chemically cured resins, which contract toward the geometric center (Fig. 5–4), light-cured resins shrink toward the light source (Fig. 5–5).

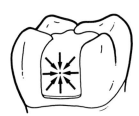

FIG. 5–4. Chemically cured composite resins shrink toward the geometric center of the mass. This leaves a small contraction gap at the gingival margin. The composite resin is strongly bonded to enamel on both the buccal and lingual walls preventing gaps at these walls, however, there may be stresses set up in both the tooth and the composite resin.

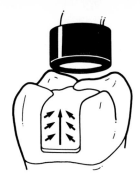

FIG. 5–5. Photocured composite resin shrinks toward the light source because the composite resin closest to the light hardens first. This, in turn, pulls the softer composite resin from the gingival areas, creating a gap. The mass of composite resin being pulled to the occlusal area is twice that found in chemically cured resins (see Fig. 5–4), hence the gingival contraction gap is roughly twice as large.

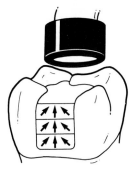

FIG. 5–6. Incremental curing reduces, but does not completely eliminate, the gingival contraction gap.

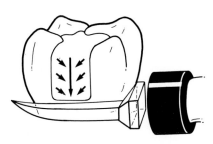

FIG. 5–7. A plastic wedge, which acts as a fiber optic extension, can pull the composite resin gingivally to minimize gap formation.

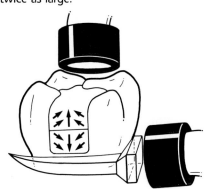

FIG. 5–8. This incremental technique, although not ideal, should reduce both the gingival contraction gap and the stresses compared to a two-increment technique involving only occlusal curing, as might be done clinically. The first layer is placed and photocured via the plastic wedge. A second layer is placed and cured occlusally. Two improvements could be made in the most gingival increment. First, regardless of tooth color, a light-colored resin should be used to ensure additional curing depth. Second, before adding the final increment, a second, occlusal cure of the first increment should be performed in order to ensure complete hardening of the mass. (Adapted from Lutz, F. et al.: Improved Proximal Margin Adaption of Class II Composite Resin Restorations. Quint 17:659, 1988.)

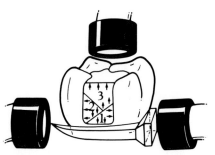

FIG. 5–9. This technique takes advantage of composite resin contraction and uses only one 11 to 13 mm curved light tip. The first increment can be pulled lingually and gingivally (via the light reflecting wedge directing light at a 90° angle to the light tip) before an additional occlusal cure. The second increment is pulled bucally and gingivally before it too receives an additional occlusal cure. The final increment is hardened occlusally after placing a ball of prepolymerized composite to act as an internal wedge. Additional occlusal increments may be necessary in large teeth. This design also minimizes pulling together of the cusps.

Because the part closest to the light hardens first, shrinkage pulls the softened mass toward the light rod. Shrinkage almost always produces leakage at the cervical margin on dentin or cementum based restorations.[22-25] Cervical enamel, when present, bonds poorly compared to occlusal enamel. Sometimes enamel prisms can actually be torn in the shrinkage toward the occlusal. Incremental curing reduces, but does not eliminate, the gingival shrinkage (Fig. 5–6). The use of a plastic wedge, which acts as a fiber optic guide,

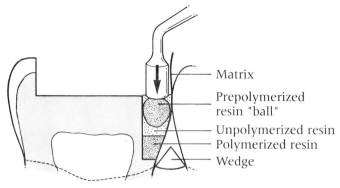

Matrix
Prepolymerized resin "ball"
Unpolymerized resin
Polymerized resin
Wedge

FIG. 5–10. Place a small egg-shaped ball of polymerized posterior composite resin into the proximal box. Push the ball into the uncured resin so that it contacts the axial wall and mylar strip and acts as an internal wedge to further tighten the contact with the adjacent tooth.

can further reduce the gap (Fig. 5–7), especially when combined with incremental placement of resin (Figs. 5–8, 5–9).[26] Gingival retention grooves are probably desirable in Class II restorations which terminate on the root because the literature is replete with reports of the benefits of these grooves in Class V situations.

Evidence exists that shrinkage can also pull cusps together, which can compound the sensitivity problem. It has been reported that cutting a finished composite resin restoration completely to the occlusal floor from mesial to distal allows the cusps to spring back, which immediately relieves sensitivity.[14] An overtightened Tofflemire retainer can also pull cusps together, compounding the sensitivity problem. Research suggests that a layering procedure can minimize cusp contraction. It is important that no increment of composite resin extends the entire buccal-lingual length in order to prevent the cusps from being pulled together during polymerization shrinkage.

Tight Proximal Contacts. In an MOD composite resin restoration, unlike an amalgam restoration, it is not necessary to place a circumferential band. First, place and wedge the band on the distal box area only. This method avoids "fighting" a thickness of the band on the mesial and a mesial wedge, and provides more mesial tooth movement.

CLINICAL TIP. As additional "insurance," a small egg-shaped ball of prepolymerized composite resin (shaped and cured on the finger) is wedged into unpolymerized composite resin at increment 3 against the axial wall and the band (Fig 5–10). The composite resin ball acts as an additional wedge, placing pressure from within on the axial wall and the mylar matrix. Use a plugger to exert active downward pressure and expose increment 3 (unpolymerized) to the curing light.

The mesial box is done in a similar manner, with the composite resins joined at the occlusal area.

CLINICAL TIP. When new composite resin is added within five minutes to existing uncontaminated cured composite resin, chemical adhesion is as strong as it would be if the two had been mixed immediately.[27,28]

Strengthening Cusps. Intuitively, a dentist may reason that given a strong enamel bond and a high tensile strength of composite resin, buccal cusps can be "tied"

to lingual cusps to strengthen the tooth, in a manner similar to that of a gold onlay. However, in vitro research on this is equivocal. One study has shown loss of reinforcement with thermal cycling.[29]

Multiple Step Buildup Technique

Armamentarium. The armamentarium is the same as that listed for a Class I restoration plus:

- Mylar matrix strip (possibly the contoured variety)
- Light reflecting wedge (Cure-Thru, Premier Dental Products Co., or Luciwedge, Coltene/Whaldent)
- Radiopaque composite or microfilled resin designed for posterior use (e.g., Heliomolar, APH, Herculite XR, P 50)

Clinical Technique

1. Cleanse the tooth with pumice and clean the proximal surface with a strip when applicable.
2. Determine the appropriate shade of the tooth while it is wet with saliva.
3. Prior to cavity preparation use articulating paper to ensure that the cavity design avoids including occlusal contacts, where possible.
4. Administer local anesthesia if necessary.
5. Place a rubber dam.
6. When warranted, the preparation may be entirely based in enamel, because extension into dentin for retention is not necessary.
7. Place appropriate liner and base.
8. Etch the enamel for 15 seconds.
9. Wash with water or a water/air spray for a minimum of 10 seconds (25 ml) for gel etchants, but not longer than 20 seconds.
10. Air-dry the preparation. (See the Clinical Tip in the section on Acid Etch Considerations)
11. Repeat if a frosty white appearance is not present.
12. Place the appropriate bonding agent.
13. Place a light-reflecting wedge from the lingual direction.

CLINICAL TIP. If the first two layers will not be part of the labial display, use a light-colored resin to ensure a more complete light penetration and subsequent polymerization.

14. Place an incremental layer of composite resin on the lingual wall. It should not touch the buccal wall. (see Figure 5−9).

CLINICAL TIP. Use bonding agent, rather than alcohol, to prevent the composite resin from sticking to the plastic instrument. (See the Clinical Tip in the section on Class I Composite Resin Restoration.)

CLINICAL TIP. Place the composite resin with a Centrix-type syringe. (See the Clinical Tip in the section on Class I Composite Resin Restoration.)

15. Cure from the lingual direction for 60 seconds.

CLINICAL TIP. Use an 11 to 13-mm angle-tipped light to ensure that the light hits the lingual surface and the wedge, optimizing light direction vectors and polymerization. (See the arrows on Figure 5−8.)

16. Cure from the occlusal direction for 60 seconds.
17. Remove the wedge from the lingual area and place it buccally.
18. Place a second layer of composite resin on the buccal wall. It should not touch the lingual wall.
19. Cure from the buccal direction for 60 seconds.
20. Cure from the occlusal direction for 60 seconds.
21. Model a small piece of posterior composite resin into an egg-shaped ball on a gloved finger and polymerize the resin.

CLINICAL TIP. Wash your gloves before beginning this procedure so that no powder remains on the surface.

22. Place the resin into the proximal box and push the ball into the uncured resin so that it contacts the axial wall and mylar strip. This acts as an internal wedge to further tighten the contact with the adjacent tooth. (See Figure 5−10.)
23. Cure from the occlusal direction for 60 seconds.
24. Add additional occlusal increments of composite resin as necessary. The shades of these increments should blend with the surrounding tooth.

CLINICAL TIP. In an MOD preparation, fill the distal box first and place the mylar strip and wedge only in the distal area. There is usually no need for the matrix band to encircle the tooth, and the absence of the band and wedge in the mesial area ensures a tighter distal contact. Then remove the distal matrix and wedge and repeat the process in the mesial area.

25. Adjust the occlusion and contour the restoration. (See the section on Finishing Considerations.)

CLINICAL TIP. It may be possible to seal marginal contraction gaps at the root surface of the proximal box of a Class II restoration with a bonding agent. This should be performed after finishing but prior to polishing.[30,31]

26. Polish the restoration. (See the section on Polishing Considerations.)

CLINICAL TIP. Cure occlusally for an additional 60 seconds after polishing to ensure complete polymerization of the deeper layers. (See the Clinical Tip in the section on Class I Composite Resin Restorations.)

Class III Composite Resin Restorations

Because a radiopaque material should be used to aid in the detection of recurrent decay in Class III restorations, only a limited number of composite resins, microfilled resins, and glass ionomer bases can be used (see Table 5−1). A sandwich technique, as described for the Class IV restoration, can be used for Class III restorations, using a radiopaque composite resin to build the lingual wall and veneering with a microfilled resin or hybrid resin labially. Alternatively, a single radiopaque microfilled or a hybrid resin can be used. This single formulation technique is rapid and useful when the restoration is completely based in enamel with the gingival enamel margin well away from the cemento-enamel junction.

The preferred approach for the removal of decay on Class III restorations is from the lingual direction. This allows for an intact labial wall and improved esthetics. If this is not possible, a labial approach with a lingually intact wall is preferred. However, extensive decay may require removal of both walls.

CLINICAL TIP. In Class III restorations, in which both the labial and lingual plate of enamel are missing, sandwich a layer of opaque composite resin between the more translucent outer layers to prevent a gray restoration.

Single Step Buildup Technique

Despite individual variations, two different techniques essentially are used in the fabrication of restorations: the single step buildup and the incremental step buildup. In most situations the incremental placement of resin is the technique of choice because it partly compensates for polymerization shrinkage; furthermore, addition of tints, color modifiers and opaques is relatively simple. The single step buildup technique, however, can be used for many types of cavities, repair of chipped teeth, diastema closures, and veneers. It is suitable for any restoration completely bounded by enamel and well away from the cemento-enamel junction (CEJ), where polymerization shrinkage cannot cause gingival gaps.

The main advantage of the single step buildup is that it is rapid. In addition, pressure from the mylar matrix eliminates composite resin pull back: preferential sticking of composite resin to the instrument rather than to the tooth. This ensures intimate adaptation of the uncured resin to the tooth contours, at least initially, and maximum contact with the bonding agent. However, contact with the dentin portions may be lost after polymerization shrinkage.

The single buildup technique makes no compensation for polymerization shrinkage, although, after initial curing, additional bonding resin or composite resin can be added. (A low viscosity resin can penetrate the gingival gap and ensure more intimate contact with the tooth.)

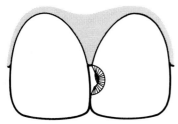

FIG. 5-11. Because the lesion is completely surrounded by enamel, the final preparation does not require an undercut. Note the bevel around the entire preparation.

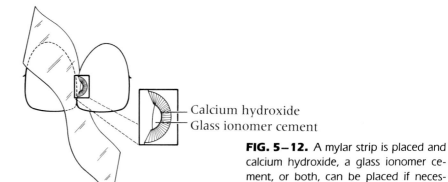

— Calcium hydroxide
— Glass ionomer cement

FIG. 5-12. A mylar strip is placed and calcium hydroxide, a glass ionomer cement, or both, can be placed if necessary.

In addition, when the gingival margin is based on or near the root surface, shrinkage can destroy the dentin bond; if the margin is on the cervical enamel, shrinkage can tear or fracture delicate gingival enamel rods.

Armamentarium. The armamentarium is the same as that listed for a Class I restoration plus:

- Mylar strip or clear crown
- Wedge (desirable if near the gingiva)
- Posterior, small particle or hybrid composite resin
- Microfilled composite resin (e.g., Silux, Durafill, Renamel)

Clinical Technique

1. Pumice the tooth and clean the proximal surface with a strip where applicable.
2. Determine the appropriate shade of the tooth while it is wet with saliva.
3. Apply local anesthesia if necessary.
4. Place a rubber dam.
5. Place a generous bevel or chamfer around the periphery of the preparation, except around the gingival area if the enamel there is thin (Fig. 5-11). This creates a gradual transition from composite resin to enamel and usually permits the creation of an invisible restoration. In addition, it minimizes the risk of damage during polishing and decreases the chance of a "white line" at the margin.
6. Place appropriate liner and base, if applicable (Fig. 5-12).
7. Etch the enamel for 15 seconds (Fig. 5-13).
8. Wash with water or a water/air spray for a minimum of 10 seconds (25 ml) for gel etchants, but not longer than 20 seconds.
9. Air-dry the preparation. (See the Clinical Tip in the section on Enamel and Enamel-Dentin Bonding Considerations.)
10. Repeat if a frosty white appearance is not present.

CLINICAL TIP. The gloved finger should be pressed firmly against the lingual mylar strip to ensure intimate contact. This minimizes subsequent lingual bite adjustment.

---

11. Place the appropriate bonding agent.
12. Adapt the mylar strip to the lingual area of the preparation. If the decay extended toward the gingiva, a wedge may be placed.
13. Rapid single step bulk placement technique is suitable when the restoration is completely contained in enamel, and when the gingival portion is well away from the CEJ. (When the restoration is close to the CEJ or on root surface, multiple step incremental placement minimizes contraction gaps at the gingival margin.) Use a radiopaque hybrid or microfilled resin for bulk placement.

CLINICAL TIP. Use bonding agent, rather than alcohol, to prevent the composite resin from sticking to the plastic instrument. (See the Clinical Tip in the section on Class I Composite Resin Restoration.)

CLINICAL TIP. Place the composite resin with a Centrix-type syringe (Fig. 5-14). (See the Clinical Tip in the section on Composite Resin Restoration.)

---

14. Use the light wand for 60 seconds labially to cure the labial area and to partially cure the lingual area (Fig. 5-15).
15. Remove the gloved finger from the mylar strip and cure from the lingual direction for 60 seconds (Fig. 5-16).
16. Contour and finish the restoration (Figs. 5-17 to 5-19). (See the section on Finishing Considerations.)

CLINICAL TIP. It may be possible to seal marginal contraction gaps in the gingival area with a bonding agent. This should be performed after finishing but before polishing.[30,31]

---

17. Polish the restoration. (See the section on Polishing Considerations.)

CLINICAL TIP. Cure labially and lingually for an additional 30 seconds after polishing to ensure complete polymerization of the deeper layers. (See the Clinical Tip in the section on Class I Composite Resin Restorations.)

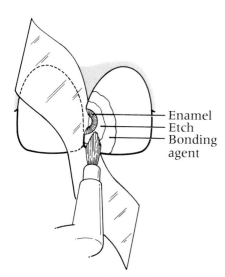

FIG. 5–13. A brush can be used to apply acid etch to enamel only, followed by a wash, dry and the use of a different brush for the application of an enamel-dentin bonding agent. Optionally, the gel etch can be applied via syringe and needle.

Enamel
Etch
Bonding agent

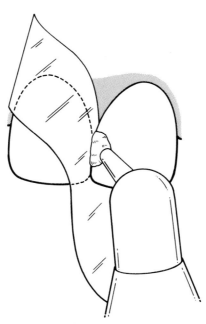

FIG. 5–14. Application of the composite resin via a syringe will minimize "pullback," which often occurs when hand instruments are used.

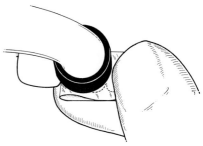

FIG. 5–15. The mylar strip is pulled tightly with finger pressure to minimize subsequent finishing. Placement of a wedge to reduce gingival composite resin excess is optional. Note that the index finger exerts labial pressure against the mylar strip. In addition to reducing composite resin excess, the labial direction of force moves the central incisors slightly labially during the polymerization. When the pressure is released the tooth springs back. This can partially compensate for the thickness of the mylar strip and ensure a tight contact area.

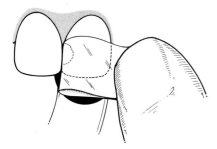

FIG. 5–16. After a 60 second labial cure, the lingual resin will have partially hardened. A 60-second lingual cure completes the process. It is impossible to overcure a composite resin. An additional 60 second cure is recommended if the tooth is dark or if a dark shade of composite resin is used. This additional cure is most beneficial after the restoration is finished to its final form.

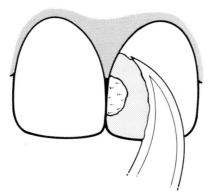

FIG. 5–17. Unbonded resin flash and small resin overhangs are removed with a Bard-Parker blade or composite resin knife prior to final polishing. The hand instrument is always moved from tooth to composite resin.

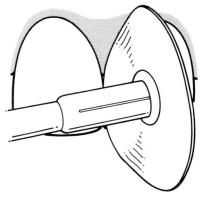

FIG. 5–18. Shaping and polishing can be done with diamonds, burs, discs, or rubber wheels. This is followed by application of composite resin polishing paste using a prophy cup or felt wheel.

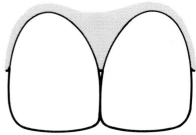

FIG. 5–19. The finished restoration.

Multiple Step Buildup Technique. Polymerization shrinkage results in gaps or strains in the restoration. It can also break dentin bonds. Gap size decreases as the restoration absorbs water, but the dentin bond will never be restored. Incremental multiple step placement reduces, but does not eliminate, the problem.

Armamentarium. The armamentarium is the same as that listed in Class IV Multiple Step Buildup Technique.

Clinical Technique. Use the same clinical technique as that described in Class IV Multiple Step Buildup Technique.

Class IV Composite Resin Restorations

Class IV restorations present free labial, incisal, and lingual surfaces and, thus, polymerization shrinkage usually is not a problem. Hybrid composite resins are ideal for Class IV restorations: they are strong and can resist occlusal stresses.

CLINICAL TIP. Consider porcelain laminate veneers, full coverage porcelain, or ceramometal crowns for patients with heavy occlusal function, and for restoring mandibular incisors. With light occlusion, hybrid composite resins can be used to restore mandibular incisors.

Hybrid composite resins tend to have good optical opacity. This often prevents the restoration from graying because of darkness from the rear of the oral cavity.

Most hybrid composite resins can receive a good surface polish, so esthetics can be good to excellent. It has been pointed out that, unlike microfilled composite resins, surface luster may need periodic renewal and repolishing.

Certain lipsticks may discolor the surface of a hybrid composite resin. This is not a stain and can be rubbed off with the tongue or paper tissue. Often it appears on natural enamel. To minimize the occurrence of this discoloration, it may be necessary to surface the hybrid composite resin with a microfilled composite resin. This can be done at the time of restoration or subsequently.

Lipstick and other discolorations clinically seem to be a function of several variables:[32]

1. The chemistry of the saliva
2. The chemistry of the discolorant and the composite resin
3. The amount of discolorant (i.e., heavy vs. light lipstick application)
4. The frequency of discolorant application (i.e., the number of times lipstick is applied per day)

Modification or alteration of one or more of the above factors may improve the situation (e.g., changing the lipstick or the composite resin or both).

Single Step Buildup Technique

The Class IV single step technique is similar to the Class III single step technique (See the preceding section for complete discussion of limitations of this technique.) It is difficult to include opaquers, which limit the gray "shine-through" from the back of the mouth, when using the single step buildup technique in Class IV restorations. With this technique it is also difficult to incorporate tints and color modifiers to the resin if that is required.

Armamentarium. The armamentarium is the same as that listed in Class III Multiple Step Buildup Technique except:

■ Clear crown form

Clinical Technique. Use the same Clinical Technique as that described in Class III Single Step Buildup Technique except a clear crown form is generally preferred.

Multiple Step Buildup Technique

Armamentarium. The armamentarium is the same as that listed for a Class I restoration plus:

■ Mylar strip
■ Posterior, small particle or hybrid composite resin
■ Optional microfilled composite resin (e.g., Silux, 3M, Inc. Durafill, Kulzer, Inc, Renamel, Cosmedent, Inc.)

Clinical Technique

1. Pumice the tooth and clean the proximal surface with a strip where applicable.
2. Determine the appropriate shade of the tooth while it is wet with saliva.
3. Administer local anesthesia if necessary.
4. Place a rubber dam.
5. To aid in finishing, place a full chamfer around the periphery of the preparation for strength, retention, and the delineation of the end of the margin. (Fig. 5–20). (This is an exception to the butt joint margin under occlusal function on lingual.)
6. Place a liner or base where appropriate (Fig. 5–21).
7. Etch the enamel for 15 seconds.
8. Wash with water or a water/air spray for a minimum of 10 seconds (25 ml) for gel etchants, but not longer than 20 seconds.
9. Air-dry the preparation. (See the Clinical Tip under the section on Enamel and Enamel-Dentin Bonding Considerations.)
10. Repeat if a frosty white appearance is not present.
11. Place the appropriate bonding agent.
12. To minimize lingual finishing, intimately adapt the mylar strip against the tooth with a gloved finger.
13. Place the posterior small particle or hybrid composite resin against the mylar strip. Place an amount that will leave sufficient room for a continuous layer of microfilled composite resin (Fig. 5–22).

CLINICAL TIP. Use bonding agent rather than alcohol to prevent the composite resin from sticking to the plastic instrument. (See the Clinical Tip in the section on Class I Composite Resin Restorations.)

---

14. Cure the composite resin from the labial direction, and then from the lingual direction. The cured

composite resin will form a strong lingual wall (Fig. 5–23).

CLINICAL TIP. Place the composite resin with a Centrix-type syringe. (See the Clinical Tip in the section on Composite Resin Restoration.)

15. Place the microfilled composite resin against the buccal wall of the previously placed composite resin (Fig. 5–24).
16. Shape the microfilled composite resin as much as possible prior to curing.
17. Cure the microfilled composite resin from the buccal direction (Fig. 5–25), and then from the lingual and incisal direction (Fig. 5–26).
18. Contour and finish the restoration (Figs. 5–27, 5–28). (See the section on Finishing Considerations.)
19. Polish the restoration. (See the section on Polishing Considerations.)

CLINICAL TIP. Cure labially, lingually, and incisally for an additional 30 seconds after polishing to ensure complete polymerization of the deeper layers. (See the Clinical Tip in the section on Class I Composite Resin Restorations.)

Class V Composite Resin Restorations
Single Step Buildup Technique

The Class V single step technique is similar to the Class III single step technique.

Armamentarium. The armamentarium is the same as that listed in Class V Multiple Step Buildup Technique except:

■ Class V cervical matrix (e.g., Cure-Thru, ESPE-Priemer Sales Corp.)

Clinical Technique. Use the same Clinical Technique as that described in Class V Multiple Step Buildup Technique except place all the composite resin in a single increment. Apply pressure with a cervical matrix and cure the resin.

Multiple Step Buildup Technique

Armamentarium. The armamentarium is the same as that listed for Class I restoration plus:

■ Composite or microfilled resin tube or syringe (see discussion)
■ Dentin and enamel bonding agents
■ Base and tinting agents (optional)
■ Finishing and polishing instruments

Clinical Technique

1. Pumice the tooth and clean the proximal surface with a strip where applicable.
2. Determine the appropriate shade of the tooth while it is wet with saliva.
3. Administer local anesthesia if necessary.
4. Place a rubber dam.
5. If the Class V restoration is entirely in enamel, place bevels or chamfers around the periphery, except at the gingival margin if the enamel there is thin. This creates a gradual transition from composite resin to enamel and usually permits the creation of an invisible restoration. In addition, it minimizes the risk of damage during polishing and decreases the chance of a "white line" at the margin.
6. If the Class V restoration ends on a root surface, place a retention groove at the gingival margin to ensure retention in the event that the dentin bonding agent fails. Beveling the gingival margin on cementum is usually undesirable.
7. Place appropriate liner and base if indicated.
8. Etch the enamel for 15 seconds.
9. Wash with water or a water/air spray for a minimum of 10 seconds (25 ml) for gel etchants, but not longer than 20 seconds.
10. Air-dry the preparation. (See the Clinical Tip in the section on Enamel and Enamel-Dentin Bonding Considerations.)
11. Repeat if a frosted white appearance is not present.
12. Place the appropriate bonding agent.
13. If the restoration is large, place composite resin in increments to minimize both stresses in the restoration and gap formation from polymerization shrinkage.[32] Place an initial pie-shaped increment entirely within the dentin on the root surface (Fig. 5–29). It is important that the bonding agent and the composite resin fill the cervical retention groove.

CLINICAL TIP. Use bonding agent rather than alcohol to prevent the composite resin from sticking to the plastic instrument. (See the Clinical Tip in the section on Class I Composite Resin Restorations.)

CLINICAL TIP. Place the composite resin with a Centrix-type syringe. (See the Clinical Tip in the section on Class I Composite Resin Restorations.)

14. Place a second increment on the occlusal enamel bevel, extending it to the axial wall, and polymerize.
15. Add a third layer to build the tooth to form.
16. Continue adding and polymerizing composite resin as necessary until the restoration is slightly overfilled.
17. Remove excess composite resin.

CLINICAL TIP. Marginal contraction gaps at the root surface can be sealed with bonding agent resin after finishing but prior to polishing.[32,33]

18. Contour and finish the restoration. (See the section on Finishing Considerations.)
19. Polish the restoration. (See the section on Polishing Considerations.)

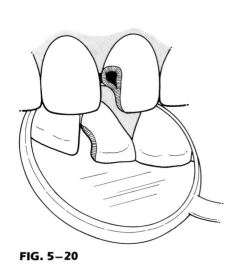

FIG. 5–20

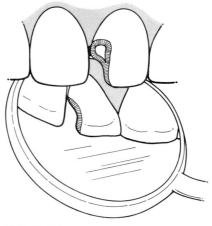

FIG. 5–21

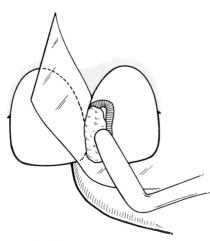

FIG. 5–22

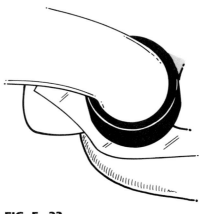

FIG. 5–23

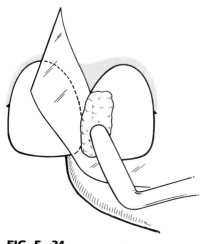

FIG. 5–24

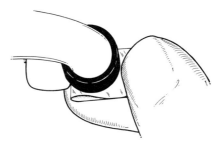

FIG. 5–25

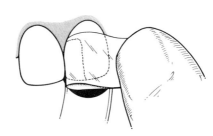

FIG. 5–26

FIG. 5–20. A chamfer bevel has been placed completely around the periphery of the restoration. Should the fracture extend to the root surface, the bevel is omitted at the gingiva, but a gingival retention groove is placed to aid retention and to minimize microleakage.

FIG. 5–21. Calcium hydroxide should be placed only in areas close to the pulp, followed by the placement of a radiopaque glass ionomer base. (Note: If the "total etch" technique is used omit the placement of glass ionomer cement.) Etch the preparation slightly beyond the chamfer. Wash, dry, and paint bonding agent beyond the area of etch.

FIG. 5–22. Pack a small increment of hybrid resin against the lingual mylar matrix (wedging optional), which is supported by the finger. This increment can be placed with the plastic instrument or a syringe.

FIG. 5–23. The increment is cured from the labial aspect first, followed by the lingual. Pressure from the finger against the mylar matrix can assure good adaption and can minimize lingual finishing.

FIG. 5–24. A second increment can be packed against the hardened lingual wall. This increment can be made of either a hybrid or a microfilled resin. If necessary, a layer of tint or opaque can be sandwiched between these two layers.

FIG. 5–25. The second increment should be cured from the labial aspect. Wrapping the matrix band around the labial surface is optional, but usually minimizes finishing and provides a realistic curve of composite resin around the interproximolabial areas.

FIG. 5–26. The lingual and incisal aspects should then be cured again. The mylar strip is removed and the occlusion adjusted. Because the surface next to the light is the hardest, it is sometimes removed during bite adjustment so a final, additional cure is advisable.

ESTHETIC DENTISTRY

FIG. 5–27. Labial flash is removed with a Bard-Parker blade or composite resin knife in an enamel-to-composite resin direction. Developmental grooves or texturing is best accomplished with micron diamonds or knife-edged discs. Finishing is accomplished with burs, diamonds, discs, and rubber cups. Final polish can be accomplished with a composite resin polishing paste.

FIG. 5–28. The final restoration.

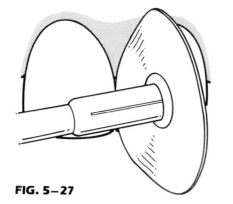

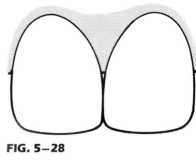

FIG. 5–28

FIG. 5–27

CLINICAL TIP. Cure labially and lingually for an additional 30 seconds after polishing to ensure complete polymerization of the deeper layers. (See the Clinical Tip in the section on Class I Composite Resin Restorations.)

CLINICAL CASES

Multiple Esthetic Problems

A 27-year-old female presented with multiple esthetic problems (Fig. 5–30). Her medical history was noncontributory. The mandibular anterior teeth had deep brown pitted discolorations, possibly caused by a childhood fever. The maxillary teeth had been incorrectly shortened to remove similar brown lesions. The canines were reduced so severely that restorations had to be placed on the incisal edges. Composite resin restorations on the maxillary anterior teeth showed amine discoloration (most likely caused by a chemically cured composite resin). In addition, the restorations were placed into retentive preparations with butt joints and not bonded; hence they exhibited a brown line around the periphery. There were many carious lesions.

First the caries were eliminated and a radiopaque composite resin was used for the Class III restoration (Fig. 5–31). Maxillary incisors were then lengthened using a hybrid composite resin. This was veneered with a microfilled composite resin because the patient preferred heavy lipstick. The mandibular anterior teeth were opaqued and restored. Fortunately, the large overjet allowed for restoration with the more brittle microfilled composite resin.

Combination Dentistry: Post Orthodontics

A 30-year-old female was referred after orthodontic therapy (Fig. 5–32). Her medical history was noncontributory. The maxillary central incisors and the mandibular right lateral incisor were slightly lingually inclined. The maxillary left lateral incisors and the mandibular right lateral incisor were too short. The mandibular incisal plane was uneven and unesthetic.

The lingually placed central incisors were brought into alignment with porcelain laminate veneers. (Fig. 5–33). Composite resins were used to build up the mandibular right lateral incisor and lengthen the maxillary left lateral incisor. Finally, cosmetic contouring was

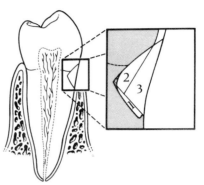

FIG. 5–29. If the preparation extends onto the root surface a gingival groove is placed to aid in retention should the dentin bond fail. Neither the first nor the second layer touches the bonded enamel, therefore, polymerization shrinkage will not place the enamel bond in competition with the dentin bond. Furthermore, use of increments ensures better light penetration and less shrinkage. The final increment, which should also be the thinnest, should cover the entire preparation to eliminate a layering effect.

used on the incisal edge and very subtly on the proximal and labial surfaces to bring the mandibular anterior teeth into an esthetic alignment.

Peg-Shaped Lateral Incisors and Diastema Closure

A 35-year-old female presented with a peg-shaped lateral incisor and a diastema, which she felt marred her smile (Fig. 5–34). The space was closed and the lateral incisor built up by placing hybrid composite resin on the lingual surface and microfilled composite resin on the labial surface (Fig. 5–35). Surface irregularities were added to the central incisors using a fine micron diamond and then polished with a composite resin polishing paste on a brush to maintain the texture.

CONCLUSION

Bonding is one of the fastest developing areas in dentistry. It has proved a boon to both the dentist and the patient. For the first time it has become possible to pro-

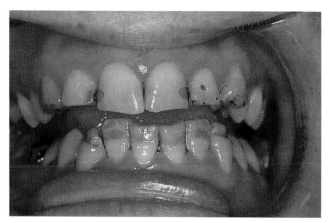

FIG. 5—30. Preoperative view of a 27-year-old female with multiple esthetic problems.

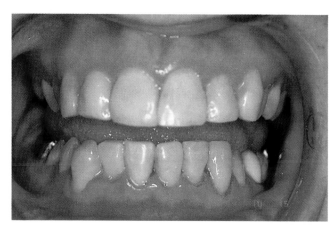

FIG. 5—31. Postoperative view following caries removal, incisal lengthening, and labial veenering.

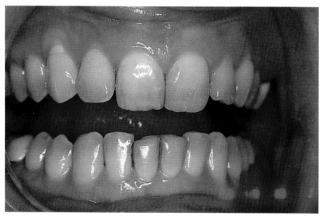

FIG. 5—32. Preoperative view of a 30-year-old female following orthodontic therapy with an unesthetic incisal architecture.

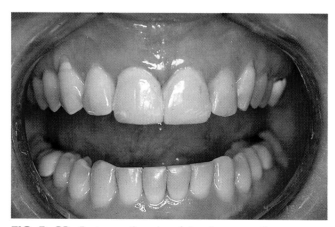

FIG. 5—33. Postoperative view following cosmetic recontouring, composite resin buildup, and porcelain laminates placement.

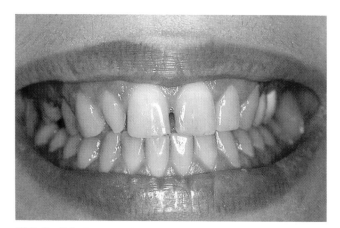

FIG. 5—34. Preoperative view of a 35-year-old female with a peg-shaped lateral incisor and a diastema.

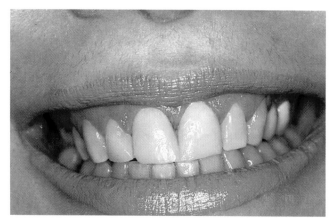

FIG. 5—35. Postoperative view following space closure and a build-up of the lateral incisor with composite resin.

duce almost invisible fillings. Furthermore, this can often be accomplished with minimal tooth reduction in contrast to amalgams, silicates, gold inlays, and foils.

Cosmetic dentistry used to consist solely of orthodontics and full coverage subgingival restorations. Bonding has made possible less costly options, often with better esthetics, less tooth reduction, and usually without invasion of the gingival sulcus. Examples include closing diastema, repairing chipped teeth, masking discolorations and changing color, replacing missing teeth, and placing tooth-colored posterior restorations.

Resins can now be bonded to enamel, dentin, composite resins, porcelain, and both etched and unetched metals. There is little doubt that resin materials will eventually be fabricated for posterior uses that not only match enamel esthetically but also exhibit the wear resistance of enamel. Bonding can be married to the new computer aided design/computer aided manufacturing (CAD/CAM) technology to lute computer-generated inlays and crowns to the teeth, in many cases in one appointment. The future of bonding looks bright.

REFERENCES

1. Davidson C.L. and DeGee A.J.: Relaxation of polymerization contraction stresses by flow in dental composites. J Dent Res 63:146, 1984.
2. Davidson, C.L. and Kemp-Scholte, C.M.: Shortcomings of composite resins in class V restorations. J Esthet Dent 1(1):1, 1989.
3. Crim, G.A.: Effect of composite resin on the microleakage of Scotchbond 2 and Gluma. Am J Dent 5(1):215, 1988.
4. Kemp-Scholte, C.M. and Davidson, C.L.: Marginal sealing of curing contraction gaps in Class V composite resin restorations. J Dent Res 67:841, 1988.
5. Crim, G.A.: Influence of bonding agents and composites on microleakage. J. Prosthet Dent 61(5):371, 1989.
6. Buonocore, M.G.: Retrospection on bonding. Dent Clin North Am 25(2):243, 1981.
7. Rowland, G.F., et. al.: The influence of topical stannous fluoride application on the tensile strength of pit and fissure sealants. J Pedodont 4:9, 1979.
8. Gwinett, A.J.: Personal communication. 1989
9. Barkemeier, W.W., et al.: Effects of 15 versus 60 second enamel acid conditioning on adhesion and morphology. Op Dent 11(3):111, 1986.
10. Baharav, H., et al.: The efficiency of liquid and gel acid etchants. J Prosthet Dent 60(5):545, 1988.
11. Mixson, J.M., et al.: The effects of variable wash times and techniques on enamel composite resin bond strength. Quint Intl 19(4):279, 1988.
12. Schulein, T.M., et al.: Rinsing times for a gel etchant related to enamel/composite bond strength. Gen Dent, July-Aug, 1986.
13. Titley, K.C., et al: Adhesion of composite resin to bleached and unbleached bovine material. J Dent Res 67(12):1523, 1988.
14. Jensen, M.E., Chan D.C.N.: Polymerization shrinkage and microleakage. Vanherle G., Smith D.C. (eds): International Symposium on Posterior Composite Resin Dental Restorative Materials. Netherlands, Peter Szulc Co., 1985.
15. Crim, G.A. and Mattingly, S.L.: Microleakage and the class V composite cavosurface. J Dent Child 47:333, 1980.
16. Feilizer, A.J., et al: Setting stress in composite resin in relation to configuration of the restoration. J Dent Res 66:1636, 1987.
17. Leinfelder, K.F., et. al.: Use of Ca(OH)2 for measuring microleakage. Dent Mat 2:121, 1986.
18. Albers, H.F.: Tooth Colored Restoratives, 7th Ed. Cotati, CA, Alto Books, 1985.
19. Ratanapridakul, K., et al.: Effect of finishing on the in vivo wear rate of a posterior composite resin. J Am Dent Assoc 118:333, 1989.
20. Lutz, F., et al.: New finishing instruments for composite resins. J Am Dent Assoc 107:575, 1983.
21. Erick, J. and Welch, F.: Dentin adhesives: do they protect the dentin from acid etching? Quint 17:533, 1986.
22. Vanharle, G., et al.: Overview of the Clinical Requirements for Post Composite Resin Restorative Materials. Netherlands, Peter Szulc Co., p. 35, 1985.
23. Jensen, M.E. and Chan, D.C.N.: Polymer shrinkage and microleakage. In Vanharle, G.: Overview of the Clinical Requirements for Post Composite Resin Restorative Materials. Netherlands, Peter Szulc Co., 1985.
24. Gross, J.D., et al.: Microleakage of post composite restorations. Dent Mat 1(1):7, 1985.
25. Lue, J.L., et al.: Margin quality and microleakage of Class II composite resin restorations. J Am Dent Assoc 14(1):49, 1987.
26. Koenigsberg, S., et al.: The effect of three filling techniques on marginal leakage around Class II composite resin restorations in vitro. Quint 20(2):117, 1989.
27. Boyer, D.B., et. al.: Buildup and repair of light cured composites: bond strength. J Dent Res 63(10):1241, 1984.
28. Boyer, D.B.: Buildup and repair of light cured composites: bond strength. Int Assoc Dent Res Abstr 949, 1984.
29. Eackle, W.S.: Effects of thermal cycling on fracture strengths of microleakage in teeth restored with bonded composite resin. Dent Mat 2:114, 1986.
30. Kemp-Scholte, C.M. and Davidson, C.L.: Marginal sealing of curing contraction gaps in Class V restorations. J Dent Res 67:841, 1988.
31. Torstenson, B., et al.: A new method for sealing composite resin contraction gaps in lined cavities. J Dent Res 64:450, 1985.
32. Leclaire, C.C., et al.: Use of a two stage composite resin fill to reduce microleakage below the cementoenamel junction. Op Dent 13:20, 1988.

Ross W. Nash, D.D.S.

COMPOSITE RESIN— INDIRECT TECHNIQUE RESTORATIONS

6

Indirect composite resin restorations can sometimes provide distinct advantages over direct composite resin restorations. Technology is continually evolving and a significant increase in the use of laboratory processed composite resin can be anticipated.

BASIC CONCEPTS

When a composite resin is cured, polymerization shrinkage takes place in the resin matrix. In the direct technique, such shrinkage can cause a marginal gap where the bond strength is the weakest, such as at the dentin-composite resin interface. When composite resin is cured in the laboratory by light, heat, or other methods, the shrinkage occurs before the restoration is bonded into place. Thus, only a thin layer of luting composite resin is subject to shrinkage at the tooth-restoration interface. This results in less marginal gap, thereby decreasing the likelihood of marginal leakage, sensitivity, recurrent decay, and staining. In addition, studies have shown that some laboratory techniques (such as techniques that use pressure or vacuum plus heat or light catalysts and those that use heat processing after or simultaneously with light) produce a greater degree of polymerization than that achieved with light alone.[1,2,3,4] Thus, the physical properties of tensile strength and hardness may be improved, providing for longer lasting and stronger restorations.[5]

Indirect techniques allow the dentist to incorporate the skills of the cosmetic dental laboratory technician. It is projected that this rapid increase in composite resin technology will provide materials that not only rival porcelain in beauty and physical properties, but that also solve the problems associated with this time proven material. Porcelain is harder than tooth structure and can cause it to wear during function. Composite resin will not cause accelerated wear of opposing natural tooth structure. After porcelain is bonded to place, it is difficult to return the surface to the original luster fol-

lowing an adjustment. Composite resin can be adjusted and repolished easily. Laboratory processed composite resin can be repaired with light-cured composite resin.

Compared to other techniques, indirect techniques may provide better control over interproximal contours and contacts and, although meticulous attention to detail is important, indirect composite resin procedures may be less technique-sensitive than direct ones.

BASIC CHEMISTRY

All composite resins are made up of filler particles in a resin matrix. The filler particles can range in size from .007 microns to over 100 microns. The filler particles provide the strength and the resin matrix binds them together and bonds them to the tooth structure. The filler can be very small silica particles, as in microfilled resins, or larger quartz or glass particles, as in small particle composite and hybrid resins. The resin matrix can be bis-GMA resin (introduced by Ray Bowen in 1962), urethane dimethacrylate, or similar polymers. Many combinations of resin and filler particles have been tried. Generally, the higher the filler content (expressed as a percentage of weight) the higher the strength; the lower the filler particle size, the higher the surface polishability.[6,7]

COMPOSITE RESIN SYSTEMS

Three types of composite resin materials are available for use in indirect techniques: microfilled resins, small particle composite resins and hybrid resins (Table 6–1). All show excellent wear resistance, but small particle composite resins and hybrid resins can be etched to produce micromechanical retention. They can also be silanated to increase the bond strength further. One manufacturer of a reinforced microfilled resin inlay/onlay system provides a special bonding agent to increase the bond strength of its material. None of the cur-

TABLE 6–1. INDIRECT COMPOSITE RESINS

NAME	MANUFACTURER	COMPOSITE RESIN CATEGORY	RESIN TYPE	CURING METHOD	TYPE OF FABRICATION	USE
Cesead	Kuraray Co., Ltd.	Hybrid	Bis-GMA	Light	Indirect	Jacket crowns Laminate veneers Veneers over metal substructure
Clearfil CR Inlay	Kuraray Co., Ltd.	Hybrid	Bis-GMA	Light and heat	Indirect	Inlays/onlays
Coltene Inlay/Onlay	Coltene AG	Hybrid	Bis-GMA	Light and heat	Indirect, direct/indirect	Inlays/onlays Laminate veneers
Concept (formerly Isosit)	Williams Dental Company, Inc.	Reinforced homogeneous microfill	Urethane dimethacrylate	Heat and pressure	Indirect	Inlays/onlays
Conquest crown and bridge	Jeneric/Pentron, Inc.	Hybrid	Polycarbonate dimethacrylate (PCDMA)	Light, heat and vacuum	Indirect	Inlays/onlays Laminate veneers Crowns and bridges Veneers over metal substructure
Dentacolor	Kulzer, Inc. USA	Microfilled	Urethane dimethacrylate	Light	Indirect	Inlays/onlays Laminate veneers
Extra Oral System (EOS)	Williams Dental Co., Inc.	Reinforced homogeneous microfilled	Urethane dimethacrylate	Light	Indirect	Inlays/onlays Laminate veneers
Herculite XRV Lab System	Kerr, Inc.	Hybrid	Bis-GMA	Light and heat	Indirect	Inlays/onlays Laminate veneers Provisional restorations
Isosit N	Williams Dental Company, Inc.	Heterogeneous microfilled	Urethane dimethacrylate	Heat and pressure	Indirect	On metal substructure of crowns and bridges
Kulzer Inlay	Kulzer, Inc. USA	Hybrid	Bis-GMA	Light	Indirect, direct/indirect	Inlays/onlays
Visio-Gem	ESPE-Premier Sales Corp.	Microfilled	Bis-GMA	Light and vacuum	Indirect	Inlays/onlays Laminate veneers Veneers over metal substructure

rent systems have proven to be vastly superior to the others and all produce good results when used properly.

Cesead (Kuraray Co., Ltd.)

Cesead is a light-cured hybrid composite resin, filled 82% by weight, which was designed for use as a crown and bridge resin to replace porcelain (Fig. 6–1). It can be used over metal copings and metal frameworks for crowns and bridges and for full composite resin jacketed crowns and laminate veneers. Cesead comes in the 16 shades corresponding to the Vita-Lumen shade guide. To produce the proper color, it is necessary to use opaque, cervical, dentin, enamel, and transparent shades, in that order. The system contains stains and opaque modifiers. It also contains opaque primer, which allows opaque resin to be strongly bonded to metal. In addition, the primer chemically cures the opaque resin, thus making it possible to promote the setting of the opaque resin even at the metal interface where it is difficult for the curing light to reach.

Light curing can be accomplished with laboratory light curing units such as the Alphalight (J. Morita USA, Inc.), the Dentacolor XS (Kulzer, Inc. USA), or a chairside visible light source, such as Quick Light or Lightel (Kuraray Co., Ltd.). Intraoral repairs can be accomplished with the Cesead composite resin.

Clearfil CR Inlay (Kuraray Co., Ltd.)

Clearfil CR Inlay is a hybrid composite resin that is filled 86.5% by weight (Fig. 6–2). Available in six shades, this light-cured composite resin has been formulated with extra body to make condensing and carving easier. Its heavier body allows for buildup and minimizes sag. The inlay is processed in the CRC-100 Curing Oven (Kuraray). Four available stains allow for final shade adaptation.

It is bonded to place with CR Inlay Cement, which is a dual-cured luting composite resin. Light irradiation for 40 seconds per surface sets the cement and stabilizes the inlay and additional chemical curing underneath the restoration assures a secure bond. It is recommended that vinyl polysiloxane impression material be used because of its low deformation. Additionally, extra-hard plaster stone is recommended for the model. Intraoral repairs can be accomplished with Clearfil Photoposterior light-cured composite resin (Kuraray, Inc. USA).

Coltene Inlay System (Coltene AG)

This system was first designed for direct/indirect application (Fig. 6–3). Separating medium is placed on a tooth prepared with divergent walls and without undercuts. A composite resin inlay is fabricated directly in the tooth, removed, and placed into a special oven which provides heat at 120° C and light for 7 minutes followed by cooling for 1 minute. The material recommended is Brilliant Dentin, a hybrid composite resin with shades corresponding to the Vita-Lumin guide.

The system has also been adapted for indirect use. An impression is made and a working model poured. A light-cured composite resin inlay, onlay, or labial veneer is fabricated on the model, heat treated, and bonded to the prepared tooth. The inlay may be fabricated in the office, thus avoiding the need for temporization, or the dentist may place a provisional restoration and have the patient return after the restoration is fabricated in the office or dental laboratory. Intraoral repairs can be accomplished with Brilliant light-cured hybrid composite resin.

Concept (Williams Dental Co., Inc.)

Concept (formerly Isosit) is a highly filled, reinforced, homogeneous microfilled resin that is heat- and pressure-cured and that produces a strong and wear resistant restoration (Fig. 6–4). It is coded to the Vita-Lumin shade guide with 7 body shades plus an incisal shade. Because it is a microfilled resin, it cannot be etched or silanated. However, a chemical agent called Special Bond is used for better wetting and penetration and, thus, increases the bond strength to rival that of composite resin to etched enamel. Special Bond should also be used when making chairside repairs with light-cured composite resin. (Heliomolar, a similar material, also is recommended.)

The system is totally indirect, requiring a final impression (preferably a vinyl polysiloxane because multiple models must be poured) and a provisional restoration.

Conquest Crown and Bridge
(Jeneric/Pentron, Inc.)

Conquest Crown and Bridge is an indirect micro-hybrid composite resin used to fabricate both all-composite resin and composite resin-cured-to-metal restorations. The material is indicated for all-composite resin short span anterior fixed bridges, full coverage crowns, inlays and onlays. The material can also be applied to any crown or fixed bridge metal substructure including titanium.

The Conquest system is available in 16 body shades, 4 incisal shades, 16 opaque shades, 2 gingival paste shades, 2 gingival powder shades (for metal coverage), an effect paste, a neck paste, and 16 opaceous dentin shades. The opaceous dentin shades retain their chroma in thin area applications such as laminate veneers and telescopic crowns.

The restorations are built up in incremental layers on a model of the prepared tooth or teeth. Each increment is individually light-cured. The entire restoration is then placed in a specially designed automated heat/vacuum chamber.

Intraoral repairs can be made with Conquest (Jeneric/Pentron) direct composite resin.

Dentacolor (Kulzer, Inc. USA)

Dentacolor is a light-cured microfilled resin crown and bridge material composed of bis-GMA resin base filled 50.5% by weight with a 0.04 microns filler particle of silicone dioxide (Fig. 6–5). Designed to be applied to metal frameworks of crowns and bridges, as well as for jackets, onlays, inlays, and laminate veneers with no metal substructure, it can also be used in partial denture fabrication. Forty-eight available shades are coded to the Vita-Lumin guide.

The Dentacolor oven cures the material with a light in the 320 to 520 nm range which generates heat at approximately 150° F, compared to intraoral light units, which cure in the 400 to 500 nm range with little or no heat. According to the manufacturer, this difference produces more polymerization than a direct intraoral composite resin restoration and results in a 20% harder and stronger restoration.

DENTACOLOR can be repaired intraorally with any visible light-cured bis-GMA composite resin.

EOS (Vivadent, Inc.)

EOS, Extra Oral System, is a complete chairside system for fabrication and cementation of light-cured compos-

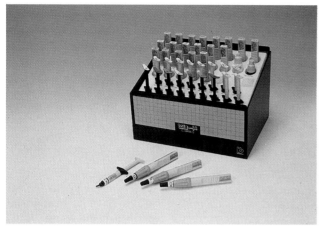

FIG. 6–1. Cesead light-cured hybrid composite resin (Kuraray Co.).

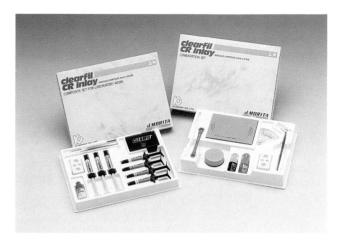

FIG. 6–2. Clearfil CR inlay hybrid composite resin (Kuraray Co.).

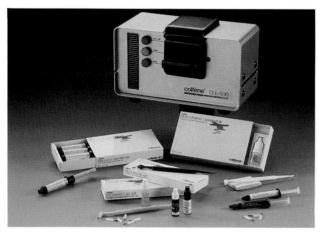

FIG. 6–3. Coltene inlay/onlay system (Coltene AG).

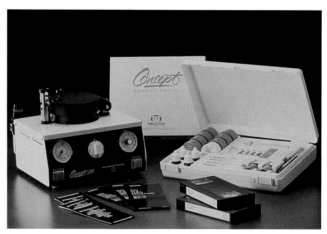

FIG. 6–4. Concept reinforced homogenous microfilled system (Williams Dental Company, Inc.).

ite resin inlays and laminate veneers in one appointment. EOS is recommended by the manufacturer as an alternative to conventional Class II amalgam and direct Class II resin restorations. The kit contains all of the materials necessary for making the impression of the preparation, and fabricating and cementing the final restoration.

The procedure involves making an impression of the prepared tooth with the Redphase-P (a fast setting silicone impression material) and injecting the Bluephase-P (a rigid setting, injectable vinyl-polysiloxane modeling material) into the impression to form a working model. EOS inlay material, a light-cured composite resin based on a variant of Heliomolar radiopaque (Vivadent), is placed into the model of the prepared tooth. It is then contoured and light-cured.

The finished restoration is cemented with Dual Cement (Vivadent), a light- and self-curing microfill resin cement. Heliomolar, Heliprogress, and Heliotints (all by Vivadent) can be used in the restoration for special esthetic effects. Intraoral repairs can be accomplished with these materials.

Herculite XRV Lab System (Kerr, Inc.)

The Herculite XRV Lab system was created to produce inlays, onlays, laminate veneers, and long-term provisional restorations using Herculite XRV, a highly filled, light-cured, micro-hybrid composite resin with an average glass filler particle size of 0.6 microns. Thirty two Vita shades (16 dentin opacity and 16 enamel opacity), 3 cervical shades, 2 incisal shades, 1 cuspal shade, and 11 color modifiers are provided.

The procedure involves fabrication of the restoration on a model poured from an impression of the prepared tooth. After the restoration is light-cured with a visible light curing unit, it is post-cured in boiling water for 10 minutes. A sophisticated curing unit is not needed because any curing light and boiling pot can be used.

Intraoral repairs can be accomplished with Herculite XRV (Kerr) micro-hybrid composite resin.

Kulzer Inlay (Kulzer, Inc. USA)

The Kulzer inlay system (Fig. 6–6) was designed to produce direct/indirect or totally indirect inlays and on-

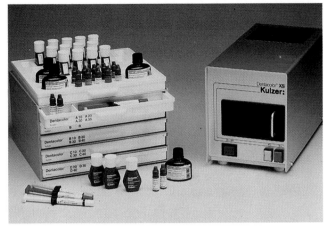

FIG. 6—5. Dentacolor light-cured microfill system (Kulzer, Inc.).

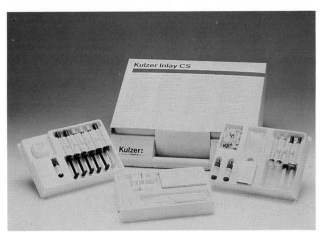

FIG. 6—6. Kulzer inlay system (Kulzer, Inc.). Either Estilux C VS or Charisma composite resin can be used.

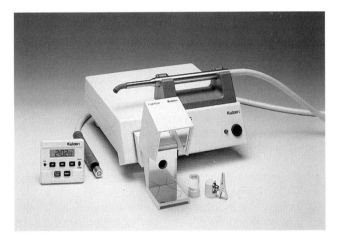

FIG. 6—7. Translux intraoral curing light (Kulzer, Inc.).

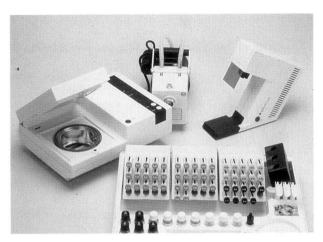

FIG. 6—8. Visio-Gem light- and vacuum-cured microfill composite resin (ESPE Premier Sales Corp.).

lays using Charisma, a hybrid composite resin with an ultra-fine radiopaque glass filler and highly dispersed silicone-dioxide micro-filler base. Because the material can be used for direct restorations, intraoral repairs also can be accomplished.

In the direct/indirect technique, Insulation Gel is applied to the entire prepared tooth with a small brush and evenly distributed with an air stream. The composite resin is placed incrementally. Each increment is light-cured for 20 seconds before adding the next layer. The restoration is then removed from the preparation and placed in a Dentacolor XS laboratory curing unit or a special light box attached to the Translux intraoral curing light (Fig. 6—7). These units subject the restoration to a highly efficient concentration of extraoral light polymerization which is reported to result in uniform hardening of the composite resin material and an increase in physical properties. The restoration is then bonded to place with a translucent, radiopaque, highly filled luting composite resin.

Indirect fabrication requires an accurate impression, a provisional restoration, the fabrication of a working model, and restoration fabrication and placement in the same manner as in the direct/indirect technique described above.

Visio-Gem (ESPE-Premier Sales Corp.)

Visio-Gem is a light- and vacuum-cured microfilled composite resin designed for laboratory fabrication over metal substructures for crown and bridge uses (Fig. 6—8). It is also recommended for indirect composite resin laminate veneers, inlays, onlays, and jacket crowns. It has been used to fabricate custom denture teeth and long-term provisional restorations. A large number of shades are available corresponding to the Vita-Lumin and Bioform shade guides.

Initial curing during buildup procedures is done with a direct visible light source, called the Visio Alpha unit. Final polymerization takes place in a light and vacuum chamber, called the Visio Beta unit. The vacuum allows complete curing of the oxygen-inhibited layer and results in greater color stability and increased physical properties.

ANTERIOR VENEERS

Indications

Indirect composite resin veneers are the treatment of choice in many situations:

1. **Abrasion considerations.** Many composite resins wear much like natural tooth structure and will not cause iatrogenic wear of the opposing dentition.
2. **Darkly stained teeth.** Indirect composite resin can cover dark color without opaquing agents, while remaining vital in appearance.
3. **Conservation of tooth structure.** Tooth preparation for composite resin laminate veneers can be more conservative than for porcelain alternatives because composite resin does not require 0.5 mm thickness as does porcelain. Composite resin can be much thinner in spots and still function well.
4. **Fabrication alternatives.** Indirect composite resin laminate veneers can be fabricated in the office or in the dental laboratory. They can be light-cured or processed. They can be made of microfilled, small particle, or hybrid composite resin. The glass in the small particle or hybrid composite resin can be etched with hydrofluoric acid providing micromechanical retention that rivals etched porcelain.
5. **Chairside repairs.** These restorations allow for repairs to be made at the chairside with light-cured composite resins.

The technique described below is for a light-cured hybrid composite resin that is heat-tempered, etched with 10% hydrofluoric acid gel, and treated with silane. The silane chemically bonds to the remaining glass particles and then to the luting composite resin, which is used to attach the veneer to the etched enamel surface of the tooth. (Note that techniques may vary between manufacturers.)

Armamentarium

- Mirror
- Explorer
- Metal "plastic" instrument
- No. 12 surgical blade
- Bard-Parker handle
- Anterior scaler
- Medium grit flame or chamfer diamond bur
- Vinyl polysiloxane impression material
- Alginate impression material
- Maxillary and mandibular full arch impression trays
- Die stone
- Hybrid composite resin
- Light-cured or dual-cured luting composite resin
- Toaster oven or Coltene oven
- 12- and 30-fluted carbide finishing burs
- Fine finishing diamond burs
- Rubber composite resin polishing cups
- Composite resin finishing discs
- Composite resin polishing paste
- 10% hydrofluoric gel
- 37% phosphoric acid gel
- Dentin/enamel bonding resin
- Silane coupling agent
- Intraoral light curing unit
- Oil-free pumice

Clinical Technique

1. Cleanse the tooth and neighboring teeth with pumice.
2. Select the desired shades of composite resin while the teeth are wet with saliva.
3. Determine the desired alignment of the teeth.
4. Prepare the eight maxillary anterior teeth by removing small amounts of enamel with a medium grit flame or chamfer diamond bur. If only minimum preparation is necessary to improve alignment and increased facial contour, remove only 0.25 to 0.50 mm of enamel from the facial area and none from the incisal area (Fig. 6–9). If incisal reduction is necessary, remove 1.0 to 1.5 mm (Fig. 6–10).

CLINICAL TIP. A definite chamfer margin is not necessary because composite resin veneers can be fabricated with feather-edged margins.

---

5. Make a full arch impression of the prepared teeth with a vinyl polysiloxane impression material. No retraction cord is needed because the margins are placed at the gingival crest.
6. Make a full arch alginate opposing impression.
7. Place a provisional restoration if needed. (See Chapter 11—Porcelain—Laminate Veneer and Other Partial Coverage Restorations).
8. Pour stone models of both the prepared and opposing arches. Veneers can be fabricated on the stone model by using a separating medium or on a flexible model as described below.
9. After the stone is fully set, soak the model of the prepared arch in water for 10 minutes and make an alginate impression of the model.

CLINICAL TIP. Soaking the stone in water prior to making the alginate impression prevents the alginate from adhering to the stone.

---

10. Inject a vinyl polysiloxane impression material (medium to heavy viscosity) into the alginate impression and form a flexible model (Fig. 6–11). This technique was first developed by Dr. K. Michael Rhyne for use in indirect composite resin inlay fabrication.

CLINICAL TIP. A flexible working model does not require a separating medium nor is it susceptible to breakage. In addition, the chance of chipping the restoration upon removal from the working model is slight.

---

11. On the flexible model, fabricate composite resin veneers using a technique similar to that described for direct intraoral application (Fig. 6–12).
12. Remove the veneers from the flexible model.
13. Contour and polish the veneers using 12- and 30-fluted finishing carbide burs in a high-speed hand-

CLINICAL TIP. To achieve a vital and natural appearance, apply layers of dentin, enamel, and incisal shades and cure each layer for 40 seconds (Fig. 6–13).

CLINICAL TIP. Fabricating every other veneer to completion before fabricating the adjacent veneer allows for good interproximal contours and contacts.

piece or porcelain contouring and polishing wheels on a lathe.

14. Place the veneers on the original stone model to check the fit and margins and adjust further if needed (Fig. 6–14).
15. Heat treat the veneers in a toaster oven at 260° F or in a Coltene unit for 10 minutes.
16. Acid etch the lingual side of the veneers with 10% hydrofluoric acid gel for 30 seconds (Fig. 6–15) and rinse thoroughly.

CLINICAL TIP. Handle hydrofluoric acid carefully because it is very caustic.

17. Evaluate the internal surfaces of the veneers to make sure an etched surface is achieved (Fig. 6–16).

CLINICAL TIP. At the delivery appointment use cheek and lip retractors to isolate the teeth. With this technique, no cotton rolls or rubber dam is needed.

18. Cleanse the teeth with No. 4 fine pumice in a prophylaxis cup, rinse, and dry with water-free and oil-free air.
19. Use 37% phosphoric acid gel to etch the enamel of the first central incisor for 15 seconds (Fig. 6–17).
20. Rinse for 30 seconds.
21. Dry with oil-free and water-free air.
22. Paint a very thin layer of dentin/enamel bonding resin onto the etched surface (Fig. 6–18).
23. Using a brush, apply silane coupling agent to the internal surface of the veneers and air dry.
24. Paint a thin layer of bonding resin onto the same surface.
25. Apply a luting composite resin to the internal surface of the veneer.
26. Place the veneer on the prepared tooth and remove excess luting composite resin using a brush dipped in bonding agent (Fig. 6–19).
27. Light-cure for 40 seconds on the facial and lingual surfaces of the tooth (Fig. 6–20).
28. Remove excess cured luting composite resin with a No. 12 surgical blade or a scaler (Fig. 6–21).
29. Place the other seven veneers in the same fashion.
30. Finish the margins with 12- and 30-fluted carbide finishing burs, fine diamonds, rubber polishing cups, finishing discs, or other composite resin finishing techniques (Figs. 6–22 to 6–24).

POSTERIOR INLAYS AND ONLAYS

Indications

Composite resin inlays and onlays are the treatment of choice in many situations.

1. **Esthetic considerations.** A bonded restoration can provide esthetics and function of high quality and may be a long lasting alternative to full coverage or the porcelain counterparts.
2. **Structural considerations.** A bonded restoration returns nearly all the original strength to the tooth and acts to hold the remaining tooth structure together.[8] An amalgam restoration that only fills a space does not strengthen the tooth but actually forms a wedge that can eventually cause fracturing of the tooth.
3. **Abrasion considerations.** Because it has been shown that some composite resins wear at about the same rate as natural tooth structure, they could prove to be the material of choice for restorative purposes. Long-term clinical data is not currently available so caution and clinical judgement should be exercised at the present time.
4. **Conservation of tooth structure.** Onlay preparations have the advantages of requiring the removal of less tooth structure than for a full crown.
5. **Supragingival margins.** Onlay preparations have supragingival margins and, therefore, infringe less on the periodontal apparatus than restorations with subgingival margins.
6. **Chairside repairs.** These restorations allow for repairs to be made at the chairside with light-cured composite resins.

With the advent of strong bonding agents and appropriate tooth-colored restorative materials, indirect composite resins can provide long lasting alternatives to full crowns or conventional cast onlays.

Direct/Indirect Technique—Fabrication

Armamentarium. The armamentarium is the same as that listed for anterior composite resin laminate veneer.

Clinical Technique

1. The preparation is similar to a gold inlay/onlay preparation, however, the divergent walls must have rounded angles and no sharp corners (Fig. 6–25).

CLINICAL TIP. No retentive grooves or parallel walls are needed because the restoration will be bonded to place (Fig. 6–26).

2. Provide at least 1.5 mm of clearance over reduced cusps or in the isthmus areas.
3. No bevels are needed and slightly tapering or butt joint margins are best.
4. Areas prepared closer than 0.5 mm to the pulp should be lined with calcium hydroxide and undercuts should be filled with glass ionomer cement, or another appropriate liner or base.

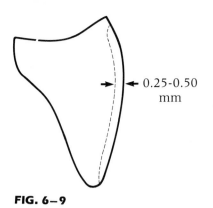

FIG. 6–9

0.25-0.50 mm

0.25-0.50 mm

1.0-1.5 mm

FIG. 6–10

FIG. 6–9. Anterior preparation without incisal reduction.

FIG. 6–10. Anterior preparation with incisal reduction.

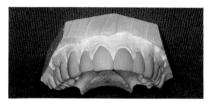

FIG. 6–11. Inject vinyl polysiloxane into an alginate impression of a stone model of prepared teeth.

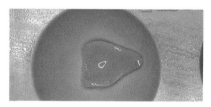

FIG. 6–12. Apply composite resin to the flexible model.

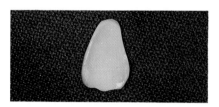

FIG. 6–13. Light-cure the composite resin veneer.

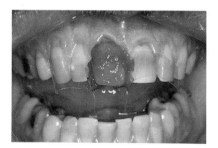

FIG. 6–14. Eight indirect composite resin veneers on a stone model.

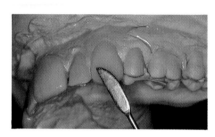

FIG. 6–15. Apply 10% hydrofluoric acid gel for 30 seconds.

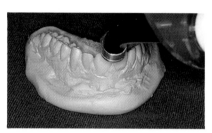

FIG. 6–16. The etched internal surface of the hybrid composite resin veneer.

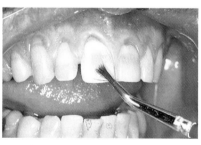

FIG. 6–17. Etch the enamel surface.

FIG. 6–18. Apply bonding resin to the etched enamel.

FIG. 6–19. Remove excess luting composite resin with a brush dipped in bonding agent.

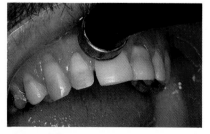

FIG 6–20.

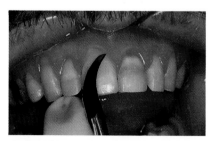

FIG 6–21.

FIG. 6–20. Light-cure the luting composite resin.

FIG. 6–21. Remove excess cured luting composite resin with a No. 12 surgical blade.

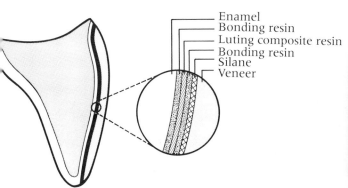

Enamel
Bonding resin
Luting composite resin
Bonding resin
Silane
Veneer

FIG. 6–22. The final anterior restoration with various layers displayed.

CLINICAL TIP. Do not use solutions containing eugenol because eugenol can interfere with the chemistry of the resins.

---

5. Apply a separating medium or glycerine to the entire tooth.
6. Place a light-cured hybrid composite resin directly into the prepared tooth using normal direct placement technique.
7. Remove the restoration from the tooth using a large spoon or other instrument.

CLINICAL TIP. Undercuts in the preparation make removal impossible, therefore carefully inspect the preparation before placing composite resin. Block out or remove undercuts.

---

8. Heat treat the inlay or onlay.
9. Place the inlay or onlay according to the placement technique described below.

Indirect Technique—Flexible Model Fabrication

A totally indirect technique that can be performed in one appointment and does not require a provisional restoration can be accomplished using a flexible model technique.

Armamentarium. The armamentarium is the same as that listed for anterior composite resin laminate veneer.

Clinical Technique

1. The first four steps are identical to those listed in the preceding section on direct/indirect technique.
2. Make an irreversible hydrocolloid impression that captures all of the margins of the preparation.
3. Inject a firm setting vinyl polysiloxane impression material into the alginate impression to form a flexible model (Fig. 6–27).
4. Fabricate a composite resin inlay using light-cured hybrid composite resin (Fig. 6–28).
5. Heat treat the restoration.
6. Place the inlay or onlay according to the placement technique described below. (Fig. 6–29).

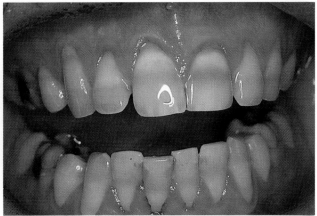

FIG. 6–23. Preoperative view of tetracycline stained teeth.

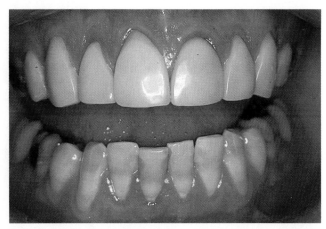

FIG. 6–24. Postoperative view of eight indirect composite resin veneers.

Placement Technique

The preparation and placement of inlays or onlays are identical regardless of whether they are fabricated in the office or at the dental laboratory using the commercial processes listed earlier.

Armamentarium. The armamentarium is the same as that listed for anterior composite resin laminate veneer.

Clinical Technique

1. Remove the provisional restorations (Fig. 6–30).
2. Place the restorations on a clean, dry surface (Fig. 6–31).
3. Place a rubber dam.
4. Thoroughly cleanse the prepared tooth with pumice.
5. Etch the enamel margins with 37% phosphoric acid gel for 15 seconds (Fig. 6–32), rinse for no more than 20 seconds, and dry with oil-free air.
6. Apply dentin primer to the dentin surface (Fig. 6–33).
7. Apply bonding resin to the dentin and enamel surfaces and the internal surface of the onlay (Fig. 6–34).

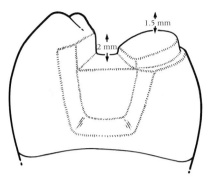

FIG. 6–25. Posterior onlay preparation. Note the rounded line angles designed to reduce internal stress.

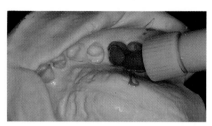

FIG. 6–26. Tooth prepared for indirect composite resin veneer.

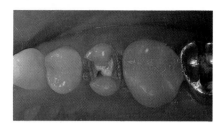

FIG. 6–27. Vinyl polysiloxane injected into an alginate impression.

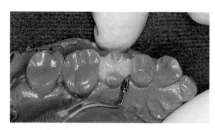

FIG. 6–28. Fabrication of the composite resin inlay.

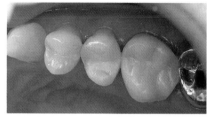

FIG. 6–29. The composite resin inlay bonded into place.

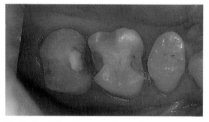

FIG. 6–30. Prepared teeth.

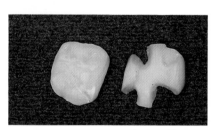

FIG. 6–31. Internal surfaces of laboratory-fabricated composite resin onlays.

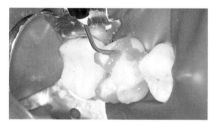

FIG. 6–32. Etch the enamel margins with 37% phosphoric acid gel.

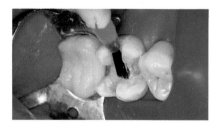

FIG. 6–33. Apply dentin primer.

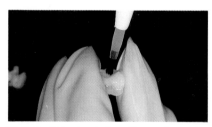

FIG. 6–34. Apply bonding resin to the internal surface of the onlay.

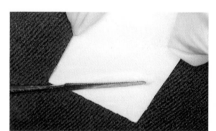

FIG. 6–35. Mix the dual cure luting composite resin.

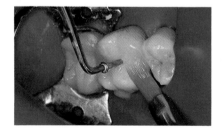

FIG. 6–36.

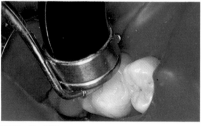

FIG. 6–37.

FIG. 6–36. Remove the excess luting composite resin with a brush dipped in bonding agent.

FIG. 6–37. Light-cure the luting composite resin with a visible light source.

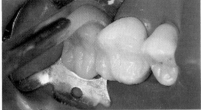
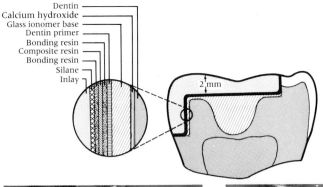

Dentin
Calcium hydroxide
Glass ionomer base
Dentin primer
Bonding resin
Composite resin
Bonding resin
Silane
Inlay

2 mm

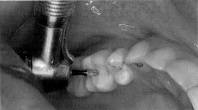

FIG. 6–38. The final posterior restoration with various layers displayed. Note the glass ionomer base is utilized to restore the preparation to the "ideal" depth.

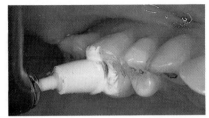

FIG. 6–39. Remove the excess cured luting composite resin with a No. 12 surgical blade.

FIG. 6–40. Adjust the occlusion with a carbide finishing bur.

FIG. 6–41. Polish the composite resin onlays with composite resin polishing paste.

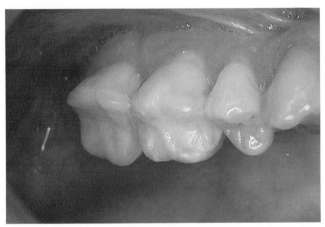

FIG. 6–42. The completed onlays.

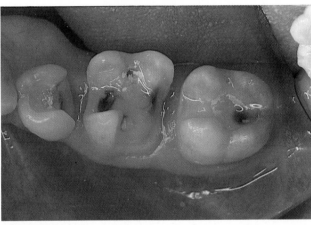

FIG. 6–43. Preparations of the mandibular arch for two inlays and one onlay.

8. Mix a dual-cured luting composite resin and apply it to the inner surface of the restoration and to the internal surface of the prepared tooth (Fig. 6–35).

9. Place the restoration and remove excess luting composite resin with a brush dipped in bonding agent (Fig. 6–36).

10. While the onlay is held in place with an instrument, run dental floss through the proximal areas, pulling in the facial or lingual direction to remove excess resin.

11. Cure the restoration for 40 seconds on the occlusal, facial, and lingual surfaces (Figs. 6–37, 6–38).

12. Excess cured luting composite resin can be removed with a surgical blade (Fig. 6–39), a scaler, or carbide finishing burs.

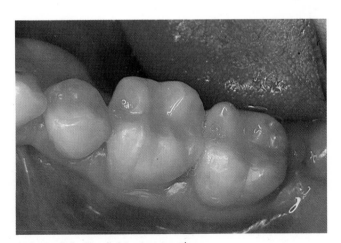

FIG. 6–44. The finished restorations.

CLINICAL TIP. The dual-cured luting composite resin will continue to cure, but finishing can begin 4 minutes after light curing.

13. Adjust the occlusion with carbide finishing burs (Fig. 6–40).
14. Polish the finished and adjusted surfaces with normal composite resin polishing techniques, including final polishing paste (Figs. 6–41 to 6–44).

THE FUTURE

The future of composite resins in dentistry is promising. Composite resin technology is progressing at a rapid rate. Composite resins that rival porcelain in every way are anticipated within the next 5 years. There will be systems available for in-office use and for laboratory use. Both esthetic and functional requirements will be met. The need for metal support will be eliminated. Bonding agents will allow strong and long-lasting adhesion to tooth structure.

REFERENCES

1. Wendt, S.L.: Time as a factor in the heat curing of composite resins. Quintessence Int 20:259, 1989.
2. Watts, D.C.: The Coltene direct inlay system. A report on the properties of the inlay composite material resulting from different curing conditions. Coltene Seminar, Sept. 1–13, 1988.
3. Duke, E.S. and Norling, B.K.: Vacuum curing of light activated composite veneering resin. USAF Medical Center and Univ of Texas HSC, San Antonio, TX.
4. Lappalainen, R.: Wear of dental restorative and prosthetic materials in vitro. Dent Mat Jan., 1989.
5. Wendt S.F.: The effect of heat used as a secondary cure upon the physical properties of three composite resins, I. Quintessence Int 18:351, 1987.
6. Ibsen R.L., Nevill K.: Adhesive Restorative Dentistry. Philadelphia, W.B. Saunders, 1974.
7. Albers, H.F.: Tooth Colored Restoratives, 7th Ed. Cotati, CA, Alto Books.
8. Simonsen R., Barouch E., Gelb M.: Cusp fracture resistance from composite resin in Class II restorations. J Dent Res 62:761, 1983.

BIBLIOGRAPHY

1. Berge, M.: Properties of prosthetic resin-veneer materials processed in commercial laboratories. Dent Mat 5:77, 1989.
2. Dimberio R.D.: A new crown and bridge veneering material. Quintessence Dent Tech 4:27, 1979.
3. Michl, R.J.: Isosit—a new dental material. Quintessence Int 9:1, 1978.
4. James, D.F.: An esthetic inlay technique for posterior teeth. Quintessence 14:725, 1983.
5. Lappalainen, R., Yll-Urpo, A., and Seppa L.: Wear of dental restorative and prosthetic materials in vitro. Dent Mat 5:35, 1989.
6. Christensen, G.J.: Tooth-colored inlays and onlays. J Am Dent Assoc 9:12E, 1988.
7. Kanca, J.: The single visit heat processed indirect composite resin inlay. J Esthet Dent 1:13, 1988.
8. Jones, R.M. and Moore, B.K.: A comparison of the physical properties of four prosthetic veneering materials. Prosthet Dent 61:38, 1989.
9. Gallegos, L.I. and Nicholls, J.I.: In vitro two-body wear of three veneering resins. Quintessence Int 20:259, 1989.
10. Miller, M., et al.: Indirect resin systems. Reality 4:52, 1989.
11. Gross, J. and Malacmacher L.: Posterior Composite Resins—the technique. Dentique 1:1, 1985.
12. Bonner, P. and Kanca, J.: Dentist reveals methods for fabricating the direct resin inlay. Cosmet Dent Gen Pract 5:1, 1989.
13. Nash, R. and Oaten R.: Indirect techniques for composites. Lab Man Today 4:35, 1988.
14. Nash, R.: Hybrid composites: excellent for veneers. Lab Man Today 4:34, 1988.
15. Nash R.: Restorative options for good aesthetics. Dent Today 3:1, 1987.
16. First Int Symp on the clinical applications of laboratory light cured composites. Valley Forge, PA, Dec. 13, 1984.

Peter R. Hunt B.D.S., M.Sc.,
L.D.S.R.C.S.Eng

GLASS IONOMER CEMENTS

7

Glass ionomer (polyalkenoic) cements have rapidly become one of the most useful materials in dentistry. Although relatively new, they are displacing many older materials and are challenging the methods that restorative dentistry has practiced for generations.[1,2] In many of the newer cosmetic techniques, the incorporation of glass ionomers may mean the difference between success and failure.

Glass ionomers have reached this high degree of acceptance for several important reasons. They release fluoride, which tends to prevent secondary decay.[3,4] They are mildly adhesive to tooth structure, and are particularly reliable when placed against dentin and cementum.[5,6] In general, they are well tolerated by the pulpal tissues.[7,8] If a veneer or overlay material covering a glass ionomer base mechanically breaks, it can be replaced without changing the base or extending the cavity because recurrent decay is extremely rare under a glass ionomer cement. With experience, glass ionomer cements are simple to use and less technique-sensitive than most other dental materials.[1,2]

Unfortunately, the rapid acceptance of glass ionomer cements has led to abuse of these materials and resulting restoration failure. It is easy to identify the clinical situations in which failure can be anticipated. These are usually when the materials are not strong enough to resist the demands placed upon them, when unrealistic esthetic expectations have been made, or when the chemistry of the setting material has been abused.

Some simple rules of handling and usage must be followed carefully for success. Most of these relate to the basic chemistry of the materials and the potential of the operator to interfere with the development of maximal strength and esthetics.

THE CHEMISTRY OF GLASS IONOMERS

The glass ionomer cements are formed by the reaction of three materials, a fluoroaluminosilicate glass powder, an ionic polymer polyacrylic acid, and water.[9,10,11] An acid-base reaction occurs between the glass powder and the ionic polymer. Water is essential because that is the medium through which ion transfer occurs. This is in sharp distinction to resin-based materials, which generally are insoluble in water and unable to tolerate any moisture contamination.

In some cements, the polyacrylic acid is a dry powder, which is reconstituted with water in the first stage of mixing.[12] These materials have a longer shelf life than those with preformulated polyacrylic acid, however, some feel that they cause more pulpal sensitivity.[13,14] The action of the acid on the glass causes the release of calcium, fluoride, and aluminum ions. In turn, these positively charged ions react with the negatively charged polycarboxylate ions to form a cross-linked network within which the remnants of the unreacted glass particles are secured. The reaction byproducts of calcium and fluoride are critical. The calcium of the tooth structure is incorporated into the reaction, which creates some adhesion.[15,16] The excess fluoride ion is absorbed by the tooth structure, thus aiding caries immunity.[17,4]

Third generation resin impregnated materials have an additional light curing mechanism, although this might be more correctly considered to be a light stabilization mechanism. Achieved by incorporating a light sensitive element, hydroxyethylmethacrylate (HEMA), a photoinitiator and a polyacrylic acid with some pendant methacryoxy groups, the light activation mechanism

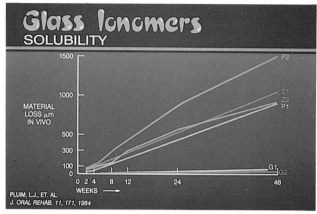

FIG. 7–1. Solubility of glass ionomers. Glass ionomers are considerably less soluble than other luting cements used in dentistry. (P = polycarboxalate cement, Z = zinc phosphate cement, G = glass ionomer cement.) (From Pluim LJ, et al.: Quantitative Cement Solubility Experiment In Vivo. J Oral Rehab 11:171, 1984.)

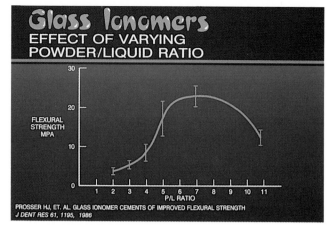

FIG. 7–2. Effect of varying powder-to-liquid ratio. The common tendency is to mix glass ionomer cements too thinly. This leads to increased solubility, decreased strength, and a slower setting time. (From Posser HJ, et al.: Glass ionomer cements of improved flexural strength. J Dent Res 61:1195, 1986.)

serves to stabilize the glass ionomer material while the conventional reaction occurs.[10] In most light-stabilized materials the percentage of light curing resin is small so that shrinkage is not significantly greater than with the conventional material. This is a true dual cure mechanism. In general, mechanical properties are enhanced while the operating procedure is facilitated. Light-cured glass ionomers are harder and stronger and bond more securely to tooth structure than conventional materials. They are also more acid-resistant and less water-soluble (Fig. 7–1). Esthetics have been greatly improved and the resin component facilitates bonding to composite resin. In addition, they are radiopaque. However, these materials are new to the market and experience with them is limited.

CLINICAL IMPLICATIONS IN THE CHEMICAL REACTION
Powder-To-Liquid Ratio

It is essential to incorporate as much powder into the mix as possible, within the guidelines of the manufacturer's recommendations (Fig. 7–2). Too little powder results in dramatically diminished strength, slower setting time, and increased susceptibility to dissolution.[18,19]

CLINICAL TIP. A high powder-to-liquid ratio increases the favorable characteristics of glass ionomer cements.

Mixing Time

The powder should be mixed into the liquid in less than 45 seconds. Otherwise, the material will thicken because of the setting reaction regardless of the powder-to-liquid ratio. The setting time with some modern materials is so rapid that the operator may not have enough working time.[20]

CLINICAL TIP. To increase the working time, mix the glass ionomer cement on a cool slab.

Working Time

The cement will become rubbery when the surface "sheen" disappears. At this stage the material will not adapt to tooth structure.

CLINICAL TIP. Material manipulation and placement must be completed before the surface "sheen" is lost.

Setting Time

When they were first introduced in the 1960s, glass ionomers were slow setting.[21] Modern materials set much faster. However, this is sometimes at the expense of esthetics because the faster setting materials tend to be more opaque.

CLINICAL TIP. Carving should begin after the "rubbery" stage has passed, when a sharp instrument removes shavings, rather than clumps, of material.

Moisture Sensitivity

After material placement, it is crucial to protect the cements from moisture contamination.[22,23,24] Early contamination causes the cement to dissolve and wash out of the cavity. Later contamination causes a milky bloom of the contaminated surface layers. Both problems can be prevented by isolating the setting material from the oral environment.

After the basic reaction has occurred and the surface is hard, but not hard enough to be carved, it is crucial to prevent moisture loss from the maturing restoration. Moisture loss creates surface microcracks, resulting in opacity.[25] This is particularly damaging when thin layers of cement are present as the microcracks spread through the entire body of the restoration. The final result is poor esthetics, increased susceptibility to leakage, rapid staining, and a severely weakened restoration. Moisture contamination can be prevented by coating the surface of the restoration with a moistureproof barrier.[26,27] Varnishes are frequently used, although research indicates that light curing composite bonding resins are much more effective.[28,29]

CLINICAL TIP. The ionomer surface should be coated as soon as the "sheen" disappears from the mix and the restoration begins to harden. When bonding resins are used, it is not necessary to light-cure the first application to prevent moisture contamination.[2] After carving and finishing the glass ionomer, apply and cure a second coat of resin to give maximal protection.

Finishing

One of the great benefits of glass ionomers over composite resins is that glass ionomer restorations can be carved without the use of rotary instruments. Sharp instruments should be used to carve from the restoration toward the tooth structure in order to place minimal stress on newly developed bonds to tooth structure.[30,31]

Contouring with a rotary instrument under a water spray is acceptable for gross shaping, although the water spray tends to dissolve out some of the matrix, leaving rough particles exposed.[32] Adequate finishing can be obtained by smoothing over the surface with a slowly rotating rubber prophylaxis cup lubricated with petroleum jelly. The shaping and finishing process should be completed rapidly in order to minimize moisture loss from the restoration surface. The surface should then be protected with the light-cured unfilled resin.

CLINICAL TIP. Restorations must not be allowed to desiccate while being finished. Either carve or finish the restoration as quickly as possible or allow it to mature fully before finishing at another appointment.

Fluoride Release

Although rates of fluoride release from the various materials are uncertain, some concepts are obvious. Fluoride is released in the initial setting reaction, creating a "reservoir" of excess fluoride that slowly leaches from the completed restoration.[33,34,35] This fluoride is absorbed by the immediately adjacent tooth structure, creating a fluorapatite complex.[17] More is absorbed by the enamel than by the dentin or cemental surfaces.

A glass ionomer restoration confers immunity against recurrent carious attack, not only in the immediate vicinity but also at a distance from the site of the restoration.[4] Those materials with additives have less fluoride available. Most of the fluoride is available immediately following the initial chemical reaction, rather than later as a slow release; however, fluoride release and caries immunity are long-term phenomena. The larger the restoration, the more fluoride available.

Some resin-based lining materials that release fluoride have recently appeared on the dental market. These have no high initial burst of fluoride release because the fluoride is not part of the chemical reaction. They are used in very thin layers, and consequently have little fluoride reserve. They also have little ability to bond to the tooth structure and are easily lost when the tooth surface is only the slightest bit contaminated with moisture, such as dentinal fluid.

Bonding To Tooth Structure

Glass ionomers develop a bond to tooth structure by chelation; the setting material is unable to differentiate the calcium of the tooth structure from that released from the silicate glass.[5] Accordingly, the bond to enamel, which has a higher calcium content than to dentin, is stronger. The dentin bond, however is more clinically reliable than that of the composite resin-based dentin bonding agents, particularly on vital dentin, which is likely to be slightly moist from the exudate of dentin fluid. The setting glass ionomer material is able to absorb small amounts of this moisture within the mix.

In order to develop an optimal bond, the surface of the tooth structure should be free of caries. In the case of erosions, the surface should be cleaned with an oil-free pumice or abraded with a fine diamond rotary instrument. A ten second application of 10 to 25% polyacrylic acid will remove the smear layer but still retain the dentinal plugs.[36–38] A smooth, clean, relatively moisture free surface will result. The polyacrylic acid further serves to chemically "prime" the surface. Once conditioned in this way, it is critical to keep the surface free of contamination from saliva or blood.

The strength of the bond is about one-third that of composite resin to enamel.[36] The limitations of bond strength are really limitations of the inherent strength of the material. Bond failures occur almost invariably within the body of the glass ionomer cement. Studies have shown that glass ionomer cements have excellent long-term retention.[6,39,40]

Lamination With Other Restorative Materials

Glass ionomers can readily be bonded to many other restorative materials, particularly composite resins.[41] Linkage to composite resins can be achieved by two means, physical or chemical. Physical linkage can be obtained by acid etching the set surface of the glass ionomer with the phosphoric acid used for bonding composite resins to enamel.[44] The ionomer surface should be treated for no more than 20 seconds or the matrix of the glass ionomer will be disrupted.

The chemical method is less well understood. Because some particular bonding agents seem to bond only with some specific glass ionomers, the manufacturer's guidelines should be followed. The light stabilized glass ionomer systems contain some composite resin to which externally applied composite resin materials can bond.

With both methods, the strength of the laminated structure is limited by the strength of the glass ionomer.[45,46] Failure invariably appears within the glass ionomer layer.

CLINICAL TIP. *Always design a glass ionomer base so that composite resin overlays are retained by an acid-etch bond to enamel.*

Strength

Glass ionomers are relatively weak and brittle.[45,46] Even the strongest materials are much weaker than composite resins and amalgam materials (Fig. 7–3).[47,48] However, because they are so simple to use, glass ionomers have been used to rebuild marginal ridges in Class II restorations and to construct cores when rebuilding teeth. This frequently results in failure. These materials are most successful when they are used in relatively stress-free environments.

CLINICAL TIP. *The strength of glass ionomer materials is often overestimated. Restorations should be designed so that loads on the glass ionomer are compressive rather than shear.*

Pulpal Compatibility

When originally developed, it was anticipated that glass ionomers would be well tolerated when placed in deep cavities.[7] The minimal shrinkage of the setting glass ionomer, when combined with the glass ionomer bond to the tooth structure, would theoretically lead to a good seal. The chemistry of the materials was such that little or no toxicity to the pulp would be expected. In

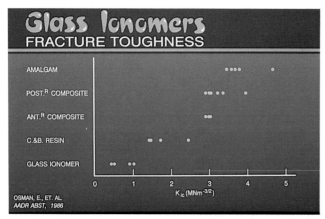

FIG. 7–3. *Fracture strength. Glass ionomers are weaker than most other restorative materials. This should be taken into account in restoration design. (From Osman E, et al.: Fracture Toughness of Several Categories of Restorative Materials. J Dent Res 65:220, 1986.)*

addition, glass ionomers have a coefficient of thermal expansion closer to that of tooth structure than any other restorative material. However, some marginal microleakage may occur with these materials.[49–51] This can be caused by various factors. The cavity floor may be contaminated, the smear layer may not be fully removed, or the flow of dentin fluid may create voids. In addition, the dentin may not be fully wetted by the restorative material and marginal finishing, acid etching, or lamination procedures may disturb the seal.

The cautious clinician should take a series of steps to minimize microleakage, particularly in deeper cavities. These include:

1. Careful eradication of all decay.
2. Cavity conditioning with an antibacterial agent (e.g., Tubulicid, Global Dental Products Co.).
3. The use of a calcium hydroxide base subliner in the portion of the cavity where the preparation is less than 1 mm from the pulp.
4. Careful injection of the glass ionomer to ensure that the whole cavity is wetted completely.
5. Allowing the material to set completely.
6. Minimizing traumatic finishing and lamination procedures.
7. Rebonding the set restoration with a composite resin bonding agent.

When these procedures are followed, glass ionomer restorations seem to be as biocompatible as any other restorative system.

Glass Ionomer Sensitivity Reactions

Particular concern exists about using glass ionomer materials for luting cements because of a curious long-term mild sensitivity reaction developed by some patients following crown cementation.[52] This sensitivity is seen mostly when the glass ionomer is used as a luting agent rather than as a base material. Generally, this problem has decreased as more operators have gained experience in the use of glass ionomer cements.[53] In particular, many operators failed to mix the cements quickly enough and did not achieve a high enough powder-to-liquid ratio. In addition, the modern cements are faster setting than earlier versions, which makes marginal washout less common. Faster set also aids in ensuring freedom from moisture contamination until the cement has set. Nevertheless, it is advisable to avoid use of glass ionomer cements on teeth that are particularly sensitive. Alternatively, the teeth should be desensitized before cementation by coating the preparation with cavity varnish. By taking these simple precautions, the incidence of reactions is minimal.

USE ORIENTED CLASSIFICATION OF GLASS IONOMERS

Although all glass ionomers have essentially the same chemistry, different forms have been developed for different situations. Accordingly, a helpful classification system for the glass ionomer materials is one based on clinical use.

Type I Materials—Luting Cements

These fine ground materials develop a film thickness of less than 25 microns, which is comparable to any alternative cementing media. Clinicians should select a material with a rapid setting time and with radiopacity. Some reports suggest that polyacrylic acid-based cements may be less sensitizing than water-based materials.[13,14]

Type II Materials—Esthetic Restorative Materials

Most of these materials are radiolucent, but radiopaque varieties are now available.[10] The use of radiopaque glasses can marginally enhance strength and speed of set, but the resultant mixture tends to have a greater visual opacity. Setting times of the new forms have declined so that the time required for placement of a glass ionomer restoration is similar to that required for a composite resin restoration.[21]

When used correctly, these materials can provide an esthetically acceptable restoration, providing care is taken in case selection. With all of the materials, there is a tendency for a somewhat opaque appearance, so their suitable use is for restorations of root surfaces.[26] The polishability and translucency of composite resin restorations is such that they are preferable when maximum simulation of enamel surfaces is required. Composite resin materials are stronger when used in high stress-bearing situations.

Type III Materials—Base and Liner Materials

Originally developed as an esthetic restorative material, glass ionomer cements are extremely useful as bases and liners (Fig. 7−4). Radiopacity is achieved with the incorporation of various metallic oxides, such as zinc oxide, or by the use of radiopaque glasses. Although zinc oxide weakens the material, it may enhance pulpal compatibility.[10]

Type III materials are the most confusing area of glass ionomer technology because so many different products are available. Careful product evaluation is required because performance varies greatly between different products.

Most conveniently, the products can be differentiated into three groups. First are relatively weak materials that have optimal pulpal compatibility because of their low acidity and high zinc oxide content. These can be used in deeper portions of a cavity, however they do not negate the need for calcium hydroxide liners. The second group consists of the stronger materials that can be used as bases to restore a substantial portion of the lost tooth substance. These are usually mixed thickly and have few additives. These materials are made stronger by mixing with stronger acids, which may reduce pulpal compatibility. Although new on the market, the third group, the light-stabilized Type III materials, have advantages over the conventional set materials. They appear stronger and are more readily placed in thin layers and are easy to "drape" over exposed dentin.

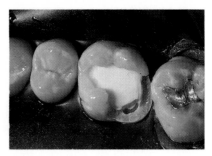

FIG. 7−4. Glass ionomers are useful as bases under most materials. This shows the base design for use under amalgam. Additional retention for the amalgam is provided by a dentin groove.

Type IV Materials—Admixtures

These materials have metallic admixtures, such as silver or amalgam filings. One process sinters the glass component of the glass ionomer to a metallic element, such as gold or silver. This is a patented process used by one company.[54] As with any process using additives, the amount of glass in the final mixture is reduced, and therefore the beneficial side effects, such as amount of fluoride released, are also reduced. However, this process greatly enhances wear resistance, probably because the metallic component is subject to some burnishing action.[56]

Another more simple process incorporates amalgam filings into the mixture of a regular glass ionomer.[57,58] Although this is another method of increasing radiopacity, it is also useful in allowing adjustment of the consistency of the final mixture. This method does not improve wear resistance, nor does it significantly alter the strength of the material. These materials have been used for cores and buildups, but as with all glass ionomer cements practitioners tend to overestimate the strength of the final restoration.[59] Glass ionomers are much weaker than the more conventional materials used for restorations and cores, and thus are contraindicated in stress bearing areas.[48] (Fig. 7−3).

CLINICAL APPLICATIONS

Final Restoration—Small, Nonstress Bearing Class III and Class V Restorations

Conventional materials, such as amalgam or composite resins, have severe drawbacks when used to restore Class III and Class V lesions (Fig. 7−5). Both situations can be visible, making amalgam increasingly unacceptable. Preparing a retentive cavity for a Class V restoration becomes increasingly unnecessary when bonding is adequate to secure the restoration (Fig. 7−6). The retention of modern third-generation dentin bonding agents, however, is generally inferior to glass ionomer restorations.[6] The composite resin restoration also tends to be more sensitizing and more prone to recurrent caries than the glass ionomer restoration. A final advantage to glass ionomers in these situations is that they are

TABLE 7–1. CLASSIFICATION OF GLASS IONOMER CEMENTS

TYPE	USE	CHARACTERISTICS	EXAMPLES
I	Luting cements	Fine ground, chemical cure materials that are generally radiopaque.	Fuji 1 (GC International Corp.) Ketac Cem (ESPE-Premier Sales Corp.)
II	Restorative materials	Generally radiolucent, currently chemically cured materials used for esthetic restorative situations.	Fuji 2 (GC International Corp.) Ketac Fil (ESPE-Premier Sales Corp.)
III-A	Bases and liners	Buffered liners that are radiopaque, weak, chemical set materials with low acidity and high zinc oxide content. Tooth-colored materials are very opaque.	GC Lining Cement (GC International Corp.) Shofu Liner (Shofu Dental Corp.)
III-B	Bases and liners	Radiopaque base materials that are stronger, chemical set materials with increased acidity. Tooth-colored materials are very opaque.	Ketac Bond (ESPE-Premier Sales Corp.) Shofu Base (Shofu Dental Corp.) GC Dentin Cement (GC International Corp.)
III-C	Bases and liners	Light stabilized materials useful as liners or bases. They are radiopaque, and are both strong and stable in thin layers. Tooth-colored materials are very opaque.	Vitrebond (3M, Inc.)
IV	Admixtures	Fine ground, chemical cure materials that are generally radiopaque.	Ketac Silver (ESPE-Premier Sales Corp.) Miracle Mix (GC International Corp.)

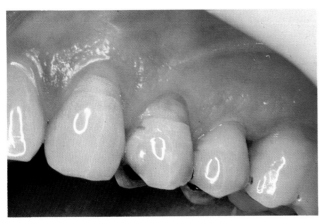

FIG. 7–5

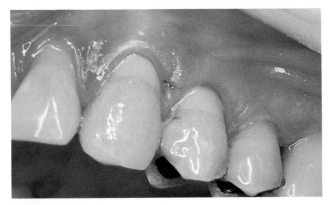

FIG. 7–6

readily carved and shaped by hand rather than by a rotary instrument.

Armamentarium

- Standard dental setup
    rubber dam
    cotton rolls
    explorer
    high-speed handpiece
    low-speed handpiece
    mouth mirror
    periodontal probe
    2 × 2 gauze
- Assorted dental burs for cavity preparation and caries removal
- Oil-free pumice
- Rubber prophylaxis cup
- 10 to 25% polyacrylic acid (e.g., Dentin Conditioner liquid, GC International Corp.)

FIG. 7–5. Cervical erosion lesion that would require extensive preparation to gain undercuts for a conventional restoration.

FIG. 7–6. Erosion lesion restored with glass ionomer cement. A type 2 restorative material has been used.

- Glass ionomer cement
  Radiopaque Type II for Class III cavity or radiolucent Type II for Class V cavity (highly visible area)
- Mylar matrix strips
- Hand instruments for carving and shaping
- Diamond finishing burs
- Composite resin bonding agent of choice (see Chapter 3—Dentin Bonding Agents)

Clinical Technique

1. Administer local anesthesia (optional).
2. Isolate the lesion with a rubber dam.
3. Cleanse the tooth with a nonfluoridated flour of pumice.
4. For Class III restorations, try to restrict the labial display. For a Class V erosion lesion, roughen the surface of the lesion with a diamond bur or with oil-free pumice in a prophy cup.
5. Prepare the cavity by removing the infected carious lesion and any grossly weakened tooth structure.
6. Treat the surface with 10 to 25% polyacrylic acid for 20 seconds to enhance the bond.
7. Once prepared, keep the tooth surface free from saliva contamination (as carefully as acid-etched enamel before the application of a bonding agent.)
8. Use a radiopaque Type II ionomer for a Class III cavity and a radiolucent Type II glass ionomer cement for a Class V cavity.
9. After application of the Type II glass ionomer material, keep the restorative material isolated from the oral environment to avoid moisture contamination as described previously.
10. After the chelation point passes (the "sheen" disappears), paint bonding liquid on the surface to prevent moisture evaporation.

CLINICAL TIP. Coat the ionomer surface with a bonding resin as soon as the "sheen" disappears from the mix and the restoration begins to harden. Begin carving after the "rubbery" stage has passed and a sharp instrument removes shavings rather than clumps of material. After carving and finishing of the glass ionomer, apply a second coat of bonding resin and cure it for maximal protection.

---

11. After carving and finishing (see the section on Finishing earlier in this chapter), apply and cure another coat of bonding resin.

Laminated Esthetic Veneers—Esthetically Demanding Class III, IV and V Restorations and Labial Veneers

When esthetic demands are high and functional stresses are significant, the glass ionomer base should be designed to replace lost dentin and to protect the dentin from acid etching used to retain a composite resin overlay to enamel. Retention of the composite resin is based on developing an adequate bond to enamel. It should not rely on the limited retention available through the glass ionomer.

Color selection of the glass ionomer is critical for the final appearance because it tends to shine through the

---

CLINICAL TIP. Glass ionomer cements are particularly well suited to replace tooth structure underneath a direct composite resin, which has the poorest coefficient of thermal expansion and the highest rate of setting contraction. The use of glass ionomer cement reduces the size of the composite resin component of the restoration, thus diminishing the impact of the undesirable characteristics of the composite resin.

---

composite resin overlay. For this reason, a Type II glass ionomer material should be used rather than a Type III, which although faster setting, tends to be unesthetically opaque.

Armamentarium. The armamentarium is the same as that listed for small, non-stress bearing Class III and Class V restoration except:

- Acid etch gel
- Glass ionomer cement
  Radiopaque Type II for Class III cavity or radiolucent Type II for Class V cavity (highly visible area)

Clinical Technique

1. Administer local anesthesia (optional).
2. Isolate the lesion with a rubber dam.
3. Cleanse the tooth with a nonfluoridated flour of pumice.
4. Prepare the cavity in a conventional manner.
5. Apply the glass ionomer according to the specifications detailed in Technique Section of Final Restoration—Small, Nonstress Bearing Class III and Class V Restorations
6. Once set, shape the surface sufficiently to allow a composite resin overlay.
7. Etch or chemically prepare the surface of the ionomer for lamination as described previously.
8. Apply the composite resin.

Bases and Liners Under Direct Placement, Stress Bearing Class I, Class II Restorations

Glass ionomers should not be used on the surfaces of Class I and Class II restorations because of their strength limitations and lack of abrasion resistance. Glass ionomer cements are ideal as a base under all restorations. They can be used to replace all missing tooth structure and restore a tooth to an ideal preparation form prior to placement of the final restoration.

Armamentarium. The armamentarium is the same as that listed for small, nonstress bearing Class III and Class V restorations except:

- Acid etch gel
- Type III resin stabilized glass ionomer cement and Centrix type syringe (optional) (e.g., Vitrebond, 3M Inc.)

Clinical Technique

1. Administer local anesthesia (optional).
2. Isolate the lesion with a rubber dam (Fig. 7–7).

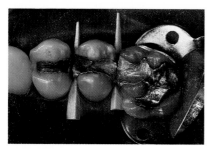

FIG. 7–7

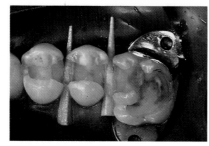

FIG. 7–8

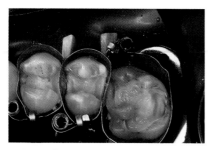

FIG. 7–9

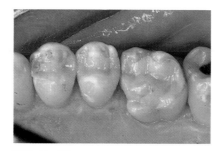

FIG. 7–10

FIG. 7–7. Defective amalgam restorations to be replaced with posterior composite resins over glass ionomer bases.

FIG. 7–8. The amalgam restorations have been removed and the cavities have been prepared for the glass ionomer bases.

FIG. 7–9. A type 3 chemically cured glass ionomer material has been used for the base. This has been injected into the cavity and tamped to place. The excess has been removed with a diamond stone, which also has been used to freshen the enamel margins. The dentin must be completely covered by the base.

FIG. 7–10. The posterior composite resins have been laminated to the glass ionomer base.

3. Cleanse the tooth with a nonfluoridated flour of pumice.

4. Prepare the cavity in a conventional manner (Fig. 7–8) except cavity preparation need only involve removal of caries and undermined dentin and enamel. It is not necessary to break the interproximal contact.

5. Completely cover the dentin with a Type III glass ionomer. Inject these base and liner materials through a syringe to ensure that the dentin surface is completely wetted and free of voids. Alternatively, the light-stabilized materials can be used. Completely cover all dentinal walls.

6. Once set, remove the excess glass ionomer from the enamel walls. Additional removal of glass ionomer may be required to ensure sufficient bulk of composite resin for strength in the final restoration (Fig. 7–9).

7. The glass ionomer can be acid etched concurrently with the walls of the enamel for a period not exceeding 30 seconds.

CLINICAL TIP. Overetching weakens the glass ionomer cement by dissolving the base and creating porosity in the material.

---

8. Apply the composite resin incrementally, filling all pits and fissures (Fig. 7–10).

Bases and Liners Under Indirect Placement, Stress Bearing Restorations—Class I and Class II Indirect Restorations

Restorative materials for inlays and onlays require considerable more bulk than their metallic counterparts. This can require deeper dentin penetration. Because these restorations are secured by composite resin luting systems, which gain adhesion by the acid-etch process, attention to dentin and pulpal protection is required. Light-stabilized glass ionomer bases and liners are the materials of choice for a number of reasons. They can easily be made to cover the dentin fully. The covering layer can be sufficiently thin to allow for sufficient bulk of the indirect restoration. The light-stabilized materials are not susceptible to breakdown under acid etching as are the conventional glass ionomer cements.

Armamentarium. The armamentarium is the same as that listed for small, nonstress bearing Class III and Class V restorations except:

- Acid etch gel
- Type III resin stabilized glass ionomer cement and Centrix type syringe (optional) (e.g., Vitrebond, 3M Inc.)

Clinical Technique

1. Administer local anesthesia (optional).
2. Place a rubber dam.
3. Prepare the tooth for the restoration.
4. Place calcium hydroxide where indicated (less than 1 mm of dentin).
5. Place a thin covering layer of light-stabilized glass ionomer (Fig. 7–11).
6. The glass ionomer can be acid etched concurrently with the walls of the enamel for a period not exceeding 30 seconds.
7. Restore the cavity with an appropriate restoration (Fig. 7–12). (See also Chapter 5—Composite Resins Fundamentals and Direct Technique Restorations, Chapter 6—Composite Resins—Indirect Technique

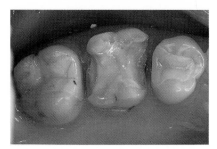

FIG. 7–11. A light-stabilized glass ionomer base has been placed. These can be used in thin layers and are easier to drape over dentin than the chemically set materials.

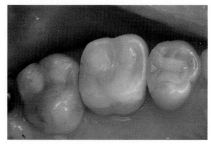

FIG. 7–12. The porcelain overlay restoration has been bonded to the base and enamel.

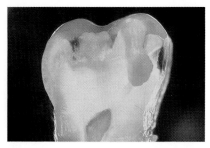

FIG. 7–13. An access approach is made toward the body of the carious lesion. (From Hunt, P.R.: Microconservative restorations for approximal carious lesions. J Am Dent Assoc 120:37, 1990.)

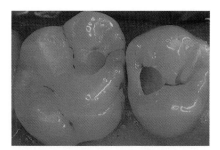

FIG. 7–14. The access opening should be placed inside the marginal ridge. (From Hunt, P.R.: The future of esthetic dentistry. J Am Dent Assoc Spec No. P:186E, 1987.)

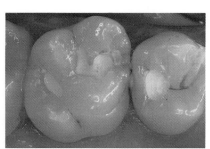

FIG. 7–15. A glass ionomer cement is injected directly onto the cavity floor so that the cement completely fills the void. (From Hunt, P.R.: The future of esthetic dentistry. J Am Dent Assoc Spec No. P:186E, 1987.)

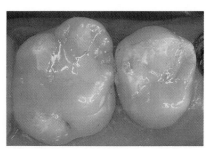

FIG. 7–16. The occlusal portion is restored with a posterior composite resin. (From Hunt, P.R.: The future of esthetic dentistry. J Am Dent Assoc Spec No. P:186E, 1987.)

Restorations, and Chapter 11—Porcelain—Laminate, Veneer and Other Partial Coverage Restorations.)

Microconservative Procedures—Internal and Miniature Box Restorations for Class II Lesions

These procedures are used to access an interproximal carious lesion without preparing a conventional box and without using a conventional dovetail, keyway, or lock to retain the restoration.[60]

Armamentarium. The armamentarium is the same as that listed for small, nonstress bearing Class III and Class V restorations except:

■ Acid etch gel
■ Glass ionomer cement
   Radiopaque type III glass ionomer cement and Centrix type syringe (optional) or glass ionomer cement in syringe dispensing system (e.g., Keta-Bond, Premier Dental Products Co.) or radiopaque Type IV glass ionomer cement

Clinical Technique

1. Make an access approach toward the body of the carious lesion (Fig. 7–13) by the most direct approach, usually from inside the marginal ridge (Fig. 7–14).
2. Examine the enamel deficiency following carious removal. If the enamel is intact but slightly porous, it may be retained and allowed to remineralize; otherwise, remove it. Often, the simplest way to do this is to create a miniature box that removes the porous or penetrated enamel and the marginal ridge lying above. Retain all the other enamel. The finished cavity preparation looks more like a Class I than a Class II preparation.
3. Select a radiopaque Type III or Type IV glass ionomer cement.
4. Inject the glass ionomer into the cavity by placing the nozzle of the syringe directly on the cavity floor so that the glass ionomer can well up and completely fill the void (Fig. 7–15).
5. Once the glass ionomer has set, freshen the enamel with a small round diamond bur prior to acid etch-

ing and restoring the occlusal deficiency with posterior composite resin material (Fig. 7–16). This provides for a stronger marginal ridge than one supported by glass ionomer alone.

Cores and Buildups

Glass ionomer strength, including that of metallic admixtures, is insufficient for cores and buildups. The core or buildup should not contain more than 40% glass ionomer. In particular, never use glass ionomers in thin sections. This restricts the use of glass ionomers to the posterior region. It is perhaps better to view them as good "block out" materials. When applying glass ionomer around posts, voids should not be present. This restricts the design of the posts to those with a simple head shape, which are readily wetted. The posts should be considered as weakening the core. Generally, the Type IV glass ionomers are used even though they are no stronger than the other types.

Cementation

Glass ionomer materials are often the materials of choice for permanent cementation of fixed restorative work. When set, they are much less water-soluble than conventional cements and the fluoride released from the cement is highly effective in preventing marginal decay.

CONCLUSION

Glass ionomer materials are useful in a wide range of situations. In particular, they should be considered the optimal material to replace lost dentin. By careful selection of suitable veneering materials, glass ionomers can satisfy almost any dental restoration demand.

REFERENCES

1. Wilson A.D. and McLean J.W.: Glass-Ionomer Cement. Chicago, Quintessence Publishing Co., 1988.
2. Mount G.W.: An Atlas of Glass Ionomer Cements, Philadelphia, B.C. Decker Co., 1990.
3. Wilson A.D., et al.: The release of fluoride and other chemical species from a glass ionomer cement. Biomat 6:431, 1986.
4. Hicks, M.J., Flaitz, C.M., and Silverstone L.M.: Secondary caries formation in vitro around glass-ionomer restorations. Quint Int 17:527, 1986.
5. Wilson A.D., Prosser H.J., and Powis D.M.: Mechanism of adhesion of poly electrolyte cements to hydroxyapatite. J Dent Res 62:590, 1983.
6. Tyas, M.J.: Latest rankings of dentine bonding agents. Dental Outlook 14:1, 1988.
7. Wilson A.D. and Prosser H.J.: Biocompatibility of the glass ionomer cement. J Dent Assoc South Am 37:872, 1982.
8. Walls A.W.G.: Glass polyalkenoate (glass ionomer) cements: a review. J Dent 14:231, 1986.
9. Wilson A.D. and Kent B.E.: A new translucent cement for dentistry. The glass ionomer cement. Br Dent J 132:133, 1972.
10. Smith, D.C.: Composition and characteristics of glass ionomer cements. J Am Dent Assoc 120:20, 1990.
11. Barry T.I., Clinton, D.J., and Wilson A.D.: The structure of a glass ionomer cement and its relationship to the setting process. J Dent Res 58:1072, 1979.
12. McLean J.W., Wilson A.D., and Prosser H.J.: Development and use of water hardening glass ionomer luting cements. J Prosthet Dent 52:175, 1984.
13. Simmons, J.J.: Post-cementation sensitivity commonly associated with the "anhydrous" forms of glass-ionomer luting cements: a theory. Tex Dent J 103:70, 1986.
14. Tobias, R.S., et al.: Pulpal response to an anhydrous glass ionomer luting cement. Endodont Dent Traumatol 5:242, 1989.
15. Wilson, A.D., Prosser, H.J., and Powis, D.M.: Mechanism of adhesion of polyelectrolyte cements to hydroxyapatite. J Dent Res 62:590, 1983.
16. Beech, D.R., Soloman, A., and Bernier, R.: Bond strength of polycarboxylic acid cements to treated dentin. Dent Mat 1:154, 1985.
17. Retief, D.H., Bradley E.L., Denton J.C., and Switzer, P.: Enamel and cementum fluoride uptake from a glass ionomer cement. Car Res 18:250, 1984.
18. Crisp S, Lewis, B.G., and Wilson A.D.: Characterization of glass ionomer cements. 2. Effect of the powder: liquid ratio on the physical properties. J Dent Res 4:287, 1976.
19. Wong, T.C.C. and Bryant R.W.: Glass ionomer cements: dispensing and strength. Aust Dent J 30:336, 1985.
20. Stokes, A.N.: Proportioning and temperature effects on manipulation of glass ionomer cements. J Dent Res 59:1782, 1980.
21. Atkinson, A.S. and Pearson, G.J.: The evolution of glass-ionomer cements. Br Dent J 159:335, 1985.
22. Saito, S.: Characteristics of glass-ionomer and its clinical application. Part I—Relations between hardening reactions and water. J Dent Med 8:4, 1978.
23. Causton, B.E.: The physio-mechanical consequences of exposing glass ionomer cements to water during setting. Biomaterials 2:112, 1981.
24. Mount G.J. and Makinson O.F.: Glass ionomer cements: clinical implications of the setting reaction. Op Dent 7:134, 1982.
25. Phillips, S., et al.: An in vitro study of the effect of moisture on glass ionomer cement, Quint Int 16:175, 1985.
26. Mount, G.: Glass ionomer cements—obtaining optimum aesthetic results. Dent Outlook 14:3, 1988.
27. Kim, K.C.: The microleakage of a glass cement using two methods of moisture protection. Quint Int 18:835, 1988.
28. Earl, M.S.A., Hume, W.R., and Mount G.J.: Effect of varnishes and other surface treatments on water movement across the glass-ionomer cement surface. Aust Dent J 30:298, 1985.
29. Earl, M.S.A., Hume, W.R., and Mount, G.J.: Effect of varnishes and other surface treatments on water movement across the glass-ionomer cement surface, II. Aust Dent J 34:326, 1989.
30. Pearson, G.J.: Finishing of glass ionomer cements. Br Dent J 155:226, 1983.
31. Pearson, G.J. and Knibbs, P.J.: Finishing an anhydrous glass ionomer cement (an in vitro and in vivo study). Rest Dent 3:35, 1987.
32. Woolford, M.J.: Finishing glass polyalkenoate (glass-ionomer) cements. Br Dent J 165:395, 1988.
33. Forsten, L.: Fluoride release from a glass ionomer cement. Scand J Dent Rest 85:503, 1977.
34. Wilson, A.D., et al.: The release of fluoride and other chemical species from a glass ionomer cement. Biomaterials 6:431, 1986.
35. Swartz, M.L., Phillips, R.W., and Clark, H.E.: Long term fluoride release from glass ionomer cements. J Dent Res 63:158, 1984.
36. Powis, D.R., Foleras, T., Merson, S.A., and Wilson, A.D.: Improved adhesion of a glass ionomer cement to dentin and enamel. J Dent Res 61:1416, 1982.
37. Duke, E.S., Phillips, R.W., and Blumershine, R.: Effects of various agents in cleaning cut dentine. J Oral Rehab 12:295, 1985.
38. Hinoura, E., et al.: Influence of dentin surface treatments on the bond strength of dentin-lining cements. Op Dent 11:147, 1986.

39. Mount, G.J.: Longevity of glass-ionomer cements. J Prosthet Dent 55:682, 1986.

40. Tyas, M.J. and Beech, D.R.: Clinical performance of three restorative materials for non-undercut cervical abrasion lesions. Aust Dent J 30:260, 1985.

41. McLean, J.W., Powis, D.R., Prosser, H.J., and Wilson, A.D.: The use of glass-ionomer cements in bonding composite resins to dentine. Br Dent J 158:410, 1985.

42. Smith, G.E.: Surface deterioration of glass-ionomer cement during acid etching: an SEM evaluation. Op Dent J 34:259, 1989.

43. Mount, G.J.: Clinical requirements for a successful "sandwich"—dentine to glass ionomer cement to composite resin. Aust Dent J 34:259, 1989.

44. Honoura, K., et al.: Tensile bond strength between glass ionomer cement and composite resin. J Am Dent Assoc 114:167, 1987.

45. Prosser, H.J., Powis, D.R., and Wilson, A.D.: Glass-ionomer cements of improved flexural strength. J Dent Res 65:146, 1986.

46. Prosser, H.J., et al.: Characteristics of glass ionomer cements. 7. The physical properties of current materials. J Dent 12:231, 1984.

47. Lloyd, L.H., and Mitchell, L.: The fracture toughness of tooth colored restorative materials. J Oral Reb 11:257, 1984.

48. Osman, E., Moore, B.K., and Phillips, R.W.: Fracture toughness of several categories of restorative materials. J Dent Res 65:456, 1986.

49. Browne, R.M. and Tobias, R.E.: Microbial microleakage and pulpal inflammation: a review. Endodont Dent Traumatol 2:177, 1986.

50. Nordenvall, K., Brannstrom, M., and Torstensson, B.: Pulp reactions and microorganisms under ASPA and concise composite fillings. J Dent Child 46:449, 1979.

51. Ucok, M.: Biological evaluation of glass-ionomer cements. Int Endodont J 19:285, 1986.

52. Council on Dental Materials: Reported sensitivity to glass ionomer luting cements. J Am Dent Assoc 120:59, 1990.

53. Christensen, G.J.: Glass Ionomer as a luting material. J Am Dent Assoc 120:59, 1990.

54. McLean, J.W. and Gasser, O.: Glass-cermet cements. Quint Int 5:333, 1985.

55. Thornton, J.B., et al.: Fluoride release from and tensile bond strength of Ketac-Fil and Ketac-Silver to enamel and dentin. Dent Mat J 2:241, 1986.

56. Moore, B.K., Swartz, M.L., and Phillips, R.W.: Abrasion resistance of metal reinforced glass ionomer cements. J Dent Res 64:371, 1985.

57. Simmons, J.J.: The miracle mixture: glass ionomer and alloy powder. Tex Dent J 100:6, 1983.

58. Simmons, J.J.: Silver-alloy powder and glass ionomer cement. J Am Dent Assoc 120:49, 1990.

59. McLean, J.W.: Cermet Cements. J Am Dent Assoc 120:43, 1990.

60. Hunt, P.: Micro-conservative restorations for approximal carious lesions. J Am Dent Assoc 120:37, 1990.

Ira D. Zinner, D.D.S., M.S.D.
Francis V. Panno, D.D.S.
Richard D. Miller, D.D.S.
Herbert M. Parker, D.D.S.
Mitchell S. Pines, D.D.S.

CERAMOMETAL—FULL COVERAGE RESTORATIONS

8

To the patient, cosmetic considerations in anterior fixed prosthodontics are as important, if not more important, than the functional aspects. The finest fitting restoration with exquisite porcelain carvings can meet with total patient dissatisfaction if it does not conform to the expected esthetic results.

BASIC CHEMISTRY

The basic chemical components of ceramometal porcelains are potassium-sodium aluminosilicate glasses (Table 8–1). In addition, combinations of metallic and nonmetallic oxides are added as opacifiers (Table 8–2).

The conventional all-ceramic and acrylic resin full and partial coverage restorations, while esthetically pleasing, can fail under heavy occlusal stresses because of low tensile and shear strengths.[1] Newer porcelain materials are stronger, but still cannot be used to create multiple unit fixed prostheses.[2] Full cast restorations offer sufficient strength, but lack the esthetic appearance required in today's society. Ceramometal dental restorations, however, offer both acceptable appearance and strength.[3]

The strength of the porcelain-to-metal bond is close to that of the tensile strength of the opaquing porcelain. Fracture usually occurs within the body of the porcelain. If this is not the case, an error in fabrication technique is usually to blame.[4,5]

Ceramic and metal alloys must have properties that allow for both physical and chemical compatibility. The fusion temperature of the ceramic (usually 100 to 150°C) is lower than the metal casting temperature, thus preventing the cast metal substructure from melting during porcelain application. Ceramometal porcelains contain more soda and potash than typical all-ceramic blends. This increases thermal expansion to a level compatible with the metal alloy. The coefficient of thermal expansion of the ceramic is between 13 and $14 \times 10^{-6}/°C$ (Table 8–3). This should be approximately 0.5 to $1.0 \times 10^{-6}/°C$ less than the coefficient of thermal expansion of the casting alloy, which places the brittle ceramic into slight compression at the ceramometal interface when it cools. Ceramic is much stronger under compression than under tension.[3] In addition, because it is brittle and it tends to form minor stress concentrating defects, the ceramic is much stronger when applied to a *rigid* metal framework. This framework, upon wetting with porcelain, reduces the internal ceramic defects and also supports the brittle porcelain, thus adding strength to the restoration.[1] Conversely, the metal of a knife-edged finishing line or a bevel contains insufficient bulk of metal to resist small deflections during seating. Porcelain should not be applied to these thin margins because if resistance to seating is encountered, flexing of the metal can cause the porcelain to flake off.[4]

Opaque porcelains, which mask the metal coping, contain metallic oxide opacifiers. New opaque porcelains can be effectively used in layers as thin as 100 microns. This opaque porcelain, however, must be covered by at least 1 mm of body porcelain to mask its reflectiveness.

Vitrification in ceramic restorations refers to a liquid phase caused by reaction or melting which, on cooling, forms a glassy phase. If this formation is disturbed by adding too much modifying oxide, devitrification (crystallization) can occur.[4] The ceramic porcelains are sensitive to devitrification because of their alkali content, which can cause clouding with additional porcelain firings. Repeated firing of high expansion ceramometal porcelains at maturing temperature increases the likelihood of devitrification.[4]

TABLE 8–1. INGREDIENTS OF DENTAL PORCELAINS

INGREDIENT	DENTAL PORCELAIN (WEIGHT %)	DECORATIVE PORCELAIN (WEIGHT %)
Feldspar	81	15
Quartz	15	14
Kaolin	4	70
Metallic Pigment	<1	1

(Adapted from Craig, R.G. (ed.): Restorative Dental Materials. St. Louis, C.V. Mosby Co., 1985.)

TABLE 8–3. PORCELAIN COEFFICIENT OF THERMAL EXPANSION

LOW COEFFICIENT	MEDIUM COEFFICIENT	HIGH COEFFICIENT
Ceramco	Pencraft	Biobond
Denpac	Duceram	Williams
Vita	Synspak	Crystar
Excelco		

TABLE 8–2. COMPOSITION OF DENTAL CERAMICS FOR FUSING TO HIGH TEMPERATURE ALLOYS

COMPOUND	BIODENT OPAQUE BG 2 (%)	CERAMCO OPAQUE 60 (%)	V.M.K. OPAQUE 121 (%)	BIODENT DENTIN BD 27 (%)	CERAMCO DENTIN T 69 (%)
SiO_2	52.00	55.00	52.40	56.90	62.20
Al_2O_3	13.55	11.65	15.15	11.80	13.40
CaO	—	—	—	0.61	0.98
K_2O	11.05	9.60	9.90	10.00	11.30
Na_2O	5.28	4.75	6.58	5.42	5.37
TiO_2	3.01	—	2.59	0.61	—
ZrO_2	3.22	0.16	5.16	1.46	0.34
SnO_2	6.40	15.00	4.90	—	0.50
Rb_2O	0.09	0.04	0.08	0.10	0.06
BaO	1.09	—	—	3.52	—
ZnO	—	0.26	—	—	—
UO_3	—	—	—	—	—
B_2O_3, CO_2 and H_2O	4.31	3.54	3.24	9.58	5.85
Total	100.00	100.00	100.00	100.00	100.00

(Adapted from Craig, R.G. (ed.): Restorative Dental Materials. St. Louis, C.V. Mosby Co., 1985.)

Ceramometal Alloys

Ceramometal alloy must be sufficiently thick to prevent deflection, (i.e., it must be rigid.) This implies that an ideal ceramometal alloy has a high modulus of elasticity. However, even though the modulus of elasticity for dental alloys varies greatly, the practical savings in using stiffer materials is minimal because even the more flexible ceramometal alloys can be reduced to the minimum coping thickness of 0.5 mm and still be clinically acceptable.[1] Ceramometal alloys should not melt during porcelain application or exhibit creep at high temperatures (see below).

CLINICAL TIP. A thin marginal apron may distort during porcelain application and result in an inaccurate fit. To avoid this, copings should be waxed with thick margins, and then thinned (after porcelain application) during final finishing.

When a ceramometal alloy is heated during porcelain firing, its modulus of elasticity must be high (rigid) enough to resist metal deformation. However, as the restoration cools, the alloy should be able to deform a small amount to relieve the stress produced by the thermal contraction of the porcelain. If the modulus of elasticity of the alloy is too high, it will be ungiving and not relieve this stress. Thus, the stress remains within the porcelain and may lead to crazing.[3]

Creep is a time-dependent strain that occurs under stress[7] and results in deformation or flow of the material. Creep is shown by a material that continues to deform even though the stress on it remains the same. This is seen in metals at temperatures close to their melting point. Creep can be controlled by avoiding extremely long firing cycles. High temperature creep is flow that occurs at elevated temperatures. For gold alloys high temperature creep occurs at about one 1800°F. It can be reduced by varying alloy composition so that a dispersion strengthening effect occurs at the high temperature.[6-8]

As required of all intraoral restorative metals, the ceramometal alloy should be resistant to tarnish and corrosion in the mouth.[3]

CLASSIFICATIONS OF CERAMOMETAL ALLOYS

There are two basic types of ceramometal alloys: the precious alloys and the base metal alloys.

Precious Alloys

Because original ceramometal restorations contained high proportions of noble metal, their clinical characteristics are well documented.[4] Noble metals exhibit good resistance to oxidation, tarnish, and corrosion. The noble metals are gold, platinum, palladium, iridium, rhodium, osmium, and ruthenium.[1] Their physical properties are all similar, although the non-gold noble alloys require a modified investment to withstand the higher casting temperatures. Ceramic alloys are very hard and strong, as compared to ADA Type I to Type III gold and are similar to Type IV golds. The coefficient of thermal expansion of ceramic alloys is less than that of Type I, II, III, or IV golds. The noble metals and silver are often referred to as precious metals.[1]

Base Metal Alloys

Base metal alloys consist of nickel, chromium, molybdenum, cobalt, and beryllium. They can be used to obtain satisfactory fit, however, laboratory procedures for base metals are much more technique-sensitive than those of the noble alloys. High casting shrinkage of the base metal alloys necessitates special investments and casting methods. When nickel-based alloys are subjected to heat treatment during the porcelain firing cycles, the strength and hardness of the alloy decreases. The control of their oxide thickness is more difficult, presenting problems with additional porcelain firings.[4]

Dental ceramometal restorative alloys may be further classified by their major constituents, as well as by the chronology of their development (Tables 8–4, 8–5).[2]

Group 1—Gold Noble, 1950s
Composition

1. 96 to 98% noble metal
   A. 84 to 86% gold
   B. 4 to 10% platinum
   C. 5 to 7% palladium
2. 2 to 3% base metal

Properties. Gold noble alloys are weaker and have less sag resistance (the property of a ceramometal alloy to resist flow under its own weight during soldering and porcelain application)[3] than the more newly developed ceramometal alloys. They are the easiest to cast and solder and have a yellow color that aids in obtaining lighter tooth color shades. These alloys are the most costly because of their high noble metal content. The Group 1 alloys were developed by both J.F. Jelenko and Co. and J. Aderer, Inc.[2]

Group 2—White Noble
Composition

1. 80% noble metal
   A. 51 to 54% gold
   B. 0% platinum
   C. 26-31% palladium
2. 14 to 16% silver

Properties. Platinum, the most costly metal, was eliminated in the Group 2 alloys. The gold content was reduced and the palladium portion increased. The overall noble metal proportion was reduced by adding silver. These alloys have improved mechanical properties with higher strength and greater sag resistance. They are easy to fabricate and are less costly than Group 1 alloys. However, the silver may cause some porcelain greening and the gray color of the alloy makes it harder to obtain lighter tooth color shades.[2] The Group 2 alloys were developed by Joseph Tuccillo in 1976 at J.F. Jelenko and Co.[9]

Group 3—Palladium-Silver Alloys
Composition

1. 53 to 60% noble metal
   A. 0% gold
   B. 0% platinum
   C. 53-60% palladium
2. 30 to 37% silver
3. 10% base metals

Properties. These alloys contain palladium, silver, and a small amount of base metals. They are easy to cast and solder, have acceptable mechanical properties, and are the least expensive of the noble alloys. The co-

TABLE 8–4. CERAMOMETAL ALLOYS

GROUP	% NOBLE METAL	CONTAINS SILVER (GREENING)	TECHNIQUE SENSITIVITY	PORCELAIN TYPE (COEFFICIENT OF THERMAL EXPANSION)	COLOR	MINIMUM THICKNESS OF METAL
1	96–98%	No	Low	Conventional	Gold	.5 mm
2	80%	Yes	Low	Conventional	White	.5 mm
3	53–60%	Yes	Medium	High	White	.5 mm
4	90%	No	Low	Low or Conventional	White	.5 mm
5	0%	No	High	Conventional	White	.4 mm
6	0%	No	Medium to High	Conventional	White	.5 mm
7	78–88%	Some contain Ag	Medium	Low or Conventional	White	.5 mm

TABLE 8–5. PROPERTIES OF CERAMOMETAL ALLOYS

GROUP	TYPE	EXAMPLE	% Au	% Pt	% Pd	% Ag	% Cr	% Ni	% Co	% Be	PROPRIETARY METALS	MELTING RANGE (°F)	CASTING TEMPERATURE (°F)	VICKERS HARDNESS	YIELD STRENGTH (PSI)	ELONGATION %	COEFFICIENT OF THERMAL EXPANSION ($\times 10^{-6}$/°C)	DENSITY (gm/cm)
1	Gold Noble	Jelenko O*	88	5	6	1					0	2,100–2,150	2,300	182	65,300	5	14.7	19.2
		Degudent†	78	10	9	1					2	2,100–2,300	2,550	200	68,150(S) 84,100(H)	7(S) 3(H)		18.0
		RxCG‡	87	7	5	1					0	2,100–2,150	2,300	165	40,000	5	14.7	18.5
2	White Noble	Cameo*	53		27	16					4	2,200–2,300	2,400	220	80,000	10	14.7	16.7
		Ceramco White‡	51		31	15					3	2,300–2,345	2,550	130(S) 220(H) 200(F)	30,450(S) 61,630(H)	35(S) 10(H)		14.5
		RxWCG‡	52		30	14					4	2,200–2,300	2,400	220	80,000	10		13.8
3	Palladium Silver	Jelstar*			60	28					12	2,250–2,380	2,500	189	67,000	20	14.8	10.7
		Degustar*			52	38					10	2,100–2,250	2,550	200(S) 250(H) 220(F)	56,550(S) 81,200(H)	25(S) 10(H)		11.2
		Rx Palladent B‡			60	28					12	2,200–2,275	2,500	165	80,000	10		10.5
4	Gold Palladium	Olympia*	52		39						9	2,320–2,380	2,450	220	83,000	20	14.1	13.5
		Deva M†	47		45						8	2,230–2,390	2,550	185(S) 275(H) 260(F)	53,650(S) 94,250(H)	31(S) 10(H)		14.4
		Sk45‡	45		45						10	2,200–2,300	2,550	250	80,000	10		13.5
5	Nickel Chromium	Rexillium‡						75	14	2	9	2,250–2,350	2,500	240	74,000	9–12		7.8
6	Cobalt	Genesis*					27		53		20	2,415–2,550	2,600	350	61,000	9	14.6	8.8
		Nouarex‡					25		55		20	2,425–2,475	2,675	260	90,000	7		8.8
7	High Palladium	Legacy*	2		85	1					12	2,020–2,360	2,450	270 260(F)	95,500(S) 83,380(H)	20	14.2	11.0
		Deguplus2†	1	1	80						18	2,110–2,355		260(S) 260(H)	83,380(S) 83,380(H)	30(S) 30(H)		11.5
		Aspen‡	6	1	75	7					11	2,115–2,275		250	80,000	21		11.0

(S) = Soft, (H) = Hard, (F) = Hardness after firing. Values are rounded to the nearest whole number. Data supplied by manufacturers. *Manufactured by J.F. Jelenko and Co. †Manufactured by Degussa Dental, Inc. ‡Manufactured by Jeneric/Penton, Inc.

efficient of thermal expansion of palladium-silver alloys is higher than that of gold alloys, necessitating the use of porcelains with a correspondingly higher coefficient of shrinkage. The silver content may cause greening of the porcelain, requiring the judicious use of metal conditioners.[2] Metal conditioner is an opaque porcelain with a high concentration of pink pigment that is used to negate the green discoloration of the porcelain caused by the silver content. These alloys can absorb gases in their liquid state, and then release the gases during solidification, which may cause bubbles to form in the porcelain during its application.[10] Palladium alloys are prone to carbon contamination, which affect the porcelain-to-metal bond; therefore, it is necessary to avoid the use of carbon blocks and graphite crucibles when using these materials. This problem can be minimized by avoiding overheating the alloy and avoiding holding the molten metal for long periods before casting. The Group 3 alloys were developed by Clyde Ingersol of Williams Gold Inc. in 1975.[11]

Group 4—Gold-Palladium Alloys
Composition

1. 90% noble metals
   A. 45 to 52% gold
   B. 38 to 45% palladium
2. 0% silver
3. 10% base metals

Properties. Both silver and platinum were eliminated from Group 4 alloys. The mechanical properties, (modulus of elasticity, yield strength, etc.), ease of fabrication, and dimensional accuracy make these the most promising of all the noble alloys. They have a lower coefficient of thermal expansion than Group 1, 2, or 3 alloys, making them compatible only with lower shrinkage porcelains. The Group 4, gold-palladium alloys were developed by Paul Cascone at J.F. Jelenko and Co. in 1978.[12] In 1985, the alloy was improved[12] by increasing the coefficient of thermal expansion, making it more compatible with conventional porcelains. These alloys are "white gold" in color.

Group 5—Nickel-Chromium Alloys
Composition

1. 0% noble metal
2. 100% base metal
   A. 60 to 82% nickel
   B. 11 to 20% chromium
   C. 2 to 9% molybdenum
   D. 0 to 2% beryllium

Properties. The use of nickel-based alloys was explored in the 1950s, but lack of a suitable investment and technique delayed their successful development. Advancements in casting investments and soaring gold prices of the 1970s spurred the acceptance of nickel alloys. These alloys are comprised of nickel, chromium, molybdenum, and beryllium. The beryllium-containing alloys, in general, cast better and have a greater porcelain-to-metal bond strength than the nonberyllium-containing alloys. This accounts for the great degree of differences in mechanical properties in this group. These alloys are the hardest, possess a very high modulus of elasticity, and have a higher melting temperature than the other alloy groups. The presence of nickel introduces the possibility of nickel hypersensitivity in allergic patients and the small amount of beryllium adds the hazard of beryllium toxicity in the dental laboratory if proper ventilation is not established. Laboratory procedures are extremely technique-sensitive.[2] These alloys produce suitable restorations when nickel hypersensitivity is not a problem and when a low cost alloy is desired. The dental laboratory should be knowledgeable in the proper handling of these alloys.

Group 6—Cobalt Base Alloys
Composition

1. 0% noble metal
2. 100% base metal
   A. 55 to 64% cobalt
   B. 25 to 34% chromium
   C. 2 to 9% molybdenum

Properties. The castability, solderability, and porcelain-to-metal bond strength of the cobalt-based alloys are, in general, not as good as the nickel-based, beryllium-containing alloys. They are harder and also more technique-sensitive than Group 5 alloys.[2]

Group 7—High Palladium Alloys
Composition

1. 78 to 88% noble metal
   A. 76 to 88% palladium
   B. 0 to 2% gold
   C. 0 to 1% silver
2. 12 to 22% base metal

Properties. The high palladium-containing alloys are extremely hard and exhibit a very high yield strength. They do not cast as well as the gold alloys and are more technique-sensitive in laboratory fabrication. These alloys are compatible with most porcelain systems.

BASIC CONSIDERATION IN FULL COVERAGE PREPARATIONS
Medicolegal Considerations

Prior to any tooth preparation, the restorative dentist should thoroughly discuss the patient's expectations and cosmetic desires. A thorough history, as well as the patient's attitude toward prior treating clinicians, should be recorded. In addition, a full series of radiographs (parallel cone technique) should be taken, using appropriate instrumentation. Ideally, two sets of diagnostic casts should be made. One set should be mounted on a semiadjustable articulator using verified oral records and the second set should be used for a diagnostic wax-up to demonstrate to the patient the desired esthetic results. If the patient's expectations are unrealistic or if the patient's opinion differs from that of the dentist, the dentist should be able to advise the patient and explain the limitations in terms of the cosmetic result. If the patient cannot accept the result set forth by the dentist, then no further dentistry should be pursued with the patient. (See Chapter 16—Esthetics and Psychology and Chapter 28—Esthetics and Dental Jurisprudence.)

Photography

Close-up photographs should be taken prior to any dental treatment as part of the patient's record. They may be used to aid communication between the dentist and the laboratory technician. Photographs should also be taken following completion of treatment and maintained as part of the patient's record. (See Chapter 17—Esthetics and Oral Photography.)

Periodontal Considerations

The presence of unesthetic, pathologic periodontal structures precludes a cosmetic result. Thus, prior to any fixed prosthodontic procedures, all periodontal tissues should be in a state of optimum health and maintained in that condition by the patient. (See Chapter 21—Esthetics and Periodontics.)

Inflammation is often caused by temporary cement or by impression material that remains in the gingival sulcus area or by placement of less than optimal provisional restorations. Areas of deficiency usually involve margins, height and width of gingival embrasures, contours, and polishing and finishing of the transitional prosthesis. Corrections should be made prior to proceeding with construction of the definitive restorations.

Diagnostic Models

Prior to tooth preparations, an irreversible hydrocolloid impression should be made of the arch to be prepared. If changes are required for cosmetic purposes an additional diagnostic cast is altered with white carving wax to create the desired effect. If soft tissue modifications are anticipated, these changes should be included on the cast using pink base-plate wax. The completed diagnostic wax-up of the desired soft and hard tissue changes may then be used by the periodontist as a guide for treatment planning and case presentation. (See Chapter 18—Esthetics and Electrosurgery and Chapter 21—Esthetics and Periodontics.)

Tooth Reduction

The laboratory technician must be provided sufficient room for both metal and porcelain, even if intentional prophylactic endodontics is necessary. Opaquing porcelain need only be 100 microns thick, but unless it is covered by an optimum thickness of surface porcelain, the final restoration appears flat and unlifelike.[13] Insufficient tooth reduction forces the laboratory technician to create either an overcontoured, periodontally unacceptable restoration or a properly contoured, unesthetically opaque restoration.[14] In either case, under-reduction in the gingival one-third precludes the proper emergence profile that is necessary to ensure gingival health.[15,16]

Over-reduction is also undesirable because it can lead to insufficient retention and resistance form as well as an increased risk of pulpal involvement. In addition, if porcelain is thicker than 1.5 mm because of inadequate tooth structure or insufficient metal buildup, the risk of porcelain failure is greater.

Provisional Restorations

The provisional restoration should serve as a guide in determining the proper esthetics and function of the definitive prosthesis. Both the dentist and the patient should select an acrylic shade. An impression of the diagnostic wax-up should be used to create a die stone cast. The designated teeth are prepared by the dentist on a second diagnostic cast. A heat-cured acrylic resin shell is fabricated in the laboratory to the desired shape and shade of the future restorations, as depicted by the diagnostic wax-up. (See also Chapter 13—Acrylic and Other Resins—Provisional Restorations for alternative methods).

An all-acrylic resin transitional restoration is appropriate only for short-term use. If provisional restorations are used for a prolonged period of time, they should be constructed of more durable materials, such as a gold thimble or less costly, nonprecious metal thimble splinted substructure casting with a heat-cured acrylic resin superstructure. The acrylic is attached to the substructure via acrylic resin retention beads. This type of restoration can withstand long-term use with the varying occlusal, functional, and parafunctional forces that may be brought to bear upon it. Also, this type of provisional restoration is used after periodontal surgery or implant placement that requires a prolonged healing period to permit evaluation of questionable teeth with a guarded prognosis. In addition, this method of provisional splinting can be utilized as a fixed orthodontic retainer following adult tooth movements for creation of a favorable esthetic and functional result.

The acrylic resin shell is usually brittle. Therefore, the dentist should cut away the interproximal sections of acrylic material with a fluted wax carving bur. This 3-fluted bur is utilized because it does not clog when carving or cutting acrylic resin. After tooth preparation, the dentist lines the entire shell with autopolymerizing acrylic resin of the same shade. The autopolymerizing resin imparts some plasticity to the restoration and reinforces the brittle shell, thereby reducing the chance of breakage.

Tooth reduction, especially that area influencing the incisal guidance, is verified with the transitional prosthesis. If the section incisal to the cingulum becomes thin or perforated then this area must be reprepared prior to impressioning the preparation. If the tooth preparation is altered, the provisional restoration is relined with autopolymerizing acrylic resin of the selected shade.

The marginal termination of the provisional fixed restoration should be at the end of the preparation. Overextension causes periodontal problems, gingival recession, and a compromised esthetic result.[17] Underextended provisional margins result in tooth sensitivity, possible pulpal damage, and the growth of gingival tissue over the shoulder of the preparation.[17]

Carvings of the provisional prostheses should simulate those of the definitive porcelain-fused-to-metal restoration in terms of size, shape, and occlusal contact. If any alterations are to be made because of either the patient's or dentist's desires, they should be performed on the provisional restoration prior to completion of the definitive fixed restoration.

For increased cosmetic effect and to simulate nature in the transitional restorations, the labial embrasures are deepened and the incisal embrasures are opened, rounded, and made to be of varying depths, and the gingival embrasures are carved to accommodate a healthy gingival papilla. A straight emergence profile should be carved in the gingival one-third of the restoration. Enhanced individuality can be created with interproximal orange-brown or brown acrylic stains. In addition, many of these restorations can be stained with decalcification or fracture lines to simulate nature in an elderly patient.

The restorations are contoured, polished, and cemented with a temporary cement. A cement is chosen that allows easy removal of the restoration and sedation of the prepared tooth. The patient is dismissed and the esthetics, tooth contours, gingival health, and the occlusion are evaluated at the next office visit.[18]

Often, more than one set of provisional restorations is necessary because of sequential alterations for creation of the desired cosmetic result. The restorative dentist should use the provisional restoration as a template, or guide, for the height, shade, and shape of the definitive prosthesis, as well as for incisal guidance.

Finishing Lines

Five kinds of finishing lines may be used for full coverage porcelain-fused-to-metal restorations:

1. a knife-edged finishing line preparation (Fig. 8–1).
2. a chamfer preparation (Fig. 8–2)
3. a full shoulder preparation (Fig. 8–3)
4. a full shoulder with a bevel preparation (Fig. 8–4)
5. a full shoulder with a bevel and a facial butt joint preparation

Knife-Edged Finishing Line. The knife-edged preparation is a tapered preparation that has maximum tooth reduction at the occlusal or incisal portion of the preparation and tapers to zero cutting at the gingival termination. Therefore, it is accomplished by inclining the cutting instrument at the occlusal end while maintaining no tooth reduction at the gingival termination of the preparation. The greater the tooth reduction, the more tapered the preparation becomes. This usually results in an overtapered preparation with insufficient tooth reduction in the gingival one-third for optimum periodontal health when using ceramometal full coverage restorations. This type of finishing line should be used only after periodontal surgery that results in long clinical crowns terminating apically onto root structure. If a shoulder and bevel were to be created at this apically positioned margin, an overprepared tooth and probable pulpal exposure is likely.

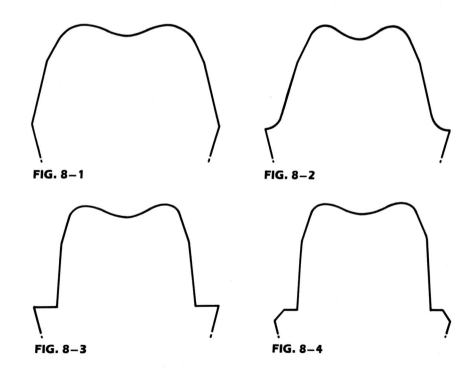

FIG. 8–1. Tapered knife edge preparation.

FIG. 8–2. Chamfer preparation.

FIG. 8–3. Full shoulder preparation.

FIG. 8–4. Full shoulder with a bevel preparation.

FIG. 8–1

FIG. 8–2

FIG. 8–3

FIG. 8–4

CLINICAL TIP. To create a knife-edged finishing line on elongated teeth, first prepare a full shoulder preparation at the cemento-enamel junction to ensure removal of adequate tooth structure. Then prepare a bevel or knife-edged finishing line to the desired gingival margin.

Chamfer Preparation. A chamfer preparation reduces more tooth structure in the gingival one-third than the knife-edged preparation. It does not, however, allow as much room as the full shoulder preparation for the buttressing of metal that is necessary to produce the rigid metallic framework for porcelain. The rounded end chamfer stone produces the same type of finishing line cut independent of the angle of handpiece placement. This allows for ease of preparation despite varying soft tissue heights, and for the creation of a consistent gingival contour. If, however, a chamfer stone is used to create a deep chamfer yielding a low stress concentration preparation, a reverse lip may be cut. A "low stress concentration preparation" is one in which the walls are more parallel than a "high stress concentration preparation" and the shoulder is between 90 and 110°, with an internal rounded line angle. Removing this lip may result in a preparation that is more subgingival than desired. A more tapered chamfer preparation results in a "high concentration type preparation." A "high stress concentration type preparation" is overly tapered and the shoulder to axial wall line angle is less than 90°. The shoulder slopes incisally. This type of preparation, as well as the knife-edged finishing line, may result in marginal metal distortion during firing, depending on the depth of the gingival portion of the preparation.

Full Shoulder Preparation. The full shoulder preparation has the same attributes as the full beveled shoulder preparation, without the disadvantages of the anterior bevel. It is used for a butt joint ceramic type restoration.

Full Shoulder with a Bevel Preparation. The ideal preparation for a porcelain-fused-to-metal restoration is a full shoulder with a bevel. The main difference

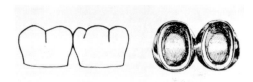

FIG. 8–5. Optimal interproximal form for biologic contours of definitive full coverage restorations. The contact area allows for an occlusal embrasure and a gingival embrasure that permits room for healthy interproximal papilla. An internal view of the castings demonstrates a beveled shoulder that has the same thickness throughout the preparation. The gingival embrasure has a wide contact area to aid in cleansibility and health of the surrounding interproximal papilla. The buccolingual embrasure enhances food deflection and periodontal health.

TABLE 8–6. SHOULDER WITH BEVEL—FINISHING LINE VARIATIONS

TYPE	INDICATIONS
Butt Joint	Anterior splints up to 6 units.
45° Facial Bevel	Esthetics is paramount. A preferred substitute for a butt joint, it is less technique-sensitive.
80° Bevel with Porcelain	Not recommended because of possible porcelain fracture.
80° Bevel without Porcelain	For short preparations to increase retention, endodontic teeth with posts, better closing angles and postperiodontally treated teeth with long clinical crowns.

between a shoulder preparation and a chamfer preparation in the gingival one-third is the additional tooth reduction necessary to create a shoulder between the horizontal and vertical line angles formed by the shoulder and the axial wall. The additional reduction provides room for additional metal, which buttresses the shoulder and supports the porcelain. The shoulder preparation may have a shoulder of 90 to 120°. The advantages of a full shoulder with a bevel preparation are:

1. The creation of adequate room in the gingival one-third for proper contouring of the restoration to maintain periodontal health with a straight emergence profile (Fig. 8–5).
2. The creation of room in the gingival one-third for proper porcelain application and esthetics.
3. The creation of a buttress of metal in the gingival area to avoid distortion of the metallic framework during the baking of porcelain and the seating of castings.
4. The creation of a more parallel, less tapered preparation enhancing retention of the restoration.[19]

Bevel Types (Table 8–6)

45° Facial Bevel. To avoid displaying a labial metal collar a facial 45° bevel and a full shoulder can be prepared. Proximally and lingually, an 80° degree bevel (Fig. 8–6) is cut. The porcelain and metal are brought to a common termination with predictable fit, contour, and color. Because the vertical amount of marginal metal is so narrow, the opaque is barely visible in the finished restoration. The 45° bevel is like a sloped shoulder and allows creation of the desired esthetic result. Also, from a laboratory viewpoint it is less technique-sensitive than a butt joint (Fig. 8–7). A porcelain margin accumulates less plaque, results in less margin exposure caused by gingival recession that occurs over a period of time, and is less objectionable cosmetically. Porcelain stacking and firing does not distort the facial margin of the 45° bevel. The 45° bevel with porcelain over the metal collar has greater esthetic potential, as

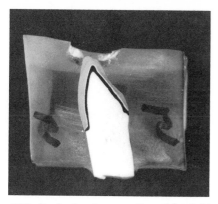

FIG. 8–6. Specimen sectioned for light microscopic examination showing a full shoulder preparation with a facial 45° bevel and a proximal and lingual 80° bevel. Black is metal; white is opaquer; gray is porcelain.

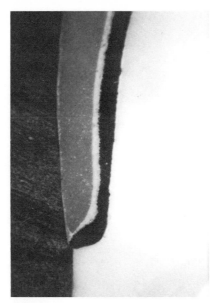

FIG. 8–7. Magnified view of a prepared tooth showing a facial margin with a 45° bevel. (Original magnification × 25.)

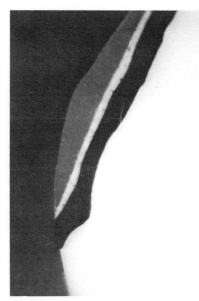

FIG. 8–8. Magnified view of a prepared tooth showing a lingual margin with an 80° bevel and a metal collar. (Original magnification × 25.)

well as the same marginal adaptation, as the 80° bevel with an all-metal collar.[20]

80° Facial Bevel with Porcelain Covering Metal Collar.
The complete bevel prepared with a plug finishing bur has an 80° or greater convergence angle (Fig. 8–8). Porcelain baked onto this labial apron will fracture off due to the flexure of the metal in the apron area.

80° Facial Bevel with Metal Collar.
For small and large splints or fixed prostheses, a full shoulder with a 360° encirclement by a bevel is required for closure at the termination of the preparation. The bevel should extend only about 0.5 mm into the labial sulcus area (Fig. 8–9). The metal collar is not a limiting factor in the fabrication of a fixed prosthesis. It can be used in a single full coverage restoration or for fixed partial prostheses.

Full Shoulder with a Bevel and a Facial Butt Joint Preparation.
The bevel is prepared on the proximal and lingual surfaces of the preparation, but not on the facial surface. The labial surface terminates in a butt joint shoulder finishing line to avoid showing a labial metal collar. In addition, for porcelain to be esthetically acceptable, 1.5 mm of thickness must be obtained for the opaque layer and body porcelain. This space does not exist at the margin of a bevel or knife-edged finishing line preparation if optimum crown contours are created. This type of finishing line is satisfactory for single or multiple unit splints of up to six units, especially when the labial gingival tissue is thin or almost transparent. For larger splints over six units, a butt joint is not recommended because of the contraction of the metal during baking of porcelain and the concomitant lack of marginal integrity.

Impression Considerations

The preferred method of impressioning full coverage preparations uses elastomeric materials. Tissue management is accomplished by preparing the teeth as described below and by creating both the bevel and room in the sulcular area for the impression material through gingival rotary curettage using a 12-fluted blunted plug finishing bur. Gingival retraction cords are not used for gingival retraction, but rather for maintaining the newly created space at the time of impressioning. If the soft tissues are healthy and the margins of the preparation were not extended more than 0.5 mm into the gingival sulcus the gingiva will not bleed during impression making. Only a No. 1 or No. 2 cord is necessary to maintain the sulcular space for the elastomeric materials (Fig. 8–10). An opposing irreversible hydrocolloid impression is also made. The dies of the individual preparations should be trimmed by the dentist, not by the technician. Prior to sectioning the cast for trimming preparation dies, the models should be mounted in an "indexed" mounting system (e.g., Accu-Trac or Pindex Systems, Coltene/Whaldent; Di-Lok System, Di-Equi Corp.) An impression of a tooth is not completed until a likeness of the prepared tooth is given to the laboratory technician for crown fabrication. If the responsibility of die preparation is given to the technician, errors in marginal placement are likely to occur. Thus, it behooves the clinician to take the time to prepare the dies prior to wax-up. Models can be returned from the laboratory with removable dies ready for trimming, or the dentist can send completed casts using a die relating system. In most cases, a cast can be poured, indexed, and the dies trimmed in the same day with little alteration in schedule. One layer of die spacer is painted over the die, down to but not including the shoulder and bevel. A

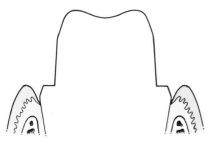

FIG. 8–9. Proper placement of the finishing line. The bevel should extend only about 0.5 mm into the labial sulcus area.

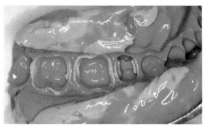

FIG. 8–10. In order to obtain adequate impressions of the gingival margin, a No. 1 or No. 2 retraction cord is necessary to maintain the sulcular space.

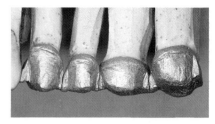

FIG. 8–11. To prevent porcelain fracture, the metal support in the crown must be adequate. The most common area of porcelain breakage is in the interproximal area, where many crowns are devoid of metal. Dies show castings with metal contacts and adequate support for porcelain.

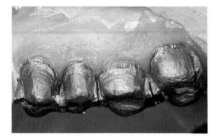

FIG. 8–12. Dies transferred to a soft tissue model for porcelain margin definition and the creation of proper crown contour.

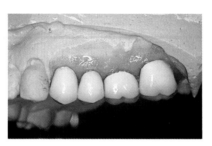

FIG. 8–13. Completed crowns with properly supported porcelain. Note that the crowns are well contoured and have adequate space for the interdental papilla.

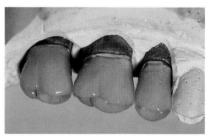

FIG. 8–14. Buccal view of maxillary second premolar and first and second molars. Optimum biologic contours enhance periodontal health. The 80° bevels are not covered by porcelain. Interproximal contact areas are placed in the occlusal one-third of the tooth. The gray color of the metal is plated with a yellow-gold color to give a softer appearance.

thin layer of cyanoacrylate is then painted in the ditched area, up to but not including the termination of the bevel, to prevent the chipping or scraping away of this area during laboratory procedures. The full-arch articulated casts with trimmed dies are then sent to the laboratory for wax-up and fabrication of the ceramo-metal castings.

Framework Considerations

One of the most important steps in the construction of the ceramometal restoration is the design of the metal framework. The metal frame must resemble the completed restoration, except the labial, lingual, and occlusal surfaces of abutments and pontics which are 1.5 mm smaller and the incisal surface is 2 mm smaller to allow for the support of porcelain and creation of a uniform shade. The connection areas are placed toward the lingual surface with adequate room for opaque, porcelain, and a deep facial embrasure in order to create individuality and the illusion of depth in the definitive porcelain-fused-to-metal restoration. If the dentist is concerned about porcelain fracture, the connection areas can be waxed, cast up to the occlusal surface posteriorly for support, and to occlusally contact the opposing teeth (Figs. 8–11 to 8–13). If the metal is gold-plated, it can mimic the interproximal occlusal embrasure space. Anteriorly, the connection areas should not interfere with the gingival embrasures or incisally with translucency or the incisal embrasure.

The work authorization should specify the placement and height of interproximal struts, the presence of metal occlusal contacts (when fabricating a posterior ceramo-metal restoration), and the type of metal desired. For anterior restorations the work authorization should also include the need for metal lingual contact, depending on the individual anterior guidance factors. The contact areas between adjacent teeth or restorations should be in metal and not in porcelain, posteriorly. If the contact point is porcelain instead of metal and the porcelain marginal ridge area fractures, a food impaction area will result and the crown will need replacement. Therefore, the interproximal metal struts on individual crowns should extend up to within 1 mm of the occlusal surface of the porcelain and should contain the contact area or point that is required. When the technician returns the ceramometal casting to the dentist, it should be tried in the mouth for gingival fit, contour, occlusion, and contact with adjacent teeth. The adaptation of the internal surface of the casting should be checked using either Cavitec cement (Kerr/Sybron, Inc.), Multiform paste, or a polysiloxane paste (e.g., Pressure Indicating Material, Coltene, Inc.), as indicating materials. Next, using a small bur, the dentist should scribe the termination of porcelain on the labial surface of the casting, at the facial gingival margin. This mark is a guide for the technician for termination of facial porcelain because no porcelain should be baked onto the apron of the crown casting; this area is thin and flexible, thus porcelain baked on it will fracture. By scribing the termination of the veneering material intraorally, allowance is made for a small gold collar or finishing line that is hidden in the sulcus area.

CLINICAL TIP. Intraoral scribing eliminates the laboratory guess work regarding the subgingival termination of the porcelain and results in maximal esthetics.

CLINICAL TIP. After the porcelain veneer has been baked and glazed, a gold-plating solution may be used to impart a yellow color to gray ceramometal casting. The gray color of the metal adds a darkness to the gingiva. The plated yellow gold color gives a softer, "self masking" appearance and thus will be more acceptable to the patient (Fig. 8–14).

Pontic Design

Sanitary Pontic. The sanitary pontic (Fig. 8–15) with no tissue contact is an alternative to the ridge lap pontic. It possesses the occlusal form and function of the tooth it replaces, but has a rounded gingival surface that does not extend to the residual ridge. This pontic is used when an esthetic replacement is not required. It, however, may be used in mandibular molar areas when desired. Maintenance of a hygienic condition of the ridge is generally satisfactory when the pontic, with rounded contours, is kept 2 to 3 mm above the ridge. When the pontic tissue clearance is less than 2 mm, it contributes to food entrapment.[13]

Ridge Lap Pontic. Ante stated "A pontic must restore the dentition to proper form and function while pre-serving the esthetic quality of the tooth it replaces, ensure its sanitation and be biologically acceptable to the tissue."[21] Ideally, a pontic would exactly duplicate the tooth it replaces. However, the residual ridge over which the pontic will be placed is usually convex.[22] Consequently, that surface of the pontic contacting the mucosa would be concave if the pontic were to recreate the natural tooth shape at the gingival area. This maximum tissue contact pontic design, known as the ridge lap or saddle pontic (Fig. 8–15), is undesirable because a concave surface is difficult to clean, resulting in soft tissue irritation with concomitant periodontal problems.[23]

Modified Ridge Lap Pontic. In the modified ridge lap design (Fig. 8–15)[24] the facial aspect of the pontic assumes the shape of the replaced tooth and contacts the soft tissue only on the buccal half of the ridge. This allows for maximum esthetics. The tissue contact is minimal and the underside of the pontic does not follow the convex anatomy of the residual ridge, as in the ridge lap design. Instead, a rounded convex surface unites with the lingual portion of the pontic in a smooth, easily cleansed design. Despite improved esthetics and control of sanitation, some problems surface soon after insertion of the fixed prosthesis.

1. Despite hygienic procedures, the concave tissue surfaces of the pontics invariably become coated with plaque and debris. The corresponding ridge surfaces usually become red and inflamed.[25]
2. The triangular area of the linguopalatal surface traps food particles and also annoys the patient's tongue.
3. The pontic may not provide adequate air seal for desired or correct phonation during speech.
4. The space that exists between pontic and ridge or pontic and abutment may permit droplets of saliva to be forced through during speech sounds causing annoyance and embarrassment.[26]

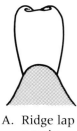 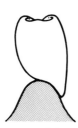 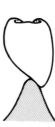 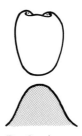 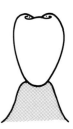

| A. Ridge lap pontic | B. Modified ridge lap pontic | C. Stein pontic | D. Sanitary pontic | E. Ovate pontic |

FIG. 8–15. Relationship of pontic design to residual ridge. A. Ridge lap pontic. This type of pontic demonstrates unacceptable excess tissue contact and is difficult to maintain hygienically. B. Modified ridge lap pontic. This type of pontic demonstrates acceptable esthetics and works best with broad edentulous ridges. C. "Stein" pontic. This type of pontic is designed for sharp edentulous ridges and exhibits minimal tissue contact and acceptable esthetics. It is contraindicated in edentulous ridges with broad buccolingual dimensions. D. Sanitary pontic. This type of pontic is 2 to 3 mm distant from the ridge. This design is easily cleaned and allows for a free flow of food beneath the pontic. It, however, exhibits unacceptable esthetics. E. Ovate pontic. This type of pontic exhibits excellent esthetics and function. It produces minimal tissue contact and is very hygienic. However, if ridge resorption occurs deterioration of esthetics results.

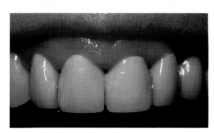

FIG. 8–16. *Illusions can be used to enhance teeth, especially when a very light shade is used. The labial surfaces are curved, the interproximal areas are stained orange-brown to enhance individuality and the incisal length and curvature follows the smile line of the lower lip. The contour of the gingival one-third presents a straight emergence profile to enhance the health of the surrounding soft tissues. Adequate interproximal room is provided for the gingival papilla and gingival embrasures.*

Stein Pontic. The Stein pontic (Fig. 8–15) is a variation of the modified ridge lap pontic. It is designed for sharp edentulous ridges, exhibits minimal tissue contact, and offers acceptable esthetics. It is contraindicated in edentulous ridges with broad buccolingual dimensions.

Ovate Pontic. The most functional and esthetic pontic is the ovate pontic (Fig. 8–15). It requires plastic reconstructive surgery of the ridge to create a concavity. In the preparation of an ovate pontic, an egg-shaped form is produced on the tissue surface that blends into the cervical one-third of the pontic and the tissue surface of the pontic is glazed and polished to a smooth finish. When properly placed, the pontic appears to emerge from the surgically created corpus of the ridge, affording a more natural and pleasing effect. Cleansing of soft tissue and the pontic is expedited and effective. A properly contoured ovate pontic automatically creates interdental papillae which fill the embrasures, thereby eliminating the dark space triangles between teeth, reducing the escape of saliva during speech, and reducing occasional lisping sounds. The ovate pontic is a necessity in patients with a high smile line. It is contraindicated in or against a knife-edged ridge. It is important that the residual ridge is capable of being augmented in buccolingual thickness to contain the ovate pontic within the body of the ridge. (See Chapter 21—Esthetics and Periodontics.)

BASIC CONSIDERATIONS IN TOOTH FORM

Patient Personality and Gender

The dentist is obligated to acquaint himself with all factors of personality that can be gleaned from the patient. Oral examination, history, and the many aspects relevant to the patient's esthetic requirements and expectations should serve the dentist well in the attempt to provide the most esthetic and functional prosthesis possible.

Endless combinations and variations of physical attributes exist in men and women, but a complete analysis also accounts for personality factors. In general, masculinity is associated with vigorous, strong, and robust qualities, whereas femininity is translated in terms of softness, delicacy, and curvature of anatomic form. (See Chapter 2—Fundamentals of Esthetics.)

By selecting and modifying a tooth form, the dentist is creating an image of the patient. By placing the two maxillary central incisors boldly in a dominating position, around which the lateral incisors are rotated and elevated slightly above the plane of occlusion, the sense of vigorous domination is established in the position of the maxillary central incisors. A small maxillary lateral incisor confers the appearance of femininity, whereas lateral incisors that are almost as broad as central incisors confer ruggedness and masculinity. A patient with a "delicate" appearance often has lighter skin and, consequently, lighter teeth.

The maxillary canines are important because they are easily visible from a frontal or lateral view, and serve as a gateway to the posterior teeth. By turning the tip of the canine inward, one may prevent a toothy, and possibly[27] anthropoidal appearance, however, the mesial aspect of the canine should not be hidden when viewed from directly in front of the patient.

An important factor to consider in all cases is the age of the patient. The dentist is seeking to create, when necessary, the desired illusion of a natural tooth in the oral environment. Age and concomitant changes bring challenges to the creative dentist trying to fabricate an artistically acceptable prosthesis. Studying changes wrought by time, and their visibility in relation to the planned porcelain restoration may suggest appropriate modifications, such as cuspal reductions caused by wear, reduction of translucent incisal edges of anterior teeth, color change, possible change in the shape of papillae and, of course, changes in chroma and value.

A study of the position of natural teeth reveals:[27]

1. Roundness of the arch form denotes femininity; squareness denotes masculinity.
2. Incisal edges of maxillary teeth of women follow the curve of the lower lip.
3. When females speak, smile, or laugh, they expose more maxillary teeth than males do. The maxillary first premolars should be contoured to conform with the canines.
4. In males, a square incisal silhouette with prominence of the maxillary central incisors and canines may indicate a bolder and more vigorous personality.

It is an inspiring challenge to the dentist to duplicate as closely as possible the qualities of the natural teeth, resulting in unobtrusive functional and harmonious restorations. (See Chapter 2—Fundamentals of Esthetics.)

Alignment of the Gingival Margins

Alignment of the gingival margins usually enhances the cosmetic result. This should be a bilaterally balanced alignment. When discrepancies are visible, refer the patient for periodontal correction before tooth preparation begins. (See Chapter 18—Esthetics and Electrosurgery and Chapter 21—Esthetics and Periodontics.)

Hue, Chroma, and Value

Preston and Bergen[28] note:

1. **Hue**. "That dimension of color used to distinguish one family of color from another." The physical hue order is, by the common names, violet, blue, green, yellow, orange, and red. It is usually defined by the color family name.
2. **Chroma**. "That quality by which one distinguishes a weak hue from a stronger, more intense hue. It is the amount of a basic hue added to gray. If more colorant is added, a stronger, more intense hue (higher chroma) results." It is also referred to as "saturation." Chroma denotes the concentration or strength of the basic hue. Intense color indicates a higher chroma or saturation.
3. **Value**. "That quality by which one distinguishes a light color from a dark color; a gray scale that extends from black to white. It has nothing to do with the amount of gray in a color—only the relative level of brightness, lightness or brilliance. It is not a quantitative, but rather a qualitative description. Value is found by comparing the chosen color to a color of similar brightness." Colors of low value are more like black; colors of high value are more like white. Value, a quality of grayness, is an important factor of color, both to the dentist and the technician, who should be able to separate value from other dimensions and detect and control differences that could prove disastrous to shade matching.

One of the simplest modifications is to raise the chroma of the dominant hue. The modification of the chroma that is too high is more difficult. If a lower chroma is needed, the color must be neutralized by its complement. The most obvious color one might use to raise value is white. The technician should be fully versed in the many ways of managing dentists' requests for modifications and characterizations and communication should be thoroughly clear. (See Chapter 2—Fundamentals of Esthetics and Appendix A, Custom Staining.)

Poor esthetics are exacerbated by the use of too light a shade, staining, and coloring which create artificiality.

The dentist should differentiate hue, value, and chroma of the patient's natural teeth and then apply these factors to the porcelain tooth or teeth to be fabricated.[29] Concentrating on these aspects for 5 second intervals helps to prevent retinal fatigue (retinal adaptation), thus permitting shade differences to be more readily detected. One of the most important factors to communicate to the technician is the type of tooth enamel being matched, i.e., opaque, translucent, dull, or highly reflective. No matter how beautifully the color has been incorporated in the porcelain restoration or how skillfully the tooth has been contoured, a high glossy glaze is incompatible with the appearance of the enamel of the surrounding teeth if the latter are comparatively dull.

Ceramometal procedures require the thinnest layer of porcelain opaquing materials that still block out the metal casting surface. Covering this opaque masking with a thin layer of translucent body and incisal porcelain permits the restoration to become highly reflective. As such, the tooth cannot be compatible with its adjacent natural teeth.

CLINICAL TIP. To compensate for high light reflection, caused by thin layers of translucent porcelain covering an opaque mask, select shades that are slightly lower in value than the surrounding teeth.[13] This should not result in reduced brightness of the restoration.

Positioning the restoration more lingually and increasing the incisal curvature directs the light in various directions away from the viewer. The contour and texture of the outer porcelain surface defines the character of the restoration and contributes vitality to its appearance. Each tooth is individualized and characterized by a distinct outline form. The incisal form and tooth position influence esthetics more than any other aspect, because the tooth is silhouetted against the dark shadow of the oral cavity.

Creation of Dental Illusions

The size of the teeth (length and width) may be influenced by contours of the teeth and the effects of light reflections (Fig. 8–16). For example, the maxillary central incisors reflect light anteriorly, superiorly, inferiorly, and laterally. By contouring the facial or labial aspects to deflect the light in directions other than forward, e.g., curving the lateral aspects into embrasures, the tooth may be made to appear narrower and longer. Reflecting light superiorly in the gingival one-third (by contouring) and inferiorly in the incisal curve, should give the illusion of a shorter and broader maxillary tooth. In the case of malpositioned teeth, it may be necessary to create the illusion of a wider tooth in a small space. This can be effected by bringing the contact points as far labially as possible and flattening the surfaces to reflect all the light labially. Similarly, a diastema can be eliminated by porcelain crowns that make contact in lingually positioned embrasure, and that have narrow facial aspects to reflect a smaller tooth. The curves moved laterally into the embrasures permit the light to be deflected away from the viewer[13] (see Chapter 2—Fundamentals of Esthetics). The facial forms of the adjacent crowns should curve into one another in the areas of the proximal contact rather than be separated by a thin straight disk.

Surface texturing that is similar to adjacent natural teeth is an important feature of the restored tooth. It produces an interplay of light and creates pleasant color matching experiences.

Horizontal and vertical lines affect the apparent width or length of the tooth being fabricated.

In addition to the variables of color and contour the technician should be informed of all aspects involving the compatibility of the porcelain with various aspects of the remaining natural teeth.

A removable bridge affords the advantage of trial

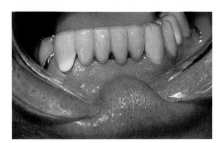

FIG. 8–17. Preoperative view of a mandibular fixed porcelain-fused-to-gold restoration that required replacement because of recurrent caries. The restorations appear as a single mass of porcelain and lacks individualization of the teeth and proper color characterization. Placing the pontics on the crest of the residual ridge creates dark spaces.

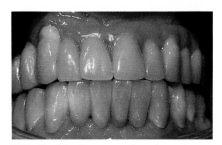

FIG. 8–18. Postoperative view shows a prosthesis that exhibits overlapping of the mandibular incisors, which greatly improves the esthetics. Brown and orange-brown staining of the interproximal and labial surfaces diffuse the reflected light and enhances the individuality within the restoration. Open gingival and incisal embrasures have been maintained and proper placement over the residual ridge creates optimal esthetics.

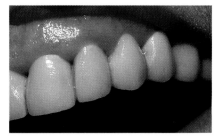

FIG. 8–19. Deep orange brown stain highlights the individuality within the restorations. Incisal embrasures are open, and curvature and incisal length follow the smile line from the central incisors to the canines.

CLINICAL TIP. Surface texturing should be slightly more emphasized on the restorations than that present on the adjacent tooth being matched because light is reflected differently from tooth enamel and glazed enamel.

---

seating in determining the size and form of the restorative teeth. Corrections can be made in wax in the process of repositioning, reshaping, or replacing the denture teeth. In fixed prosthodontics, temporary acrylic resin coverage serves a similar diagnostic step. By adjusting the plastic, the dentist may satisfy the patient's esthetic expectations. An impression and a poured stone model may serve as further instructional guidance for the laboratory technician.

A valuable aid in creating esthetic restorations is to place a degree of importance on the personality of the patient. Esthetic factors usually correlate with the patient's facial form and degree of facial symmetry. Rounded, blunt, or sharp distoincisal line angles of incisor teeth will greatly vary the visual perception of facial esthetics. Incisal embrasures should vary from one side of the tooth and arch to the other. The degree of space from the mesiolabial incisal line angle must contain both horizontal and vertical variations of this space.

Extrinsic staining and shading will highlight or illuminate the cosmetic result only when all the above factors have been satisfied. Incisal translucency, enamel hypocalcifications, enamel crazing line, and areas of wear can be accurately created in an esthetic restoration. Overcharacterization can mar the result and produce an unwanted, unsightly effect.

Poor esthetics occur when the teeth lack individuality. Poor esthetics are exacerbated by shade, staining, or coloring that is too light as well as by a lack of proper embrasures, surface texture, and contours. When all the above occur, the restoration appears flat, unindividualized, and of uniform color, giving the appearance of a single mass of porcelain, or what is known as "chicklets" (Figs. 8–17, 8–18). An acceptable cosmetic result is obtained in the following ways.

1. Avoid flatness by optimum fabrication of the curvature of the labial surfaces, which reflect light differently.
2. Use deep orange-brown stain interproximally to enhance the individuality of the prosthesis (Fig. 8–19).
3. Create deep incisal embrasures for individuality; the length and curvature of the incisal surfaces should follow the smile line of the lower lip.
4. Avoid gingival inflammation by providing adequate interproximal space for the papillae and gingival embrasures. The gingival terminations must not be overextended or shy of the margin, or too bulky which results in gingival problems. The labial gingival heights must be the same. The porcelain-fused-to-metal restorations should aid in maintenance of an optimal periodontal environment.[30]

MANAGEMENT OF MALALIGNED TEETH

Diastemata

Several methodologies may be used to create a favorable cosmetic result when diastemata are present or when teeth are rotated. The optimum method of treatment is to employ adult orthodontics, whether minor tooth movement or full banded complete therapy (see Chapter 22—Esthetics and Orthodontics).

CLINICAL TIP. If porcelain-fused-to-metal restorations are fabricated to close existing diastemata without prior orthodontics and if the occlusogingival height is not great, the resultant crowns will appear short and square. This may create a more unfavorable esthetic result than maintaining the diastemata.

ESTHETIC DENTISTRY

After tooth movement is complete, the teeth are held in place for at least 6 months by a fixed retainer. If the teeth are to be covered eventually, metal and acrylic resin fixed provisional restorations may be used as the fixed retainer. The major problem with adult orthodontics for closure of diastemata or correction of rotated or overlapped anterior teeth is the common need for splinting the teeth to maintain their positions after tooth movement, since they have a tendency to revert to their original positions.

Protruded Teeth

When a tooth is labially protruded, the surrounding facial soft tissue is thin. This is especially common with the maxillary canines. Orthodontic therapy is the treatment of choice (see Chapter 22—Esthetics and Orthodontics). If this tooth is to be covered with a restoration for realignment and cosmetics without orthodontic treatment, sufficient tooth structure must be removed to allow not only for metal and porcelain, but also for the realignment. Prophylactic endodontic therapy is often necessary. Second, the facial margin of the restoration cannot be carried subgingivally without the risk of gingival recession due to the thinness of this facial soft tissue. In addition, a pronounced labial bulge at the gingival margin of the definitive restoration cannot be avoided because of the facial angulation of the underlying root.

CLINICAL TIP. The patient must know the risks and the problems, as well as the anticipated cosmetic result of porcelain-fused-to-metal restorations placed without prior orthodontic treatment on malaligned or spaced anterior teeth. These problems can be demonstrated to the patient on a diagnostic wax-up before performing any irreversible dental procedures.

Tooth Reduction

Armamentarium

- Standard dental setup
    Explorer
    Mouth mirror
    Periodontal probe
    Appropriate anesthesia
    High-speed handpiece
    Low-speed handpiece
    Suitable size impression trays
- Diamond burs
    A football-shaped diamond stone, coarse or medium (e.g., 63-68-023 large or 63-68-016 small Brasseler USA).
    A shoulder diamond stone or a cylinder stone (e.g., 835-010, Brasseler USA).
    A 1-mm diameter shoulder diamond with a 3° taper (e.g., 6847-016, Brasseler USA) for molars or the smaller 811-033 (Brasseler USA) for premolars). The 45° bevel is formed with the Premier two striper DCB.5.

Clinical Technique

1. Administer the appropriate anesthesia.
2. Create two 1-mm 3° taper labial guide cuts with the shoulder diamond bur. The first cut follows the facial angle from the height of contour to the incisal edge. The second cut parallels the long axis of the tooth from the gingival margin to the height of contour. This ensures sufficient removal of tooth structure and a 3° taper.
3. For anterior teeth, prepare a third depth guide cut on the lingual surface from the gingival margin to the height of the cingulum, using the same shoulder diamond stone as for the labial surface. Prepare a fourth depth guide cut from the height of the cingulum to the incisal edge with a 1.2-mm shoulder stone.
   For posterior teeth, prepare two depth guide cuts on the lingual surface as described for the facial surface. Create an additional depth cut at least 1.5 mm deep on the occlusal surface to ensure adequate occlusal reduction.

CLINICAL TIP. To ensure sufficient room for incisal or occlussal porcelain and to prevent a restoration from being too protrusive, remove at least 1.5 mm of tooth structure from the incisal one-third of the labial surface.

4. Finish the preparation, except for the area incisal to the cingulum of anterior teeth, by following the depth guiding grooves.

CLINICAL TIP. Follow the height of contour of the soft tissues labially, lingually, and proximally. If the preparation extends too deeply within the sulcus, the sulcular epithelium and gingival attachment will be damaged, resulting in gingival inflammation and recession. Preparations extending too far subgingivally in the interproximal portions and those that do not follow the contour of the soft tissues may result in interproximal inflammation, as well as facial gingival recession.

5. For anterior teeth, reduce the height of the incisal edge by at least 2 mm.
6. For anterior teeth, prepare the area from the incisal edge to the cingulum with a football-shaped stone. The depth of preparation in this area must accommodate for the incisal guidance created in the diagnostic wax-up, as well as provide room for the metal, opaque, and porcelain of the restoration. If the pulp is large, a metal lingual surface may have to be used to avoid pulp exposure.
7. For the anterior teeth, verify tooth reduction, especially that area influencing the incisal guidance, with the transitional prosthesis. If the section incisal to the cingulum becomes thin or perforated, reprepare this area or alter the treatment plan (e.g., metal lingual, intentional endodontics, or selective grinding of opposing teeth) prior to impressioning the preparation.
8. Contour and polish the provisional restorations, and cement them with a sedative temporary cement. (See Chapter 13—Acrylic and Other Resins—Provisional Restorations.)
9. Dismiss the patient and evaluate the esthetics, tooth

contours, gingival health, and occlusion at the next office visit.

Bevel Placement

Once the esthetics of the provisional restorations are acceptable to both the dentist and the patient, create a finishing line.

Armamentarium

- Standard dental setup (see the preceding section on Tooth Reduction)
- Blunted 12-fluted steel finishing bur (e.g., GTB 300.11-14, Brasseler USA) which is manufactured with a blunted tip, or a fine diamond bur (e.g., 8863-012, Brasseler USA)

Clinical Technique. Prepare a bevel on the mesial, palatal, and distal margins with a blunted 12-fluted steel plug or fine diamond finishing bur (Figs. 8–20 to 8–23). Use a clockwise direction for beveling and a counterclockwise rotation for gingival curettage. Hold the bur parallel to the path of insertion. The bevels and subgingival buccal shoulder must not violate the biologic width (see Chapter 21– Esthetics and Periodontics).

Tissue Management and Impressioning

Armamentarium

- Standard dental setup (see the section on Tooth Reduction)
- No. 1 gingival retraction chord
- No. 2 gingival retraction chord
- Suitable impression material

Clinical Technique

1. Bevel placement, creates adequate room in the sulcular area for the impression material.

CLINICAL TIP. Gingival retraction cords are not used for gingival retraction at the time of impressioning, but rather to maintain the space created while beveling.

---

2. There should be no gingival bleeding at the time of impression making. If the soft tissues are healthy and were managed without extending the margins of the preparation more than 0.5 mm into the gingival sulcus, the gingiva will not bleed.
3. Only a No. 1 or No. 2 cord is necessary to maintain the sulcular space for the impression material.
4. The single strand of cord should be fully visible when in place. It is not used for retraction, but rather to maintain the prepared sulcus.
5. Make a final impression of the preparations.
6. Make an irreversible hydrocolloid impression of the opposing arch.
7. Prior to sectioning the cast for trimming preparation dies, the models should be mounted in an "indexed"

mounting system (e.g., Accu-Trac or Pindex Systems, Coltene/Whaldent; Di-Lok System, Di-Equi Corp.).

8. After securing the dies, trim and ditch them below the end of the preparation.

CLINICAL TIP. To ensure proper delineation of the margin, the individual dies should be trimmed by the dentist. Models can be returned from the laboratory with removable dies ready for trimming or the dentist can send completed casts using an "indexed" mounting system (e.g., Accu-Trac or Pindex Systems, Coltene/Whaldent; Di-Lok System, Di-Equi Corp.). With practice, casts can usually be poured, indexed, and the dies trimmed in one day, with little alteration in the practitioner's schedule.

Die Trimming and Preparation
Armamentarium

- Denture vulcanite bur
- No. 6 handpiece round bur
- Die spacer-0.25 mm thickness (George Taub Products)
- Cyanoacrylate

Clinical Technique

1. Trim the die first with a vulcanite bur.
2. Ditch below the bevel with a No. 6 round bur.
3. Paint a single layer of die spacer over the entire die, except for auxiliary grooves, at the shoulder and bevel.
4. Paint a thin layer of cyanoacrylate over the termination of the bevel to prevent chipping or scraping away of this area during laboratory procedures.
5. Articulate the full-arch casts (with trimmed dies) and send instructions to the laboratory for wax-up and fabrication of the ceramometal castings.

Work Authorization

The work authorization should specify the placement and height of interproximal struts, metal occlusal contacts (when fabricating a posterior ceramometal restoration), and the type of metal that the dentist desires. For anterior restorations, the work authorization should also include the need for metal lingual contact, depending on the individual anterior guidance factors. Emphasize to the laboratory that the contact areas between adjacent teeth or restorations should be in metal and not in porcelain, posteriorly.

CLINICAL TIP. If the contact point is in porcelain instead of metal and the porcelain marginal ridge area fractures, a food impaction area results and the crown will have to be remade. Therefore, the interproximal metal struts on individual crowns should extend up to within 1 mm of the occlusal surface of the porcelain and should contain the contact area or point that is required.

Try-In of Castings
Armamentarium

- Standard dental setup (see the section on Tooth Reduction)

FIG. 8–20. Preoperative view of unesthetic right central incisor requiring a full coverage restoration.

FIG. 8–21. The tooth is prepared with a labial butt joint and a mesial, distal, and lingual full shoulder with an 80° bevel.

FIG. 8–22. Palatal view of the patient shown in Figure 8-20.

FIG. 8–23. The provisional restoration is contoured, polished, and cemented with a sedative temporary cement. A gingivectomy was performed to improve soft tissue esthetics.

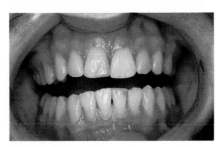

FIG. 8–20

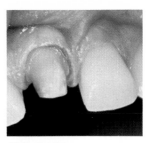

FIG. 8–21

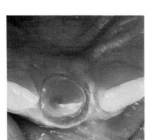

FIG. 8–22

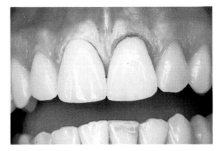

FIG. 8–23

- Indicating paste
  Cavitec cement (Kerr/Sybron, Inc.) or Multiform paste (Surgident, Corp.) or polysiloxane material (e.g., Pressure spot indicator, Coltene/Whaldent)
- No. 1 round bur

Clinical Technique

1. Check the adaptation of the internal surface of the casting using either Cavitec cement, Multiform paste, or a polysiloxane material, as indicating materials.
2. Check the castings in the mouth for gingival fit, contour, occlusion, and contact with adjacent teeth.
3. Using a small bur, scribe the desired location of the termination of porcelain on the labial surface of the casting, at the facial gingival margin.

CLINICAL TIP. A scribed line serves as a guide for the technician for the cervical termination of facial porcelain and allows the thin metal collar or finishing line to be hidden in the sulcus area.

Soft Tissue Models and Shade Selection

CLINICAL TIP. Crown contours are critical for establishing esthetics and maintaining gingival health. A soft tissue cast is helpful in this regard, especially in anterior teeth. Create the soft tissue model after the castings are tried in and found to be clinically acceptable.

Armamentarium

- Standard dental setup (see the section on Tooth Reduction)
- Suitable luting agent
- Autopolymerizing acrylic resin (e.g., Duralay, Reliance Corp.)

- Suitable impression material, e.g., irreversible hydrocolloid
- Metal retention device, e.g., flat headed screws or bent dowel pins
- Soft Denture Reline Acrylic (ex. Coe Soft, Kerr Manufacturing Co.)
- Self-curing pink acrylic (e.g., Jet Pink Acrylic, Lang Dental Manufacturing Co., Inc.)
- Yellow stone

Clinical Technique

1. Lute the castings together intraorally with red autopolymerizing acrylic resin.
2. Make an overall irreversible hydrocolloid impression with the castings reseated firmly into the index.
3. Flow a soupy mix of red autopolymerizing acrylic resin into the occlusal two-thirds of the casting and insert a flat headed screw or bent dowel pin into the stone cast for retention.
4. Cover the gingival area surrounding the castings with a mixture of two parts resilient autopolymerizing denture liner and one part hard pink autopolymerizing acrylic resin.[31]

CLINICAL TIP. Apply the mixture with a standard disposable syringe. Then sprinkle acrylic beads onto the surface to facilitate union with the subsequent die stone cast.

---

5. Make an irreversible hydrocolloid impression of the provisional restoration and send models to the laboratory.
6. Select a shade and prepare a proper laboratory prescription, including required characterization. (See the sections on Basic Considerations in Tooth Form,

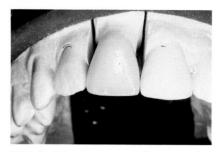

FIG. 8-24. The crown is inspected for marginal fit, porcelain imperfections, and proper esthetics.

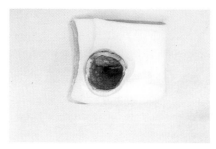

FIG. 8-25. The internal aspect of the crown shows a clearly defined finishing line and labial porcelain.

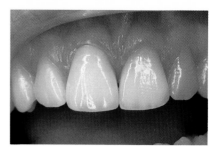

FIG. 8-26. The final restoration.

and Hue, Chroma, and Value; see also Chapter 2—Fundamentals of Esthetics.)

CLINICAL TIP. With a small No. 1 round bur, scribe the porcelain termination line on the labial surface of the casting at the facial gingival margin. This line will serve as a guide for the technician for the cervical termination of the facial porcelain and allow the thin metal collar or finishing line to be hidden within the sulcus area.

CLINICAL TIP. Use intrinsic, rather than extrinsic, stains because intrinsic staining will not be eliminated when the crown is reshaped by the clinician or technician. In addition, intrinsic stains have a more realistic appearance than surface stains.

Porcelain Try-In

Armamentarium

- Standard dental setup (see the section on Tooth Reduction)

Clinical Technique

1. The laboratory should only use low-speed handpiece fine green stones or fine diamond stones to recarve the bisque bake porcelain.
2. Correct the points or areas of contact until unwaxed extra fine dental floss just snaps through.
3. Refine the crown contours intraorally with appropriate high-speed diamond stones and copious amounts of water to avoid overheating and fracturing the veneering material.
4. Refine the occlusion. If the cast is inaccurate, make another impression. If the articulation is incorrect, remount the case prior to returning it to the laboratory.

CLINICAL TIP. Perform extensive additions directly on the model, using ivory wax. Take an irreversible hydrocolloid impression of these altered restorations and make a cast. This creates a guide for the technician to make the required alterations.

---

5. When splinting a posterior quadrant, the metal interproximal struts can be maintained up to and including the occlusal surface for maintenance of occlusal

stability in patients with a high risk of porcelain fracture. (See the section on Framework Considerations.) Correct centric occlusal discrepancies on the articulator, on which the casts had been previously mounted according to verified maxillomandibular recordings.
6. Correct small discrepancies in eccentric movements intraorally.
7. Return the bisque bake restoration to the laboratory with the proper work authorization, including the required alterations and a shade guide tab or a drawing of the selected color indicating placement of gingival, body, and incisal shades, and character variations (Figs. 8-24, 8-25).

CLINICAL TIP. To maintain a natural appearance and surface texture, use the natural glaze of the porcelain, rather than painting on a low temperature glaze after applying surface stains.

CLINICAL TIP. If the original bisque bake does not match the selected color, return the chosen shade guide tab to the laboratory. Alternatively, an acrylic shade guide tab can be modified to the correct shade of the provisional restoration using an acrylic resin stain kit (e.g., Minute Stain, George Taub Products).

Trial Cementation and Final Cementation

Use a trial cementation on multiple unit cases for final evaluation of esthetics, occlusion, and other potential processing errors. Then place the restoration with the definitive cement (Fig 8-26).

CONCLUSION

The procedures described in this chapter involve newer concepts and techniques. The diagnostic phase permits consultation and treatment planning between two disciplines. The introduction of new surgical and prosthetic techniques permits the solution of more problems with greater patient satisfaction.

The clinician should discuss treatment plans and esthetic goals directly with the patient in order to achieve a satisfactory result. The surgeon is responsible for ensuring that all prosthetic and esthetic goals are clearly defined. Thus, preprosthetic and presurgical planning and joint consultations should occur as frequently as needed to determine the resolution of problems that may affect the result. Such problems may include the feasibility of the design of the pontics, the design of the provisional prosthesis, the nature of the ridge deformity and potential reconstruction, and unexpected complications.

REFERENCES

1. Craig, R.G.: Restorative Dental Materials, 7th Ed. St. Louis, C.V. Mosby Co., p. 354, 1985.

2. Asgar, K: Casting materials. International State-of-the-Art Conference on Restorative Dental Materials. Natl Inst Health, pp. 105–123, 1986.

3. Phillips, R.W.: Skinners Science of Dental Materials, 8th Ed. Philadelphia, W.B. Saunders Co., p. 520, 1982.

4. McLean, J.W.: The Science and Art of Dental Ceramics, Vol. II. Bridge Design and Laboratory Proceedings in Dental Ceramics. Chicago, Quintessence Publishing Co. Inc., 1980.

5. Cascone, P.J.: The theory of bonding for porcelain-to-metal systems. In Yamaha, H. and Grenoble, P.: Dental Porcelain. The State of the Art. University of Southern California Conference Proceedings, 1977.

6. Williams, D.F.: Materials in Clinical Dentistry. New York, Oxford University Press, 1979

7. Avner, S.H.: Introduction to Physical Metallurgy, New York, McGraw Hill, 1974.

8. Vickery, R.C. and Badinelli, L.A.: Nature of attachment forces in porcelain-gold systems. J Dent Res 47:683, 1968.

9. Tuccillo, J.J.: Dental restorations combining dental porcelain and improved white gold alloy. U.S. Patents 3,961,420 and 3,981,723, 1976.

10. Tuccillo, J.J.: Comments at the International State-of-the-Art Conference on Restorative Dental Materials. Natl Inst Health, pp. 151–155, 1986.

11. Ingersoll, C.: Tarnish resistant palladium base dental casting alloy. U.S. Patent 113,929,474, 1975.

12. Cascone, P.J.: Low dental alloy. U.S. Patents 4,523,262, and 4,539,176, 1978, 1985.

13. Eissman, H.S., Rudd, K.D., and Marrow, R.M.: Dental Laboratory Procedures in Fixed Partial Dentures, Vol. 2. St Louis, C.V. Mosby Co., 1980.

14. Perel, M.L.: Periodontal considerations of crown contours. J Prosthet Dent, 26:627, 1971.

15. Wheeler, R.C.: Complete crown form and the periodontium. J Prosthet Dent 11:722, 1961.

16. Yuodelis, R.A., Weaver, J.D., and Sapkos, S.: Facial and lingual contours of artificial crown restorations and their effects on the periodontium. J. Prosthet. Dent 29:61, 1973.

17. Schwartz, H.: Anterior guidance and aesthetics in prosthodontics. Dent Clin North Am 31:323, 1987.

18. Zinner, I.D., Trachtenberg, D.I., and Miller, R.D.: Provisional restorations in fixed prosthodontics. Dent Clin North Am, 33:355, 1979.

19. Panno, F.V.: Preparation and management to full coverage restorations for combination fixed removable prostheses. Dent Clin North Am 31:505, 1987.

20. Panno, F.V., Vahidi, F., Gulker, I.A., et al: Evaluation of the 45-degree labial bevel with a shoulder preparation. J Prosthet Dent 56:655, 1986.

21. Ante, I.H.: The fundamentals principals, designs and construction of crown and bridge prosthesis. Dent Items Interest 1:215, 1928.

22. Abrams, H., Kopczyk, R., and Kaplan, A.: Incidence of anterior ridge deformities in partially edentulous patients. J Prosthet Dent 57:191, 1987.

23. Stein, R.S.: Pontic-residual ridge relationships: a research report. J Prosthet Dent 16:251, 1966.

24. Langer, B. and Calagna, L.: The subepithelial connective tissue graft. J Prosthet Dent 44:363, 1980.

25. Hirschberg, S.M.: The relationship of oral hygiene to embrasure and pontic design—a preliminary study. J Prosthet Dent 27:26, 1972.

26. Seibert, J.S. and Cohen, D.W.: Periodontal Considerations in Preparation for Fixed and Removable Prosthodontics. Dent Clin North Am 31:529, 1987.

27. Heartwell, C.M. and Rahn, A.O.: Syllabus of Complete Dentures, 4th Ed. Philadelphia, Lea & Febiger, 1986.

28. Preston, J.D. and Bergen, S.F.: Color Science and Dental Art. St. Louis, C.V. Mosby Co., 1980.

29. Pincus, C.L.: Achieving the Ultimate Esthetic Smile. Proceedings of the Second International Congress of Prosthodontics, 1979.

30. Seide, L.J. (ed.): A Dynamic Approach to Restorative Dentistry. Philadelphia, W.B. Saunders, 1980.

31. Pameijer, J.H.N.: Periodontal and Occlusal Factors in Crown and Bridge Procedures. Amsterdam, Holland, Dental Center for Postgraduate Courses, 1985.

Vincent Celenza, D.M.D.

CAST GLASS CERAMIC—FULL COVERAGE RESTORATIONS

9

The contemporary dental practitioner is faced with an ever-increasing assortment of restorative materials for use in single tooth rehabilitation. Technology in dental ceramics has led to new materials which, in selected situations, rival or surpass the conventional "standard" porcelain-fused-to-metal restoration.

HISTORY

Years of research in adapting "pyroceram," a well known industrial glass ceramic developed by Corning Glass Works, to dentistry culminated in the introduction of Dicor, a cast "glass ceramic," by Peter Adair and David Grossman in 1984.[1] Having properties of both glass and ceramic, pyroceram has been developed into literally thousands of chemical variants for production use.[2] Microchips, computer parts, cookware, and high temperature enduring automobile and aircraft engine parts, are some of the uses of pyroceram, which can be custom formulated to meet a wide variety of physical requirements. For dental purposes, Dicor cast glass ceramic has been developed as a restorative material that is strong, physically stable, nonabrasive, biocompatible, can be custom colored, and has thermal insulation properties (Table 9–1).[3-7]

CHARACTERISTICS

Creation of a cast glass ceramic restoration involves four fabrication steps (Fig. 9–1).

1. full anatomic wax-up
2. casting to a glassy state
3. "ceramming" to a crystalline glass ceramic
4. applying external colorants

The expected comparison of cast glass ceramic materials to conventional all-porcelain and porcelain-fused-to-metal systems reveals some distinct differences.

Chemistry

Chemically, many of the oxides of conventional feldspathic porcelains, such as silicon dioxide, potassium oxide, magnesium oxide, aluminum oxide, and zirconium oxide, are also used to make glass ceramic. However, the percentage amounts, the standardization of component chemical compounds, and the method of fabrication, make these materials completely dissimilar. Batch to batch variations are nearly eliminated with glass ceramic because large quantities are manufactured under strict quality control in an effort to produce a consistent material. Conventional feldspathic porcelain systems are many and varied in composition, properties, and technical handling characteristics. An experienced ceramist must be able to master all the variables relevant to a particular manufacturer's ceramic product, including manipulation of opaquing, body and incisal porcelains and color modifiers, compatibility with various metal substructures, firing temperatures, and much more. Cast glass ceramic fabrication involves a full contour anatomic wax-up that is sprued, invested, burned-out, and cast in a manner similar to that used in conventional crown and bridge metal casting techniques.[5,8]

Strength

The strength of conventional porcelain-fused-to-metal restorations has been relied upon for years. Nevertheless, problems occur. Traditional all-porcelain jacket crown systems are even more subject to fracture, crazing, and chipping, and therefore are considered too weak for posterior applications.[9] Griffith flaws, microscopic defects created during the sintering process of porcelain fabrication, are present in all fired porcelain and are largely responsible for crack propagation.[10] Subsurface porosity, discoloration (greening or graying), cracking, and bond failure may also occur.[9] Glass

TABLE 9–1. PROPERTIES OF METALS

PROPERTY	CAST CERAMIC*	ENAMEL†	DENTIN†	PORCELAIN*	COMPOSITE RESIN†	GOLD ALLOY†	AMALGAM†
Density g/cm^3	2.7	3.0	2.2	2.4	2.0	14.0	11.0
Refractive Index	1.52	1.65	—	—	—	0	0
Translucency	0.56	0.48	—	0.27	.55–.70	0	0
Thermal Conductivity cal/sec/cm^2/C/cm	.0040	.0022	.0015	.0030	.0026	.7	.055
Thermal Diffusivity mm^2/sec	.800	.469	.183	.640	.675	119	9.6
Coefficient of Expansion $\times 10^{-6/C}$	7.2	<11.4>	—	8.0	26–40	14.4	22–28
M.O.R. MPa	152	10.3	51.7	75.9	45.5	448	69
Compressive Strength MPa	828	400	297	172	194	—	379
Modulus of Elasticity MPa	70.3	84.1	18.3	82.8	16.3	90	62
Microhardness KHN$_{100}$	362	343	68	460	30	90–220	110

*Internal measurements from the Physical Properties Department, Corning Glass Works, Corning, NY.
†Data from Craig, R.G. (ed.): Restorative Dental Materials. St. Louis, C.V. Mosby Co., 1980.
(Adapted from Dicor Clinical Instructions for Dicor Restorations and the Use of the Dicor Light Activated Cementation Kit, Dentsply/York Division. Lab Products Dentsply International Inc., York, PA, 1988.)

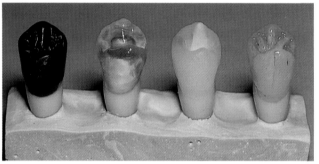

FIG. 9–1. The four laboratory steps involved in the fabrication of a cast glass restoration. From left to right: (1) full anatomic wax-up, (2) casting to a glassy state, (3) "ceramming" to a crystalline glass ceramic, and (4) external application of colorants.

ceramics, however, have compressive strengths greater than all-porcelain systems and can be used both anteriorly and posteriorly.[11,12] The crystalline structure of this material lessens the likelihood of crack propagation because the lattice structure is able to absorb compressive forces.[10] An adequate thickness (1.0 mm axially and 1.5 to 2.0 mm occlusally) of glass ceramic minimizes fracture susceptibility from excessive lateral or tensile forces from which the material is most vulnerable.[8,12,13] Nevertheless, restoration fracture may occur in the molar region and ceramometal restorations are better able to resist these compressive forces.

Abrasiveness

Porcelains can wear opposing natural, metal, or porcelain surfaces.[9,14,15,16] Rough, improperly glazed and finished surfaces are particularly abrasive, but even well finished porcelain surfaces can cause significant tooth wear. Metal occluding surfaces can minimize this effect, however, patient's often request esthetic porcelain oc-clusions. A carefully adjusted and finished porcelain occlusal surface is nevertheless considered a reasonable risk in the absence of parafunctional activity.[17] The hardness coefficients, and thus wear characteristics, of cast glass ceramic materials are similar to those of human enamel.[18] However, because the glass ceramic crowns can only be colored on the external surface, occlusal wear or adjustment after permanent cementation result in loss of color. This may not be an esthetic problem in the posterior teeth, depending on tooth position, the degree of color loss, and the patient's desires. Wear on the lingual surface of maxillary anterior teeth poses no esthetic problem. Thinning of the glass from severe ceramic abrasion could significantly weaken the restoration. Any patient who demonstrates bruxism, however, should be considered a candidate for an occlusal guard appliance, regardless of the restorative material selected.

Light Absorption and Refraction

The metal component of porcelain-fused-to-metal restorations prevents the transmission of light. Even diffusion of light through the porcelain is diminished where metal is present beneath the veneering porcelain.[9] Often, the marginal soft tissues adjacent to subgingivally placed metal collars appear dark, especially if the gingival tissues are thin. This effect may occur in porcelain-fused-to-metal restorations with labial butt joint designs because the small amount of porcelain covering the metal is opaque and creates a shadow of the root surface by blocking the normal transmission of light through the labial gingival tissues.[19]

Porcelain jackets, cast glass ceramic crowns, and natural teeth all allow light transmission because of the absence of a metal coping. However, dental porcelains refract light differently than cast glass ceramic and enamel.[9,12] The unorganized, random crystalline form of porcelain refracts approximately 25% of the available

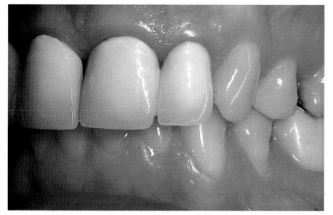

FIG. 9–2. Preoperative view of anterior porcelain-fused-to-metal crowns to be replaced for esthetic reasons.

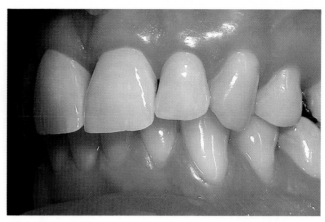

FIG. 9–3. Postoperative view of cast glass ceramic lateral and central incisors.

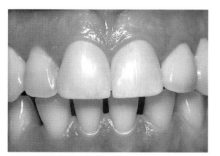

FIG. 9–4. The two central incisors are cast glass ceramic restoration. The patient's left lateral incisor is part of a three-unit porcelain-fused-to-metal bridge.

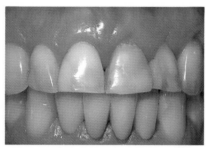

FIG. 9–5. These four maxillary incisors were repeatedly restored with composite resin. Note the gingival clefting produced by overly aggressive dental flossing.

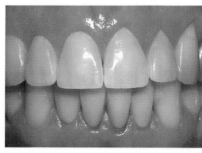

FIG. 9–6. Final restorations in cast glass ceramic.

FIG. 9–7. These cast glass ceramic crowns have been in place for 2 years. The excellent soft tissue response here is not uncharacteristic.

FIG. 9–8. These two central incisors are cast glass ceramic restorations finished at the level of the soft tissue.

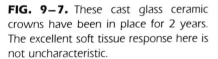
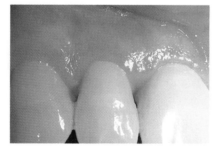

FIG. 9–7

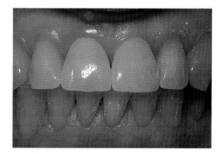

FIG. 9–8

light and opacifying porcelain refracts even less. Glass ceramic refracts 75% of entering light because its organized crystalline form has a refractive index similar to that of enamel.[4,7,12,13] With proper coloration, cast glass ceramic crowns can be extremely lifelike (Figs. 9–2 to 9–6).

Biocompatibility

Rough, uneven, porous surfaces may encourage the colonization of many forms of bacteria. Poorly fitting metal margins, improperly glazed porcelains, and rough acrylics can result in gingival inflammation.[20-29]

A recent study showed that cast glass ceramics exhibit less surface plaque accumulation than enamel, cementum, or any other restorative material.[30,31] This may result from the extremely smooth surface, low surface tension, and electrostatic repulsion of the cast glass ceramic.[29-31] Clinically, gingival response and esthetics are consistently excellent because of superb marginal fit, control of margin placement, and proper light refraction (Figs. 9–7, 9–8).

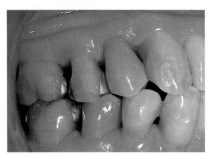

FIG. 9–9

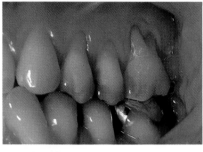

FIG. 9–10

FIG. 9–9. The maxillary first premolar and the mandibular second premolar are cast glass ceramic restorations.

FIG. 9–10. The maxillary first molar is finished far from the gingival margin. Note how the gray color seems to be absorbed from the amalgam restoration in the second premolar.

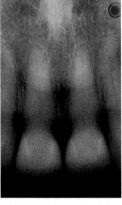

FIG. 9–11. Radiograph of the crowns shown in Figure 9–8 luted with a radiopaque dual cure urethane dimethacrylate translucent shade cement.

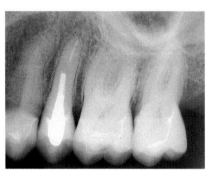

FIG. 9–12. Radiographic appearance of posterior cast glass ceramic restorations cemented with zinc oxyphosphate cement. (Courtesy of Dr. Harold Litvak.)

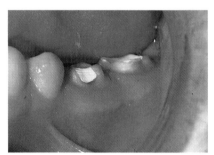

FIG. 9–13. After preparation, these teeth exhibit unsuitable axial wall height for cast glass ceramic restorations. Surgical crown lengthening procedures are indicated.

Control of Margin Placement

The gingival extent of the interproximal shoulder of a full crown restoration may be deeper than the ideal because of caries or a pre-existing deep restoration. A bevel extends the preparation further subgingivally. Deep subgingival margins complicate retraction, impression techniques, and margin evaluation. Biological width violation and compromised oral hygiene access can result in gingival inflammation, pocket formation, and other periodontal problems.[12,20,27,32-35] Elimination of the bevel would decrease the depth of the finishing line by an amount equal to the length of the bevel. This, however, compromises the marginal integrity of a ceramometal crown because the "slip-joint" effect of the cast metal bevel to the prepared bevel tooth surface is lost.[36-39] Retention also is decreased.

Investment materials and casting techniques for cast glass ceramic allow consistently accurate casting to butt joint or rounded shoulder preparations, thus eliminating the need for a bevel. These somewhat technique-sensitive procedures, however, leave little or no room for error for either the clinician or the laboratory technician.

Coloration

Glass ceramic colorants are applied and oven fired in multiple layers. These colorants contain less primary opacifiers (dioxides of titanium, zirconium, and tin) than conventional body porcelains. By selecting the color (hue) and varying the intensity (chroma) at various locations of the restoration (i.e., cervical and incisal areas and line angles) shading can be accurately developed. Light entering through the porcelain colorants into the glass ceramic crown is scattered in many directions by the crystalline form and demonstrates an optical quality similar to opalescence. Cast glass ceramic can absorb light from other teeth and filling materials creating a "chameleon" effect[12] (Figs. 9–9, 9–10). In addition, some degree of color modification and enhancement may be effected with colored luting agents.[8]

The glass ceramic crown will not discolor or distort from multiple firings because the coloring and glazing temperatures do not approach the casting or cerarming firing cycle temperatures. Therefore, an unlimited number of oven firings may be used to add or change color.

Radiographic Density

Cast glass ceramic crowns are radiolucent and allow radiographic examination of margin integrity, cement thickness, bases, and post and cores (Figs. 9–11, 9–12).

CAST GLASS CERAMIC PROCEDURES

Adequate axial wall height is necessary for retention of the restoration. Proper occlusal reduction is necessary for correct anatomic form and strength. Anteriorly, the criteria used for other all-porcelain systems applies when considering cast glass ceramics as a restorative material. Interproximal axial wall height becomes increasingly more important posteriorly in the mouth because greater masticatory forces may be generated and teeth are generally shorter. Periodontal surgical crown lengthening procedures should be employed when adequate axial wall height does not exist.[20,27,32-35,39,40] If such procedures are not possible, restoration with cast glass ceramic is contraindicated (Fig. 9–13).

If a large core buildup is necessary to replace missing tooth structure in an endodontically treated tooth, a metallic core is recommended. Large composite resin cores should not be used because of insufficient deformation resistance. Some practitioners use cores (*not* post-cores) of cast ceramic because of their inherent stiffness and ability to be etched and bonded in place.[41]

Tooth Preparation for Full Coverage Anterior and Posterior Cast Glass Ceramic Restorations

Armamentarium

- Standard dental setup
  explorer
  mouth mirror
  periodontal probe
  suitable anesthesia
  high-speed handpiece
  low-speed handpiece
- Diamond burs
  Wheel-shaped gross reduction bur (e.g., 5909-040 or 909-055, Brasseler USA)
  Tapered rounded end medium grit diamond bur, 1 mm at tip (856L-018, Brasseler, USA)
  Tapered rounded end fine diamond bur, 1 mm at tip (856L-020, Brasseler, USA)
  Football-shaped diamond for anterior cingulum reduction (e.g., 379-023, Brasseler, USA)
  Large round bur for posterior occlusal reduction (e.g., 801-035, Brasseler USA) or round end taper (e.g., 30006-106, Brasseler USA)
  End-cutting diamond to eliminate the "lip" at the external aspect of the shoulder or square end diamond stone (smaller diameter than the rounded bur and stone used for axial reductions)
- No. 0 and No. 1 Gingabraid (Van R) nonimpregnated retraction cord
- Hemostatic agent (e.g., Hemodent)
- Occlusal reduction measuring device 1.5 mm/2.0 mm (Dentsply International, Inc.)
- Scissors
- Gingettage packing instrument No. 1 (Pollard, Vic Dental Products, Inc.)

Clinical Technique (Figs. 9–14 to 9–25)

1. **Anterior preparation.** Reduce the tooth a minimum of 1.0 mm labially and axially, 1.5 mm incisally, and 1.5 mm palatally (Fig. 9–26) in order to allow for sufficient bulk of material to resist tensile (lateral) loads (Fig. 9–27). Axial reduction on the labial surface follows two planes. (See Chapter 8—Ceramometal—Full Coverage Restorations.) All prepared tooth surfaces should be smooth, rounded, and flowing, avoiding sharp corners where stress concentrations may occur.[8,42]

   Posterior Preparation. Reduce the tooth a minimum of 1.2 to 1.5 mm axially[43,44] and 1.5 to 2.0 mm occlusally (Fig. 9–28) in order to allow for sufcient bulk to resist tensile (lateral) load. Axially reduction on the buccal and lingual surfaces follows two planes. (See Chapter 8—Ceramometal—Full Coverage Restorations.) All prepared tooth surfaces should be smooth, rounded, and flowing, avoiding sharp corners where stress concentrations may occur.

CLINICAL TIP. Careful case selection is important when full coverage cast glass restorations are used because of fracture potential in the molar area. Ceramometal restorations are better able to resist these compressive forces.

CLINICAL TIP. Posterior occlusal reduction should be "scooped-out" buccolingually. This ensures adequate occlusal thickness while not sacrificing axial wall height or restricting the ceramist in creating anatomic groove carving (Figs. 9–29 to 9–31).

CLINICAL TIP. Deep carvings may weaken the glass ceramic because the material may begin to cleave at these grooves (Fig. 9–32) unless adequate strength is ensured by appropriate occlusal reduction, which permits sufficient thickness of material. The thickness of the material is more important than the amount of occlusal reduction.

---

2. Marginal design may be either a shoulder or rounded shoulder with even reduction all around the tooth for strength (Fig. 9–33). Inadequate reduction may lead to failure caused by flexure movement during function (Fig. 9–34).

CLINICAL TIP. Do not place any bevels because they produce inherent weakness in the glass and increase the risk of chipping.

---

3. The finishing line of the preparation must terminate entirely on sound tooth structure.[26] Ending on cements, bases, or metallic substructures does not ensure a positive seal against microleakage. Crown lengthening procedures alone or in combination with forced eruption procedures[45,46,47] can help enhance marginal integrity while avoiding violations of biologic attachment dimensions.

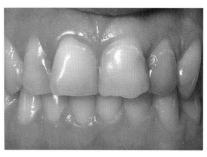

FIG. 9—14. Large class III composite resin restorations with recurrent decay preceeded four full coverage restorations for these incisors.

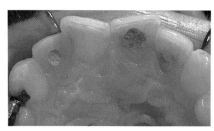

FIG. 9—15. Three of these teeth required endodontic therapy.

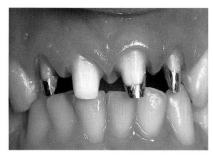

FIG. 9—16. Indirect cast posts and cores were fabricated to replace lost tooth structure. The final restorations must "mask" these post and cores.

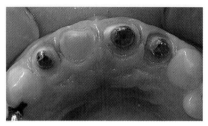

FIG. 9—17. The deep interproximal lesions led to deeply placed shoulders and difficult impressioning. Here a double-cord technique for retraction is used. The first cord placed is thin, No. 0 size, and nonimpregnated. It will remain in place beneath the shoulder during impressioning. The second cord is a No. 1 size Gingabraid. It will be removed prior to impressioning.

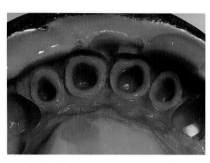

FIG. 9—18. The hydrocolloid impression. Note that although the right central incisor has a labial indentation, even reduction is maintained.

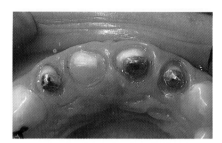

FIG. 9—19. Invagination of soft tissue tags under the provisional restorations must be removed or retracted prior to cementation to avoid trapping them and to insure marginal integrity.

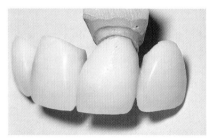

FIG. 9—20. Provisional restorations with open margins allow soft tissue proliferation. Placing the provisional restoration on the die demonstrates the problem.

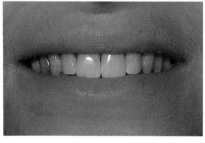

FIG. 9—21. Final crowns in place. Note that it is possible to block out underlying gold posts and cores through development of opacity.

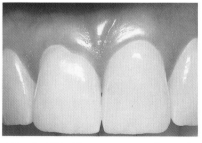

FIG. 9—22. Close-up several weeks later showing soft tissue adaptation and acceptance. Note labial indentation on the right central incisor, as previously noted.

FIG. 9—23. Preoperative photograph of central and lateral incisors to be prepared for cast glass ceramic restorations.

FIG. 9—24. Postoperative photograph at the time of cementation. Note the cast post and core in the lateral incisor is sufficiently masked.

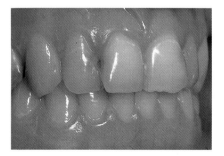

FIG. 9—23

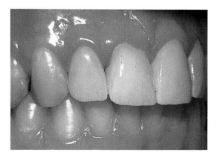

FIG. 9—24

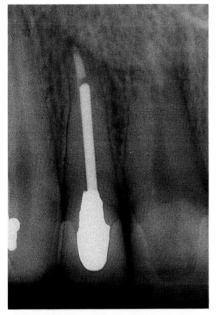

FIG. 9—25. Radiograph of crowns that were cemented with a radiolucent glass ionomer cement. The crowns were not intrinsically etched.

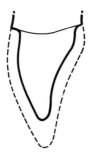

FIG. 9—26. Tooth preparation for cast glass ceramic restoration showing acceptable finishing lines. All preparations require rounded internal line angles.

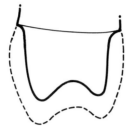

FIG. 9—28. Tooth preparation for cast glass ceramic restoration showing acceptable finishing lines. All preparations require rounded internal line angles.

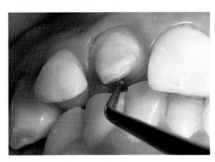

FIG. 9—27. A 1.5-mm cingulum reduction is necessary anteriorly to provide enough strength to resist tensile forces.

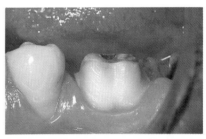

FIG. 9—29. Posterior occlusal reduction should be "scooped-out" buccolingually. This ensures adequate occlusal thickness while not sacrificing axial wall height or restricting the ceramist during anatomic groove carving.

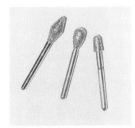

FIG. 9—30. The right two burs are round-ended and are well suited for posterior occlusal reduction. A conventional diamond shaped bur (left) is not.

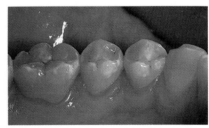

FIG. 9—31. Adequate occlusal reduction has allowed deep anatomic occlusal carvings to be made, while maintaining a 1.5 mm to 2.0 mm thickness of cast glass ceramic material.

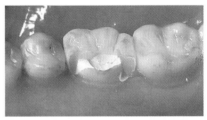

FIG. 9—32. The crown made for this clinically short tooth was further weakened by deep anatomic grooves. A 2.0 mm reduction was achieved, however, carving created thinner areas.

FIG. 9—33. Internally rounded shoulder preparation with even reduction circumferentially.

FIG. 9—34. Tooth flexure or crown bending during function is the most reasonable explanation for this fracture failure.

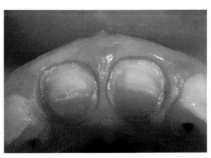

FIG. 9—33

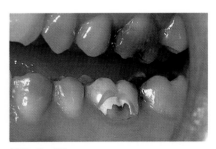

FIG. 9—34

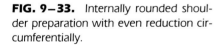

Tooth Preparation for Cast Glass Ceramic Onlays and Inlays

Armamentarium

- Standard dental setup (see the section on Tooth Preparation for Full Coverage Anterior and Posterior Cast Glass Ceramic Restorations
- Football-shaped medium grit diamond bur (e.g., 379-023, Brasseler, USA)
- 1-mm diameter tapered shoulder diamond bur (e.g., 846-016, Brasseler, USA)

Clinical Technique

1. Prepare the tooth (Figs. 9–35 to 9–37) following standard partial coverage principles for gold restorations with the modifications for glass ceramic. Occlusal reduction where cuspal coverage is necessary must be at least 1.5 mm flowing into axial areas of 1.0 mm reduction or more (Figs. 9–38, 9–39).
2. All internal surfaces should be smooth, rounded, and continuous, avoiding sharp corners that create areas of stress concentration.[42]
3. Cavosurface bevels are contraindicated because they produce inherent weakness in the glass and increase the risk of chipping.[8]
4. Avoid preparation designs with large bulky areas that flow into thinner areas because heat-sinking may occur during the firing and cooling stages resulting in crack propagation.

Veneers

Cast glass ceramic veneers exhibit superior fit when compared to the veneers made from feldspathic porcelains. The ability to custom color repeatedly is an advantage over conventional porcelain laminates veneers, which are often fabricated with foil matrices. The major drawback of cast glass ceramic veneers is limited postinsertion adjustment flexibility. Occlusal adjustment or shortening of incisal edges and labial contour after luting will result in loss of surface colorant. This is particularly relevant in mandibular situations. Similarly, marginal finishing consists only of luting agent removal using rotary instrumentation with the utmost care.

Impressioning—Double Cord Retraction

The butt joint or rounded shoulder preparation design allows little or no room for error in reading the final preparation in die material. Therefore, the entire extent of prepared tooth structures must be clearly visible in the impression.

Armamentarium

- Standard dental setup (see the section on Tooth Preparation for Full Coverage Anterior and Posterior Cast Glass Ceramic Restorations)
- Gingettage packer No. 1 (Van R)
- No. 0 gingival retraction cord
- No. 1 gingival retraction cord
- Suitable hemostatic agent
- Scissors
- Suitable impression material

Clinical Technique

1. Gently place a nonimpregnated No. 0 Gingabraid cord in the sulcus.
2. Place a second cord over the No. 0 cord. Use a No. 0 nonimpregnated cord if connective tissues are firm and tight; Use a No. 1 nonimpregnated cord for other cases.
3. Remove only the second cord prior to impressioning.

CLINICAL TIP. To avoid interference with full shoulder capture in the impression, it is essential that the remaining cord lie just beneath the shoulder level (see Fig. 9–17).

4. Make the impression with any standard impression material (see Fig. 9–18).

Supragingival preparation designs simplify impression procedures and whenever possible are the designs of choice from both restorative and periodontal standpoints.[24,25,28] Consider supragingival preparations when axial wall height is sufficient and esthetic demands permit.

Provisional Restorations. Properly contoured and well fitting provisional restorations may be regarded as templates for final restorations (see Chapter 13—Acrylic and Other Resins—Provisional Restorations). These provisional restorations should act to protect prepared tooth structure and maintain the tooth's position in the arch. Fit becomes critical when margins of prepared teeth have been subgingivally placed because slight openings or short margins allow gingival tissues to proliferate and invaginate into any acrylic opening (see Fig. 9–19). Undercontouring of the provisional restoration allows soft tissue overgrowth circumferentially (see Fig. 9–20). These shortcomings will be realized at the try-in appointments and will invariably result in trapping of soft tissue tags. Soft tissues that interfere with full seating at the final case delivery visit should be retracted prior to cementation procedures (see Figs. 9–24, 9–25). Failure to remove these tags, which prevent full seating of the crown and create an area of potential marginal leakage, can result in restoration failure (Figs. 9–40 to 9–42).

CLINICAL TIP. Impressions of provisional restoration may be made to preserve information regarding tooth length, width, emergence profile, contour, esthetic arrangement, occlusion, and incisal guidance (discclusion). This information may be very helpful to laboratory technicians in the fabrication of final restorations, especially in the anterior region.[49-51]

CLINICAL TIP. Eugenol-containing cements are contraindicated for cementation of temporary restorations because they interfere with the polymerization process of the composite resin luting agent used for final cementation.

Occlusal Registrations

Minimimal occlusal adjustments at insertion is a reasonable objective for any restorative material. Conventional occlusal registration procedures that work well and are familiar to the operator may also be used for restoration with cast glass ceramic. However, unlike feldspathic restorations, if a great deal of occlusal adjustment is necessary, much of the colorant can be lost. This may necessitate additional oven firings or an additional visit to recreate a naturally colored restoration.

CLINICAL TIP. For posterior restorations use the "occlusal index" technique,[52] a stone index of an equilibrated provisional restoration.

Crown Try-In and Placement

It is important to have a uniform, uninterrupted skin layer prior to coloration procedures.[53] The skin layer is an opaque white surface layer that forms during the ceramming stage. If it is lost during grinding, a sharp decrease in value and a corresponding increase in translucency results (Fig. 9–43). Alterations to labial contour after ceramming or coloration lead to streaky, uneven loss of the skin layer or color. Should this loss occur, it is difficult, especially in lighter shades, to recreate a natural blend of colors without creating a blotchy, patchy effect. The most predictable method to correct this situation is to cut back the labial surface and fire a feldspathic porcelain (e.g., Vitadur-N, Dicor-Plus or Dicor

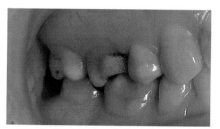

FIG. 9–35. Preoperative view of the maxillary first molar to be prepared for a full cast glass ceramic crown.

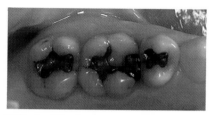

FIG. 9–36. Occlusal view of the maxillary first molar to be prepared for a full cast glass ceramic crown.

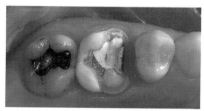

FIG. 9–37. The final preparation with etched enamel and glass ionomer base. Note the even axial reduction around the mesiolingual cusp.

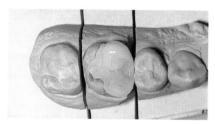

FIG. 9–38. This partial coverage restoration of cast glass ceramic has the advantage of being etchable internally.

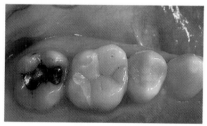

FIG. 9–39. The final restoration bonded to place.

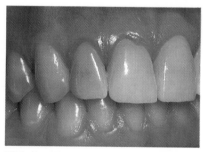

FIG. 9–40. Extrinsic graying of the lateral incisor. Since only one tooth is affected, the problem does not appear to involve the superficial colorant but is suspected to lie underneath.

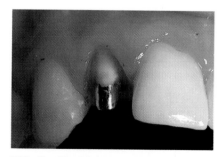

FIG. 9–41. Moisture contamination of the glass ionomer cement leading to cement washout and discoloration is thought to be the problem.

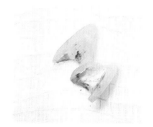

FIG. 9–42. Marginal leakage and decay were evident at the mesial aspect once this crown was removed.

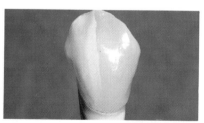

FIG. 9–43. The skin surface layer, which forms after ceramming, was removed from the right side of this demonstration crown. While the right side appears gray and translucent, the left side has developed opacity. Both were colored identically.

add-on porcelains) with subsequent coloration. In fact, this technique has evolved into a standard clinical procedure called the "Willi's Glas Crown,"[13] which incorporates the advantages of both cast glass and feldspathic porcelains.

In this technique, a cast glass coping is waxed and cerammed followed by veneering with feldspathic porcelain labially and lingually (Figs. 9–44, 9–45). In this way, the excellent fit and transillumination properties of the cast glass ceramic are retained, combined with the more familiar techniques for feldspathic porcelain buildups. However, the disadvantage of the adverse wear characteristics of feldspathic porcelain is now introduced. State of the art polishing techniques for glazed porcelain surfaces can serve to decrease or minimize this effect.[54] A further development designed to address this issue is the "Bioven crown." Based on studies that support the low abrasive quality of cast glass ceramic, especially in the noncolored state, lingual surfaces are full contoured and the labial surface's cutback to allow for porcelain veneering (Figs. 9–46 to 9–48).

Another option to eliminate the gray effect caused by the loss of the skin layer is to attempt to "color it out" with porcelain stains and opaquers. This is easier to accomplish with darker teeth. Attempts at receramming crowns to restore the skin layer have been successful, however, no research exists to support this procedure.

CLINICAL TIP. If major modifications have been made, and the placement of a layer of feldspathic porcelain is not desired, it is usually easier to recast a new unit to the proper contour than to attempt to recolorize the crown.

CLINICAL TIP. To avoid coloration problems, fit, contour, and adjust multiple anterior restorations at the cast glass noncerammed state (Fig. 9–49).

Posteriorly, glass ceramic restorations are usually brought to completion if the number of units is small. A try-in visit at the glass stage is usually unnecessary if occlusal registration techniques are accurate.

Contacts

Armamentarium

- Standard dental setup (see the section on Tooth Preparation for Full Coverage Anterior and Posterior Cast Glass Ceramic Restorations)
- Colored spray powder (e.g., Occlude, Pascal Co., Inc.)
- Unwaxed dental tape
- Polishing wheels (e.g., Brasseler porcelain polisher white 0301-220 and pink 0306-220)

Clinical Technique

1. Try in the final crowns with gentle finger pressure.
2. Check margins with an explorer tip to confirm full seating.
3. Check contact areas with floss while holding the crown in place.

4. Locate areas of tight contacts by applying a light powder mist of Occlude (Pascal, Co., Inc.). indicator powder to the interproximal surfaces of the crown.
5. Reseat the crown, remove it, and observe the interrupted powder area created by the tight contact.
6. Adjust the "mark" with polishing wheels.
7. Reseat the crown and check the contact area with floss.
8. Recheck the margin with an explorer.
9. If the contact is light, make corrections by firing add-on porcelains.

Internal Fit

Because the color of conventional silicones or indicator pastes closely approximates the internal color of cast ceramic, they are ineffective in detecting areas where the castings bind. However, because the occlusal surface and all axial surfaces have been die-spaced, the only area of the casting that may interfere with full seating is the unspaced shoulder. This explains why castings made on a spaced die frequently completely seat on a second unspaced die.

Armamentarium

- Standard dental setup (see the section on Tooth Preparation for Full Coverage Anterior and Posterior Cast Glass Ceramic Restorations)
- Colored indicator spray (e.g., Occlude, Pascal Co., Inc.)
- Fine diamond bur to be used at low speed for internal adjustment (e.g., Brasseler 247F-009)

Clinical Technique

1. Spray the internal aspect of the castings with a thin mist of a colored spray, specifically on the unspaced shoulder (Fig. 9–50).
2. Try in the crowns with gentle finger pressure.
3. Remove the crowns and carefully inspect the shoulders for rub marks.
4. Gently adjust the binding areas with a fine diamond using a slow-speed handpiece (Fig. 9–51).
5. Repeat, if necessary.
6. Check the margins with an explorer tip to confirm full seating.

Adjustments

Once interproximal contacts and internal fit are satisfactory, make occlusal corrections.

Armamentarium

- Standard dental setup (see the section on Tooth Preparation for Full Coverage Anterior and Posterior Cast Glass Ceramic Restorations)
- Two-color double-sided articulating paper (Accufilm II)
- Fine diamond burs, football-shaped and small fine (e.g., Brasseler 8368-016)
- Rubber wheels (e.g., Brasseler porcelain polishers, white 0301-220 and pink 0306-220)
- Green stones (e.g., IC3 and IC1 Shofu Dental Corp.)

Clinical Technique

1. With two color, double-sided articulating paper in place, have the patient gently "tap" his (dry) teeth into occlusion.
2. Remove the paper.
3. Have the patient close his mouth again. This causes a superimposition of the opposing occlusal markings. In this way, the thickness of the paper is compensated for and only "true" contacting surfaces superimpose. Other marks are erroneously caused by the thickness of the paper and should not be adjusted.

CLINICAL TIP. The red side of the articulating paper marks the arch where the restoration is being made and the opposing occlusal contact (in black) is superimposed. It is more difficult to read if done in reverse.

4. Adjust the restoration with fine diamonds and rubber wheels, where necessary. Color will be lost where changes have been made, revealing the grayish-glass color of the cast ceramic (Fig. 9–52). If this is determined to be an esthetic problem, the crown may be refired with a single, thin layer of colorant in these areas.

FIG. 9–44. Thimbles or copings of cast glass ceramic allow the use of more conventional porcelain application techniques.

FIG. 9–45. The "Willi's glas crown technique" combines the advantage of cast glass ceramic in the area of marginal fit with familiar porcelain buildup systems.

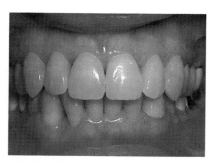

FIG. 9–44

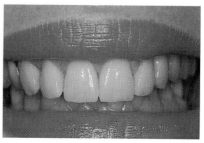

FIG. 9–45

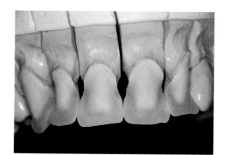

FIG. 9–46. Full contour anatomic wax-ups are cut back labially only before casting, to create room for porcelain veneer materials. (Courtesy of Dr. Mauro Fradeani.)

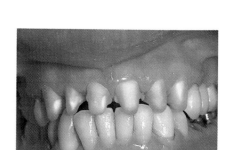

FIG. 9–47. Occluding areas are designed to be on noncolored cast glass ceramic surfaces only. (Courtesy of Dr. Mauro Fradeani.)

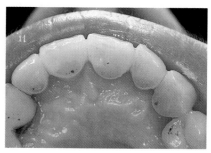

FIG. 9–48. Conventional porcelains used to veneer over the glass ceramic in the final restorations. (Courtesy of Dr. Mauro Fradeani.)

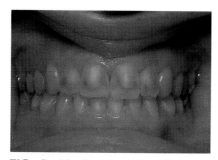

FIG. 9–49. Anterior restorations are usually tried in the mouth at the cast glass "green" state. Here, the crowns are considered too long incisally and will be adjusted (shortened) at chairside using green stones in a low speed handpiece.

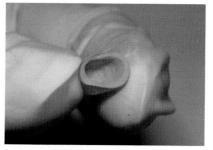

FIG. 9–50. "Occlude" (Pascal Co, Inc.) powder sprayed on the shoulder to mark binding or high spots.

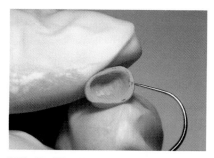

FIG. 9–51. After crown seating, binding areas are revealed. These may be very carefully adjusted using a fine diamond stone in a slow speed handpiece.

CLINICAL TIP. The crown expands approximately 1.6% after casting, but this is neutralized by a 1.6% shrinkage that occurs after ceramming. This usually results in incomplete contact areas that must be built up. In cases involving many teeth, it is best to try the restoration in the mouth after ceramming and contacts have been added. In this way, all contact areas and internal fit adjustments may be made prior to re-mounting (Figs 9–53 to 9–55).

Coloration

The coloration steps that follow do not appreciably alter the size of the cerammed glass crown. Unlimited oven firings may be undertaken to add color in layers and to improve light filtration and characterization.

Luting

A dual-cured light-activated cement of urethane dimethacrylate composite resin is currently the luting agent of choice for cast glass ceramic restorations.[55-61] Translucent, opaque, and several shades are available, which may be used to subtly influence the final esthetic outcome. Water soluble try-in pastes are available if it is necessary to preview the final result of these subtle variations. These cements have film thicknesses of 10 microns for translucent cements to 25 microns for shaded cements. High compressive strengths of 20,000 to 36,000 psi and tensile strengths of 3,500 to 5,000 psi may be achieved. They are biocompatible and, once cured, water insoluble.[8]

Armamentarium

- Standard dental setup (see the section on Tooth Preparation for Full Coverage Anterior and Posterior Cast Glass Ceramic Restorations)
- Nonmetallic (plastic) spatula
- Mixing pad
- 35% phosphoric acid gel
- Polyacrylic acid (e.g., Dentin Conditioner, G.C. International Corp.)
- Cavidry (Parkell, Inc.)
- Dentin bonding agent (e.g., All-Bond, Bisco, Inc.)
- Urethane dimethacrylate luting composite resin (e.g., Dicor light-activated, Dentsply International Inc. cementation kit or Biomer cement, Caulk/Dentsply)
- Gingival margin trimmer

Clinical Technique

1. Etch the internal aspect of the glass ceramic crown in the laboratory or at chairside with an acid specifically formulated by the manufacturer for this purpose (Fig. 9–56).
2. Silane coupling agent is added by the laboratory to increase bond strengths and add a measure of protection from most contaminants to the etched restoration surface (Fig. 9–57).

3. Prior to luting procedures, clean all tooth surfaces with Cavilax on a cotton pellet (Figs. 9–58, 9–59).
4. If the tooth is vital, it may be necessary to apply anesthesia, especially if a polycarboxalate or other strong cement was used during temporization and must be removed with an ultrasonic cleaner (e.g., Cavitron, Dentsply International, Inc.).
5. Dry the tooth with Cavidry and then with oil-free air.
6. Etch any enamel in the preparation (Fig. 9–60).
7. Place a dentin bonding agent on all exposed dentin surfaces. (See Chapter 3, Dentin Bonding Agents.)
8. Gently retract any soft tissue that interferes with the complete seating of the crown (Fig. 9–61).

CLINICAL TIP. Avoid exposing the cement to light.

9. Load the crown with cement and seat the restoration with finger pressure, lightly tapping the occlusal to confirm full seating.
10. Leave some excess cement in place as curing proceeds to protect the critical cement at the finishing line (Fig. 9–62).

CLINICAL TIP. If the excess cement is removed with a brush prior to light curing, shrinkage during set increases the likelihood that crevicular fluids could contaminate the cement at the finishing line. This could lead to premature cement breakdown, exposure of dentinal tubuli, and subsequent dentinal sensitivity in vital teeth.

11. Cleave off cured excess cement with a sharp interproximal carver.
12. Carefully inspect with a sharp explorer tip to confirm that there is no excess cement (Fig. 9–63).
13. Floss the contact with dental tape.

CLINICAL TIP. Occasionally, excess cement may cure at a proximal contact area preventing the passage of floss tape. To break the bond of the cement to the adjacent tooth, have the patient bite on a wood stick placed on the occlusal surface of the restoration only; then on the adjacent tooth only. If floss still cannot be passed through the contact and the only excess cement is at the contact area, have the patient return to the office in a few days. Normal masticatory function will undoubtedly solve the problem.

CONCLUSION

Lifelike esthetic restorations can be produced with cast glass ceramics. Their superb marginal integrity and strength makes them an excellent alternative to porcelain-fused-to-metal for single unit restorations. Additional research and experimentation will give rise to even stronger materials. This, coupled with improved technology in luting and dentin bonding agents, will further expand the indications and applications of cast glass ceramics.

The author is grateful to Mr. Marino Patrk for his assistance and technical support in fabricating all the cast glass ceramic restorations that appear in this chapter.

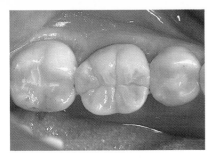

FIG. 9–52. Occlusal adjustment was necessary after final placement of this mandibular molar restoration. Note that colorant has been lost and areas of adjustment appear gray. (Mesiobuccal, buccal, and mesiolingual inner inclines of the first molar.)

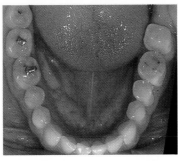

FIG. 9–53. This bulemic patient required a complete reconstruction. The preoperative view of the mandible exhibited characteristic "islands of amalgam".

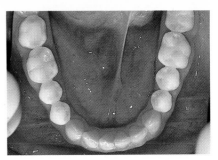

FIG. 9–54. Because of the number of units involved, this case was tried in at the cerammed state to adjust interproximal contacts. Remounting procedures to adjust occlusion followed.

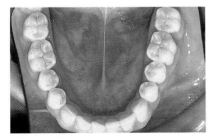

FIG. 9–55. The final restoration of multiple single unit cast glass ceramic.

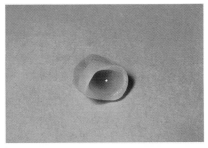

FIG. 9–56. Cast glass ceramic is internally etched using a liquid etchant.

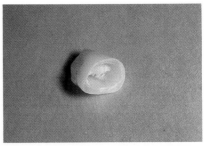

FIG. 9–57. Typical internal appearance of a cast glass ceramic crown after etching and silane coupling treatments.

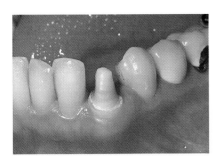

FIG. 9–58. Tooth preparation with temporary cement residue.

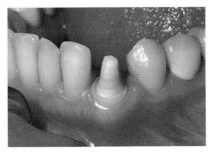

FIG. 9–59. Residue removed by scrubbing with a cotton pellet soaked in an alcohol-based solvent.

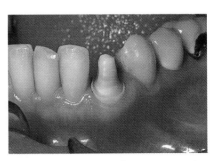

FIG. 9–60. Enamel, if present, may be etched. The smear layer may be removed with polyacrylic acid treatment.

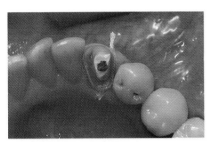

FIG. 9–61. Soft tissue that may interfere with crown placement is retracted.

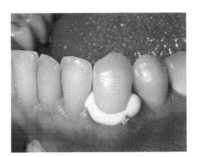

FIG. 9–62. The crown is seated, leaving excess cement in place.

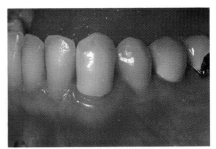

FIG. 9–63. The final crown after cement removal and inspection.

REFERENCES

1. Adair, P.J. and Grossman, D.G.: The castable ceramic crown. Int J Periodont Res Dent 4:32, 1984.
2. Grossman, D.G.: The science of castable glass ceramics. *In* Preston J.D. (ed.): Perspectives in Dental Ceramics. Chicago, Quintessence Publishing Co., p. 117, 1988.
3. Adair, P.J. and Hoeksta, K.E.: Fit Evaluation of a Castable Ceramic. J Dent Res 61:345, 1982.
4. Adair, P.J. and Grossman, D.G.: Esthetic properties of lost tooth structure compared with ceramic restorations. J Dent Res 61:292, 1982.
5. Adair, P.J., Bell, B.H., and Pameijer, C.M.: Casting techniques of machinable glass ceramics. J Dent Res 59:475, 1980.
6. Adair, P.J., Sackett, P.B., and Commarato, V.T.: Preliminary clinical evaluation of cast ceramic full crown restorations. J Dent Res 61:292, 1982.
7. Grossman, D.G., Adair, P.J., and Pameijar, C.H.: Evaluation of the color of a cast ceramic restorative material. J Dent Res 59:542, 1980.
8. Dicor Clinical Instructions for Dicor Restorations and the Use of the Dicor Light Activated Cementation Kit, Dentsply/York Division. Lab Products Dentsply International Inc., York, PA, 1988.
9. McLean, J.: The Science and Art of Dental Ceramics, Vol. II. Bridge Design and Laboratory Procedures in Dental Ceramics. Chicago, Quintessence Publishing Co., 1980.
10. Griffith, A.A.: The phenomena of rupture and flow in solids. Philos Trans R Soc Lond A221:63, 1920.
11. Malament, K.A.: Considerations in posterior glass-ceramic restorations. Int J Periodont Res Dent 8:33, 1988.
12. Malament, K.A.: The cast glass-ceramic crown. *In* Preston J.D. (ed.): Perspectives in Dental Ceramics. Chicago, Quintessence Publishing Co., 1988.
13. Grossman, D.G.: Cast Glass Ceramics. Dent Clin North Am 29:725, 1985.
14. Woda, A., Gourdon, A.M., and Faraj, M.: Occlusal contact and tooth wear. J Prosthet Dent 57:85, 1987.
15. Ellison, J.A.: Bioven crown. Presented to American Association of Dental Research, March 15, 1989.
16. Palmer, D.S., Barco, M.T., Peller, B., and McKinney, J.E.: Wear of human enamel against dicor. Presented to American Association of Dental Research, March 15, 1989.
17. Seligman, D.A., Pullinger, A.G., and Solberg, W.K.: The prevalence of dental attrition and its association with factors of age, gender occlusion and TMJ symptomatology. J Dent Res 67:1323, 1988.
18. Corning Glass Works: Internal Measurements, Physical Properties Department. Corning, NY, 1984.
19. Geller, W. and Kwiatkowski, S.: The Willi's Glas Crown: a new solution in the dark and shadowed zones of esthetic porcelain restorations. Quint Dent Tech 11:233, 1987.
20. Flores-de Jacoby, L., Zafiropoulos G.G., and Ciancio, S.: The effect of crown margin location on plaque and periodontal health. Int J Periodont Res Dent 9(3), 1989.
21. Silness, J.: Periodontal conditions in patients treated with dental bridges, III. The Relationship Between the Location of the Crown Margin and the Periodontal Condition. J Periodont Res, 5:225, 1970.
22. Dragoo M.R. and Williams, G.B.: Periodontal tissue reactions to restorative procedures. Int J Periodont Res Dent 1:9, 1981.
23. Waerhaug, J.: Presence or absence of plaque on subgingival restorations. J Dent Res 83:193, 1975.
24. Silness, J.: Fixed prosthodontics and periodontal health. Dent Clin North Am 24:317, 1980.
25. Wilson, R.D.: Intracrevicular Restorative Dentistry. Int J Periodont Res Dent 3:40, 1983.
26. Nevins, M. and Skuron, H.M.: The intercrevicular restorative margin, the biologic width, and the maintenance of the gingival margin. Int J Periodont Res Dent 4:30, 1984.
27. Nevins, M.: Interproximal periodontal disease—the embrasure as an etiological factor. Int J Periodont and Res Dent 2(6) 9–28, 1982.
28. Waerbaug, J.: Tissue Reactions Around Artificial Crowns. J Periodont 54:172, 1983.
29. Sorenson, J.A.: Rationale for comparison of plaque-retaining properties of crown systems. J Prosthet Den. 62:264, 1989.
30. Savitt, E.D. and Melament, K.A.: Effects on colonization of oral microbiota by a cast glass-ceramic restoration. Int J Periodont Res Dent 7:22, 1987.
31. Savitt, E.D.: Clinical applications of oral microbiology in restorative dentistry. *In* Perspectives in Dental Ceramics: Proceedings of the Fourth International Symposium on Ceramics. Chicago, Quintessence Publishing Co., 1988.
32. Ingber, J.S., Rose, L.F., and Coslet, J.G.: The biological width—a concept in periodontics and restorative dentistry. Alpha Omegan 10:62, 1977.
33. Kramer, G.M.: A consideration of root proximity. Int J Periodont Res Dent 6:8, 1987.
34. Kramer, G.M.: Rational of periodontal therapy. *In* Goldman, M.M., et al.: Periodontal Therapy, 6th Ed. St. Louis, C.V. Mosby Co., 1980.
35. Gargiulo, A.W., Wentz, F.M., and Orban, B.: Dimensions and relations of the dentogingival junction in humans. J Periodont 32:261, 1961.
36. Shillingburg, M.T., Jacobi, R., and Brockett, S.E.: Fundamentals of tooth preparation. Chicago, Quintessence Publishing Co., 1987.
37. Panno, F.V., Vahidi, F., Gulkea, I., et al.: Evaluation of the 45° labial bevel with a shoulder preparation. J Prosthet Dent 56:655, 1986.
38. Rosner, D.: Furcation placement and reproduction of bevels for gold casting. J Prosthet Dent 13:1160, 1963.
39. Wagenburg, B.D., Eskow, R.N., and Langer, B.: Exposing adequate tooth structure for restorative dentistry. Int J Periodont Res Dent 9:323, 1989.
40. Rosenberg, E.S., Garber, D.A., and Evian, C.: Tooth lengthening procedures. Compend Cont Dent Ed 1:3, 1980.
41. Malamet, K.: Personal communications, 1989.
42. Kelly, J.R., Campbell, S.D., and Bowen H.K.: Fracture-surface analysis of dental ceramics. 62:536, 1989.
43. Friedlander, L.D., Mundz, C.A., et al.: The affect of tooth preparations designed on the breaking strengths of Dicor crowns, Part 1. Int J Prosthet Dent 3:159, 1990.
44. Doyle, M.G., Mundoz, C.A., et al.: The effects of tooth preparation design on the breaking strength of Dicor crowns, Part II. Int J Prosthet Dent 3:241, 1990.
45. Ingber, J.S.: Forced eruption. Part I, a method of treating one and two wall intrabony osseous defects—rationale and case reports. J Periodont 45:199, 1974.
46. Ingber, J.S.: Forced eruption. Part II, a method of treating nonrestorable teeth—periodontal and restorative considerations. J Periodont 47:203, 1976.
47. Pontoriero, R. and Celenza F. Jr.: Rapid extrusion with fiber resection, a combined orthodontic-periodontic treatment modality. Int J Periodont Res Dent 7:30, 1987.
48. Dentsply: Personal communication, 1990.
49. Skurow, H.M. and Nevins, M.: The rationale of the preperiodontal provisional biologic trial restoration. Int J Periodont Res Dent 8:1, 1988.
50. Rieder, C.E.: The use of provisional restorations to develop and achieve esthetic expectations. Int J Periodont Res Dent 9:2, 1989.
51. Shavell, H.: Mastering the art of tissue management during provisionalization and biologic final impressions. Int J Periodont Res Dent 3:25, 1988.

52. Celenza, F.V. and Litvak, H.: Oral management in conformative dentistry. J Prosthet Dent 36:164, 1976.

53. Patrk, M. and Celenza, V.: Cast glass ceramics: a closer look at color. Unpublished research presented before World Congress of Dental Technology, New York, 1986.

54. Winter, R.: Paper presented to Northeast Gnathological Society, May 11, 1990.

55. Grossman, D.G. and Nelson, J.W.: The bonded dicor crown. J Dent Res, 66:206, 1987.

56. Eden, G.T. and Kacicz, J.M.: Dicor crown strength improvement due to bonding. J Dent Res 66:307, 1987.

57. Malament, K.A. and Grossman, D.G.: Clinical application of bonded dicor crowns: two-year report. Abstract of Dental Research (in print).

58. Jensen, M.E., Sheth, J.J., and Tolliver, D.: Etched porcelain resin bonded full-veneer crowns: in vitro fractures resistance. Comp Contin Ed Dent 10:337, 1989.

59. McInes-Ledoux, P.M., Ledoux, W.R., and Weinberg, R.A.: Bond strength study of luted castable ceramic restorations. J Dent Res 68:823, 1989.

60. Shotall, B.D.S., Fayyad, M.A., and Williams, J.D.: Marginal seal of injection molded ceramic crowns cemented with three adhesive systems. J Prosthet Dent 61:24, 1989.

61. Rosenstiel, S.F.: Apparent fracture toughness of all-ceramic crown systems. J Prosthet Dent 62:529, 1989.

Charles Lennon, D.M.D.

PORCELAIN—FULL COVERAGE RESTORATIONS

The introduction of new all-ceramic, ceramometal, and cast glass restorations has complicated the selection of the ideal restoration for any given clinical situation. However, knowledge of the materials, the indications and contraindications, and the particular clinical techniques required for each restoration will simplify the selection process.

THE HISTORY OF PORCELAIN

Kaolinite, potash, feldspar, and quartz were used to produce porcelain from the end of the eighteenth century to the early 1960s. These materials could match tooth color, but failed to recreate the natural translucency of dentin and enamel. The early porcelain restorations lacked vitality because of porosity trapped between irregular crystals, which created considerable opacity.

As the level of translucency has come closer to that of natural tooth structure, porcelain restorations better simulate enamel and dentin. Translucency has been increased in several ways. The proportions of kaolinite, potash, feldspar, and quartz in porcelain were reduced, and glass modifiers were added. In the late 1940s vacuum sintering produced finer, more regularly shaped porcelain crystals. Improved porcelain buildup and condensation techniques and the use of the vacuum oven both contributed to an increase in translucency. Paradoxically, the translucent porcelain created the need for opaque porcelains. Early all-porcelain restorations used weak opaques to allow color contribution from the underlying tooth structure. Presently, opaque or core porcelains can approximate the shade of the overlying dentin and enamel porcelain. High concentrations of opacifying oxides produce a highly reflective surface. Consequently, sufficient thickness of the overlying dentin and enamel porcelain is necessary to prevent areas of brightness emanating from the opaque or core porcelain.

In the early 1960s dental porcelains were developed with higher coefficients of thermal expansion, which allowed compatibility with dental casting alloys. This enabled the fabrication of porcelain-fused-to-metal restorations. The porcelain is fused to the metal by both a chemical and a mechanical bond. The chemical bond is developed primarily from oxides produced by the casting alloys. The mechanical bond is developed from the surface texture of the metal and the design of the supporting metal framework. This design produces compressive stresses that are much stronger than the tensile stresses when loaded.[1] Tensile stresses cause most fractures in dental porcelain.[2]

Porcelain fused to a metal substructure can be used for single and multiple restorations. The all-porcelain restoration is predominately limited to single unit restorations. The "Hollywood" bridge has been updated and uses all-porcelain acid etched retainers in combination with all-porcelain pontics. The main concern is the strength of the interproximal connection. Addressing this problem by increasing the incisogingival height of the connection often encroaches upon the interproximal tissue space. Full coverage all-porcelain bridges with high alumina rods reinforcing the pontic and interproximal area have been reported in the literature.[3] Research, development, and testing of all-porcelain multiple restorations is currently underway, however, laboratory and clinical results concerning the strength and long-term success of both types of restorations are inconclusive at this time.[3]

CLINICAL PROPERTIES OF ALL-PORCELAIN RESTORATIONS

Elimination of a metal substructure is a method of addressing the critical requirements for esthetic anterior restorations. Porcelain alone, (porcelain "jacket" crowns) can produce excellent esthetics and offer some distinct advantages over ceramometal restorations.

Advantages

1. **Better esthetic results.** The inherent translucency of all-porcelain restorations and the absence of an underlying metal substructure, which would have to be masked, produces excellent esthetic results. (See Chapter 9, Cast Glass Ceramic—Full Coverage Restorations.)
2. **Biocompatibility.** Glazed porcelain produces a nonporous surface, which is the most biocompatible of all restorative materials.[4] Potential metal allergies or toxicity reactions are avoided.
3. **Periodontal health.** A butt joint margin design places less material subgingivally when compared to the beveled margin design of the ceramometal restoration. (The subgingival depth of the restoration is reduced by an amount equal to the length of the bevel.) (See Chapter 9, Cast Glass Ceramic—Full Coverage Restorations.)
4. **Transillumination of the gingiva.** These translucent materials allow light to be transmitted into the tooth and do not cause tissue darkening adjacent to the restoration. (See Chapter 9, Cast Glass Ceramic—Full Coverage Restorations.)

Disadvantages

1. **Low compressive strength.** All-porcelain restorations are inherently weak and have high fracture rates.
2. **Limited placement.** All-porcelain restorations are limited primarily to the restoration of anterior teeth, although some manufacturers (e.g., Cerestore and Dicor) claim the materials can be used posteriorly.
3. **Limited ability to create multiple units.** Except in special cases, all-porcelain systems are limited to single units.
4. **Adequate remaining tooth structure is required for ideal preparation form.** All-porcelain restorations require uniform reduction for equal distribution of internal stresses. Therefore, these restorations cannot compensate for extensive loss of tooth structure. The metal component of ceramometal restorations, on the other hand, can be fabricated to provide optimum porcelain support (Figs. 10–1, 10–2).
5. **Marginal integrity is laboratory technique-sensitive.** Good marginal integrity is technically more difficult to achieve with the porcelain butt joint as compared to a metal margin.

6. **Wear of opposing tooth structure.** Porcelain, especially unglazed porcelain, causes wearing of opposing enamel, dentin, and metal. When the opposing tooth structure exhibits areas of wear, metal occlusal surfaces should be used to minimize destruction. Cast glass restorations show great promise because studies indicate that they wear at the same rate as tooth structure.[5]
7. **Inability to esthetically attach a removable partial prosthesis.** Currently, no precision or semiprecision attachment is available to adhere to the all-porcelain restoration. In addition, splinting is not possible.

One porcelain cannot answer the needs of all restorative systems. The physical and chemical properties of porcelain are altered to fit the needs of a particular restorative system.

ALUMINA-REINFORCED CROWN

The alumina-reinforced crown was introduced by McLean and Hughes in 1965. Alumina crystals reinforce a core, which serves as the substructure onto which the porcelain is fired (Figs. 10–3, 10–4).

Advantages

1. **Strength.** Alumina-reinforced crowns have a higher modulus of elasticity and double the compressive strength[6] of regular feldspathic porcelain.
2. **Esthetics.** Alumina-reinforced crowns exhibit excellent esthetics because they transmit light better than ceramometal restorations.
3. **Biocompatibility.** (See the section on Clinical Properties of All-Porcelain Restorations.)
4. **Periodontal health.** (See the section on Clinical Properties of All-Porcelain Restorations.)
5. **Transillumination of the gingiva.** (See the section on Clinical Properties of All-Porcelain Restorations.)

Disadvantages

1. **Microcracks.** Internal surface microcracks invariably occur in alumina-reinforced crowns. They are caused by the inability to adequately wet the foil.
2. **Limited to anterior tooth placement.** (See the section on Clinical Properties of All-Porcelain Restorations.)
3. **Limited ability to create multiple units.** (See

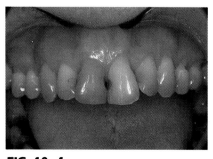

FIG. 10–1

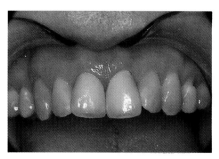

FIG. 10–2

FIG. 10–1. Previous endodontic treatment of the maxillary central incisors necessitated a full coverage restoration. If the remaining tooth structure is limited, all-porcelain restorations are not recommended.

FIG. 10–2. Conservative cast posts and cores and ideal tooth preparation provided maximum support for these all-porcelain restorations.

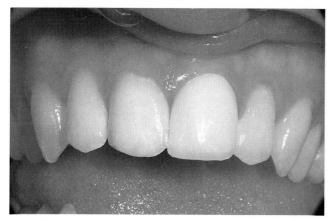

FIG. 10−3. A patient presented with a defective feldspathic porcelain crown on a maxillary left central incisor. The tooth exhibited both poor esthetics and gingival inflammation.

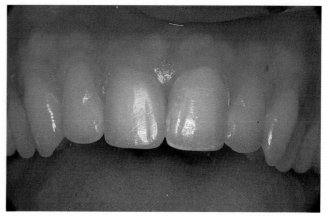

FIG. 10−4. An alumina-reinforced crown was used to replace the existing crown. Note the improved gingival health. Overall esthetic success was enhanced by reshaping the natural tooth structure on the lateral incisors and restoring the incisal edge of the right central incisor with composite resin.

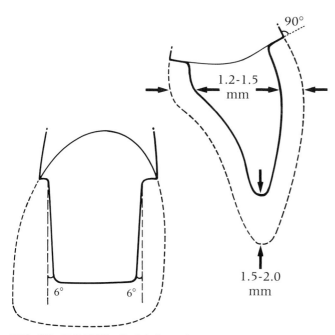

FIG. 10−5 (LEFT). Facial view of anterior preparation.

FIG. 10−6 (RIGHT). Lateral view of anterior preparation.

the section on Clinical Properties of All-Porcelain Restorations.)

4. **Adequate remaining tooth structure is required for ideal preparation form**. (See the section on Clinical Properties of All-Porcelain Restorations.)
5. **Marginal integrity is laboratory technique-sensitive**. (See the section on Clinical Properties of All-Porcelain Restorations.)
6. **Wear of opposing tooth structure**. (See the section on Clinical Properties of All-Porcelain Restorations.)
7. **Inability to esthetically attach a removable partial prosthesis**. (See the section on Clinical Properties of All-Porcelain Restorations.)

Clinically, these restorations have not shown superiority over conventional porcelain jacket crowns esthetically, periodontally, or in terms of strength.

Indications

These restorations are indicated for:

1. Individual anterior teeth when excellent esthetics or biocompatibility is required.
2. Preparation criteria can be met (see below).

Contraindications

These restorations are contraindicated for:

1. Patients with heavy occlusion or bruxism.
2. Patients with short clinical crowns.
3. Patients requiring splinting of teeth.
4. When the preparation criteria can not be met (see below).

Preparation Criteria

1. The preparation of the axial walls should result in an overall 6°-taper (Fig. 10−5).
2. The preparation should result in at least 1.2 to 1.5 mm of reduction and should be two-thirds the length of the anatomic crown of the tooth (Fig. 10−6).
3. The incisal edge of the final preparation should be vertically aligned beneath the incisal edge of the restoration. (See Fig. 10−6).
4. The shoulder should be slightly rounded at the juncture of the axial wall and gingival floor and should end in a sharp line angle at the outer cervical margin (see Fig. 10−6).
5. The junction between all surfaces should be rounded to reduce any stresses at these points (except at the external margin)(see Fig. 10−6).
6. The width of the shoulder should be at least 1 mm around the entire tooth. (See Fig. 10−6.)

Tooth Preparation for Alumina-Reinforced Crowns

The alumina-reinforced crown requires a butt joint margin. Although this type of preparation is mechanically sound, problems may arise from the use of porcelain at the butt joint margin. The somewhat inconsistent and uncontrollable shrinkage of porcelain is largely responsible for the relatively poor marginal fit when compared to the marginal accuracy that can be developed with cast metal systems. The technical skill of the ceramist in handling the various porcelains is as important as the technical skill of the dentist in minimizing these discrepancies.

Armamentarium

- Standard dental setup
  explorer
  mirror
  periodontal probe
  suitable anesthesia
- High-speed handpiece
- Low-speed handpiece
- High-speed burs
  No. 2 high-speed round carbide or equivalent diamond bur (1-mm diameter)
  Round-ended tapered coarse diamond bur with an end diameter of 1 mm.
  Round-ended tapered fine diamond bur with an end diameter of 1 mm.
  Elliptical (football-shaped) medium diamond bur
- Hand instrument, including a double-ended chisel
- No. 0 and No. 1 braided gingival retraction cord (nonepinephrine)

Clinical Technique

1. Create three 1.2-mm vertical depth guide grooves on the labial surface by placing a No. 2 round carbide or diamond bur into the surface of the tooth to slightly greater than its full diameter. The grooves should divide the labial surface into thirds.
2. Create three 2-mm incisal depth guide grooves by placing the bur to twice its diameter into the incisal edge.
3. Place three 1.2-mm depth guide grooves on the lingual surface in a manner identical to the labial guide grooves.
4. Prepare the incisal edge with the tapered coarse diamond bur. Reduction of the incisal edge first eases axial reduction.
5. Remove the remaining labial tooth structure between the depth guide grooves with the tapered round-ended coarse diamond bur and prepare the surface in two planes. First prepare the incisal portion of the labial surface by holding the tapered diamond bur parallel to its surface. Then prepare the gingival portion.
6. Prepare the interproximal surface with the round-ended tapered diamond bur, establishing a 1.2-mm shoulder and 6° of overall taper. The shoulder should follow the contour of the interproximal gingiva.

7. Prepare a 1.2-mm lingual shoulder and establish a gingival one-third axial wall with the round-ended coarse tapered diamond bur. Establishing a sufficient lingual axial wall is important for retention. The lingual axial wall should have 6° of taper when compared to the prepared labial axial wall. Reduce the remaining lingual portion with the elliptical diamond bur to the depth of 1.2 mm.

CLINICAL TIP. If esthetics do not permit supragingival margins (which are desirable for periodontal health) create a subgingival margin and place braided retraction cord in the gingival sulcus slightly below the margin of the preparation. The ends of the chords should not overlap. The shoulder can now be finished just below the free marginal gingiva without trauma.

---

8. Refine and smooth the entire preparation with the fine tapered round-ended diamond bur, rounding all axial line angles. The shoulder should smoothly continue from the labial, to the proximal, to the lingual surfaces, following the free gingival contour. Verify that the labial and interproximal shoulder placement is slightly subgingival if desired. The round ended diamond bur may leave a slight lip at the outer aspect of the shoulder which, with the cord in place, can be easily removed with the diamond bur or with hand instruments.

CLINICAL TIP. Place the retraction cord below the margin and leave it in place during impressioning to create a space for the impression material so that a portion of the *unprepared* tooth structure is captured in the impression.

---

9. The techniques for impressioning, provisional restorations, occlusal registrations, crown try-ins and placements, adjustments of contacts, adjustments of internal fit, and luting are identical to those described in Chapter 9 for Cast Glass Ceramic, Full Coverage Restorations.

PLATINUM BONDED ALUMINA CROWNS

Fabrication of the platinum bonded alumina crowns involves the use of a thin (0.05 mm) platinum foil matrix, which is burnished directly to a die and is bonded with alumina-reinforced porcelains. The microcracks that occur on the internal surface of porcelain crowns and alumina-reinforced crowns are virtually eliminated by the increased ability of the porcelain to wet and bond to the platinum foil. Upon completion of the porcelain laboratory stages, but prior to cementation procedures, the platinum foil matrix is removed. Problems arose from this technique because the incisal edge lengths and occlusion often are altered when the foil is removed. Refiring after the foil is removed is difficult because overall distortion of the crown is no longer controllable.

A "twin foil" technique has been developed to overcome these shortcomings and to ensure an accurate porcelain butt joint fit. Initially, two layers of platinum foil are burnished to the die and the crown is fabricated.

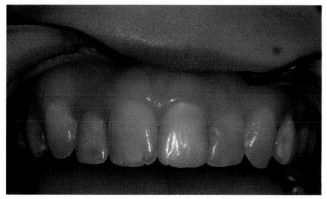

FIG. 10-7. This patient required replacement of the porcelain-fused-to-metal restoration on the right maxillary lateral incisor and the left maxillary central incisor, which had failed esthetically because of poor shade selection and excess opacity.

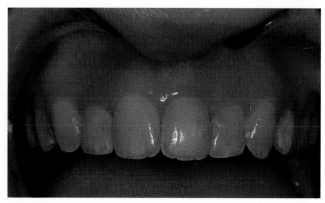

FIG. 10-8. The final restoration in place. A "twin" foil technique was used because it allowed greater control of the incisal length and the necessary repeated firings for proper shade, characterization, contour and texture match.

Upon completion, only one foil is removed and, if an additional oven firing is needed, it can now be accomplished. Repeated firings of the porcelain restoration may result in dimensional changes (Figs. 10-7, 10-8).

Advantages

Platinum bonded alumina restorations offer all the advantages of alumina-reinforced crowns (see the preceding section) and:

1. Elimination of internal surface microcracks produced at the internal surface.
2. Improved marginal integrity.
3. "Twin foil" technique improves the predictability of the final fit and allows firing of porcelain after the first foil is removed.

Disadvantages

Platinum bonded alumina restorations have all the disadvantages of alumina-reinforced crowns. (See the preceding section.) and:

1. Require additional laboratory time.
2. Single layer technique precludes the ability to refine the restoration following the removal of the single layer of foil.

Indications

The indication for the use of platinum bonded alumina crowns are identical to those of alumina-reinforced crowns. (See the preceding section.)

Contraindications

The contraindications for the use of platinum bonded alumina crowns are identical to those of alumina-reinforced crowns. (See the preceding section.)

Clinical Technique

The preparation for this restoration is the same as for an alumina-reinforced crown. (See the preceding section.)

ALUMINOCERAMIC CROWN

Porcelain fused to an aluminoceramic core (Cerestore, Johnson & Johnson Professional Dental Care Co.) was introduced in 1982 by the Coors Biomedical Corporation. This core replaces the metal coping and opaque porcelain of the ceramometal restoration. It eliminates the potential marginal and internal surface flaws of the porcelain jacket restoration.

The core begins as a wax pattern fabricated on an accurate epoxy die. After plaster investing, the wax is boiled out leaving the investment and epoxy die. An aluminoceramic thermoplastic pellet is heated and injection molded under pressure into the remaining void in the investment. This molded coping is the substructure to which porcelain is applied. The coping has an excellent fit because the core is fabricated directly on the epoxy die and, unlike metal copings, these ceramic cores can maintain better marginal integrity with the repeated firings of veneering porcelains.[7] Because of the strength of the ceramic core, this restoration can be used to restore teeth that have a less than ideal prepared tooth structure, but not to the extent that ceramometal restorations can replace lost tooth structure.

The final preparation design is either a butt joint or, preferably, a heavy chamfer with the core material brought out to the external margin. Core modifiers can be used to prevent brightness and opacity in the cervical one-third. The amount of reduction is 1.5 mm axially and 1.5 mm occlusally.

The porcelain buildup is the same as for an aluminous porcelain jacket crown with the same ability to build color intrinsically, however, internal faults in the porcelain are reduced. The aluminoceramic core differentiates the Cerestore restoration from the aluminous porcelain jacket crown.

Although laboratory tests showed excellent results with aluminoceramic crowns, these restorations exhibited a high clinical failure rate.[8] This caused the Cerestore system to be taken off the market and reevaluated. The system is to be reintroduced and hopefully the clinical results will match those of the laboratory.

Advantages

1. Excellent esthetics.
2. Biocompatibility.
3. Coping maintains excellent marginal integrity under repeated firings.
4. Can be used to restore anterior and posterior teeth.

Disadvantages

1. Limited to single units.
2. Requires extensive tooth preparation.
3. Wears opposing tooth structure.
4. Initial cost of laboratory equipment.

Indications

The indications for the use of these crowns include those of alumina-reinforced crowns (see the preceding section), and in addition the restoration of posterior teeth.

Contraindications

The contraindications for the use of these crowns are identical to those of alumina-reinforced crowns. (See the preceding section.)

Clinical Technique

The preparation for this restoration is the same as for alumina-reinforced crowns (see the preceding section), but requires 1.5 mm of axial reduction.

NONCAST METAL CERAMIC SYSTEM

The noncast metal ceramic restoration known commercially as the Renaissance Crown System permits the fabrication of metal ceramic restorations without waxing, investing, and casting the metal coping. A prefabricated pleated gold palladium metal foil is adapted to the die by crimping, burnishing and swedging. After adaptation, the foil is heat treated, forming a rigid gold-ceramic alloy. The foil is extremely thin (0.15 mm), allowing more room for porcelain than traditional cast metal. The metallic foil does not oxidize, therefore, a mechanical bonding material is used to create retention. The gold colored bonding material adequately masks the silver colored foil and helps in shade matching.

The porcelain is applied using conventional techniques. The prepared foil is readily wetted with the porcelain reducing the possibility of internal flaws occurring at the porcelain-foil interface. This results in a restoration with greater strength than the aluminous porcelain jacket restoration. The restoration can be successfully completed with as little as 0.7 mm reduction, but the preparation must be ideal.

The margin design can be an all-metal, shoulder-bevel, feather-edge or chamfer preparation for a thin metal margin or butt joint porcelain.

Advantages

1. Excellent esthetics.
2. Conventional metal coping fabrication is eliminated.

3. Greater strength than aluminous porcelain restoration.
4. Reduced tooth preparation is especially advantageous in restoring mandibular anterior and labially protruded teeth.
5. Fewer laboratory steps.

Disadvantages

1. Limited to single anterior teeth.
2. Requires ideal tooth preparation.
3. Wears opposing tooth structure.

Indications

The indication for the use of these crowns are identical to those of alumina-reinforced crowns (see the preceding section).

Contraindications

The contraindications for the use of these crowns are identical to those of alumina-reinforced crowns (see the preceding section).

Clinical Technique

The preparation for this restoration is the same as for an alumina-reinforced crown (see the preceding section) if an all-porcelain margin is desired, although reduction can be as little as 0.7 mm. A long chamfer, shoulder-bevel, or feather edge preparation is necessary for a metal margin.

CONCLUSION

The current technology of the all-porcelain restoration produces a lifelike result. Success of these restorations depends on sufficient remaining tooth structure, familiarization by both the dentist and laboratory technician with the appropriate techniques, and a knowledge of proper selection criteria.

REFERENCES

1. Saachi, N. and Paffeubarner, C.C.: A simple technique for making dental porcelain jacket crowns. J Am Dent Assoc 54:366, 1957.
2. Wilson, H.J. and Whitehand, F.I.N.: Comparison of some physical properties of dental porcelain. Dent Pract 17:350, 1967.
3. McLean, J.: High alumina ceramics for bridge pontic construction. Br Dent J 123:571, 1968.
4. Eichner, K.: Einflusse von Bruckenjwishengliedein auf die Gingiva. DtschZahnarztl Z 30:639, 1975.
5. Grossman, D.C.: The science of castable glass ceramics. In J.D. Preston (ed.): Perspective in Dental Ceramics. Proceedings of the Fourth International Symposium on Ceramics. Chicago, Quintessence Publishing Co., 1988.
6. McLean, J.W. and Hughes, T.N.: The reinforcement of dental porcelain with ceramic oxides. Br Dent J 119:251, 1965.
7. Sozio, R.B. and Riley, E.J.: The shrink-free ceramic crown. J Prosthet Dent 49:132, 1983.
8. Donovan, T.E.: A longitudinal study of the Cerestore crown, unpublished.

Kenneth W. Aschheim, D.D.S.
Barry G. Dale, D.M.D.

PORCELAIN—LAMINATE VENEERS AND OTHER PARTIAL COVERAGE RESTORATIONS

In the nineteenth century, porcelain inlays were introduced as an esthetic alternative to metallic restorations. These inlays were formed by either grinding a solid porcelain block[1] or more commonly by fusing porcelain chips to a platinum-gold foil matrix.[2] Extremely brittle restorations, they were contraindicated in high stress areas. Their imprecise fit resulted in a visible cement line and caries susceptibility because of cement wash out. In addition, the absence of an adhesive cement limited these restorations to preparations that provided sufficient frictional retention.

Porcelain use decreased following the introduction of silicate cements in 1908. Although silicates, a combination of silica alumina and calcium fluoride, showed significant solubility in salivary fluids, the fluoride component provided anticariogenicity. Acrylic resins, introduced in 1946, immediately replaced silicate resins as the "esthetic material of choice." Although they exhibited better long-term retention, they did not contain fluoride, which resulted in an increased incidence of recurrent decay. Advances in acrylic resin systems compared to earlier restorations controlled some of the polymerization shrinkage but they still exhibited poor overall dimensional stability. In addition, like silicates, acrylic resins required mechanical retention. The introduction of the acid-etch technique and filled composite resins further diminished the use of porcelain as an internal restorative material. Porcelain, in the form of all-porcelain and porcelain-fused-to-metal restorations, was relegated to full coverage restorations.

In the late 1970s, direct and indirect laminate veneers were introduced. Direct veneers, which used light-cured composite resin to overlay the entire facial surface, allowed great flexibility in both shaping and shading teeth, but they were time-consuming and required substantial artistic skill. In addition, they exhibited poor color stability and wear resistance.

Indirect or preformed veneers attempted to overcome some of these limitations.[3] Composed of acrylic, they were treated with ethyl acetate, methylene chloride, or methyl methacrylate and then luted to the etched tooth with a composite resin. Although they exhibited greater color stability and stain resistance than early direct composite resin veneers, the composite resin-to-laminate veneer bond proved to be a fatal weak link.[4] The acrylic veneer also exhibited a dull and monochromatic appearance, poor abrasion resistance,[5] and resulted in unsatisfactory gingival inflammation.

Porcelain-Bonded Restorations

Early research[6] indicated that it was possible to chemically bond silica to acrylic or bis-GMA using a silane coupling agent (see below). Most research[7-9] focused on the direct chemical bonding of porcelain teeth to acrylic denture bases. Early silane bonds prevented seepage of oral fluids between the porcelain-acrylic interface.[10] However, differences in the coefficient of thermal expansion between porcelain and acrylic caused bond deterioration during bench cooling of the heat-cured acrylic.

The need for a technique to repair ceramometal restorations with debonded porcelain prompted interest in the composite resin to porcelain bond. It was discovered that no bond formed between the glazed porcelain and composite resin, even with silane,[11-13] unless the surface was roughened.[14]

In 1983, the porcelain laminate veneer was introduced.[15] It combined the esthetic and positive tissue response of porcelain with the adhesive strength of acid-etch retained restorations and the convenience of a laboratory fabricated restoration. Since that time, posterior inlays and onlays, multiple units for splinting, and even all-porcelain bridges have been advocated.[16-18]

TABLE 11–1. STRENGTH OF RESTORATIVE MATERIALS COMPARED TO ENAMEL

MATERIAL	MODULUS OF RUPTURE (PSI)	COMPRESSIVE STRENGTH (PSI)	MICROHARDNESS (KNH)
Enamel	1,550	58,000	343
Composite Resin	6,600	35,000	30
Porcelain	11,000	25,000	460
DICOR	22,000	120,000	362
OPTEC	25,000	150,000	405

(From Calamia, J.R.: Etch porcelain veneers, the current state of the art. Quintessence Int, 16:5, 1985.)

TABLE 11–2. PROPERTIES OF HIGH STRENGTH PORCELAINS

MATERIAL	STRENGTH FACTOR	OPACITY	MULTIPLE UNITS (PER MANUFACTURER)
Dicor	Mica	Translucent	No
Cera Pearl	Oxylaptite	Translucent	No
Hi-Ceram	Aluminum Oxide	Opaque	No
Optec	Leucite	Translucent	Yes
Cerinate	Unknown	Translucent	Yes

(Adapted from Calamia, J.R.: High strength porcelain bonded restorations: anterior and posterior. Quintessence Int, 20:717, 1989.)

TABLE 11–3. EFFECTS OF ETCHING AND SILANE ON BOND SHEAR STRENGTH

GROUP	ETCH	SILANE	BOND SHEAR STRENGTH
A	Yes	No	2907±SD165
B	Yes	Yes	3485±SD340
C	No	No	564±SD140
D	No	Yes	978±SD390

(Adapted from Hsu, C.S., Stangel, I., and Nathanson, D.: Presentation at the 63rd session of the International Association of Dental Research)

TABLE 11–4. SILANE COUPLING AGENTS

Gamma aminoproppyltriethoxysilane
Vinyltriethoxysilane
Methylacryloxypropyltrimethoxysilane

BASIC CHEMISTRY

The porcelain-bonded restoration consists of four components:

1. an internally etched porcelain veneer
2. an acid etched enamel surface
3. a silane coupling agent
4. a composite resin luting cement.

Porcelain

Dental porcelains are composed of naturals feldspars (both potassium and sodium aluminosilicate glasses).[19] Early porcelain laminate veneers utilized the same porcelains used in all-porcelain restorations. In recent years, high-strength porcelains specifically designed for bonded restorations have been introduced. These materials have greater strength than conventional porcelain, enamel, or composite resin. In addition, they have a hardness more comparable with that of enamel (Table 11–1).[17]

Some manufacturers claim that high-strength porcelains have sufficient strength for use as all-porcelain bridges.[17] Individual composition and properties vary among different manufactures, with some materials exhibiting cast glass characteristics (Table 11–2). (See Chapter 9—Cast Glass Ceramic—Full Coverage Restorations.)

Acid Etching

Retention of the acid-etch retained porcelain restoration is accomplished by the creation of microporosites in both the porcelain and enamel. Porcelain porosities are derived from treating the internal surface of the restoration with a 10% acid solution, such as hydrofluoric acid (HFA). Studies show that etching with or without the use of a silane coupling agent greatly increases bond shear strength,[20] which can even surpass resin-enamel bond strength (Table 11–3).[21] This strength does not diminish over extended periods of time.[21]

Salivary contamination of the etched porcelain can significantly reduce bond strength, even after cleaning with acetone.[22] Application of 37% phosphoric acid for 15 seconds has been shown to restore the etched surface.[22] The etched surface is stable over extended periods. One study[22] demonstrated that a 7-day delay between etching and silane application/veneer cementation did not reduce bond strength when the laminate veneers were kept in a dry environment (e.g., a simple plastic box).

Silane Coupling Agents

The function of a coupling agent is to alter the surface of a solid to facilitate either a chemical or physical process.[10] Numerous silane coupling agents exist and are used in dentistry to increase the shear strength of the porcelain-to-composite resin bond (Table 11–4).

It is believed that these agents are capable of chemically bonding to silica in both the porcelain laminate veneer and the composite resin matrix. Scanning electron micrographs reveal that silane eliminates the polymerization contraction gap, which forms in both etched, nonsilanated and unetched-silanated restorations, by allowing the resin to better wet the surface.[21]

Composite Resin Luting Cements

Initially, laminate veneers were retained with auto-curing composite resins. Light-activated composite resin luting cements provided increased working time.[23] Most resin cements are thinned versions of previously available restorative resins.[24] (See Chapter 5 – Composite Resin Fundamentals and Direct Technique Restorations.)[24] Numerous viscosities are available, with medium viscosity being the most popular. Different shades and opacities allow for color modification of the restoration.

Light-activated resins are ideally suited for most laminate veneers. However, because they require sufficient light to initiate curing, they should not be used when the light must travel through more than a 3-mm thickness of porcelain.[21] This is particularly problematic in the gingival floor and axial wall areas of the interproximal box of porcelain inlays or onlays. Since the light source cannot be positioned perpendicular to the interproximal surface because of the approximating tooth, light rays entering this region at an angle would be required to penetrate 4 to 8 mm of porcelain.[21] In both these cases, a dual-cured composite resin luting system should be utilized.

BASIC LABORATORY TECHNIQUE

Porcelain laminate veneers can be fabricated by the laboratory in one of three ways:

1. **Platinum foil backing.** This method is also used to construct the all-porcelain crown. A very thin layer of platinum foil is placed on the die. The porcelain is layered on the foil. Then the porcelain-foil combination is removed from the die and fired in an oven. Prior to try in, the foil is removed and the porcelain is etched.[17]

   The use of platinum foil permits the porcelain to be repeatedly removed from and replaced onto the die during restoration fabrication. This permits easier access to the proximal margins. In addition, the thickness of foil creates a space for opaques and tinting agents.

   A disadvantage of the platinum foil technique is the gap created when the platinum foil is removed. The clinical significance of this space is uncertain.

2. **Refractory models.** The use of refractory models is the most commonly used method of porcelain lami-

nate veneer fabrication. The restoration is fired directly on a refractory die. This eliminates the platinum layer but makes repeated firings difficult once the laminate veneer has been removed from the die.

   The advantages of the refractory model include tighter contacts and the absence of the gap created by the use of platinum foil. The disadvantages are less room for coloring agents and more difficulty in adjusting proximal areas by the technician.

3. **Direct castings.** Cast glass ceramic restorations are fabricated using the "lost wax" technique. This eliminates the need for multiple firings but requires extrinsic staining for coloration. (See Chapter 9 – Cast Glass Ceramic – Full Coverage Restorations.)

ADVANTAGES

The main advantages of bonded porcelain restorations are:

1. **Excellent esthetics.** Porcelain offers unsurpassed esthetics and inherent color control. In addition, unlike direct laminate veneers, the porcelain laminate veneers depend less on the esthetic skill of the dentist.
2. **Excellent long-term durability.** Porcelain is both abrasion-resistant and color-stable. In addition, porcelain has excellent resistance to fluid absorption.
3. **Inherent porcelain strength.** Porcelain exhibits excellent compressive, tensile, and shear strengths when bonded to enamel.
4. **Marginal integrity.** Porcelain restorations bonded to enamel exhibit exceptional marginal integrity.
5. **Soft tissue compatibility.** Properly polished porcelain is highly biocompatible with gingival tissue.
6. **Minimal tooth reduction.** In anterior restorations, enamel reduction of 0.5 mm or less is adequate for the fabrication of a laminate veneer in many cases.

DISADVANTAGES

The main disadvantages of bonded porcelain restorations are:

1. **Time.** Multiple visits are required.
2. **Cost.** Laboratory involvement and additional chair time are required when compared to direct restorations, resulting in higher costs to the patient.
3. **Fragility.** Although strong when bonded to the tooth, bonded porcelain restorations are extremely fragile during the try-in and cementation stages.
4. **Lack of repairability.** Porcelain restorations are difficult, if not impossible, to repair.
5. **Difficulty in color matching.** Although porcelain restorations are color stable, precise matching of a desired shade tab or an adjacent tooth can be difficult. In addition, shade alteration is impossible after cementation.
6. **Irreversibility.** Unlike bleaching, tooth reduction, although minimal, is required.

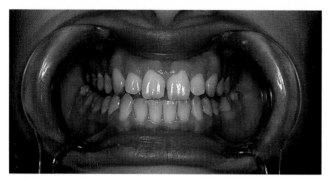

FIG. 11—1. The patient presented with a midline diastema. She also thought her teeth were too long.

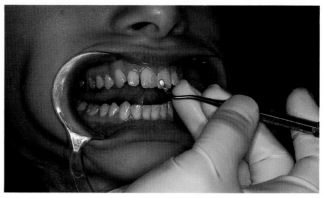

FIG. 11—2. The wax is refined with a plastic instrument.

7. **Inability to trial cement the restoration.** Unlike traditional indirect restorations, bonded porcelain restorations cannot be temporarily retained with a provisional cement for evaluation purposes.

INDICATIONS

Porcelain laminate veneers are indicated in areas traditionally restored with single crowns or composite resin veneers for:

1. Correcting diastemata.
2. Masking discolored or stained teeth.
3. Masking enamel defects.
4. Correcting malaligned or malformed teeth.

Porcelain inlays and onlays are indicated in areas traditionally restored with amalgams, single unit cast restorations, and composite resins:

1. For the esthetic restoration of large posterior teeth with adequate tooth structure.
2. As a conservative esthetic alternative to full coverage restorations in teeth requiring onlaying of cusps.
3. As a more durable alternative to posterior composite resin restorations.
4. As a less periodontally invasive alternative to full coverage restorations with subgingival margins.
5. In "amalgam phobic" patients.

CONTRAINDICATIONS

Porcelain laminate veneers are contraindicated for:

1. Patients who exhibit tooth wear due to bruxism.
2. Short teeth.
3. Teeth with insufficient or inadequate enamel for sufficient retention (e.g., severe abrasion).
4. Existing large restorations or endodontically treated teeth with little remaining tooth structure.
5. Patients with oral habits causing excessive stress on the restoration (e.g., nail biting, pencil biting).

Porcelain inlays and onlays are contraindicated for:

1. Patients who exhibit bruxism.
2. Short teeth.
3. Insufficient or inadequate enamel for sufficient retention.

4. Exceedingly thin buccal or lingual walls.
5. Endodontically treated teeth with little remaining tooth structure.
6. Patients with oral habits causing excessive stress on the restoration (e.g., nail biting, pencil biting).

DIAGNOSTIC AND TREATMENT PLANNING AIDS

Porcelain laminate veneers can be used to change any or all of the following characteristics of a single tooth or multiple teeth:

1. Color (including characterizations and degree of polychromaticity)
2. Size
3. Shape
4. Position within the arch.

Wax and Paint Simulation

White orthodontic wax and acrylic paint provide an extremely effective diagnostic and patient education aid. This is especially helpful when evaluating the treatment of single or multiple diastemas, and fractured, misshaped, or malpositioned teeth. The wax can be used to quickly and inexpensively simulate (and thereby "preview") the effects of porcelain laminate veneer placement.

CLINICAL TIP. Prediction of the anticipated outcome of porcelain laminate veneer placement without the use of a preliminary wax simulation is deceptively difficult even for the experienced dentist. A wax "preview" often reveals a favorable prognosis for a clinical situation that initially appears unmanageable with porcelain laminate veneers.

Armamentarium

- White orthodontic tray wax (Hygienic Corp.)
- Mars Black artist's acrylic paint (Liquidtex, Inc.)
- Plastic instrument (Plastic Instrument PF4, Schein, Inc.)
- One-piece lip retractor (e.g., Self-Span, Ellman International Manufacturing Co. or Expandex, Parkell)
- Cotton-tipped applicator

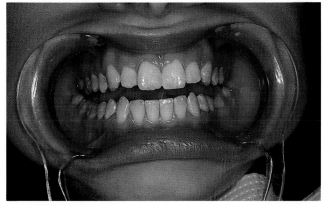

FIG. 11–3. The diastema is closed with white orthodontic tray wax.

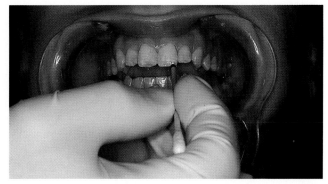

FIG. 11–4. Mars black acrylic paint is applied to the teeth with the wooden end of a cotton-tipped applicator.

Clinical Technique

1. Isolate the teeth with a one-piece lip retractor (Fig. 11–1).
2. Dry thoroughly with an air syringe.

CLINICAL TIP. Squeeze a one-eighth inch strip of orthodontic wax between the thumb and index fingers. This will quickly form a thin "veneer-shaped" piece of wax.

---

3. Apply the wax to the teeth and grossly mold to shape with the index finger.
4. Refine the wax with the plastic instrument (Figs. 11–2, 11–3).

CLINICAL TIP. Shortening of the teeth can be simulated by applying an appropriate amount of black artist's acrylic paint to the dried tooth surface using the wooden end of a cotton-tipped applicator, (Fig. 11–4), turning off the examination light, and having the patient separate the teeth until they do not exhibit vertical overlap (Fig. 11–5). Squinting will augment the illusion.

Computer Imaging

Computer imaging provides a two-dimensional prediction similar to the three-dimensional preview provided by wax simulation and acrylic paint. This system has the added advantage of previewing the effects of color and characterization changes and providing a more lifelike prognostication. Computer imaging systems can also provide instant photographs of the predicted changes. (See Chapter 29 – Esthetics and Advanced Technology).

PATIENT EDUCATION
Photography

One of the most effective patient education tools is a book or photograph album containing before and after images of representative cases. These educational materials can be purchased commercially or produced by the dentist. (See also Chapter 17 – Esthetics and Oral Photography.)

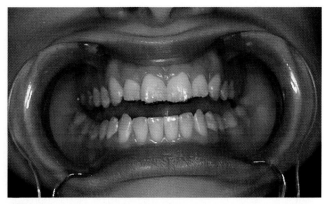

FIG. 11–5. The black acrylic paint helps the patient envision the esthetic effect of shortening the teeth.

Demonstration Models

Sample porcelain laminate veneers fabricated to fit on prepared denture teeth or stone models are valuable patient education aids. They effectively demonstrate the conservative nature of this technique and the lifelike appearance of the final restorations.

TOOTH PREPARATION

The outline form of the porcelain laminate veneer tooth preparation depends largely on the degree of desired color alteration. This consideration particularly influences the location of the interproximal and gingival finish lines.

Static Area of Visibility vs. Dynamic Area of Visibility

The entire labial tooth surface, including the gingival area and the area immediately labial to the contact area with the adjacent tooth (the labial embrasure), is visible if the available light and the perspective of the viewer is optimal. This static area of visibility occurs when the patient is seated in the dental chair under adequate lighting and with the lips fully retracted. The static area of visibility significantly differs from the actual dynamic area of visibility exhibited during normal function.

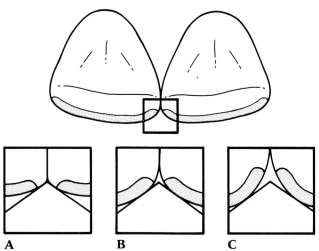

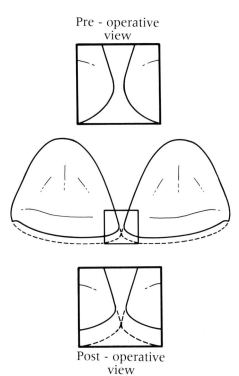

FIG. 11–6. The dynamic area of visibility of the labial embrasure is influenced by the depth of the embrasure space and by the shadow cast by surrounding structures including the tooth itself. A. The entire embrasure space is visible. The margins of the laminate veneers illustrated in the figure will be visible. In order to hide this margin the finishing line must be placed into the contact area. B. The embrasure space is only partially visible. The margins of the porcelain laminate veneers illustrated in the figure are just within the nonvisible area. C. The majority of the embrasure space is not visible. The margins of the porcelain laminate veneer illustrated in the figure need not have been placed as deeply into the interproximal area.

Pre - operative
view

Post - operative
view

FIG. 11–7. Feather-edged proximal finishing lines are used in proximal areas adjacent to diastemata.

The dynamic area of visibility of the labial embrasure is partially a function of viewing perspective. It is particularly influenced, however, by shadows cast from surrounding structures. The lip, adjacent tooth contour and position, and gingival architecture, as well as the contour, shade, and position of the tooth under observation are all important factors (Fig. 11–6).

The dynamic area of visibility of the gingival area is governed by the position of the lip during maximal smiling (the high smile line).

Minimal or No Color Change

Proximal Finishing Lines. A proximal chamfer finishing line is preferred except when diastemata are present. Proximal areas adjacent to diastemata should receive a feather-edged finishing line (Fig. 11–7).

Proximal Contact Area. When the shade difference between the tooth *following* preparation and the desired final restoration is minimal, proximal chamfer finish lines are placed slightly labial (approximately 0.2 mm) to the contact areas of the adjacent tooth. This provides for:

1. ease in evaluating marginal fit during the try-in stage.
2. access for performing and evaluating finishing procedures.
3. access for home care (margins in "self-cleansing" area).
4. ease in evaluating marginal integrity during follow-up maintenance visits.

The major disadvantage of this design is the possibility of eventual staining at the tooth-restoration interface. However, the factors influencing the dynamic area of visibility often negate this disadvantage. (See the preceding section on Static vs. Dynamic Area Of Visibility.)

Proximal Subcontact Area. The proximal subcontact area (PSCA) consists of the interproximal tooth structure which is immediately gingival to the contact area with the adjacent tooth. This area is usually not visible from a direct frontal view of the tooth (Fig. 11–8) and is, therefore, often left underprepared or totally unprepared. It is visible, however, from an oblique view. Therefore, preparation of the PSCA is essential[25] and is particularly crucial when the final restoration significantly differs in shade from that of the unprepared tooth structure (Figs. 11–9 to 11–12).

CLINICAL TIP. View the preparation of the PSCA from all oblique angles to assure adequate extension into this often overlooked area.

Diastemata. The proximal area adjacent to a diastema should receive a feather-edged finishing line (see Figure 11–7). This finishing line extends from the incisal edge to a point adjacent to the height of the gingival papilla.

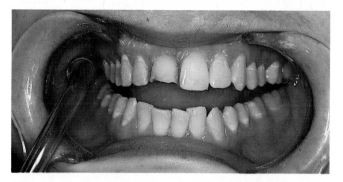

FIG. 11–8. A partially prepared tooth shows that the proximal subcontact area is not visible when the tooth is observed from a direct frontal view.

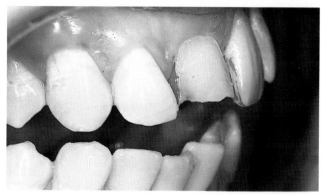

FIG. 11–9. The same preparation as shown in Figure 11–8, viewed from an oblique angle. The proximal subcontact area is often overlooked during tooth preparation. The red dye on the proximal surfaces delineates the area that must be reduced in order to hide the margin of the subsequent restoration.

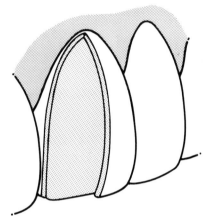

FIG. 11–10. The proximal subcontact area is visible only from an oblique perspective and is often left unprepared or underprepared.

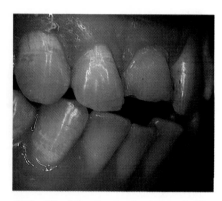

FIG. 11–11. The tooth shown in Figure 11–8 following removal of the red dye and tooth reduction in the proximal subcontact area.

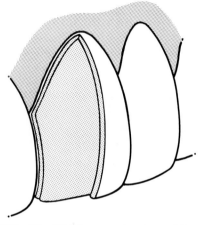

FIG. 11–12. Proper extension of the preparation into the proximal subcontact area.

Gingival Finishing Lines. A chamfer is preferred for all gingival finishing lines. Supragingival finishing lines provide the same advantages as proximal finishing lines which terminate labial to the contact areas. In addition, impressions are easier to make with supragingival preparations as compared to subgingival preparations. Supragingival finishing lines also increase the likelihood that restoration margins will end on enamel. The major disadvantage, however, is that any subsequent staining or color changes at the restoration margin will be visible. Therefore, supragingival margins are limited to clinical situations when this area remains concealed by the lip during maximum smiling (high lip line).

When the entire clinical crown is included in the labial display, the gingival margin should be placed 0.1 mm below the free gingival margin. If gingival recession is anticipated, the gingival finishing line can be extended deeper subgingivally provided the biologic width is not violated.

CLINICAL TIP. The position of the lip during maximum smiling (the high lip line) may be deceptive. Patients with unattractive smiles often habitually adapt a high lip line position which is significantly less revealing of tooth structure than is anatomically possible. After porcelain laminate veneers are placed, the high lip line may significantly elevate because the psychological barriers inhibiting full smiling have been removed. Therefore, this lip position must be critically evaluated before supragingival finishing lines are planned.

Incisal Preparation. Incisal reduction should ideally provide for 1 mm of porcelain thickness. Therefore, if the incisogingival height of the final restoration is to be 0.5 mm longer than the existing tooth, only 0.5 mm of incisal reduction is required. If the preoperative teeth are to be lengthened by 1 mm, only a rounding of the incisal edge and placement of a finishing line is required.

A butt joint finishing line provides for the proper thickness of porcelain at the margin to prevent restoration fracture. The finishing line should slope slightly

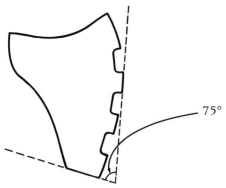

FIG. 11–13. A butt joint incisal finishing line should slope approximately 75° gingivally from the labial to provide for adequate thickness of porcelain at the margin to prevent restoration fracture and displacement.

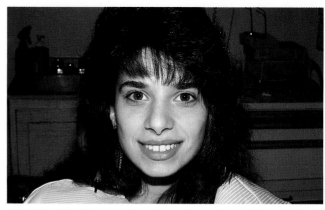

FIG. 11–14. Preoperative view of a patient with multiple diastemata and discolored teeth.

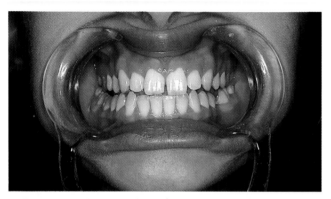

FIG. 11–15. Close-up view of the patient in Figure 11–14.

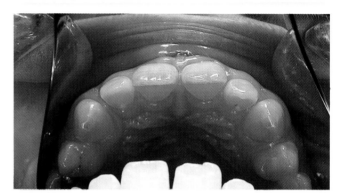

FIG. 11–16. Incisal view of the patient in Figure 11–14.

gingivally (approximately 75° from the labial). This augments resistance to labial displacement of the final restoration due to long-term composite resin fatigue (Fig. 11–13).

After ideal preparation, the incisal outline of the tooth, when viewed from the labial aspect, should be identical to the incisal outline of the proposed final restoration, except for a 1-mm incisal reduction. This allows for an even thickness of porcelain. Incisal line angles must be rounded to reduce internal restoration stresses.

Labial Depth Reduction. A labial reduction of approximately 0.5 to 0.7 mm is sufficient for most maxillary teeth and 0.3 mm for smaller teeth, such as mandibular incisors, if adequate thickness of enamel is present. Inadequate thickness of enamel, such as in the gingival one-third of the tooth, may require a more conservative tooth reduction. Teeth or portions of rotated tooth surfaces that are in lingual version require proportionately less reduction. Preparation into dentin is sometimes necessary, however, this should involve less than 50% of the prepared surface.[20] The entire finishing line should ideally remain in enamel.

Major Color Change

In addition to considerations of preparation design for minimal color changes (see the preceding section on

Minimal or No Color Change), major color differences between the prepared tooth and the desired final restoration may also require extension of the interproximal finishing line into the contact area to a depth of approximately one-half the labiolingual dimension of the contact area if the area is visible during function (see the preceding section on Static vs. Dynamic Area Of Visibility). The gingival finishing line can be extended 1 mm subgingivally provided the biologic width is not violated. Supragingival margins are indicated, however, if this area remains concealed by the lip during maximal smiling (high smile line). (See the preceding Clinical Tip.) The preparation depth may be increased to approximately .7 mm if sufficient thickness of enamel is present. This will allow for an increased thickness of porcelain or additional layers of die spacer to increase the available space for an opaque cement.

CLINICAL TIP. Tetracycline discoloration occurs in the dentin. The prepared tooth may be darker in color than the original tooth shade because the deep tooth preparation that is often necessary in these cases removes a significant amount of the "masking" enamel.

Armamentarium

■ Basic dental setup
  Explorer
  High-speed handpiece

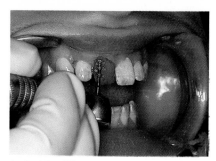

FIG. 11-17

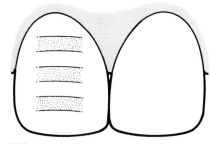

FIG. 11-18

FIGS. 11-17 AND 11-18. Three horizontal depth cuts are prepared in the labial surface.

Low-speed handpiece
Mouth mirror
Periodontal probe
Suitable anesthesia (if necessary)
- One piece lip retractor (e.g., Self-Span, Ellman International Manufacturing Co. or Expandex, Parkell)
- High-speed (friction grip) diamond three-tiered depth cutting burs (e.g., LVS-1 (0.3 mm depth cut) and LVS-2 (0.5 mm depth cut), Brasseler)
- High-speed (friction grip) two-grit burs (LVS-3, LVS-4, Brasseler)
- High-speed (friction grip) diamond wheel bur (e.g., 5909, Brasseler)
- Unwaxed regular dental floss
- Interproximal abrasive strips (Sof-Flex Strips No. 1954 coarse/medium, 3M, Inc.)
- Sharp pencil
- Retraction cord packer (e.g., Fischer's Ultrapak Packer, Ultradent Products, Inc.)
- Nonimpregnated gingival retraction cord (e.g., Ultrapak No. 0 or No. 1, Ultradent Products, Inc.; Gingibraid No. 0 or No. 1, Van R)
- Gingival retraction instrument (e.g., Zekrya, Foremost Dental Manufacturing, Inc.)(optional)
- Pencil

Clinical Technique

1. Evaluate the high lip line. (See the Clinical Tip in the preceeding section on Gingival Finishing Lines.) (Figs. 11-14 to 11-16)
2. Administer suitable anesthesia (if necessary).
3. Prepare three horizontal surface depth cuts in the

labial surface with a friction grip three-tiered LVS-1 or LVS-2 depth cutting diamond (Figs. 11-17, 11-18). Depth cuts should be 0.5 to 0.7 mm deep for "ideal" teeth, and 0.3 mm deep for mandibular incisors. Lingually positioned teeth and those with thin enamel require less reduction. (See the preceding section on Labial Depth Reduction.)

CLINICAL TIP. When the three-tiered depth cutting bur is held tangentially to the surface of the tooth, only the middle section of the bur penetrates to its entire depth. This is due to the tooth's convex labial surface (Figs. 11-19, 11-20). In order to avoid underpreparation, the bur must be positioned two additional times to assure complete penetration of each section of the bur (Figs. 11-21 to 11-24).

4. Prepare three incisal depth cuts with an LVS-3 or LVS-4 diamond bur (Figs. 11-25, 11-26). (The incisal reduction should create a preparation that is 1 mm shorter than the desired final restoration.)
5. Using the depth cut as a guide, prepare the incisolingual finishing line to a modified butt joint with the diamond wheel bur (Figs. 11-27, 11-28). The labioincisolingual angle should be approximately 75°. (See Fig. 11-13.)

CLINICAL TIP. In order to prevent over-reduction, pencil lines can be drawn into the prepared enamel guide cuts (Fig. 11-29). Labial reduction is complete immediately after the pencil lines are removed by the action of the reduction bur.

6. Using the depth cuts as a guide, prepare the labial surface with an LVS-3 or LVS-4 diamond bur (Figs. 11-30, 11-31).
7. Prepare the proximal chamfer finishing lines.
   A. For *diastema*
      (1) Prepare a feather-edged finishing line with an LVS-3 or LVS-4 diamond bur. The finishing line should terminate as far to the lingual aspect as possible without creating an undercut area, and should extend from the incisal edge to the point adjacent to the height of the gingival papilla (Fig. 11-32, see also Fig. 11-7).
   B. *For minimal or no color change and no diastema* (See the preceding section on Minimal or No Color Change)
      (1) Prepare the proximal chamfer finishing line with an LVS-3 or LVS-4 diamond bur to approximately .2 mm labial to contact area (Figs. 11-33, 11-34).
      (2) Prepare the proximal subcontact area with an LVS-3 or LVS-4 diamond bur (Fig. 11-35).
   C. *For major color change and no diastema* (See the preceding section on Major Color Change)
      (1) Prepare the proximal chamfer finishing line with an LVS-3 or LVS-4 diamond bur to a depth of one-half the labiolingual dimension of the interproximal contact area (Figs. 11-36, 11-37).

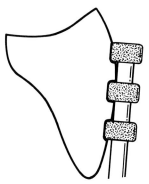

FIG. 11–19. When the three-tiered depth cutting bur is held tangentially to the surface of the tooth, only the middle section of the bur penetrates to its entire depth.

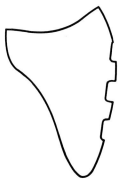

FIG. 11–20. Only the middle section of the tooth is prepared to the full depth because of the convex labial surface. The incisal and gingival portions of the tooth are underprepared.

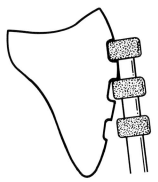

FIG. 11–21. The bur is angled a second time to complete the gingival depth cut.

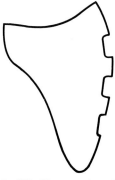

FIG. 11–22. The tooth after two depth cuts. The incisal portion of the tooth remains underprepared.

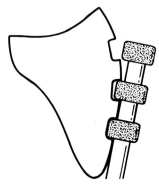

FIG. 11–23. The bur is angled for the third time to complete the incisal depth cut.

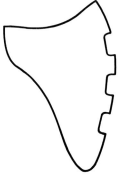

FIG. 11–24. The three depth cuts are equally deep.

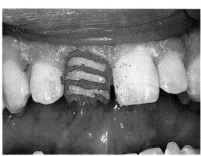

FIGS. 11–25 AND 11–26. Three vertical depth cuts are prepared in the incisal edge.

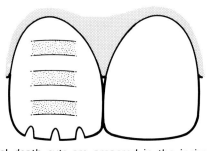

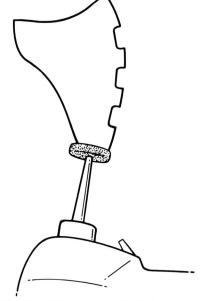

FIG. 11–27. The incisolingual finishing line was prepared to a modified butt joint using the depth cut as a guide.

FIG. 11–28. An incisal butt joint angled approximately 75° from the labial provides for adequate thickness of porcelain at the margin and resistance to displacement of the restoration.

FIG. 11–29. In order to prevent over-reduction, pencil lines can be drawn into the prepared enamel guide cuts. Labial reduction is complete immediately after the pencil lines are removed by the action of the reduction bur.

FIGS. 11–30 AND 11–31. The labial surface is prepared using the horizontal depth cuts as a guide.

FIG. 11–32. The feather-edged finishing line is prepared adjacent to the diastemata. (See incisal view Figures 11–7 and 11–47.)

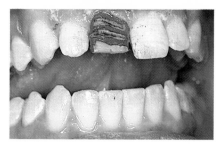

FIG. 11–29

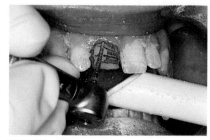

FIG. 11–30

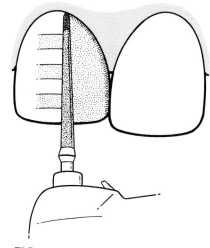

FIG. 11–31

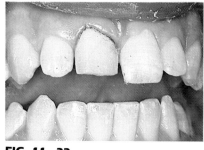

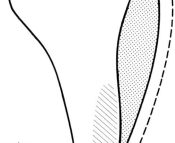

FIG. 11–32

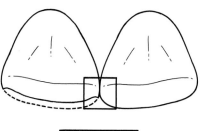

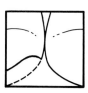

FIG. 11–33. If the final porcelain laminate veneer will be similar in color to that of the prepared tooth, the proximal finishing line terminates 0.2 mm labial to the contact area.

FIG. 11–34. Proximal representation of porcelain laminate veneer preparation prior to reduction of the proximal sub-contact area. The proximal finishing line terminates 0.2 mm labial to the contact area because the final porcelain laminate veneer will be similar in color to that of the prepared tooth. The contact area is indicated with diagonal lines.

FIG. 11–35. Proximal representation of porcelain laminate veneer preparation shown in Figure 11–34 after proper reduction of the proximal subcontact area.

FIG. 11–36. If the final porcelain laminate veneer will significantly differ in color from that of the prepared tooth, the proximal finishing line terminates within the interproximal contact area at a depth of one-half the labiolingual dimension of the contact area.

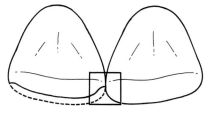

FIG. 11–34   **FIG. 11–35**

FIG. 11–36

(2) Prepare the proximal subcontact area with an LVS-3 or LVS-4 diamond bur (Fig. 11–38).

CLINICAL TIP. Be certain that unprepared tooth structure in the proximal subcontact area is not visible from all oblique viewing perspectives. (See the Clinical Tip in the preceeding section on Proximal Subcontact Area and Figures 11–8 and 11–12.)

---

8. Prepare the gingival finishing line:
   A. *For supragingival preparations*
      (1) Prepare the gingival finishing line to the desired location.
   B. *For subgingival margins*
      (1) Gently place gingival retraction cord (Fig. 11–39). The cord should extend into the sulcus of the interproximal papillae beyond the proximal finishing line (Fig. 11–40).

CLINICAL TIP. For subgingival preparations, draw a line with a sharpened pencil at the present location of the gingival cavosurface margin (currently at the level of the free gingival margin).

CLINICAL TIP. When retraction cord is placed, the gingiva will not only be retracted labially, but usually also gingivally (Fig. 11–41).

---

9. Extend the gingival finishing line (for subgingival preparations only) approximately 0.1 mm subgingivally with an LVS-3 or LVS-4 diamond bur (Fig. 11–42). Use the pencil line (see above Clinical Tip) as a guide. Severely discolored teeth may require a 1-mm subgingival extension of the finishing line.

CLINICAL TIP. The gingiva can be gently retracted with the gingival retraction instrument (Fig. 11–43).

---

10. Round the incisal line angles with an LVS-3 or LVS-4 diamond bur. The thinner LVS-5 or LVS-6 diamond burs may be necessary to access line angles that are close to adjacent teeth (Figs. 11–44 to 11–48).

CLINICAL TIP. Rounding the incisal line angles reduces the internal stress, and thereby the fracture potential, of the final restoration.[26]

IMPRESSIONING

Armamentarium

- Retraction cord packer (e.g., Fischer's Ultrapak Packer, Ultradent Products Inc.)

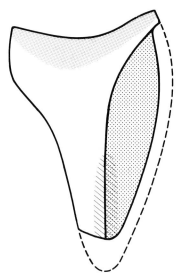

FIG. 11–37. Proximal representation of porcelain laminate veneer preparation prior to reduction of the proximal subcontact area. The proximal finishing line terminates within the interproximal contact area at a depth of one-half the labiolingual dimension of the contact area because the final porcelain laminate veneer will be significantly different in color from that of the prepared tooth.

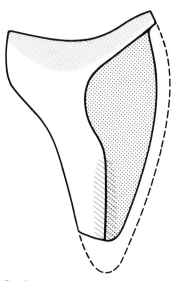

FIG. 11–38. Proximal representation of porcelain laminate veneer preparation shown in Figure 11–37 after proper reduction of the proximal subcontact area.

- Nonimpregnated gingival retraction cord (e.g., Ultra-pak No. 0 or No. 1, Ultradent Products, Inc.; Gingi-braid No. 0 or No. 1, Van R)
- Scissors
- Elastomeric impression material

Clinical Technique

1. Gently place a retraction cord in the sulcus unless previously placed during preparation.

> **CLINICAL TIP.** It is essential that the cord is positioned just beneath the finishing line to avoid interfering with capturing the entire gingival margin in the impression.

2. Make the impression with any accurate elastomeric impression material.

> **CLINICAL TIP.** The retraction cord should be left in place during impressioning. It is usually removed in the impression. However, be certain that all remaining cord is removed prior to proceeding to the next step (Fig. 11–49).

PROVISIONAL RESTORATIONS

The placement of provisional restorations is usually unnecessary because of the conservative nature of porcelain laminate veneer preparations (Figs. 11–50, 11–51). A patient's desire for provisional restorations is often based on expectations or previous experience with crown and bridge procedures, rather than actual esthetic necessity. In many cases the improved contour of the prepared teeth and the possible removal of surface discolorations after preparation results in enhanced esthetics when compared with the preoperative appearance. These considerations, as well as any additional fees for provisional restorations, should be discussed in the initial consultation.

If a provisional restoration is deemed necessary, the gingival termination of the provisional restoration should not impinge upon the gingival tissue in order to prevent gingival inflammation or recession.

Provisional restoration fabrication involves the use of a template and light-cured composite resin. A preoperative study model is made from an irreversible hydrocolloid impression. If the preoperative tooth contours are esthetically unacceptable, appropriate recontouring or wax buildup is accomplished. The modified model is duplicated and a clear plastic matrix is fabricated by either the Ellman Press-Form system or a vacuum former unit. (See Chapter 13 – Acrylic and Other Resins—Provisional Restorations.) An alternate method involves the fitting of individual celluloid (clear) crown forms over the prepared teeth. (See Chapter 13 – Acrylic and Other Resins—Provisional Restorations). The appropriate palatal and proximal surfaces of the crown form or matrix are then removed.

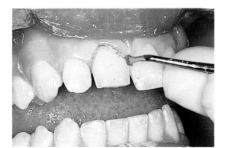

FIG. 11–39. Retraction chord is placed.

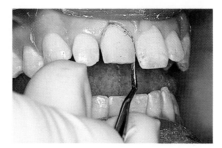

FIG. 11–40. The cord should extend into the sulcus of the interproximal papillae beyond the proximal finishing line.

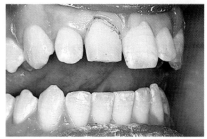

FIG. 11–41. When retraction cord is placed, the gingiva will not only be retracted labially, but usually also gingivally as the pencil line demonstrates. The pencil line was drawn at the level of the free gingival margin prior to cord placement (see Fig. 11–32).

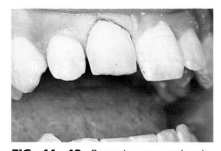

FIG. 11–42. Properly prepared subgingival finishing line.

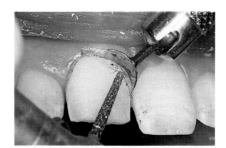

FIG. 11–43. The gingiva can be gently retracted with the gingival retraction instrument.

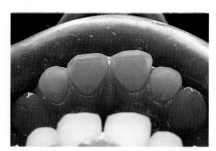

FIG. 11–44. The incisal line angle is rounded to prevent internal stresses within the porcelain laminate veneer.

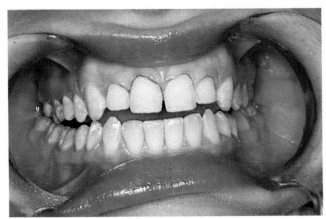

FIG. 11—45. Teeth prepared for porcelain laminate veneers. The proximal subcontact area is not visible from this direct frontal view.

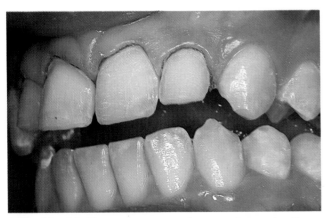

FIG. 11—46. The same preparation as shown in Figure 11—44 viewed from an oblique angle. The proximal subcontact area chamfer preparation between the maxillary left central and lateral incisor has been properly extended. The proximal chamfer finishing line terminates approximately 0.2 mm labial to the contact area between these two teeth. All incisal edges have been rounded.

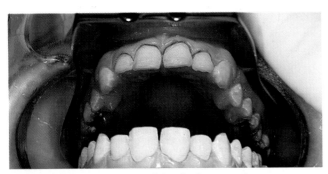

FIG. 11—47. Incisal view of the final preparations.

CLINICAL TIP. The retention of the restoration is solely mechanical in nature. Therefore, a single multitooth provisional restoration will be more effectively retained than separate single tooth provisional restorations.

Armamentarium

- Basic dental setup (See preceding section on Armentarium under Major Color Change.)
- Plastic matrix or celluloid crown forms (see above)
- Sable brush (No. 0)
- Bonding agent
- Hybrid composite resin (e.g., Multifil VS, Kulzer, Inc.)
- Fine diamond finishing burs (e.g., ET Burs, Brasseler; Micron Finishing System, Premier Dental Products Co.)

Clinical Technique

1. Fit the plastic matrix over the prepared teeth (Fig. 11—52).

CLINICAL TIP. The matrix margins should allow for easy removal of excess composite resin.

2. Remove the matrix and place the appropriate shade of composite resin into the matrix.

CLINICAL TIP. It is unnecessary to etch the enamel, prime the dentin surfaces, or place bonding agent on the teeth before composite resin placement. Retention of the provisional restoration is solely mechanical.

3. Place the matrix and resin onto the prepared teeth. (If multiple celluloid crown forms are used, all should be placed before curing; after curing, the restoration will be a single solid unit.)
4. Remove excess composite resin from the *entire* buccal, lingual, and proximal surfaces (Fig. 11—53).

CLINICAL TIP. Dip a sable brush or cotton pellet in bonding agent and wipe off all excess composite resin before curing. The composite resin should also be feather-edged on the palatal surfaces with the wetted brush. Precise, smooth marginal adaptation will assure minimal adjustment after curing and prevent gingival inflammation.

5. Light-cure all surfaces for a minimum of 60 seconds each.

CLINICAL TIP. Light-cured resin cannot be damaged by excessive light exposure. It is therefore preferable to err on the side of longer exposure times.

6. Verify and correct the occlusion with high-speed diamond finishing burs.

CLINICAL TIP. Adjustments of the provisional restoration must not alter the previously prepared tooth. If this would not be possible, remove the entire restoration and place a new restoration, making certain that all excess composite resin is removed prior to curing.

7. Recontour with high-speed diamond finishing burs (if necessary).
8. Instruct the patient that the provisional restoration is for esthetic purposes only and that careful limited function is required (Figs. 11—54, 11—55).

CLINICAL TIP. If the provisional restoration dislodges it can be re-cemented with a noneugenol temporary cement. Alternatively, a 1-mm diameter area of midlabial surface enamel can be etched and the provisional restoration can be luted into place with a low viscosity resin cement.

9. Remove the provisional restoration with a hemostat at the try-in appointment. Break the brittle composite resin into smaller fragments if it cannot be removed in one piece.

LABORATORY COMMUNICATIONS
Natural vs. Idealized Artificial Appearance

Natural teeth are polychromatic and characterized. Canines are usually slightly lower in value or higher in chroma than incisors and premolars. These can be disturbing insights for patients who often desire an idealized artificial appearance (monochromatic, white "chicklets"). Both of these alternatives, and the myriad options in between, should be discussed before a final shade selection is made. It may be helpful to elicit the opinion of the patient's friend or family member.

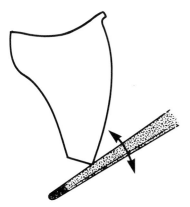

FIG. 11–48. Incisal view demonstrating clearly defined palatal finishing lines.

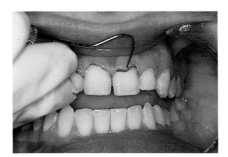

FIG. 11–49. Retraction cord should be removed immediately after impressions are made.

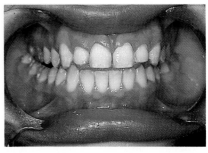

FIG. 11–50. The placement of provisional restorations is usually unnecessary because of the conservative nature of porcelain laminate veneer preparations.

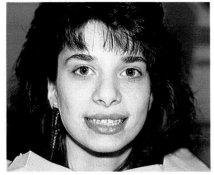

FIG. 11–51. Full face view of patient in Figure 11–50.

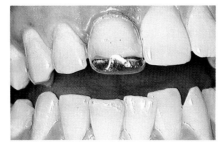

FIG. 11–52. A patient with a single prepared maxillary incisor who required a provisional restoration. A trimmed celluloid crown form is positioned over the prepared tooth.

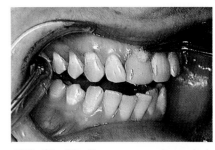

FIG. 11–53. Excess composite resin is removed with a cotton pellet moistened with bonding agent.

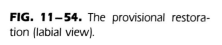

FIG. 11–54. The provisional restoration (labial view).

FIG. 11–55. The provisional restoration (incisal view).

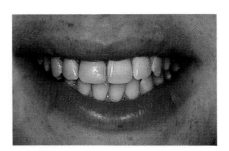

FIG. 11–54

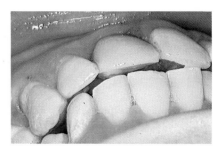

FIG. 11–55

Shade

CLINICAL TIP. Include in the laboratory prescription both the shade of the tooth after tooth reduction and the desired final restoration shade. This will allow the laboratory technician to compensate for the underlying discoloration.

In order to achieve the desired shade change, the percentage of opaquing porcelain and the amount of die spacer can be appropriately adjusted by the dental laboratory technician. The specific ratios vary depending on the type and brand of materials used. Close communication with the dental laboratory technician is essential in this regard.

CLINICAL TIP. It is easier to "darken" (lower the value and increase the chroma) than to "lighten" a porcelain laminate veneer by use of internal modification with luting resin. Therefore, when in doubt about a final shade, select the "lighter" alternative. (See Chapter 2 – Fundamentals of Esthetics and Appendix A – Custom Staining).

Shape

Indicate the desired shape and size of each individual porcelain laminate veneer. As a general rule, feminine teeth are more rounded, less textured, and smaller than masculine teeth, however, this is not always appropriate nor is it always desired by the patient. (See Chapter 2—Fundamentals of Esthetics.) Therefore, specific characterizations should be specified diagrammatically, or in writing, on the laboratory prescription.

Texture

Texturing scatters reflected light and produces a more natural appearance. If not all of the teeth in the labial display are to be restored, the laboratory should be instructed to match the texture of the adjacent teeth.

CLINICAL TIP. Lack of texturing can produce an artificial appearance because scattering of light is diminished or absent.

Characterization of Porcelain Laminate Veneers

Characterization and polychromaticity of porcelain laminate veneers can be accomplished by the laboratory technician through the use of different shades of porcelain or by surface staining. Additional modifications can also be accomplished by the dentist at the time of cementation through the use of internal color modifying agents.

A combination of composite resin color modifiers, opaquers, and different shades of luting cements can be layered between the prepared tooth and the restoration in order to create a polychromatic effect. However, it is difficult to maintain continuity from tooth to tooth with this technique. Even slight variations in the ratios and relative positioning of these agents and differences in the spacing between the porcelain and the tooth surface can influence the final appearance. This is further complicated because the uncured shade-modifying materials are spread by compression from the seating of the porcelain laminate veneer and not by direct manual placement and subsequent curing before overlaying (as with direct composite resin laminate veneers).

Characterization and polychromaticity of porcelain laminate veneers, including body, gingival, and incisal shading and the degree of opacity, is therefore best incorporated directly into the porcelain by the laboratory technician. Internal resin shading should be limited to the minor changes that can be accomplished through the use of a single homogeneous shade of luting cement.

TRY-IN CONSIDERATIONS

The porcelain laminate veneers should be tried in and evaluated either with water-soluble, noncuring try-in paste (if available) or with the actual luting agent.

The water-soluble, noncuring try-in paste has the advantage of allowing unlimited time to evaluate the effect of the differing shades. If desired, a number of porcelain laminate veneers, each with a different shade of try-in paste, may be simultaneously evaluated. The pastes will approximate the color of the corresponding luting cement.

The actual luting cement can be used to evaluate the effects of different shades. However, the evaluation must be performed quickly so that the material does not begin to cure.

Whether water-soluble, noncuring try-in paste or the actual luting agent is used, the final result may vary from that which is visualized during this evaluation procedure. This occurs for the following reasons:

1. The shade of the try-in paste may not precisely match that of the corresponding luting resin.

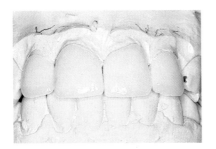

FIG. 11–56

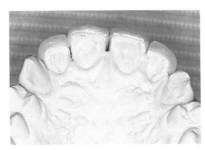

FIG. 11–57

FIG. 11–56. The porcelain laminate veneers positioned on the laboratory model (labial view).

FIG. 11–57. The porcelain laminate veneers positioned on the laboratory model (palatal view).

2. The shade of the luting resin may change immediately following curing.

3. The shade of the cured resin may change over time.

To partially compensate for these phenomena, a sample of each shade of luting resin should be bench-cured and placed in water and any relative changes noted. These changes can be recorded and considered at the time of try-in to help predict the eventual appearance of the final restoration. For example, if the chosen shade of uncured luting agent or try-in paste is higher in value than the corresponding cured sample, the final restoration will probably be similarly affected and appropriate compensation should be considered. However, other factors, such as the metameric influence (see Chapter 2 – Fundamentals of Esthetics) of the porcelain and dentin, the thickness of the luting agent layer, and the degree of opacity of the porcelain will further complicate this assessment. These considerations are generally more significant when attempting to match unprepared or previously restored adjacent teeth than when an entire anterior arch is being restored.

Armamentarium

- Oil-free pumice
- Water-soluble try-in paste or composite resin luting cement (Insure, Cosmedent)
- Extra-fine diamond bur for adjusting porcelain laminate veneers during try-in (Laminate Veneer Kit, Brasseler; Micron Finishing System Diamond Burs MF1, MF2, MF3, Premier Dental Products Co.)
- Cotton-tipped applicators
- Acetone or alcohol
- Double-sided clear adhesive tape (e.g., double-sided tape 3M, Inc.)

Clinical Technique

1. Inspect the porcelain laminate veneers for cracks and imperfections. Place the veneers on the model and verify appropriate fit individually and collectively (Figs. 11–56, 11–57).

CLINICAL TIP. Although the porcelain laminate veneers will be cemented with an appropriately shaded luting cement, precise restoration margins are necessary to minimize the exposure of the composite resin cement, which may discolor over time.

2. Pumice all areas of the prepared teeth (Fig. 11–58). Rinse thoroughly with water and leave wet.

CLINICAL TIP. Prophylaxis pastes contain oil that may contaminate the tooth surface. Therefore, do not substitute prophylaxis pastes for oil-free pumice.[27]

3. Moisten the teeth and the internal surfaces of the porcelain laminate veneers with water. Glycerin, a more viscous liquid, may be used if greater retention of the porcelain laminate veneer is desired during this stage.

4. Place the porcelain laminate veneers on the teeth and evaluate for proper fit and color (Fig. 11–59). Adjustments to the fit can be made with a fine diamond bur.

CLINICAL TIP. Whenever possible, adjustments should be delayed until after the porcelain laminate veneers are bonded into place because of the fragile nature of these restorations prior to bonding. Therefore, only adjustments that are necessary for proper seating of the restorations should be performed at this time. Porcelain laminate veneers are much less susceptible to fracture after bonding.

5. Verify shade.
   A. *If the shade is correct:* verify that untinted luting resin will be acceptable by placing untinted water-soluble try-in paste or the actual resin luting cement into the internal surface of the porcelain laminate veneers and placing the veneers on the teeth. This step is often unnecessary if adjacent unprepared teeth or previously restored teeth will not be visible and therefore need not be matched.

CLINICAL TIP. If the resin luting cement is used to preview the final result, care must be taken to work quickly so that the material does not begin to cure.

CLINICAL TIP. Because the shade of the resin luting cement can change immediately upon polymerization and after time, the final choice of resin cement should be correlated with bench-cured shade samples. (See the preceding section on Try-In Considerations)

   B. *If the shade must be altered:* place the appropriate shade of water-soluble try-in paste or the actual resin luting cement into the internal surface of the procelain laminate veneers and place the veneers on the teeth.

FIG. 11–58. All areas of the prepared teeth are pumiced.

FIG. 11–59. The porcelain laminate veneers are placed on the prepared teeth and evaluated for proper fit and appearance.

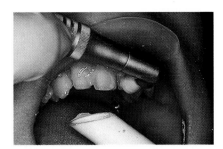

FIG. 11–58

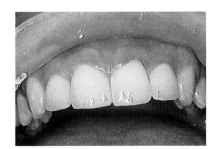

FIG. 11–59

CLINICAL TIP. If the resin luting cement is used to preview the final result, care must be taken to work quickly so that the material does not begin to cure.

CLINICAL TIP. If different shades are evaluated simultaneously in adjacent porcelain laminate veneers, comparisons can be easily visualized (Fig. 11–60). This is best accomplished with try-in pastes that allow unlimited working time.

CLINICAL TIP. Because the shade of the resin luting cement can change immediately upon polymerization and after time, the final choice of resin cement should be correlated with bench-cured shade samples. (See the preceding section on Try-In Considerations.)

CLINICAL TIP. If an acceptable shade cannot be obtained, the laminate veneer can be custom stained in the office (see below) or by the laboratory.

6. Clean the internal surfaces with a cotton-tipped applicator followed by a water spray, and finally in an ultrasonic cleaner with acetone or alcohol. Apply 37% phosphoric acid for 15 seconds to remove any salivary contamination from the etched surface.

CLINICAL TIP. The "etching" of the etched porcelain surface of a porcelain laminate veneer is much more durable than the "etching" of etched enamel. Cleaning (as described in the preceding step) will not damage the etched surface.

7. Clean the teeth again with oil-free pumice (Fig. 11–61); wash and dry with oil-free air (Fig. 11–62).
8. Clean proximal surfaces with a finishing strip (Fig. 11–63); wash and dry thoroughly with oil-free air.

CUSTOM LABORATORY STAINING

Large discrepancy in hue or chroma will require custom staining either at chairside or by the laboratory technician. Most laminate veneers are fabricated on a refractory model, which is destroyed when the veneer is removed, so a new model must be fabricated.[28]

Armamentarium

- Basic dental setup (See the section on Armamentarium under Major Color Change)
- Low-speed green stone
- Basic custom shading setup (See Appendix A—Custom Staining)
- Porcelain laminate investment material
- Sandblaster (e.g., Microetcher, Danville Engineering)
- Porcelain etch (10% hydrofluoric acid)

Clinical Technique

1. Mix investment material and carefully place a small

amount of investment on the lingual aspect of the porcelain laminate veneer.
2. Shape the remaining investment into a block and place the porcelain laminate veneer on this block with the labial side of the restoration facing out.
3. Trim excess investment to completely expose the labial surface. This is best done before the investment sets.
4. Carefully remove the glaze on the buccal surface with a low-speed green stone.
5. Modify the porcelain laminate veneer as necessary and fire. (See Appendix A—Custom Staining.)
6. After "bench-cooling," carefully remove the porcelain laminate veneer from the investment.
7. Carefully sandblast the internal aspect of the porcelain laminate veneer to remove any remaining investment material.
8. Try-in the porcelain laminate veneer. If the shade is still not acceptable, repeat steps 1 through 7.
9. Re-etch the internal aspect of the porcelain laminate veneer as per the manufacturer's instructions. Do not allow the etchant to contact the external surfaces.

CEMENTATION

Armamentarium

- Basic dental setup (See the section on Armamentarium under Major Color Changes)
- Oil-free pumice
- Interproximal abrasive strips (Sof-flex Strips, 3M, Inc.)
- Dentin disclosing agent (e.g., Dentin Detector Gel, Caulk/Dentsply)
- Dead soft matrix strips (e.g., Dead soft metal matrix strip, Den-Mat) or clear plastic matrix strips (e.g., Clear Mylar Strips, Healthco, Inc.)
- Silane coupling agent (often included in porcelain laminate veneer cementing kit)
- Dentin bonding agent (e.g., Gluma, Columbus Dental Corp.)
- Set of shaded resin luting cement
- Composite resin carving instruments (e.g., TCA, TCB, TCD, American Dental Manufacturing)

Clinical Technique

CLINICAL TIP. Placement of a porcelain laminate veneer on an incorrect tooth can easily occur after the luting cement is applied. This is particularly true for canine teeth restorations, which can easily be transposed. To avoid this, draw and label circles on the bracket table cover (Fig. 11–64) or a mixing pad, or affix the laminate veneers to double-sided clear adhesive tape in the correct order.

1. Apply silane coupling agent to the internal surface of all the porcelain laminate veneers according to the manufacturer's instructions (Figs. 11–65, 11–66).

CLINICAL TIP. Some silane coupling agents require acid for activation.

CLINICAL TIP. Restore both central incisors simultaneously, then proceed distally. Should minor errors in porcelain laminate veneer positioning occur they will thereby be located as far from the midline as possible, where any necessary compensatory adjustments will be less visible.

2. If the tooth surface has been contaminated, pumice the labial and lingual tooth surfaces again.
3. If dentin exposure is a possibility:
   A. Apply dentin disclosing agent.
   B. Condition the exposed dentin with dentin bonding agent according to the manufacturer's instructions.
4. Place matrix strips between the first teeth to be restored and the adjacent teeth (Fig. 11–67).
5. Etch the enamel with 37% phosphoric acid for 15 seconds (Fig. 11–68).

CLINICAL TIP. Controlled positioning of the 37% phosphoric acid is facilitated by the use of a gel. This is particularly useful if etching of any exposed dentin is not desired.

6. Wash for a minimum of 10 seconds (25 ml) but no more than 20 seconds using water or water and air spray (Fig. 11–69).
7. Dry the preparation with oil-free air (Fig. 11–70).
8. Repeat steps 6, 7, and 8 if frosted white appearance is not present.
9. Discard interproximal matrix strips.
10. Replace with new matrix strips (Fig. 11–71).
11. Apply bonding agent to the internal surface of the porcelain laminate veneers as per the manufacturer's instructions (Fig. 11–72).
12. Apply preselected shade of luting cement to the internal surface of the porcelain laminate veneer (Fig. 11–73).

CLINICAL TIP. Place the porcelain laminate veneers underneath an opaque cup to prevent premature curing of the resin.

13. Place appropriate bonding agent onto the tooth as per the manufacturer's instructions (Fig. 11–74).
14. Carefully place the porcelain laminate veneers onto the teeth, and fully seat to place.

FIG. 11–60. If different shade modifications are evaluated simultaneously in adjacent porcelain laminate veneers, comparisons can be easily visualized.

FIG. 11–61. The teeth are pumiced to remove all traces of the try-in paste or luting agent.

FIG. 11–62. Following a thorough water wash, the teeth are dried with oil-free air.

FIG. 11–63. Proximal surfaces are cleaned with a finishing strip.

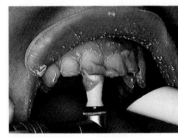

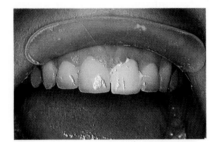

FIG. 11–60

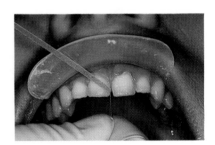

FIG. 11–61

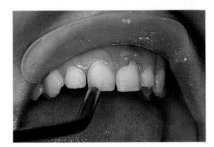

FIG. 11–62

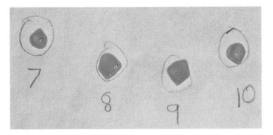

FIG. 11–63

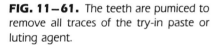

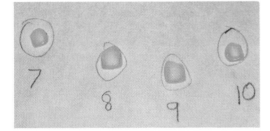

FIG. 11–64. Placement of a porcelain laminate veneer on an incorrect tooth can easily occur after the luting cement is applied. To avoid this, draw and label circles on the bracket table cover.

FIG. 11–65. Some silane coupling agents require acid etch activation of the porcelain surface.

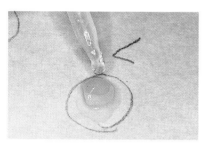

FIG. 11–66. Silane coupling agent is applied to the internal surface of the porcelain laminate veneer according to the manufacturer's instructions.

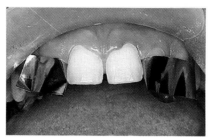

FIG. 11–67. Matrix strips are placed between the first teeth to be restored and the adjacent teeth.

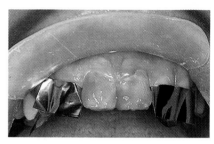

FIG. 11–68. The enamel is etched with 37% phosphoric acid for 15 seconds.

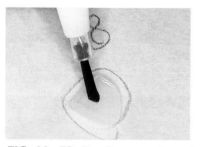

FIG. 11–69. The etchant is removed with water.

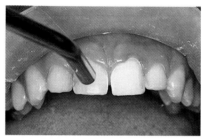

FIG. 11–70. The preparation is dried with oil-free air.

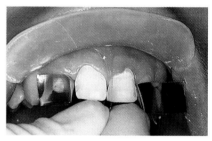

FIG. 11–71. Fresh matrix strips are placed into all interproximal areas.

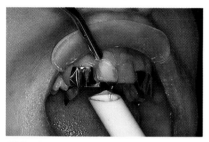

FIG. 11–72. Bonding agent is applied to the internal surface of the porcelain laminate veneers as per manufacturer's instructions.

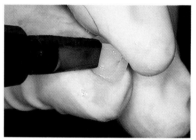

FIG. 11–73. The preselected shade of luting cement is applied to the internal surface of the porcelain laminate veneer.

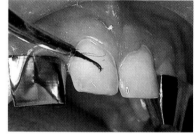

FIG. 11–74. Bonding agent is applied to the tooth structure according to the manufacturer's instructions.

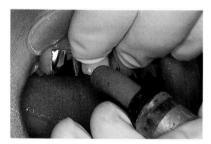

FIG. 11–75. The restoration is carefully seated onto the prepared tooth and the incisal tip is cured from the incisolabial direction for 10 seconds.

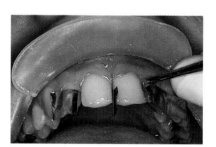

FIG. 11–76. The excess luting agent is removed from marginal areas with a sable brush moistened with bonding agent.

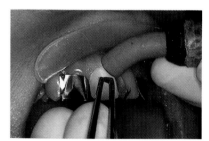

FIG. 11–77. The luting cement is cured from the buccal directions.

CLINICAL TIP. In order to insure proper seating of the porcelain laminate veneer, first use finger pressure with a pulsing motion on the incisal edge in an incisogingival direction. Then press with a pulsing motion on the labial surface in a labiolingual direction.

15. Hold the porcelain laminate veneer in place and cure the incisal tip from a labial direction for 10 seconds (Fig. 11–75).
16. Remove excess luting cement with a sable brush moistened with bonding agent (Fig. 11–76).

CLINICAL TIP. Dipping the brush into bonding agent before removing excess cement prevents "pulling" of the cement, which could create marginal voids.

17. Cure the remaining luting cement from the buccal, lingual, and incisal directions (Figs. 11–77, 11–78).

CLINICAL TIP. Light-cured resin cannot be damaged by excessive light exposure. It is therefore preferable to err on the side of longer exposure times.

18. Remove the matrix strips.
19. Remove excess flesh with composite resin carving instruments (Figs. 11–79, 11–80).
20. Repeat steps 2 to 19 for the remaining porcelain laminate veneers. Two adjacent teeth can be placed simultaneously.

CLINICAL TIP. It is essential to try-in the remaining restorations at this stage. Even minimal amounts of excess luting agent can prevent the proper seating of the porcelain laminate veneer (Figs. 11–81, 11–82).

FINISHING AND POLISHING

Marginal discrepancies immediately after cementation of indirect restorations are, to some degree, inevitable. Postcementation intraoral finishing of both porcelain and resin at the tooth-restoration interface can be accomplished with rotary instruments. Scanning electron microscope and spectrographic reflectance analyses reveal that adjusted porcelain can attain a surface smoothness that is superior to that of glazed porcelain if a specific protocol is followed.[29] This protocol is outlined below and involves the use of progressively finer abrasives. Finishing and polishing instruments include diamond burs, a 30-fluted carbide bur, and a 2- to 5-micron particle size diamond polishing paste on a webbed rubber prophylaxis cup.

It is possible that the degree of surface smoothness attained by this protocol is clinically unnecessary and that omitting some steps may be acceptable. In this case the gingival tissue response can probably serve as an appropriate indicator of the need for further polishing.[30] No controlled clinical studies, however, have investigated this premise.

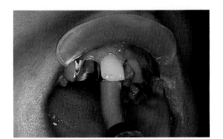

FIG. 11–78. The remaining luting cement is cured from the palatal direction.

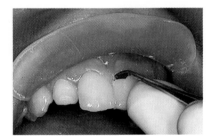

FIG. 11–79. Excess cured composite resin is initially removed from the marginal areas with composite resin carving instruments.

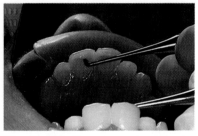

FIG. 11–80. Excess cured composite resin is removed from the palatal marginal areas.

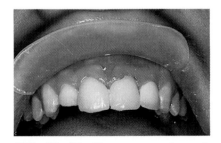

FIG. 11–81. The open margin at the gingival area on the maxillary left lateral incisor restoration indicates improper seating, which is caused by excess luting cement on the distal aspect of the maxillary left central incisor restoration.

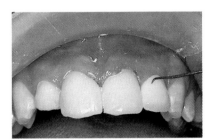

FIG. 11–82. After removal of the interference the maxillary left lateral incisor restoration seats properly.

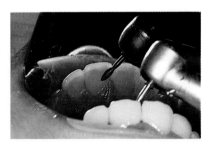

FIG. 11–83. Palatal margins are finished with a football-shaped diamond bur.

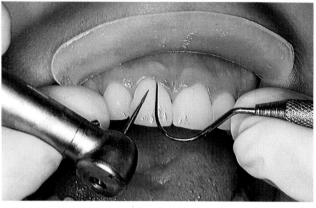 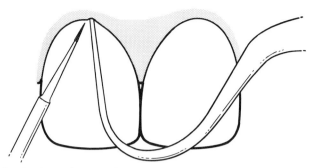

FIGS. 11—84 AND 11—85. The finishing instrument is held in the dominant hand while the explorer is held in the other hand. Two-handed instrumentation allows for efficient repetitive alternation between the evaluation instrument and the finishing instrument. This expedites the tedious, repetitive "margin polishing/margin evaluation" process.

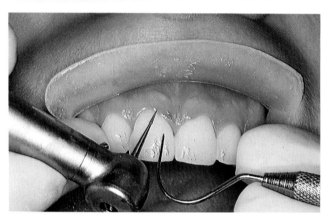 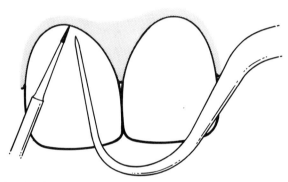

FIG. 11—86 AND 11—87. The polishing instrument is held in the dominant hand while the explorer is held in the other hand. Two-handed instrumentation can expedite the tedious "margin polishing/margin evaluation" process.

Armamentarium

- Composite resin carving instruments (e.g., TCA, TCB, TCD, American Dental Manufacturing)
- Diamond finishing burs (Micron Finishing System Diamond Burs MF1, MF2, MF3, Premier Dental Products Co.)
- 30-fluted carbide bur (e.g., ETUF6 and 379-UF, Brasseler)
- Interproximal abrasive strips (Sof-Flex Strips, 3M, Inc.)
- Unwaxed regular dental floss
- Porcelain polishing paste (ex. Truluster, Brasseler; Instaglaze, George Taub Products)
- Webbed rubber prophylaxis cup

Clinical Technique

1. Carefully finish the facial margins with the M1 finishing diamond in a high-speed handpiece at low speed (regulated by applying appropriate pressure on the rheostat) with water coolant.
2. Finish the lingual areas with a fine "football-shaped" diamond (Fig. 11—83).
3. Dry the marginal areas to evaluate for smoothness and repeat steps 1 and 2 if necessary.

CLINICAL TIP. Hold the finishing instruments (composite resin carving instruments or the handpiece) in the dominant hand (right hand for right-handed dentists, left hand for left-handed dentists) and the evaluation instrument (explorer) in the other hand. This allows for efficient repetitive alternations between the evaluation instrument and the finishing instruments. If all instruments are held with only the dominant hand, repeated instrument transfers can become tedious, resulting in inadvertent overlooking of restorative material overhangs (Figs. 11—84 to 11—87).

4. Evaluate the occlusion with articulating paper in both centric occlusion and in all eccentric excursions. Adjust porcelain, if necessary, with an extra-fine "football-shaped" diamond bur.
5. Repeat steps 1 through 4, substituting first an M2 finishing diamond, then an M3 finishing diamond, and lastly, a 30-fluted carbide bur.

CLINICAL TIP. A 9- or 12-fluted carbide bur tends to chip or cleave the porcelain and should not be substituted for the recommended 30-fluted carbide bur.[30]

CLINICAL TIP. Whenever possible centric occlusion stops and excursive movements should be on natural tooth surfaces. This may not be possible with certain occlusal schema, such as canine-protected occlusion (Figs. 11–88 to 11–90).

6. Finish and polish the proximal areas with interproximal abrasive strips (Fig. 11–91).
7. Evaluate the interproximal contact areas with unwaxed dental floss (Fig. 11–92) and repolish if necessary.
8. Polish with a diamond polishing paste on a prophylaxis cup using intermittent pressure to prevent heat buildup (Fig. 11–93).

CLINICAL TIP. Cosmetic recontouring should be deferred, if possible, for approximately 1 to 2 weeks following porcelain laminate veneer placement. The initial dramatic cosmetic change can elicit in the patient a psychological ambivalence and a desire to re-establish the previous appearance. (This familiar response is commonly seen following the creation of a drastically new hairstyle.) Recontouring at this time, therefore, may result in overcorrection.

9. Re-evaluate the finishing and polishing procedures in approximately 1 to 2 weeks for additional marginal discrepancies that may have been obscured by gingival bleeding or may result from subsequent water sorption by excess luting resin (Figs. 11–94 to 11–98).

POSTERIOR PORCELAIN INLAYS AND ONLAYS

Porcelain inlay and onlay cavity design is similar to that used for gold inlays and onlays, except that all line angles other than finishing lines must be rounded and bevels are contraindicated. In addition, adequate thickness must be provided to prevent porcelain fracture. Unlike gold restorations, frictional retention is unnecessary since porcelain restorations are bonded into place.

Clinical Technique—First Visit (Fig. 11–99)
Armamentarium

Same as the basic setup for porcelain laminate veneers (see the section on Armamentarium under Major Color Change) plus:

- Burs: medium grit tapered diamond bur (e.g., 6847-016, Brasseler), medium grit flame or chamfer diamond bur (e.g., 6856-018, Brasseler)
- Retraction cord packer (e.g., Fischer's Ultrapak Packer, Ultradent Products, Inc.)
- Nonimpregnated gingival retraction cord (e.g., Ultrapak No. 0, No. 1, or No. 2, Ultradent Products, Inc.; Gingibraid No. 0, No. 1, or No. 2, Van R.)
- Suitable hemostatic agent (optional) (e.g., Astringedent, Ultradent Products, Inc.)

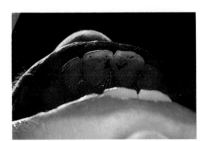

FIG. 11–88. Centric occlusion and excursive movements are evaluated for prematurities.

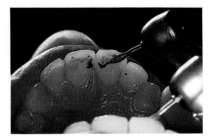

FIG. 11–89. Prematurities are removed with a football-shaped diamond.

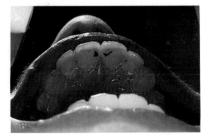

FIG. 11–90. Whenever possible, the centric occlusion stop should only be on natural tooth structure and the restoration should be out of occlusion during excursive movements. This is particularly important if the opposing teeth are not restored with porcelain.

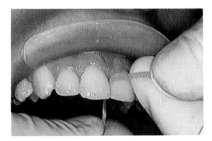

FIG. 11–91. The proximal areas are finished with finishing strips.

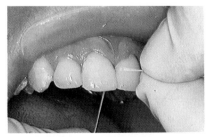

FIG. 11–92. The interproximal contact area is evaluated with unwaxed dental floss.

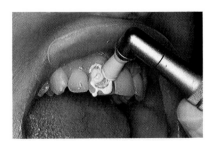

FIG. 11–93. The restoration is polished with diamond polishing paste on a webbed prophylaxis cup.

- Scissors
- Elastomeric impression material

Clinical Technique

1. Administer suitable anesthesia.
2. Prepare the tooth in a manner similar to a gold inlay or onlay preparation. Provide divergent walls and *round* all internal line angles to reduce stress (Fig. 11–100).

CLINICAL TIP. Because the restoration will be bonded into place, no retentive grooves or parallel walls are needed.

3. Provide 1.5 mm of occlusal clearance.

CLINICAL TIP. Since the occlusion can only be adjusted after cementation, it is often difficult at the try-in stage to predict if there will be an adequate thickness of porcelain after occlusal adjustment of the bonded restoration. Therefore, verification of adequate occlusal reduction must be done at the time of preparation. This will prevent the need for overadjustment, and subsequent increased fracture susceptibility, because of inadequate occlusal clearance.

CLINICAL TIP. Beveled finishing lines create thin areas of porcelain, which may result in porcelain fracture, and are therefore contraindicated. Use butt joint margins.

4. Areas prepared closer than 0.5 mm to the pulp should be lined with calcium hydroxide.
5. Cover all exposed dentin and undercut areas with a glass ionomer cement. After base placement, the cavity preparation should attain ideal form.

CLINICAL TIP. Materials containing eugenol should not be used because eugenol can interfere with the chemistry of the bonding resins.

6. Verify that there are no undercuts in the preparation.
7. Gently place a nonimpregnated No. 0 Gingibraid retraction cord in the sulcus.
8. Place a No. 1 or No. 2 cord over the No. 0 cord.
9. Remove only the second cord prior to impressioning.

CLINICAL TIP. It is essential that the remaining cord lie beneath the finishing lines in order to avoid interfering with the capture of the entire gingival margin in the impression.

10. Make the impression with any accurate crown and bridge impression material.
11. Make a counterimpression and obtain a suitable bite registration.
12. Place a provisional restoration and dismiss the patient. Materials containing eugenol are contraindicated.
13. Send the impressions and models to the laboratory for fabrication of the restoration.

CLINICAL TIP. The first retraction cord is left in place during the impressioning procedure. It is usually removed by the impression material. However, be certain that all remaining cord is removed prior to proceeding with the next step.

Clinical Technique – Second Visit

Armamentarium

- Basic dental set-up (see the section on Armamentarium under Major Color Changes.)
- Colored spray powder (e.g., Occlude, Pascal Co., Inc.)
- Pumice
- Extra-fine diamond burs for adjusting porcelain inlays and onlays during try-in (Laminate Veneer Kit, Brasseler; Micron Finishing System Diamond Burs MF1, MF2, MF3, Premier Dental Products Co.)
- Cotton-tipped applicators
- Acetone or alcohol
- Interproximal abrasive strips (Sof-Flex Strips, 3M, Inc.)
- Silane coupling agent (often included in laminate veneer cementing kit)
- Dentin bonding agent (e.g., Gluma, Columbia Dental Corp.)
- Composite resin carving instruments (e.g., TCA, TCB, TCD, American Dental Manufacturing)
- Dead soft matrix strips (e.g., Den-Mat, Inc.) or clear plastic matrix strips (e.g., Healthco, Inc.)
- 30-Fluted carbide burs (Brasseler)
- Unwaxed regular dental floss
- Porcelain polishing paste (e.g., Truluster, Brasseler, Instaglaze, George Taub Products, Inc.)
- Webbed rubber prophylaxis cup

Clinical Technique

1. Remove the provisional restoration and thoroughly cleanse the tooth.
2. Gently try-in the restoration and adjust the internal aspects and contact areas to allow for complete seating.

CLINICAL TIP. The unbonded porcelain restoration is very fragile. Care must be taken in order to prevent inadvertent breakage. Do not use a bite stick or have the patient use biting pressure to seat the restoration.

CLINICAL TIP. If the restoration is difficult to manipulate with fingers, it can be temporarily luted on the occlusal surface with sticky wax to a small amalgam plugger. This is particularly helpful when preparing the internal surface for final cementation.

CLINICAL TIP. Use a colored spray powder (e.g., Occlude) to reveal binding areas.

3. Verify that the restoration is completely seated and that all the margins are adequately sealed. A radio-

graph is helpful to assure proper interproximal seating and marginal adequacy.

4. Use dental floss to verify the accuracy of the contact areas.

CLINICAL TIP. Do not adjust the occlusion at this time. Occlusal adjustment must be performed after cementation.

5. Shade evaluation and adjustment are accomplished in a manner similar to that for porcelain laminate veneers. (See the preceding section on Try-In Considerations.)

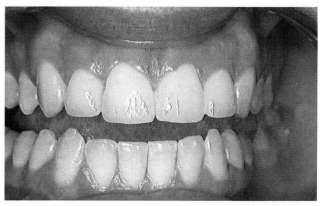

FIG. 11–94. The final porcelain laminate veneer restorations.

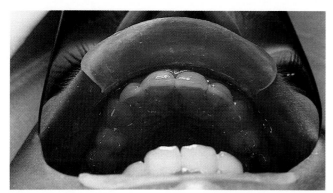

FIG. 11–95. Incisal view of the patient shown in Figure 11–94.

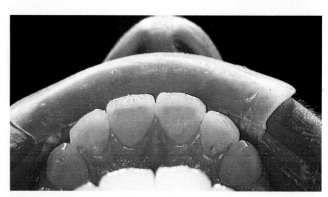

FIG. 11–96. Palatal view of the patient shown in Figure 11–94.

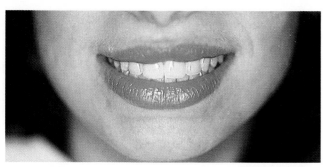

FIG. 11–97. Anterior view of the patient shown in Figure 11–94.

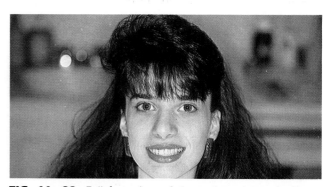

FIG. 11–98. Full face view of the patient shown in Figure 11–94.

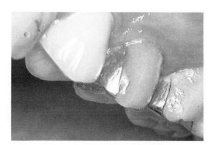

FIG. 11–99. The inlay in the second premolar presented with an unesthetic labial display of gold. (Courtesy of Dr. Brian Pollack.)

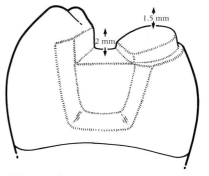

FIG. 11–100. The tooth is prepared in a manner similar to that for a gold inlay/onlay preparation. Divergent walls and rounded internal line angles reduce stress in the restoration.

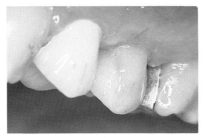

FIG. 11−101. A porcelain onlay was fabricated to replace the gold onlay shown in Figure 11−99. (Courtesy of Dr. Brian Pollack.)

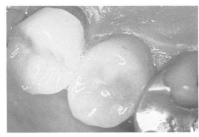

FIG. 11−102. Occlusal view of porcelain onlay. (Courtesy of Dr. Brian Pollack.)

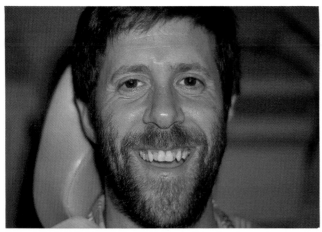

FIG. 11−103. Patient presented with anterior crowding. The patient refused orthodontic treatment.

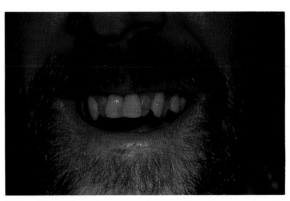

FIG. 11−104. Close-up view of patient shown in Figure 11−103.

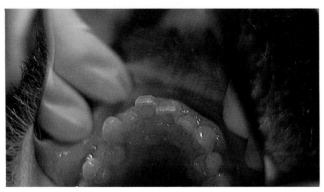

FIG. 11−105. Incisal view of patient shown in Figure 11−103.

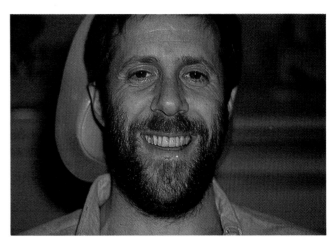

FIG. 11−106. Full face view of the patient shown in Figure 11−103 three years following porcelain laminate veener placement on the four maxillary incisors and the left first premolar.

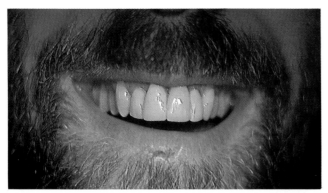

FIG. 11−107. Close up view of the patient shown in Figure 11−106.

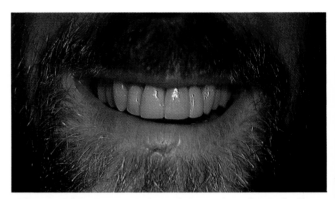

FIG. 11−108. Close-up view of the patient shown in Figure 11−106 showing a high smile line.

6. Clean the internal surfaces of the restoration with a cotton-tipped applicator followed by a water spray, and finally, in an ultrasonic cleaner with acetone or alcohol. Etch the surface for 15 seconds with 37% phosporic acid.

7. Place a rubber dam. Place an interproximal matrix strip.

8. Place the restoration on a clean, dry surface.

9. Apply silane coupling agent to the internal surface of the restoration according to the manufacturer's instructions.

CLINICAL TIP. Some silane coupling agents require acid for activation.

---

10. Thoroughly clean the prepared tooth with pumice.
11. Etch the enamel with 37% phosphoric acid for 15 seconds.
12. Wash for a minimum of 10 seconds (25 ml), but no longer than 20 seconds, using water or water and air spray.
13. Dry the preparation with oil-free air.
14. Repeat steps 12 and 13 if a frosted white appearance is not present. Replace the matrix strip.
15. Apply dentin primer to any dentinal surfaces not covered by glass ionomer cement.
16. Apply bonding resin to the glass ionomer cement, dentin, enamel, and internal surface of the restoration according to the manufacturer's instructions.
17. Mix a dual-cured luting composite resin and apply it to the internal surface of the restoration.

CLINICAL TIP. A dual-cured luting cement must be used because the light source may not penetrate all internal surfaces.

---

18. Place the restoration on the tooth and seat with finger pressure using a pulsing motion; remove excess luting composite resin with a brush dipped in bonding agent.

CLINICAL TIP. Dipping the brush into bonding agent before removing excess cement prevents "pulling" of the cement which could create marginal voids.

---

19. While the onlay is held in place with an instrument, run dental floss through the proximal areas and pull to the facial or lingual aspect to remove excess resin.

20. Cure the restoration on the occlusal, facial, and lingual surfaces for 40 seconds each. Remove matrix strips.

21. Excess cured luting composite resin can be removed with a surgical blade, scaler, composite resin carving instruments, or with diamond finishing burs.

22. Adjust the occlusion with diamond finishing burs.

23. Finish and polish in a manner similar to that for porcelain laminate veneers (Figs. 11–101, 11–102). (See the preceding section on Finishing and Polishing.)

CLINICAL CASE STUDY 1

A 43-year-old male presented with malpositioned maxillary anterior teeth (Figs. 11–103 to 11–105). His medical history was noncontributory. The patient refused orthodontic care, which was presented as the treatment of choice.

An initial chairside wax-up predicted a favorable prognosis for treatment with porcelain laminate veneers. The veneers were placed on the maxillary left first premolar and the four incisors. The patient's slight mandibular prognathism permitted the palatally positioned teeth to be significantly "brought labially" with the porcelain laminate veneers without creating a class II appearance (Figs. 11–106 to 11–109).

CLINICAL CASE STUDY 2

A 33-year-old male presented with discolored maxillary teeth and a midline diastema (Fig. 11–110). His medical history was noncontributory. The incisors were restored with porcelain laminate veneers (Fig. 11–111).

CONCLUSION

Significant advances in porcelain technology have permitted increased versatility in its use as a restorative

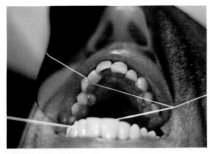

FIG. 11–109. Three year post-operative incisal view of the patient shown in Figure. 11–105. Floss is easily negotiated through all contact areas.

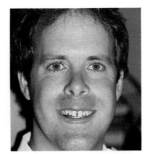

FIG. 11–110. This patient exhibited discolored teeth and a midline diastema.

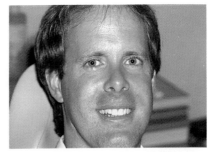

FIG. 11–111. The four incisors were restored with porcelain laminate veneers.

material. When combined with acid-etch bonding techniques, porcelain laminate veneers and partial coverage restorations have become a more conservative and highly esthetic alternative to full coverage restorations.

REFERENCES

1. McGehee, W.H., True, H.A., and Inskipp, E.F.: A Textbook of Operative Dentistry, 3rd Ed. New York, The Blakiston Co., 1950.
2. Fauce, F.G.: Tooth restorations with preformed laminated veneers. J Tex Dent Assoc, 53:30, 1977.
3. Boyer, D.B. and Chalkley, Y.: Bonding between acrylic laminates and composite resins. J Dent Res, 61:489, 1982.
4. Cannon, M.L., Marshall, G.W. Jr., Marshall S.J., Cooley, R.O.: Surface resistance to abrasion of preformed laminate resin veneers. J Prosthet Dent 52:323, 1984.
5. Bowen, R.L.: Report 6333. Development of silica resin direct filling material. Washington D.C., National Bureau of Standards, 1958.
6. Paffenberger, G.C., Sweeney, W.T., and Bowen, R.L.: Bonding porcelain teeth to acrylic denture bases. J Am Dent Assoc, 74:1018, 1967.
7. Semmelman, J.O. and Kulp P.R.: Silane bonding of porcelain teeth to acrylic. J Am Dent Assoc, 76:69, 1968.
8. Meyerson, R.L.: The effects of silane bonding of acrylic resin to porcelain on porcelain structures. J Am Dent Assoc, 78:113, 1969.
9. Quinn, F., McConnell, R.J., and Byrne, D.: Porcelain laminates: a review. Br Dent J, 161:61, 1986.
10. Newbury, R. and Pameijer, C.H.: Composite resin bonded to porcelain with silane solution. J Amer Dent Assoc, 96:288, 1978.
11. Highton, R.M., Caputo, A.A., and Matyas, J.: The effectiveness of porcelain repair systems. J Prosthet Dent, 42:292, 1979.
12. Barreto, M.T. and Bottaro, B.F.: A practical approach to porcelain repair. J Prosthet Dent, 48:349, 1982.
13. Jochen, D.G. and Caputo, A.A.: Composite repair of porcelain teeth. J Prosthet Dent, 38:673, 1977.
14. Simonsen, R.J. and Calamia, J.R.: Tensile bond strength of etch porcelain. J Dent Res, 62:297, 1983.
15. Jordan, R.E., Suzuki, M., and Senda, A.: Clinical evaluation of porcelain laminate veneers: a four year recall report. J Esthet Dent, 1:126, 1989.
16. Calamia, J.R.: Etch porcelain veneers: the current state of the art. Quintessence Int 16:5, 1985.
17. Jenkins, C.B.G. and Abousch, Y.E.Y.: Clinical durability of porcelain laminate over 8 years. J Dent Res 67:1081, 1987.
18. Phillips, R.W.: Skinner's Science of Dental Materials, 7th Ed. Philadelphia, Saunders, 526, 1973.
19. Hsu, C.S., Stangel, I., and Nathanson, D.: Shear bond strength of resin to etch porcelain. J Dent Res, 64:296, 1985.
20. Garber, D.A., Goldstein, R.E., and Feinamn, R.E.: Porcelain Laminate Veneers. Chicago, Quintessence Publishing Co., 1988.
21. Nichols, J.I.: Tensile bond of resin cements to porcelain veneers. J Prosthet Dent, 60:443, 1988.
22. Horn, H.R.: Porcelain laminate veneers bonded to etched enamel. Dent Clin North Am 27:671, 1983.
23. Christenson G. (Ed.): Porcelain veneers, Cementation kits. Clin Res Assoc Newsletter, 12:7:3, 1988.
24. Plant, C.G. and Thomas, G.D.: Porcelain facings, a simple clinical and laboratory method. Br Dent J, 163:231, 1987.
25. Nixon, R.L.: Tooth preparation for porcelain veneers. Forum Esthet Dent, 4:5, 1986.
26. Highton, R., Caputo, A.A., and Mátyás, J.: A photoelastic study of the stresses on porcelain laminate preparations. J Prosthet Dent, 58:157, 1987.
27. Calamia, J.R.: Materials and techniques for etch porcelain facial veneers. Alpha Omegan, 4:81, 1988.
28. Scharf, J.: In-office custom staining of porcelain laminate veneers. Dentistry Today, 9:28, 1990.
29. Haywood, V.B., Heymann, H.O., Kusy, R.P., et al: Polishing porcelain veneers: an SEM and specular reflectance analysis. Dent Mat, 4:116, 1988.
30. Heymann, H.O.: Personal communication, April, 1991.

Morton Wood, D.D.S., M.Ed.
Van Thompson, D.D.S, Ph.D.

ADHESIVE RESIN BONDED CAST RESTORATIONS

12

Conventional ceramometal fixed prosthodontics require the removal of substantial amounts of tooth structure so that the resulting restorations are strong, appropriately contoured, and esthetic. Alternatives that remove less tooth structure have always been desirable.

The primary goal of the resin bonded prosthesis is conservation of tooth structure. In addition, a bonded restoration may be more esthetic than conventional ceramometal fixed partial dentures because the facial enamel of the abutment teeth is not prepared. Original designs for bonded bridges had minimal, if any, preparation of enamel. The latest designs incorporate a more detailed preparation of enamel, but are still highly conservative and do not involve the facial enamel.

HISTORICAL PERSPECTIVE AND PHILOSOPHY

Bonded Pontics

Early attempts to conserve tooth structure when replacing missing anterior teeth with a fixed restoration led to the use of acid etched retained pontics. Limited to short anterior spans, these pontics were attached to the adjacent abutment teeth with composite resin that was bonded to etched enamel in the approximal contact areas and was mechanically retained within the pontic. A variety of techniques and materials had been advocated, including the use of acrylic denture teeth (with and without retentive pins),[1] composite resin,[2] and the patient's natural extracted tooth.[3] These pontic replacements preserved vital tooth structure, however the failure rate was extremely high and they now are used only as temporary replacements.[4]

Cast Perforated Bridges (Mechanical Retention)

Rochette[5] first introduced the cast perforated resin bonded periodontal splint in 1973. Castings were re-

tained by a "sandwich" of unfilled acrylic resin that bonded to etched enamel and mechanically locked into flaring perforations in the metal (Fig. 12–1). This gross mechanical attachment provided improved retention when compared to the bonded pontic replacements because the metal framework engaged a much broader surface area for enamel bonding.

This design could be adapted to include a porcelain-fused-to-metal pontic.[6] Initially, patients who had little or no opposing arch occlusal contact were selected. In addition, no tooth modifications were performed and the framework was extended to cover a maximum amount of the lingual surface. The restorations were bonded using a heavily filled composite resin as a luting medium.

Livaditis[7] later used cast perforated bridges placed in full occlusion to replace posterior teeth. He extended the perforated retainer framework from the lingual surfaces over the occlusal surfaces and into the interproximal surfaces adjacent to the edentulous areas. He advocated minimal enamel preparation to increase the surface area for retention and develop an occlusogingival path of insertion free from undercuts. The path of insertion was obtained by lowering the proximal and lingual height of contour on the abutment teeth.

Although cast perforated bridges showed promise, several disadvantages accompany their use.

1. The mechanical retention of resin to metal perforations was often weaker than the resin to enamel bond.[8] The retention of retainers was, therefore, only as strong as the resin to metal mechanical bond.
2. Perforations weakened the framework, resulting in cracking between the holes and flexing of the retainers. To compensate, an undesirably thick metal wing was required.
3. The resin in the exposed perforations was subject to wear, stain, and plaque accumulation, requiring periodic replacement of the surface layer of composite resin.

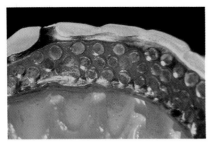

FIG. 12–1. This perforated cast periodontal splint was designed with a rest seat for the lingual plate of a removable partial denture. The resin locks into the perforations, which flare outward from the tooth surface. Wear and staining of the resin in the area of the perforations is common.

FIG. 12–2. This incisal view diagram noticeably outlines the proximal preparation design for anterior teeth. The "proximal wrap around" is a two-plane reduction that follows the natural contour of the teeth. The dotted line shows the outline of the porcelain that will cover the metal framework.

Etched Cast Resin Bonded Bridges (Micromechanical Retention)

Based on the work of Tanaka, et al.,[9] on pitting corrosion for retaining acrylic resin facings, Thompson and Livaditis developed a technique for the electrolytic etching of nickel-chromium (Ni-Cr) and chromium-cobalt (Cr-Co) alloys.[10] The lack of perforations to serve as escape vents for the composite resin required a new "cementing type" of composite resin (e.g., Comspan, Caulk/Dentsply). A moderately filled (60% by weight) composite resin, with a film thickness of approximately 20 microns allowed good strength and full seating of the cast retainers.[11]

Etched cast retainers provide several advantages over cast perforated restorations:

1. Retention is improved because the resin to etched metal bond is twice as strong as the resin to etched enamel bond.
2. The absence of perforations allows for thinner retainers which resist flexing.
3. The oral surface of the cast retainers are highly polished, resist plaque accumulation, and are impervious to wear.

Guidelines for optimum design were empirically derived. The first generation of etched cast designs included an "interproximal wrap around" concept developed to resist occlusal forces and provide a broader area for bonding. Enamel preparations consisted of creating occlusal clearance, placing occlusal and cingulum rests, and lowering the lingual and proximal height of contour, thus creating proximal extensions. Frameworks seated in an occlusogingival direction and resisted faciolingual displacement (Fig. 12–2).

The current, second-generation design combines the basic concepts of earlier techniques with the addition of parallel grooves in the interproximal areas and shallow but distinct gingival chamfers.

Second-generation mouth preparations, in an effort to minimize failures, do not preserve as much tooth structure as their predecessors; nevertheless, they still do not extend into dentin and are true to conservative design principles.

BASIC PRINCIPLES
Adhesion Bridges (Chemical Bonding)

One limitation of the etched cast resin bonded technique is that the etching process is limited to Ni-Cr and Cr-Co alloys. The etching of these alloys requires strict attention to details and has been a problem for many dental laboratories.[12] An improved adhesive system allows bonding directly to a casting alloy without the need for etching or incorporating gross mechanical retention.[13] Panavia (Kuraray Co. Ltd.) is an adhesive liquid and powder mixture bis-GMA based composite resin that eliminates laboratory etching procedures and expands the number of alloys that can be used for resin bonded restorations. Panavia has shown excellent bonds to air abraded Ni-Cr and Cr-Co alloys, as well as to tin-plated gold, tin-plated ceramic gold, and tin-plated gold palladium-based alloys.[14,15] Another adhesive resin is Super Bond C&B (Sun Medical), based on a methyl methacrylate polymer powder and methyl methacrylate liquid modified with the adhesion promoter, 4-methacryloxyethyl trimellitie anhydride (4-META). It requires a tri-n-butylborane (TBB) catalyst system. Super Bond has the highest initial bond strengths to base metal alloys of any adhesive resin system, but there is some concern about hydrolytic stability and the possible resultant loss of bond strength over time.[16]

Panavia has a tensile bond strength to etched enamel (10 to 15 MPa) that is comparable to the bond strengths of traditional bis-GMA low film thickness composite resins, such as Comspan (Cault/Dentsply) and Conclude (3M, Inc.) The combination of etching metal and using the adhesive Panavia does not improve the strength of the tensile bond to the alloy; this bond strength is actually slightly lower than that of bonds to air abraded alloys[17] because the etching removes some of the oxides essential for the chemical bonds. Tensile bond strengths of Panavia to tin-plated high gold ceramic alloys are lower than either the etched or air abraded nickel-chromium-beryllium (Ni-Cr-Be) alloys (18 to 30 MPa), but still greater than the bond to etched enamel.

Although the adhesive materials have not yet shown the same degree of long-term clinical bonding (since 1983 in Japan) as the conventional composite resins (1980 in the United States), the laboratory data supports their efficacy by demonstrating stable bond strengths upon aging in water.[14,15]

Recently, some have advocated a new adhesive method for bonding resin to metal that involves the flame application of a silica-carbon layer to the metal surface. A silane can be coated onto this treated metal, which provides a surface to which composite resin will bond. The system, which involves a burner-aspirator-timer system and associated chemistry, has been marketed to the dental laboratory industry as the Silicoater (Kulzer, Inc. USA).[18] In the laboratory, the strength of the bonds to base metal alloys with this system are high and appear stable, while the strength of the bonds to noble metal, although initially high, may degrade with thermal cycling.[19] Clinical trials using this bond system for the metal are in progress.

Changing the method of attachment of the resin to the metal framework does not change the design of the framework itself, because the short-term limiting factor in the system is still the bond of resin to enamel and the long-term limiting factor is the fatigue strength of the luting composite resin. Mechanical retention based on the framework design is necessary to limit the stress on the bond interfaces and the composite resin.

Maximum Enamel Coverage

The University of Maryland Dental School criteria for resin bonded cast restorations includes coverage of maximum enamel surface, provided that occlusion, esthetics, and periodontal health are not compromised. Retention, despite the overall success, is only as strong as the resin to enamel bond.[20,21] Because the strength of the resin to enamel bond cannot be increased, it is critical to add mechanical retention for long-term success.[22] Bond failures in the first or second year usually result from inadequate enamel coverage, contamination of the enamel during bonding, or improper etching of the metal. Bridges that debonded at 5 to 7 years seemed to demonstrate a variety of failure causes, which has led to the speculation that long-term failures may result from possible fatigue failure of the composite resin. Failure is evident by separation at either the resin to enamel interface or the resin to metal interface, or a cohesive failure may occur through the resin itself. The fatigue phenomenon in composite resin is well known and the strength of composite resin is reduced to approximately 60% of its original strength following load cycling (similar to occlusal loading).[23] It is, therefore, inappropriate to rely solely upon bonding to lingual enamel for retention of the prosthesis.

CLINICAL TIP. When it comes to mechanical retention (i.e., surface area of covered enamel, retention grooves), more is better than less.

Gingival Chamfer

The gingival chamfer should be no greater than 0.2 to 0.5 mm and should not extend into dentin. The resulting preparation allows a slight bulk of metal in the gingival one-third. This lowers stress in the resin to enamel bond,[24] by limiting metal flexing and providing a positive gingival stop. It also provides a useful guide for the laboratory technician when developing finishing lines and establishing proper contour in this area.

Cingulum and Occlusal Rests

Rests serve the same function as the gingival chamfer in terms of positive seating, a gingival stop, and a guide for the laboratory technician.

Interocclusal Clearance

Interocclusal clearance of 0.5 mm in all excursions is required to ensure adequate thickness of the metal framework.

Retention Grooves

Retention grooves, placed only in enamel, protect against rotational forces in the same way that the grooves in a three-quarter cast crown do. The placement of grooves is especially critical when abutment teeth have short clinical crowns, when the occlusion is heavy, or when esthetics or occlusion prevents adequate surface area to be included. Grooves in anterior abutment teeth should be designed with minimal proximal extension to the facial surface (Figs. 12–3, 12–4).

Path of Insertion

The existing heights of contour can be visualized by examining surveyed casts. Lowering the lingual and proximal heights of contour allows the restoration to cover a greater surface area. After performing this and other aspects of tooth preparation, a distinct incisal (occlusal)/gingival path of insertion, which is free of undercuts, should exist.

Provisional Restorations

Because provisional restorations are not required, resin bonded bridges should be fabricated as soon as possible to prevent tooth movement.

CLINICAL TIP. To prevent supereruption of opposing teeth against the lingual or occlusal preparation, place "composite resin spacers."

Reversibility

The second generation preparation is retentive and conservative, but not as reversible as earlier designs. Reversibility, however, becomes less significant as clinical studies continue to demonstrate the long-term success of these restorations.

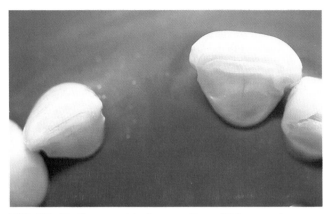

FIG. 12–3. The completed preparation of this second generation design includes a chamfer margin in the cingulum area and a shallow tapered groove just lingual to the proximal contact area. The marginal ridge distal to the edentulous area is reduced and a second groove placed in an accessible area. When a groove and chamfer finishing line are incorporated, a cingulum notch is not required.

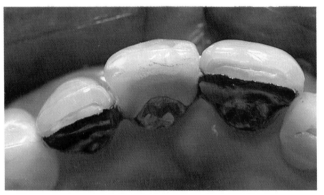

FIG. 12–4. The postoperative view of the bonded prosthesis demonstrates adequate retention, open embrasure form, and a retentive design that should resist dislodgement.

Unit Size

The same principles that are used in determining the number of abutments needed for proper periodontal support of conventional fixed bridges are applied to bonded prostheses. It is not necessary to add abutments merely to increase the size of the bonded area. Sufficient retention can be created by preparing the abutment teeth with retention components, such as grooves and rests (or, as in the case of short clinical crowns in the posterior region, by onlaying). The replacement of two missing anterior teeth can be considered routine. Replacement of two maxillary central incisors requires double abutting, using both the lateral incisors and the canines for the requisite periodontal support. Replacement of more than two missing maxillary anterior teeth should be approached with caution. Replacement of all mandibular incisors is routine and can be accomplished with only the canines as abutments if the occlusion is limited.

Posterior restorations should be limited to one pontic using bonded retainers unless inlaying or onlaying the abutment teeth is planned. When multiple posterior pontics are present, the forces of occlusion can create high stresses on the resin and the resin to enamel bond unless extensive mechanical retention is used to dissipate these forces.

Adhesive Systems vs. Etch Systems

Adhesive systems offer clinical convenience but require base metal or tin-plated noble metal. Base metal must be air abraded (50 micron alumina at a minimum of 60 psi of air pressure) to allow bonding. Surface contamination with saliva during try-in reduces the bond strength by up to 50%. The bond strengths can be returned to normal by repeated air abrading of the metal surface or by the use of hot detergent solution. An air abrasive instrument in the dental office is almost a requisite for the adhesive system. This system can be used with palladium- or gold-based alloys, provided that they are properly tin-plated. In addition, gold- or palladium-based metal frameworks must be thicker than those of base metals to compensate for the relatively lower elastic modulus and yield strength of these alloys.

Salivary contamination does not appreciably degrade the bond of the etched metal system. The micromechanical retention is not compromised by a salivary protein coat, as is the case in the chemical bond adhesive system. The disadvantage of the etch system is the requirement for careful and critical laboratory techniques involving strong acids. Also, no chairside etching techniques provide an adequate degree of three-dimensional relief on the base metal alloy surface for good bonding. Good laboratory support is mandatory. In addition, not all base metal alloys can be used in this technique.

Tooth Mobility

Mobile teeth should be avoided as abutments for resin bonded prostheses because of their tendency to debond. However, if mobile teeth must be incorporated into the design, they should be prepared with as much retention as possible. In order to prevent faciolingual displacement, the retainer should cover as much enamel surface as possible and incorporate retentive designs (e.g., distinct grooves, multiple rests, incisal hooks).[26] In general, when the framework is seated, the abutment teeth must not be displaced out of the framework by the occlusion in any direction. This requirement is particularly important on mobile teeth. In addition, the connector to retainer transitional area should be thick to prevent fatigue failure of the metal framework on mobile abutment teeth. It is possible for splints to fail with the bonding remaining intact because of metal fatigue.

TOOTH PREPARATION
Anterior Preparations
Armamentarium

- Standard dental setup
  explorer

mouth mirror
periodontal probe
high-speed handpiece
low-speed handpiece
- Surveyed and articulated study models
- Diamond burs
  Round-ended, tapered (small and medium diameter with carbide tips)
  Bullet- or football-shaped
  Round
- Carbide burs
  No. 6 round
  No. 35 inverted cone
  No. 169 and No. 169L
  No. 700 and No. 701
- Tapered and ovoid 12-fluted finishing burs
- Custom or stock impression trays
- Impression materials
- Anterior restorative composite resin kit

Clinical Technique

1. Prior to any tooth reduction, survey and evaluate the models to determine where to create retention, lower the height of contour, place proximal extensions, position cingulum rests, and locate proximal grooves, as well as where to provide occlusal clearance.

CLINICAL TIP. Interocclusal clearance should be at least 0.5 mm to 1 mm in both centric and eccentric movements of the mandible. In the maxillary anterior, the clearance can usually can be obtained by reducing the lingual enamel of the abutment teeth. If enamel is thin or if the abutment teeth are sensitive, obtain clearance by reducing the incisal edges of mandibular anterior teeth. Depending on the anatomy of the teeth, use a tapered, ovoid, or football-shaped diamond bur to create the lingual clearance (Fig. 12–5). Verify the clearance visually or with wax (Fig. 12–6).

2. Because no provisional restorations are used, bond a light-cured composite resin to the incisal edges of the opposing anterior teeth to maintain the clearance. The resin can be easily removed for try-in appointments or after bonding procedures. Mandibular anterior abutment teeth seldom need incisal clearance because the framework engages only the lingual and proximal areas.
3. Using a small tapered diamond bur, create a shallow lingual chamfer within 1 mm of the gingival crest. The chamfer should be approximately 0.25 mm deep, without penetrating into dentin or creating a subgingival margin (Fig. 12–7).
4. Using the same diamond bur, create proximal extensions as far to the facial aspect as esthetics allow.

CLINICAL TIP. If a standard framework design would allow metal to be visible in the labial display, modify the technique to cover the area with porcelain. The preparation should allow the metal framework to be fabricated shy of the facial area. The proximal area of the porcelain pontic is etched, silanated, and bonded to the etched enamel of the abutment teeth with the cementing composite resin.[25]

5. When a tooth has a distinct cingulum, place a well defined cingulum rest with an inverted cone bur,

CLINICAL TIP. The proximal reduction is a critical aspect of the preparation. It determines the path of insertion and the amount of "wrap around" that can be achieved, especially when combined with a retainer design that is extended over the marginal ridges on tooth surfaces not adjacent to the edentulous space (Fig. 12–8).

running from mesial to distal marginal ridges. When this retentive notch is used, the chamfer can be eliminated from the preparation. This has been verified in photoelastic model studies.[24] When lingual anatomy is shallow or not distinct, use proximal grooves and a chamfer.

6. Proximal grooves are best used when abutment teeth are short or subject to excessive occlusal forces. To properly prepare the groves, place a No. 169L bur just lingual to the contact area and parallel to the long axis of the tooth (Fig. 12–9) toward the facial. The bur should penetrate no deeper than the diameter of the bur, otherwise the metal of the final restoration will creat a gray shadow through the enamel. Place tapered, parallel grooves on both the proximal area and the marginal ridge opposite the edentulous area (Fig. 12–10). The preparation should resemble a shallow three-quarter crown preparation (Fig. 12–11).

Posterior Preparations

Conceptually, anterior and posterior preparations are similar, except that the design and retentive features for posterior teeth are more extensive because of tooth morphology and the need to resist forces of posterior occlusion. Extensive occlusal clearance is usually not required because framework extensions to the occlusal surface are usually limited to the rest seat areas and lingual slope of the lingual cusp.

Armamentarium. The armamentarium is the same as that listed for anterior preparations (see the preceding section).

Clinical Technique

1. Prior to tooth reduction, survey and evaluate the models to determine where to create retention, place interproximal extensions, position occlusal rests, and locate grooves, as well as where to provide occlusal clearance.
2. Use a No. 6 round bur for molars or a No. 4 round bur for premolars. Penetrate the fossa next to the marginal ridge and reduce the tooth sufficiently to obtain 0.5 to 1.0 mm of occlusal clearance in the marginal ridge area. Angle the bur gingivally toward the center of the tooth and, although it does not penetrate to the dentin, the resulting rest seat should have distinct walls that provide retention and resistance form. In addition, occlusal rest seats aid in providing a positive seating for the casting. These rests resemble those for removable partial dentures but are more distinct (Figs. 12–12, 12–13).
3. Use a tapered diamond bur to reduce the lingual and proximal heights of contour and establish the occlu-

sogingival path of insertion. The lingual finishing line should be no less than 1.0 mm above the crest of the gingiva. The proximal "wings" of the casting should be approximately 3.0 to 5.0 mm in occlusogingival length and should never impinge on the soft tissue. Increase this occlusogingival height whenever possible by extending the casting as high toward the occlusal surface as the opposing occlusion will allow. Thus, the casting will extend up the lingual slope of the lingual cusp. By following these guidelines, castings should not be overcontoured and the embrasure form should allow ease of cleansing.

4. To improve retention, prepare a groove or a shallow slot in the proximal surface buccal to the occlusal rest seat. Place a No. 700 bur along the long axis of the tooth and penetrate to a depth of one-half the bur. When abutment teeth are short or if additional retention is needed, place a second groove similarly

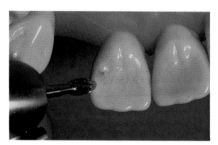

FIG. 12–5. The occlusal contact is marked with articulating paper so that only a minimal amount of enamel is removed for lingual clearance. An ovoid diamond or 12-fluted carbide bur can be used for this reduction.

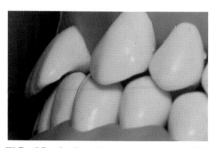

FIG. 12–6. The ideal clearance is 0.5 to 1.0 mm. The clearance can be verified visually or confirmed with wax. Check for adequate clearance in centric occlusion and in excursive movements.

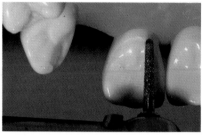

FIG. 12–7. Using a tapered diamond- or carbide-tipped bur (No. 383–012 Brasseler) the lingual chamfer can be created. This chamfer finishing line extends from the mesiolingual line angle to the distal marginal ridge.

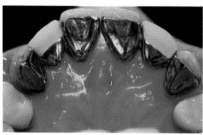

FIG. 12–8. These restorations are still successfully bonded after 7 years, partly because the frameworks had maximum extension especially over mesial and distal marginal ridges.

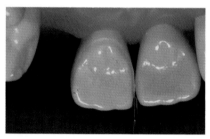

FIG. 12–9. Using a 169L bur, create the proximal groove, making sure that it does not extend too far to the facial aspect or penetrate into dentin.

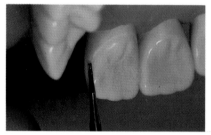

FIG. 12–10. The groove should be parallel with the long axis of the tooth and also parallel to the groove that will be placed on the canine.

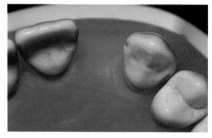

FIG. 12–11. The completed preparations on both the central incisor and the canine resemble modified three-quarter crown preparations.

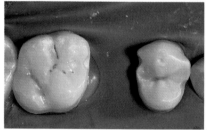

FIG. 12–12. An occlusal view of these completed posterior preparations demonstrate the placement of multiple occlusal rest seats. The premolar has mesial and distal rests, whereas the molar has rests on the mesial and lingual surfaces. Note the distinct chamfer finishing line that extends from the facial extent of the edentulous area to the opposite lingual proximal line angle.

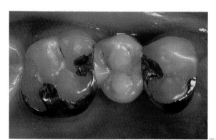

FIG. 12–13. The occlusal view of the completed restoration highlights the placement of multiple occlusal rests.

on the linguoproximal line angle opposite the initial groove. All grooves must be shallow, distinct, and parallel. If the grooves are not parallel, they can be realigned by using a No. 701 to one-half its depth. Alternatively, a second occlusal rest can be placed distal to the edentulous space on the abutment tooth (see Fig. 12–12).

Miscellaneous Preparations

Ideal abutment teeth are not always available for use in resin bonded restorations. Abutment teeth commonly have existing restorations, are rotated or tilted, and are sometimes too short to have an adequate retentive design.

When an existing restoration is present, it must be evaluated for overall quality and marginal integrity. If it is not adequate, it should be replaced before the restoration is fabricated. Small Class III composite resins that appear to be sound can be incorporated into the design, provided that the framework fully covers the restoration and the resin is roughened just before bonding. If anterior teeth have extensive Class III or Class IV composite resin restorations, they should not be used as abutment teeth.

Posterior teeth with amalgam restorations often require variations in basic techniques. Small or moderate Class I amalgams seldom cause a serious problem because alternative sites for rest seats can usually be found.[26] Large Class I or small two-surface Class II amalgams adjacent to the edentulous area require the amalgam to be partially removed and the remaining walls flared to accept an inlay component (Figs. 12–14, 12–15). The remaining amalgam functions as a base and the surrounding enamel walls provide adequate resin bonding surface area. Again, it is important that the amalgam restoration be completely covered by the framework. The amalgam functions as a high elastic modulus base for the metal; a glass ionomer would be inadequate in this regard. The luting resin Panavia has a moderate bond to dental amalgam as a result of the high tin composition of the amalgam.

If the existing dental amalgam restoration is defective, it can be removed and replaced with a posterior composite resin restoration. The shallow inlay preparation for the bonded retainer should still be incorporated in the design.

When teeth have extensive restorations or are tilted, a bonded onlay can be routinely used (Figs. 12–16, 12–17). The enamel must be reduced by 1.0 mm and verified in excursive movements of the mandible. Composite resin is bonded to the opposing cusp tips to prevent supereruption or mesial drifting of the onlayed tooth. A shallow chamfer helps to define the gingival margin and later helps provide a definitive finishing line for the metal.

Impressions

Impression techniques for resin bonded restorations are similar to those used for conventional crown and bridge restorations, except that anesthetics and retraction cords are seldom used.

Armamentarium

- Standard dental setup (see the section on Anterior Preparations)
- Suitable impression agent, i.e., reversible hydrocolloid, rubber base, condensation silicone, vinyl polysiloxane, or polyether

Clinical Technique

1. Inject a light body or syringe material around the abutment teeth using great care to capture any grooves, slots, or rests.

CLINICAL TIP. *Use only accurate elastomeric impressions, i.e., rubber base, condensation silicone, vinyl polysiloxane, polyether, or reversible hydrocolloid. Irreversible hydrocolloid is not indicated and should be avoided as a final impression material.*

2. Load a heavy body or tray material into a custom or stock tray and seat it. Because all finishing lines are supragingival, details of each abutment tooth should be easily captured.

CLINICAL TIP. *The low tear strength of vinyl polysiloxane and polyether is a limitation when taking impressions of multiple abutment teeth. Often these materials tear in the interproximal embrasure and the finishing line may be lost. The high tear strength of polysulfide rubber is generally more convenient in this regard, particularly for periodontal splint impressions.*

Laboratory Techniques. Impressions can be poured in an investment material to develop a refractory cast, however, most technicians prefer to work with stone models.

CLINICAL TIP. *Conventional trimmed and indexed dies are not recommended. The model is, therefore, very stable and allows the technician to develop anatomic contours with open and cleansible embrasure form.*

The outline should be drawn lightly with a wax pencil in a color that contrasts with the pattern (Fig. 12–18) and an acrylic resin pattern fabricated. The completed pattern can be sprued with a runner bar and auxiliary sprues, or with one large sprue with a reservoir attached to the pontic.[27]

Base metal alloys historically have been used for resin bonded prostheses because of their etching characteristics. However, the etching conditions for each alloy vary and each requires different acids, current densities, or etching times. These alloys are contraindicated in patients with known metal sensitivities.

CLINICAL TIP. *Review the patient's medical history concerning reactions to metals. For patients with pierced ears this is particularly important. If they can tolerate only pure gold posts they likely have a nickel sensitivity. Inexpensive gold posts are nickel plated and then coated with a thin gold layer. The nickel diffuses through the gold and sensitizes some individuals.*

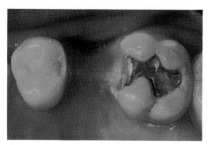

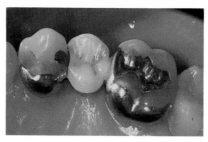

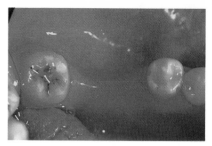

FIG. 12–14. The completed preparation demonstrates the removal of part of the two-surface amalgam in the molar. Not only does the inlay form itself provide retention, but also, the enamel walls provide additional surface for resin bonding.

FIG. 12–15. The completed restoration demonstrates the outline form for the inlay, as well as the conventional lingual extension. This design is extremely retentive even though the bond of resin to amalgam is not as strong as resin to etched enamel.

FIG. 12–16. Because of the shortness and mesial tilting of the molar, an onlay retainer was designed to extend over the entire occlusal surface as well as portions of the buccal, lingual, mesial, and distal surfaces. The premolar was also short and, as a result, it has mesial and distal grooves and a distinct disto-occluso rest seat.

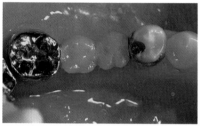

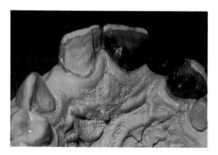

FIG. 12–18. This cast demonstrates a pencil outline on the right side and a completed pattern on the left. The outline covers a broad area of enamel and extends just facial to the proximal grooves. Because the teeth are short and the surface area for bonding is limited, the retainers extend closer to the gingiva than is ideally desirable.

FIG. 12–17. Postoperative view of the bonded bridge.

Gold- and palladium-based alloys may be selected if the dental laboratory has the facilities for tin-plating (see below) or "silicoating."

CLINICAL TIP. Enter the composition of the alloy used by the laboratory and the brand name into the patient's record.

CLINICAL TIP. In cases involving longer spans, or postorthodontic or periodontal splinting, a metal framework try-in is essential to verify the fit and occlusion prior to porcelain application.

Because of the wide variability and quality of commercial laboratory work, the etching work is often performed less than ideally.[12] The adhesive system that uses Panavia resin (or Silicoater, Kulzer, Inc. USA technique) provides more consistent results and eliminates the need for a chemical or electrolytic etching process. If an adhesive bonding system is selected, the framework only requires air abrasion after each firing of porcelain or if contaminated by saliva.

Esthetic Try-In

When Comspan (Caulk/Dentsply) was first introduced in 1980, it was a very translucent composite resin that allowed the darkened etched metal to cause graying or dark shadowing in the incisal area of anterior teeth. The graying was not always visible when the bridge was tried in, but was often evident following bonding. As a result of the graying problem, most of the commonly used bis-GMA composite resins now contain opaquers to mask the color changes.[28] Despite the use of opaquers, obtaining a pleasing esthetic result necessitates an esthetic try-in with a simulated bonding.

Armamentarium

- Standard dental setup (see the section on Anterior Preparations)
- Stones and burs to adjust the metal and contour the porcelain
- Composite resin bonding kit that includes translucent *and* opaque resins
- Air brush (optional) (e.g., Micro Etcher, Danville Engineering)
- Eugenol or glycerine
- Plastic filling instrument
- Porcelain staining kit
- Acetone in a glass beaker
- Ultrasonic bath
- Alcohol wipes
- Battery operated tin plating device (e.g., Micro Tin, Danville Engineering)
- Panavia Kit (J. Morita USA, Inc., Kuraray Inc. USA)

Clinical Technique

1. Alter the metal framework where necessary before using the cementing resins.

CLINICAL TIP. If the framework does not fit, do not rely upon the composite resin cement to fill the gaps. Bond only well adapted retainers.

---

2. If the interproximal metal is visible, reduce it toward the lingual surface. The porcelain can be etched to provide retention in these areas.
3. Evaluate the lingual and gingival extension of the framework and reduce or recontour where necessary.
4. To preview the final esthetic result and determine whether the resin has adequate opacity to mask the gray metallic shadowing, trial bond the restoration with an inhibited composite resin (see below). Both translucent and opaque resins should be available in a composite resin bonding system so that the amount of opacity can be regulated.

CLINICAL TIP. Translucent resins should be used in the interproximal area because most opaque resins will leave a visible, high value line in this area.

CLINICAL TIP. Although opaque resins are effective in preventing incisal graying, too much opaqueness can increase the color value of the abutment teeth and make them appear lighter than the pontic.

---

5. Using a spatula dipped in eugenol, mix the opaque catalyst and base resins in equal proportions. Eugenol is a powerful inhibitor of the setting reaction of composite resins; the mix will not set, but will remain quite viscous. Eugenol only partially inhibits the setting reaction of Panavia, therefore, mix Panavia powder with glycerine rather than with the Panavia liquid. Load the metal retainers with the inhibited resin and seat the bridge on the *unetched* abutment teeth.
6. Most resins mask the gray metal at a thickness of 25 to 50 microns. If, however, the mixture is too opaque and the abutment teeth appear too light, make a second inhibited mix incorporating some of the translucent resin with the opaque resin.

CLINICAL TIP. Use opaque resins for all posterior restorations so that any excess flash can be visualized and removed.

---

7. Trial and error will determine the correct proportion of translucent to opaque resin.

CLINICAL TIP. Esthetic anterior restorations are best created by using opaque and translucent resins for the lingual and interproximal areas, respectively. The Panavia system is excellent because it contains both an opaque Panavia and a translucent Panavia TC.

---

8. Remove the inhibited resin from the metal retainers by rinsing in acetone or placing in an ultrasonic bath with acetone.
9. Clean the teeth of the eugenol/resin mix by wiping them thoroughly with gauze dipped in alcohol.
10. Once the ideal ratio of translucent to opaque resins is obtained, record it in the patient's record so that it can be used during the actual bonding.

CLINICAL TIP. Simulated bonding can be used to control the color value of the abutment teeth in conjunction with characterization and staining of the porcelain-fused-to-metal pontic. After placing the correct combination of inhibited resins, apply porcelain stains to the pontic section to produce the most natural color blend. Remove the inhibited composite resin from the interproximal area of the pontic. The resin that remains on the metal surface does not have to be washed away with acetone because it will be burned off in the porcelain oven when the pontic is glazed.

Preparation of the Bridge for Final Cementation

After the bridge is glazed, the inner surface of the metal is air abraded and the oral side polished. If using an etched bridge, the metal is either chemically or electrolytically etched at this stage. When using an adhesive system and a metal framework cast in a base metal alloy, a freshly air abraded surface is necessary for good bonding. Laboratory systems are available for tinplating the gold- or palladium-based casting alloys. The laboratory masks the area not to be plated and then, using conductive tweezers, places the bridge in the tin-plating bath. The automatic system then indicates when the tin-plating is completed. The tin-coated surface is only slightly lighter in color than the air abraded surface. Coating that is too thick is light gray to white in color and will lower bond strength. The strength of the bond of Panavia or Superbond to the tin-plated surface is not as high as that for base metal alloys, but it is very stable in water.

CLINICAL TIP. If the esthetics are acceptable at the esthetic try-in stage and if an adhesive system is to be used with a base metal alloy, the restoration does not have to be returned to the laboratory. After cleaning, abrade the metal with an air brush and cement the restoration.

CLINICAL TIP. A small microprocessor controlled, battery operated system for tin-plating in the dental office is available (Micro Tin, Danville Engineering).

BONDING

The most essential prerequisite for bonding is maintaining a dry field. Many early failures of resin bonded bridges are attributed to enamel contamination following etching and prior to the application of bonding agents. To ensure consistent and predictable results rubber dam isolation is essential.

CLINICAL TIP. When punching holes in the rubber dam, leave extra material in the pontic area so that the bridge can fully and passively seat without tension from the dam acting to unseat it.

Panavia Bonding

Armamentarium

- Standard dental setup (see the section on Anterior Preparations)
- Rubber dam setup
- Mylar matrix strips
- Panavia Kit (J. Morita/Kuraray, Inc.)

Clinical Technique

1. Place a rubber dam, taking care to invert it at all gingival margins and making certain that it will not impinge on bonded areas.
2. Pumice the abutment teeth; rinse, and dry.
3. Protect the adjacent teeth by lightly wedging mylar strips between them and the abutment teeth.
4. Etch the teeth for 60 seconds (90 seconds if the enamel is unprepared).

CLINICAL TIP. Once teeth are etched, proceed *immediately* to bonding.

5. Rinse the abutment teeth for 20 seconds.
6. Air-dry the teeth with an oil-free air spray. Apply the air until the area is dry and the teeth appear frosty. Either the dentist or assistant maintains a dry area until ready to paint the teeth with a thin layer of the cementing resin (Fig. 12–19).
7. The assistant mixes the liquid and powder according to the manufacturer's directions. Be certain to gently fluff the powder prior to dispensing it on the mixing pad and to use only a level scoop. Incorporate the powder rapidly into the liquid until the mixture is creamy.

CLINICAL TIP. Panavia is extremely oxygen inhibited because it sets anaerobically. Keep it in thin layers to provide a long working time (Fig. 12–20).

8. With a flat brush the assistant paints the inside of the castings with a *thin* layer of the resin. From the same mix, the dentist lightly coats the bonded area of the abutment teeth. Do not use an unfilled resin with Panavia (Fig. 12–21).
9. Apply the opaquer to the full lingual area of the metal and then apply the Panavia TC to the interproximal area of the retainer.
10. Apply the remainder of the opaquer to the lingual area of the etched, rinsed and dried abutment teeth.
11. Holding the bridge by the pontic, quickly transfer it

CLINICAL TIP. Coordinate the bonding sequence with the dental assistant so that each stage proceeds efficiently.

from the assistant to the dentist, who seats it and holds it in place.
12. With a second stiff pointed brush, wipe away the excess resin. The thin layer of resin that flows beyond the casting margins does not easily set unless it pools. Continue wiping until the metal, tooth, embrasure areas, and soft tissues are free of cementing resin (Fig. 12–22).

CLINICAL TIP. When removing the excess, be careful not to wipe the opaquer through the facial embrasure.

13. Inject the "blue-green" Oxyguard gel (polyethylene glycol) around the margins of the castings (Fig. 12–23). This gel seals the area from air, resulting in a complete setting of the resin. Hold the restoration in place for approximately 5 minutes.
14. Wipe and rinse the gel from the teeth.
15. Because excess resin can be removed effectively before it sets, there should be little hard resin to remove. Excess resin can be removed using scalers, currettes, and finally rotary instruments. Finishing burs or composite resin finishing stones are effective for this purpose.

CLINICAL TIP. If rubber points are used, avoid overheating the metal because this may soften the resin and lead to debonding.

16. Remove the rubber dam and verify the occlusion. Provide patients with instructions on using floss threaders or other periodontal aids to keep the tissues healthy (Fig. 12–24).

Adhesive Bonding

Armamentarium. The armamentarium is the same as that listed for Panavia bonding except:

- Adhesive bonding system (e.g., Comspan Caulk/Dentsply)
- Dentinal bonding systems (e.g., Scotchbond 2, 3M, Inc., or Tenure Den-Mat)

Clinical Technique. Use the same Clinical Technique as that described for Panavia bonding except:

1. When dentin is exposed, etch the enamel as usual and use a dentinal bonding system on the de   n and surrounding enamel.
2. Light-cure the bonding agent.
3. Apply the luting resin in a normal fashion. When using Tenure, mix bottles A and B and apply the normal luting resin directly to the coated dentin.
4. Be careful not to contaminate the gingival and lingual bonding surfaces with saliva or crevicular fluid. If there is any question, re-etch the enamel to avoid compromising the bond to enamel.

CLINICAL TIP. Do not rely on dentin bonding unless an exposed dentin area is surrounded by enamel.

Followup Visits

Patients should be seen on a regular basis to check for debonding or other problems with the restoration. Educate patients to notify the dentist if they become aware of changes in feel or fit of the bridge. Early detection of debonding is critical.

If debonding (full or partial) is detected, remove the entire restoration and rebond it or make a new one. To remove a bonded restoration, take advantage of the low shear strength of the cementing composite resin and direct a controlled high-impact blow along the path of insertion on each abutment tooth.

CLINICAL TIP. To best remove a bonded restoration, place a straight chisel at the occlusal or incisal edge of the retainer at the metal-enamel interface (Fig. 12–25). With a rubber tipped gold foil mallet, direct several sharp blows along the long axis of the tooth. During the tapping procedure, make sure that either the dentist or the assistant supports the tooth to ensure safe removal of the restoration. (Fig. 12–26).

FIG. 12–19. With a rubber dam properly inverted, the abutment teeth are etched, rinsed, and dried, revealing the characteristically frosty-appearing enamel.

FIG. 12–20. When Panavia is properly mixed, it should have a smooth creamy appearance. When kept in *thin* layers on the mixing pad, the material has an extended working time. The thin film of Panavia should be applied to the framework using a disposable brush.

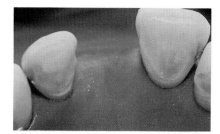

FIG. 12–19.

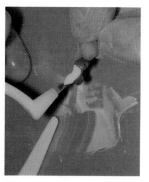

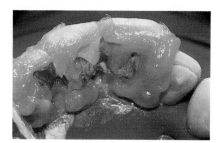

FIG. 12–20.

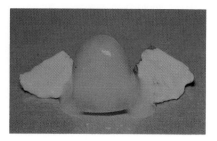

FIG. 12–21. When combining the opaque and translucent resins, place the opaque resin on the body of the retainer and use the translucent resin in the interproximal areas so that there will not be a visible opaque line on the facial surface.

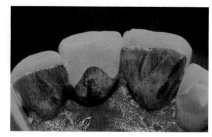

FIG. 12–22. After seating the restoration, use a clean pointed brush to wipe away all excess resin. The framework should be held in place so the debridement process does not dislodge the restoration before it is bonded.

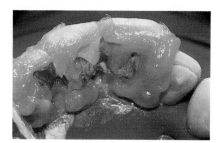

FIG. 12–23. After all excess resin is removed place *liberal* amounts of Oxy-Guard over all exposed margins. The gel seals the resin from the air, permitting it to set quickly.

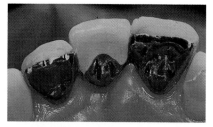

FIG. 12–24. After all excess resin is removed, the rubber dam is removed and the occlusion verified.

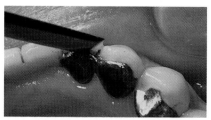

FIG. 12–25. A bonded restoration can be easily removed when using a mallet and directing sharp taps along the long axis of the tooth at the incisal aspect of the metal-enamel junction.

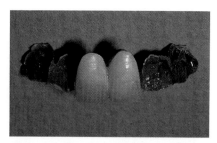

FIG. 12–26. Observation of the removed bridge reveals that the resin is still attached to the etched metal. This is typical of partial debond failures, which are the result of enamel contamination during the bonding process.

CONCLUSION

Resin bonded prostheses can be used for a wide variety of clinical situations. They provide long-term esthetically pleasing restorations when proper case selection, design, and bonding conditions are followed. Although resin bonding is less complicated than conventional fixed prosthodontics, the procedures are technique-sensitive and demand careful attention to details.

The authors wish to thank Mr. Victor Stryzak, CDT, for his technical and laboratory assistance.

REFERENCES

1. Ibsen, R.L.: One-appointment technique using an adhesive composite. Dent Surv 37:28, 1973.
2. Portnoy, J.: Constructing a composite pontic in a single visit. Dent Surv 49:30, 1973.
3. Ibsen, R.L.: Fixed prosthetics with a natural crown using an adhesive composite. J South Cal State Dent Assoc 41:100, 1973.
4. Jordan, R.E., et al.: Temporary fixed partial dentures fabricated by means of the acid-etch resin technique: a report of 86 cases followed up to three years. J Am Dent Assoc 96:994, 1978.
5. Rochette, A.L.: Attachment of splint to enamel of lower anterior teeth. J Prosthet Dent 30:418, 1972.
6. Howe, D.F. and Denehy, G.E.: Anterior fixed partial dentures utilizing the acid etch technique and a cast metal framework. J Prosthet Dent 37:28, 1977.
7. Livaditis, G.J.: Cast metal bonded bridges for posterior teeth. J Am Dent Assoc 101:926, 1980.
8. Williams, V.D., Drennon, D.G., and Silverstone, L.M.: The effect of retainer design on the retention of filled resin in acid-etched fixed partial dentures. J Prosthet Dent 48:417, 1982.
9. Tanaka, T., et al.: Pitting corrosion for retaining resin facings. J Prosthet Dent 42:282, 1979.
10. Livaditis, G.J. and Thompson, V.P.: Etched casting: an improved retentive mechanism for resin bonded retainers. J Prosthet Dent 47:52, 1982.
11. Levine, W.A.: An evaluation of the film thickness of resin luting agents. J Prosthet Dent 62:175, 1989.
12. Hussey, D.L., Gratton, D.R., McConnell, R.J., and Sands, T.D.: The quality of bonded retainers from commercial laboratories. J Dent Res 68:919, 1989.
13. Yamashita. A.: A dental adhesive and its clinical application, Vol. II. Tokyo, Quintessence Publishing, 1983.
14. Omura, I., Yamauchi, J., Jarda, I., and Wada, T.: Adhesive and mechanical properties of a new dental adhesive. J Dent Res 63:233, 1984.
15. Thompson, V.P., Grolman, K.M., and Liao, R.: Bonding of adhesive resins to non-precious alloys. J Dent Res 64:314, 1985.
16. Ohno, H., Araki, Y., Sagara, M., and Yamane, Y.: The adhesion mechanism of dental adhesive resin to the alloy—experimental evidence of the deterioration of bonding ability due to adsorbed water to the oxide layer. Dent Mat J 5:211, 1986.
17. Thompson, V.P.: Cast bonded retainers. In S.H.Y. Wei (ed.): Pediatric Dentistry: Total Patient Care. Philadelphia, Lea & Febiger, 1988.
18. Hansson, O.: The silicoater technique for resin-bonded prostheses: clinical and laboratory procedures. Quint Int 20:85, 1989.
19. Ruyter, I.E. and Waarli, M.: The Adhesion Mechanism of the Silicoating Technique. J Dent Res 68:891, 1989.
20. Thompson, V.P., Wood, M., and de Rijk, W.G.: Bonded bridge recalls and Weibull distributions: results averaging seven years. J Dent Res 68:920, 1989.
21. Verzijden, C.W. and Creugers, N.H.: Survival rate of resin-bonded bridges: a 5-year evaluation. J Dent Res 68:920, 1989.
22. Crispin, B.J., Fisher, D.W., and Avera, S.: Etched metal bonded restorations: three years of clinical follow-up. J Dent Res 65:311, 1986.
23. Draughn, R.F.: Fatigue and fracture mechanics of composite resin. In G. Vanherle and D.C. Smith (eds.): International Symposium on Posterior Composite Resin Dental Restorative Materials. St. Paul, MN, 3M Co., 1985.
24. Seto, B.G., and Caputo, A.A.: Photoelastic analysis of stresses in resin-bonded cingulum rest seats. J Prosthet Dent 56:460, 1986.
25. Williams, H.A., Caughman, W.F., and Pollard, B.L.: The esthetic hybrid resin-bonded bridge. Quint Int 29:623, 1989.
26. Wood, M.: Etched castings an alternative approach to treatment. Dent Clin North Am 29:393, 1985.
27. Wood, M., Thompson, V.P., and Mager, L.S.: Etched casting resin bonded retainers: design and fabrication (I). Quint Dent Tech 7:409, 1982.
28. Wood, M. and Thompson, V.P.: Masking tooth color changes of etched castings. J Dent Res 62:305, 1983.

David Federick, D.M.D., M.Sc.D.

ACRYLIC AND OTHER RESINS—PROVISIONAL RESTORATIONS

Achievement of esthetic and functional excellence in fixed prosthodontics is the reward for meticulous attention to detail at each stage of treatment. The quality provisional restoration is crucial to this success. The interim crown or bridge must be a mirror image of the definitive restoration, the only variable being the material (Figs. 13–1, 13–2). When this goal is not realized, failure often includes periodontal damage, pulpal irritation, occlusal aberrations, and patient dissatisfaction (Fig. 13–3).

BASIC CONCEPTS

The provisional (treatment) restoration provides for the following:

1. **Pulp protection and sedation** of the prepared abutments while the cast restorations are being fabricated. An adequate thickness of acrylic resin and good marginal integrity affords protection against thermal insult and bacterial and salivary invasion of the dentinal tubules.
2. **Evaluation of the tooth preparation** and of parallelism of abutments. When the treatment restoration is designed to be similar to the final cast restoration, the operator has an immediate opportunity to critique (and correct if necessary) tooth preparation for undercuts, inadequate bulk removal, and mutual paths of insertion.
3. **Immediate replacement** of missing or extracted teeth. The inclusion of pontics in the provisional restoration provides immediate replacements for edentulous spaces. This aids in stabilizing and preventing drifting of abutments.
4. **Improvement of esthetics** in interrupted and debilitated dentition. The provisional restoration provides coverage with an esthetic resin crown for malaligned, eroded, discolored, poorly restored, and fractured abutments.

5. **A healthy environment for the periodontium.** Crowded and malaligned abutments, overhanging margins of existing restorations, and areas of erosion or abrasion are replaced with properly contoured resin crowns compatible with periodontal health.
6. **A means of evaluation** and reinforcement of the patient's oral home care in maintaining an interim fixed restoration as a prerequisite to the permanent restoration. The patient's dexterity and motivation may be determined inadequate to provide the meticulous daily preventive maintenance necessary to care for a fixed splint. In this case, placing a removable prosthesis may be prudent.
7. **Facilitation of periodontal therapy** by providing access to and total visibility of surgical sites. Removal of the provisional restoration gives the periodontist an unobstructed surgical field in which to perform soft and hard tissue corrective procedures.
8. **Stabilization of mobile teeth** during and after periodontal therapy. The splinting action of joining two or more teeth increases resistances to an applied force and offers a stabilizing effect and reorientation of stress vectors.[1] This is important when fibers of the periodontal ligaments are in the process of reattaching to the cementum of a periodontally treated abutment. A tooth made "still" by a splinting procedure may undergo a reinsertion of periodontal fibers, whereas a mobile abutment has little chance of reattachment.[2]
9. **Facilitation of development and evaluation of occlusal scheme.** Many occlusal schemes and excursive guides may be evaluated by adding or deleting acrylic resin to the occlusion and contours of the provisional restoration.
10. **Evaluation of vertical dimension, phonetics, freeway space and esthetics.** The information gleaned during the alteration and finalization of the

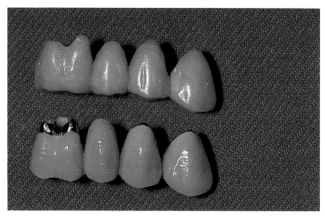

FIG. 13–1. Note the similarity between the acrylic resin maxillary provisional splint (top) and the porcelain-fused-to-gold bridge (bottom).

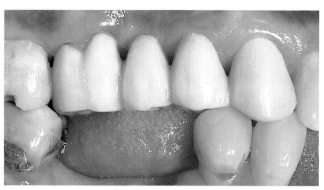

FIG. 13–2. The four-unit acrylic resin provisional splint (canine through first molar) viewed intraorally.

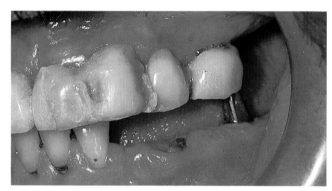

FIG. 13–3. An unacceptable provisional restoration exhibiting poor contour, open margins, gingival impingement, and unacceptable esthetics.

interim splints can be used to develop the subsequent cast splints.

11. **Aid in determining the prognosis** of questionable teeth. Changes in mobility patterns, osseous graft "takes," redefined lamina dura, periodontal ligament thickness, success of endodontic therapy, success of hemisection and bicuspidization procedures, pocket-depth decreases, and alleviation of signs and symptoms of periodontal disease may be determined during the provisional restorative phase of therapy. This will aid the operator in decisions about retaining a questionable abutment.

REQUIREMENTS FOR THE PROVISIONAL RESTORATION

The interim acrylic resin restoration must maintain gingival health. The basic requirements of a morphologically correct and physiologically acceptable provisional restoration are as follows:

1. **Good marginal adaptation.** This is achieved by careful attention to the details of the acrylic margins and reline/remargination procedures, when necessary.
2. **Good retention.** A temporary cement must always be used to ensure a barrier to intrusion of saliva and bacteria. Thick layers of cement will not correct a poorly made, ill-fitting restoration.
3. **Strength and durability.** An acrylic resin must stand the test of time if an extended period of service becomes necessary.
4. **Nonporous and dimensional stability.** A good grade of acrylic resin that is properly polymerized provides a superior restoration capable of extended service.
5. **Esthetics.** Attention to anatomic details encourages a patient's cooperation and acceptance of the provisional restoration.
6. **Physiologic contours and embrasures.** Adequate sluiceways and deflecting contours (avoiding overcontour) enhance the health of the periodontium.

7. **Ease of refinement.** This is especially important in a patient with a periodontal prosthesis when the provisional splint is fabricated and delivered before periodontal surgery. The healing periodontium usually exhibits controlled gingival recession for pocket elimination. It then becomes necessary to alter the abutments by apically extending the finishing lines and by relining the original provisional splint to cover the newly exposed tooth surfaces.
8. **Biologic occlusion.** The occlusal scheme developed in the provisional restoration must include a stable centric occlusion, acceptable vertical dimension of occlusion, unobstructed excursive movements, and proper cusp-fossae development for efficient mastication.
9. **Kindness to supporting tissues.** Rough unpolished margins, overcontoured crowns, impinged embrasures, and poor fit must be avoided in the provisional restoration to ensure periodontal health.
10. **Ease of cleaning by the patient.** The patient must be able to maintain a plaque-free environment using routine preventive home care devices and techniques. Advise patients that extended use of chlorhexidine oral rinses will stain acrylic resin restorations.

TABLE 13-1. PROPERTIES OF ACRYLIC RESINS FOR CROWN AND BRIDGE TEMPORIZATION

MATERIAL	STRENGTH	COLOR STABILITY	DIMENSIONAL STABILITY	POLYMERIZATION TIME	EXOTHERMIC HEAT	COST
Polymethyl methacrylate	Good	Good	Fair	Long	High	Low
Polyethyl methacrylate	Fair	Fair to Low	Good	Long	Moderate to High	Low
Polyvinyl methacrylate	Fair	Fair to Low	Good	Long	Moderate to High	Low
Iso-butyl	Fair	Fair	Good	Long	Low	Low
Bis-GMA (Auto-cured)	Good	Excellent	Very good	Moderate to Long	Very low	High
Bis-GMA (Dual-cured or Light-cured)	Good	Excellent	Very good	Moderate	Very low	High

BASIC CHEMISTRY

Auto-Cured Resin in Provisional Restorations

Acrylic polymers were introduced to dentistry in 1937, primarily as a denture base material. Polymethyl methacrylates are supplied in powder and liquid components. The powder (polymer) is polymethyl methacrylate plus benzoyl peroxide (initiator). The liquid (monomer) is methyl methacrylate [$CH_2 = C(CH_3) - COOCH_3$] plus hydroquinone (inhibitor). Other temporization materials are supplied in powder/liquid or paste/paste form.

The selection of an acrylic resin used for crown and bridge temporization is based on many factors. Shade availability, handling ease, polymerization time, and exothermic heat production are major considerations. The operator may choose an extended putty stage resin to facilitate manipulations and may prefer a rapid set resin for repairs. One should evaluate various types of resins before selecting a "favorite." Table 13-1 presents a comparison of properties of the various classes of acrylic resins available for crown and bridge temporization.

Light-Cured Resin in Provisional Restorations

Contemporary restorative materials, such as microfilled and hybrid light-activated composite resins, have definite applications in crown and bridge temporization. Unlimited working time and favorable manipulative properties make light-cured composite resins a popular alternative to conventional auto-curing crown and bridge resins. Light-cured resins may also be used:

1. For intraoral repair of fractured provisional bridges.
2. For re-establishing proximal and contact areas.
3. For remargination procedures.
4. For veneering conventional acrylic resin provisional crowns and bridges to provide an exceptionally esthetic and durable restoration.

Stages of Setting Auto-Cured Resin

1. **Doughy or putty stage.** At this stage a mixture of acrylic resin can be hand manipulated, it sticks to nonlubricated fingers, and all surface gloss has dissipated.

2. **Rubbery stage.** At this stage the resin is about 60 to 70% set, and can be removed from the mouth. The excess is easily trimmed with sharp scissors, and *immediately* repositioned over the abutments for complete polymerization.

TECHNIQUES AND MATERIALS

Preformed Crowns and Crown Forms

An acceptable interim restoration may be produced using polycarbonate, celluloid strip, or metallic crowns. Although, this concept may result in gingival abuse if improperly performed (Figs. 13-4 to 13-6), the cautious clinician, allotting adequate time, can produce a serviceable restoration (Table 13-2).

Polycarbonate Crowns (Anterior)

To achieve adequate retention and physiologic contours, the preformed crown must be altered, relined, and recontoured prior to cementation.

Armamentarium

- Standard dental setup (Tables 13-3 to 13-5)
    Cotton rolls
    Dappen dish
    Explorer
    High-speed handpiece
    Low-speed handpiece
    Mouth mirror
    Periodontal probe
    2 × 2 Gauze
- Petroleum jelly or silicone liquid
- Acrylic resin of choice (Table 13-6)
- Polycarbonate crown kit
- Polycarbonate crown mold guide
- Boley gauge (optional) (Henry Schein, Inc.)
- 1/2 Hollenback carver
- Acrylic bur setup—low-speed straight handpiece
    - Low-speed tapered carbide bur—rounded tip 4 mm base (e.g., H79E-040 carbide "E" cutter, Brasseler USA)
    - Low-speed tapered carbide bur—rounded tip 2.3 mm base (e.g., H261D-023 carbide "D" cutter, Brasseler USA)
    - Low-speed "Christmas tree" diamond bur—pointed tip 3.7 mm base (e.g., 852-037 medium grit diamond cutter, Brasseler USA)

TABLE 13–2. PREFORMED CROWNS AND CROWN FORMERS

TYPE	BRAND	MANUFACTURER
Polycarbonate	ION crown (Anterior) SDI crowns	3M, Inc. Svenska Dental Instrument
Plastic or Acetate (clear)	Caulk crown forms	L.D. Caulk/Dentsply
	Crown forms (Anterior/Posterior) Odus pella Crown forms	Den-Mat Corp. E.C. Moore Co., Inc. Interstate Dental Equipment and Supply, Inc.
Metal	Aluminum crowns Isoform (Posterior) Unitek crowns Gold anodized Java crown (epoxy-coated aluminum) Stainless steel and aluminum crowns	Parkell 3M, Inc. 3M, Inc. 3M, Inc. Java Crown, Inc. Denovo

TABLE 13–3. MISCELLANEOUS MATERIALS AND DEVICES

BRAND	MANUFACTURER
Duoloid Impression System	Cadco
Burlew Dry Foil	J.F. Jelenko and Co.
Concise Core Resin	3M, Inc.
Bond-Wand	Demetron Research Corp.
Aquapres	Lang Dental Mfg. Co., Inc.
Binocular Loupes	Almore International, Inc.
Triad VLC System	Dentsply International, Inc.
Metal/Mesh Reinforcing Bars	Ellman International Mfg. Co.
Hand Instruments Crown scissors Crown crimping pliers Crown contouring pliers	3M, Inc.
Perfectone Molds	George Taub Products
Novatech Collection Cement spatulas Cement placement instruments Cement removal instruments	Hu-Friedy Co.
Flexible Dappen Dish	George Taub Products Pulpdent Corp. Healthco International, Inc.
Dr. David Federick Temporization Kit	Brasseler USA
Electric Dental Engines 5,000-35,000 RPM	Bell International
	Weissman Tech International
Aluminum or Stainless Steel Para Post Plus	Coltene-Whaledent

TABLE 13–4. CROWN REMOVERS

BRAND	MANUFACTURER
Kline Crown Remover	Brasseler USA
Baade Pliers	S.S. White Burs, Inc.
Wynman Crown Gripper	Premier Dental Products Co.
Morrell Crown Remover	Premier Dental Products Co.
Crown Remover	Ellman International Mfg. Co.
Automatic Crown Removers	J.S. Dental Manufacturing, Inc.
Richwell Crown Removers	Almore International, Inc.

TABLE 13–5. SILICONE LUBRICANT (LIQUID)

BRAND	MANUFACTURER
High Spot (spray)	Cadco
Mizzy (spray)	Buffalo Dental Mfg. Co., Inc.
Crown and Bridge Lube.	Cadco

- Low-speed round carbide (No. 10) bur—rounded tip 2.7 mm head (e.g., H1-027 carbide cutter, Brasseler USA)
- Low-speed straight carbide bur (No. 557)—flat tip 1.0 mm base (e.g., H31-010 carbide cutter, Brasseler USA)
- Low-speed inverted cone carbide bur (No. 34)—flat tip 0.8 mm base (e.g., H2-008 carbide cutter, Brasseler USA)
- Acrylic finishing setup (See section on Finishing Procedures later in the chapter.)
- Shade correction setup (optional) (See the section on Color Correction and Shade Characterization later in the chapter.)
- Temporary cementation setup (See the section on Cementation of Provisional Restorations later in the chapter.)

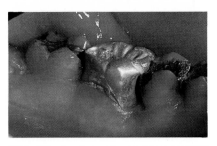

FIG. 13—4. A poorly adapted metallic provisional crown on the mandibular molar.

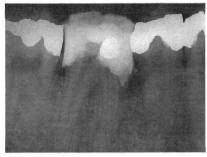

FIG. 13—5. Radiograph of the metallic provisional crown seen in Figure 13—4. Marginal irregularities have contributed to periodontal damage.

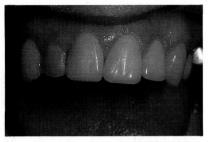

FIG. 13—6. Relined stock polycarbonate crowns cemented on the prepared left maxillary lateral incisor and both maxillary central incisors. Surface color correction has been applied.

TABLE 13—6. SELECTED ACRYLIC RESINS

TYPE	BRAND	MANUFACTURER
Methyl Methacrylate	Duralay	Reliance Dental Mfg. Co.
	Jet	Lang Dental Mfg. Co., Inc.
	Tab	Kerr Manufacturing Co.
	True	Harry J. Bosworth Co.
	Alike (Radiopaque)	Coe Laboratories, Inc.
	Cold-Pac	Matloid Dental Mfg. Co.
	Duracryl	Masel Orthodontics, Inc.
Ethyl Methacrylate	Temporary Bridge Resin	L.D. Caulk/Dentsply
	Splintline	Lang Dental Mfg. Co., Inc.
Vinyl Ethyl Methacrylate	Snap	Parkell
	Trim	Harry J. Bosworth Co.
	Provisional C & B Resin	Cadco
	Dura-Seal	Reliance Dental Mfg. Co.
Bis-GMA Auto-cured	Kind	Den-Mat Corp.
	Pro-Temp II	Premier Dental Products Co.
	Super-T	American Consolidated Mfg.
Bis-GMA Light-cured	Mirage	Chameleon Dental Products, Inc.
	Triad (Light-cured)	Dentsply International, Inc.
	GC Unifast LC	GC International Corp.
	Astron LC (Dual-cure)	Astron Dental Corp.
Iso-butyl	Temp Plus	Ellman International Mfg. Co.
	Aristocrat HTC Resin	Healthco International, Inc.

1. Select the correct size crown from the kit. A mold guide or Boley (Henry Schein, Inc.) gauge will facilitate selection (Fig. 13—7).
2. Adjust the crown gingivally and proximally with a low-speed diamond or carbide bur (e.g., H79E040, H261D023, 852037, Brasseler USA) and remove a thin layer of internal acrylic with a handpiece round bur (02710, Brasseler USA) so that it fits over the prepared tooth and prevents binding (Figs. 13—8, 13—9).
3. Protect the dentin and adjacent soft tissue with a layer of petroleum jelly or silicone liquid.
4. Fill the crown shell with a mixture of acrylic resin. Wait until the surface monomer dissipates (surface sheen disappears) and then carefully seat it on the preparation. As a guide to proper seating, note that the incisal edge relates correctly to the adjacent teeth.
5. When the reline acrylic resin achieves the rubbery stage, trim excess away from the margin with a No. 1/2 Hollenback carver (Fig. 13—10).

CLINICAL TIP. While the acrylic is setting, remove and replace the temporary crown. This will:
1. Protect the tooth from the exothermic reaction of the setting material.
2. Prevent the temporary crown from locking into undercuts in the prepared tooth or into undercuts between adjacent teeth.
3. Prevent the temporary crown from locking onto the tooth because of shrinkage during the setting reaction.

6. Remove the unit when the reline material has set.
7. Trim and smooth.
8. Reline or remarginate, if necessary. (See the section on remargination later in the chapter.)
9. Finish and polish the restoration. (See the section on Finishing Procedures later in the chapter.)
10. Custom stain or characterize, if necessary. (See the section on Color Correction and Shade Characterization later in the chapter.)
11. Cement. (See the section on Cementation of Provisional Restorations later in the chapter.) (Fig. 13—11).

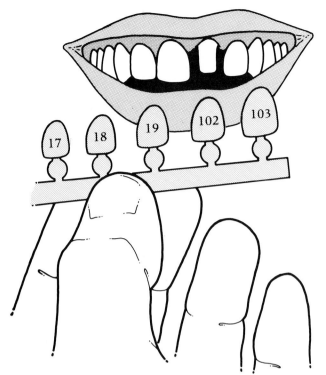

FIG. 13-7. The mold guide used to select stock preformed polycarbonate crowns.

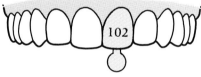

FIG. 13-8. A polycarbonate crown shell has been adjusted to fit over the preparation and to align with the adjacent teeth.

Celluloid (Clear) Strip Crown (Anterior)

Armamentarium

- Standard dental setup (see the preceding section on Preformed Crowns and Crown Forms.)
- Petroleum jelly or silicone liquid
- Acrylic resin of choice (see Table 13-6)
- Celluloid crown kit
- Boley gauge (optional)
- Crown and bridge scissors (e.g., No. 325, Brasseler USA)
- 1/2 Hollenback carver
- Acrylic bur setup (see section on Preformed Crowns and Crown Forms earlier in the chapter.)
- Acrylic finishing setup (see the section on Finishing Procedures later in the chapter.)
- Shade correction setup (optional) (see the section on Color Correction and Shade Characterization later in the chapter.)
- Temporary cementation setup (see the section on Cementation of Provisional Restorations later in the chapter.)

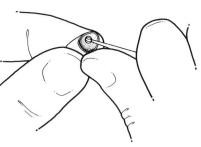

FIG. 13-9. A large H.P. (Hand Piece) round carbide bur is used to remove the internal layer prior to relining.

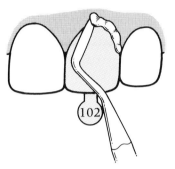

FIG. 13-10. A No. 1/2 Hollenback carver is used to trim excess reline resin at the putty stage.

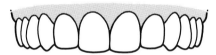

FIG. 13-11. The completed restoration.

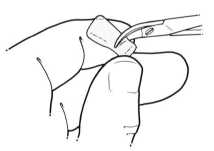

FIG. 13-12. Gingival adjustment using a curved crown and bridge scissors.

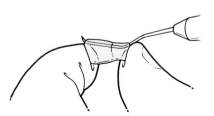

FIG. 13-13. The incisal edge is perforated with an explorer.

FIG. 13–14. The occlusal surface is left 1.0 mm in superocclusion. The metal margin extends at least 1.0 mm apical to the preparation margin.

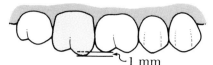

FIG. 13–14

FIG. 13–15. A preformed metal crown has been altered to serve as a matrix for the acrylic resin.

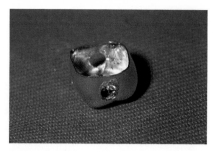

FIG. 13–15

FIG. 13–16. The altered metal preformed crown carrying acrylic resin.

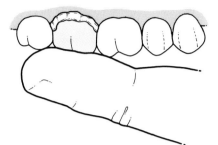

FIG. 13–17. An esthetic acrylic resin provisional crown made with the metal preformed crown matrix technique.

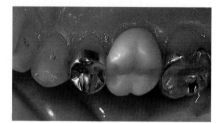

FIG. 13–16

FIG. 13–17

Clinical Technique. The Clinical Technique is similar to that described earlier for polycarbonate crowns with the following exceptions:

1. Trim the appropriate strip crown with scissors to achieve the correct length (Fig. 13–12).
2. Perforate the incisal edge with an explorer, penetrate through to the tyne hub, and open the proximal surfaces with a No. 6 round bur so the acrylic resin establishes proximal contacts (Fig. 13–13).

CLINICAL TIP. While the acrylic is setting, remove and replace the temporary crown. (See the preceding Clinical tip.)

3. After the acrylic resin has set, remove the restoration, cut away the celluloid shell, and finish.

Modified Metal Crown (Posterior)

Manufactured metallic shell crowns present a challenge to the restorative dentist. They are seldom morphologically accurate and require considerable alteration to achieve even minimal acceptability. Cutting, bending, and crimping the metal often results in a ragged, thick margin that readily retains plaque. The metal occlusal surface is not easily corrected to obtain a functional occlusal relationship. An esthetic result is impossible. These crowns are best used as a matrix only.

Armamentarium

- Standard dental setup. (see the section on Preformed Crowns and Crown Forms earlier in this chapter)
- Petroleum jelly or silicone liquid
- Acrylic resin of choice (see Table 13–6)
- Metal crown kit
- Crown and bridge scissors (e.g., No. 325, Brasseler USA)
- 1/2 Hollenback carver

- Acrylic bur setup (see the section on Preformed Crowns and Crown Forms earlier in the chapter)
- Acrylic finishing setup (see the section on Finishing Procedures later in the chapter)
- Shade correction setup (optional) (see the section on Color Correction and Shade Characterization later in the chapter.)
- Temporary cementation setup (see the section on Cementation of Provisional Restorations later in the chapter)

Clinical Technique

1. Select a metal crown that is one size too large for the available space.
2. Trim the gingival contour with a curved crown and bridge scissors so that the crown is 1 mm above the occlusion of the adjacent teeth when seated. (Use marginal ridge relationships as a guide.) Leave the metal at least 1 mm apical to the tooth preparation margin (Fig. 13–14).
3. Using a large round carbide, cut a window of approximately 6 to 8 mm diameter, from inside the metal crown, into each proximal surface. This will establish proximal contacts with the adjacent teeth. The preformed metallic crown is now ready to serve as a matrix for the acrylic resin (Fig. 13–15).
4. Protect the dentin and adjacent soft tissue with a layer of petroleum jelly or silicone liquid.
5. Mix the appropriate shade of acrylic resin in a dappen dish and fill the altered metal crown.

CLINICAL TIP. Use a rubber or silicone dappen dish rather than glass for easier cleanup (acrylic will not stick to rubber or silicone).

6. When the acrylic is doughy, seat the metal crown 1.0 mm in superocclusion onto the prepared tooth (Fig. 13–16).

7. Remove excess resin at the margins and at interproximal areas with a sharp Hollenback carver.
8. When the acrylic is fully polymerized, remove the metallic crown and resin reline.
9. Strip off the metal shell. Do not leave the metal crown over the acrylic resin. Use the metal crown only as a matrix in the development of the interim acrylic resin crown.
10. Trim and smooth.
11. Reline or remarginate, if necessary. (See the section on Remargination later in the chapter.)
12. Finish and polish restoration. (See the section on Finishing Procedures later in the chapter.)
13. Custom stain or characterize, if necessary. (See the section on Color Correction and Shade Characterization later in the chapter.)
14. Cement. (See the section on Cementation of Provisional Restorations later in the chapter.)

This technique yields an esthetic, well contoured provisional crown that is significantly superior to a crudely adjusted, unesthetic, ill-fitting, preformed metallic crown (Fig. 13–17).

Direct Preparation/Impression Technique

The use of an impression is the most popular method of positioning polymerizing acrylic resin over tooth preparations to produce a multiunit provisional splint. Any elastic impression material in a stock impression tray is acceptable. Either the direct or indirect method may be performed.

Armamentarium

- Standard dental setup (see the section on Preformed Crowns and Crown Forms earlier in this chapter)
- Petroleum jelly or silicone liquid
- Acrylic resin of choice (see Table 13–6)
- Impression material: irreversible hydrocolloid or silicone impression material
- No. 15 scalpel
- Acrylic bur setup (see the section on Preformed Crowns and Crown Forms earlier in the chapter)
- Acrylic finishing setup (see the section on Finishing Procedures later in the chapter)
- Shade correction setup (optional) (see the section on Color Correction and Shade Characterization later in the chapter)
- Temporary cementation setup (see the section on Cementation of Provisional Restorations later in the chapter)

Clinical Technique

1. Make an impression of the unprepared abutments using irreversible hydrocolloid or silicone impression material in a stock tray.

2. Remove unnecessary elastic material from the impression (e.g., interproximal tags, border extensions) to make reseating easier.
3. Store until tooth preparation is completed.
4. Prepare teeth.
5. Protect the prepared abutments with petroleum jelly or silicone emulsion.
6. Pour a mixture of acrylic resin into the impression and, when no sheen is present, carefully insert the impression to assure full and accurate seating over the preparations.
7. Remove the splint at the rubbery stage and trim any excess resin with sharp scissors.
8. Return the splint to the impression and position the tray over the preparations.
9. When fully set, remove the splint and finish in the usual manner.
10. Reline or remarginate, if necessary. (See the section on Remargination later in the chapter.)
11. Finish and polish the restoration. (See the section on Finishing Procedures later in the chapter.)
12. Custom stain or characterize, if necessary. (See the section on Color Correction and Shade Characterization later in the chapter.)
13. Cement. (See the section on Cementation of Provisional Restorations later in the chapter.)

Indirect/Direct Technique

If the patient presents with coronally debilitated teeth or with edentulous spaces, secure preoperative diagnostic casts. The cast can be "corrected" to ideal anatomic form using inlay wax, resin, denture teeth, or preformed polycarbonate or metallic crowns. The "corrected cast" now serves as the model, which is impressed. The impression is used to position the polymerizing acrylic resin onto the prepared teeth (Figs. 13–18, 13–19).

Armamentarium. The armamentarium is the same as that listed for Direct Technique.

Clinical Technique. Use the same Clinical Technique as that described for Direct Technique except use an altered model as the source of the impression.

Plastic Matrix Technique

Some clinicians feel that elastic materials are inadequate and inaccurate for carrying acrylic resin during the fabrication of provisional splints. Disadvantages include:

1. **Voids and bubbles** that are not easily detected until the polymerization of the resin is complete, yielding a porous, unesthetic surface.
2. **Occlusal discrepancies** caused by distortion or incomplete reseating of the impression.
3. **Cumbersome procedures** allowing minimal or no visibility or access to the polymerizing resin.

The use of a clear plastic matrix (Table 13–7) to carry acrylic resin eliminates the above disadvantages and provides additional advantages:

TABLE 13–7. STENT FORMERS

TYPE	BRAND	MANUFACTURER
Vacuum Type	OmniVac	Howmedica Corp.
	StaVac	Buffalo Dental Mfg. Co., Inc.
	Dentiformer	Healthco International, Inc.
Manual Type	Press-Form Kit	Ellman International Mfg. Co.

1. The clear matrix serves as a tooth preparation (reduction) guide.
2. Acrylic resin polymerizes to a smooth, void-free surface against the plastic.
3. The matrix is reusable for fabrication of replacement splints.
4. The matrix is easily made by auxiliary personnel.
5. The matrix is inexpensive to produce.

Ellman Press-Form System (Fig. 13–20)

Armamentarium

- Standard dental setup (see the section on Preformed Crowns and Crown Forms earlier in this chapter)
- Petroleum jelly or silicone liquid
- Acrylic resin of choice (see Table 13–6)
- Diagnostic cast
- Press-Form System (Ellman International Mfg., Co.)
- Plastic sheets (various sheet thickness): 0.020 in. for short spans, 0.040 in. for medium spans, 0.060 in. for long spans
- Blue inlay wax (optional)
- Denture or metallic crown forms or polycarbonate crowns (optional)
- Acrylic bur setup (see the section on Preformed Crowns and Crown Forms earlier in the chapter)
- Acrylic finishing setup (see the section on Finishing Procedures later in the chapter)
- Shade correction setup (optional) (see the section on Color Correction and Shade Characterization later in the chapter)

- Temporary cementation setup (see the section on Cementation of Provisional Restorations later in the chapter.)

Clinical Technique

1. Prepare a stone or plaster cast.
2. Make any necessary corrections to the tooth structure (Fig. 13–21).

CLINICAL TIP. If it is necessary to correct coronal anatomy with inlay wax, duplicate the cast in plaster or stone before adapting the heated plastic sheet. However, if resin denture teeth or preformed crowns are used to correct the original cast, it is not necessary to duplicate the cast prior to adapting the heated plastic.

3. Blockout peripheral undercuts with clay or Mortite (Mortite, Inc.) stripping.
4. Select the appropriate plastic sheet. Use a 0.020 in. plastic sheet for a 1 to 6 unit splint. For longer spans use a 0.040 to 0.060 in. thick sheet.
5. Securely insert the plastic sheet into the frame.
6. Use silicone spray to coat the cast and both sides of the plastic sheet.
7. Heat the plastic sheet on one side until opacity begins to disappear (3 to 5 seconds).

CLINICAL TIP. Do not allow the sheet to overheat or sag excessively, causing it to tear or buckle. This provides a distorted, inaccurate matrix which may also adhere to the cast.

8. Place the plastic sheet on the cast and aggressively apply putty for 10 seconds to mold the sheet to the cast.
9. Allow the sheet to cool for 20 seconds; peel away the putty and lift the sheet off the cast.
10. Trim the plastic sheet with scissors.

CLINICAL TIP. Trim the borders to within 2 to 3 mm of the gingival margins (Fig. 13–22). Include one tooth mesial and one tooth distal to the terminal abutments of the bridge. If no teeth are adjacent to terminal preparations, leave a 5 mm "drape" of plastic covering the distal soft tissue area. Carefully round all sharp corners of the matrix to avoid intraoral tissue laceration.

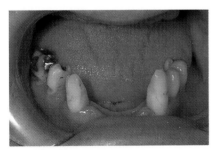

FIG. 13–18. The mandibular dentition prior to rehabilitation.

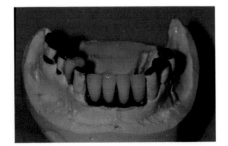

FIG. 13–19. The "corrected" diagnostic cast. Prior to making the elastic impression inlay wax and denture teeth were used to restore occlusal anatomy, increase the vertical dimension of occlusion, and replace missing teeth.

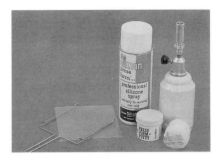

FIG. 13–20. Components of the Ellman Press Form Kit.

11. Prepare the teeth.
12. Protect the prepared abutments with petroleum jelly or silicone emulsion.
13. Pour a mixture of acrylic resin into the matrix.

CLINICAL TIP.
1. Place wet paper towel "wads" into the stent adjacent to the terminal abutments (Fig. 13–23). This confines the resin until it reaches the putty stage.
2. Place the acrylic in the stent (Fig. 13–24).
3. When the surface sheen disappears remove the paper "wads" (Fig. 13–25).
4. Carefully seat the stent and acrylic over the preparation in the correct path of insertion.

---

14. Carefully position the plastic sheet carrying the acrylic resin over the preparations to assure full and accurate seating.
15. Remove the matrix and resin at the rubbery stage so excess resin can be trimmed with sharp scissors.
16. Return the splint to the plastic sheet and reseat both over the preparation.

CLINICAL TIP. While the acrylic is setting, remove and replace the matrix/resin or direct a stream of water over the matrix containing the polymerizing acrylic resin. (See the Clinical Tip in the section on Preformed Crowns and Crown Forms.)

---

17. When fully set, remove the splint and finish in the usual manner.
18. Remarginate, if necessary. (See the section on Remargination later in the chapter.)
19. Finish and polish the restoration. (See the section on Finishing Procedures later in the chapter.)
20. Custom stain or characterize, if necessary. (See the section on Color Correction and Shade Characterization later in the chapter.)
21. Cement. (See the section on Cementation of Provisional Restorations later in the chapter.)

Vacuum Former Unit (Fig. 13–26)

The vacuum former unit is particularly suited to producing long-span matrices. This technique is more time consuming than the hand molded method and yields a closely adapted sheet.

Armamentarium. The armamentarium is the same as that listed for the Ellman Press-Form System with the exception of a vacuum forming unit (e.g., Dental Vacuum Forming Unit, Buffalo Dental Mfg. Co., Inc.)

Clinical Technique

1. Prepare a stone or plaster cast.

CLINICAL TIP. The coronal anatomy can be corrected on the model. (See the Clinical Tip in the section on Plastic Matrix Technique.)

---

2. Preheat the unit by activating the calrod element.
3. Drill a hole of 1 in. diameter in the center of the palate of a maxillary cast. A mandibular cast should be horseshoe-shaped.

4. Block out peripheral undercuts with clay or Mortite (Mortite, Inc.) stripping.
5. Spray the cast with silicone.
6. Select the plastic sheet. Use a 0.020 in. plastic sheet for a 1 to 6 unit splint. For longer spans use a 0.040 to 0.060 in. thick sheet.
7. Secure the plastic sheet into the frame and reposition the frame upward to the highest position just below the calrod.
8. Allow the plastic sheet to sag only 0.5 in. before guiding the frame with the sheet down over cast.

CLINICAL TIP. Do not allow the sheet to overheat or sag excessively causing it to tear or buckle. This provides a distorted, inaccurate matrix.

---

9. Quickly lower the frame over the cast.
10. Activate the vacuum.

CLINICAL TIP. Leave the calrod element on for an additional 30 seconds and vacuum for 1 minute. This allows for proper adaptation and cooling of the plastic.

---

11. When the sheet has cooled, remove it from the cast. Cut away the excess sheet material to aid in removal.
12. Trim the plastic sheet (Figs. 13–27, 13–28).

CLINICAL TIP. Trim the borders to within 2 to 3 mm of the gingival margins. (See the Clinical Tip in the section on Plastic Matrix Technique.)

---

13. Prepare the teeth.
14. Protect the prepared abutments with petroleum jelly or silicone emulsion.
15. Pour a mixture of acrylic resin into the impression. (See Figs. 13–23 to 13–25.)

CLINICAL TIP. Place wet paper towel "wads" into the stent on the teeth adjacent to terminal abutments. (See the Clinical Tip in the section on Plastic Matrix Technique.)

---

16. Carefully position the plastic sheet carrying the acrylic resin over the preparations to assure full and accurate seating.
17. Remove the matrix and resin at the rubbery stage so the excess resin can be trimmed with sharp scissors.
18. Return the splint to the plastic sheet and reseat both over the preparation.
19. When fully set, remove the splint and finish in the usual manner.
20. Reline or remarginate, if necessary. (See the section on Remargination later in the chapter.)
21. Finish and polish restoration. (See the section on Finishing Procedures later in the chapter.)
22. Custom stain or characterize, if necessary. (See the section on Color Correction and Shade Characterization later in the chapter.)
23. Cement. (See the section on Cementation of Provisional Restorations later in the chapter.)

Indirect Technique

When a clinician prefers to avoid direct contact of freshly cut dentin with the acrylic resin monomer or to avoid the potentially damaging effect of the exothermic heat of polymerization on pupal tissue, the indirect technique may be employed. This method should also be considered when long span splints of six or more units are made, if fresh extraction sites are present, or to decrease chair time. It involves securing an impression of the prepared teeth, preparing a quick-set plaster cast, and making the acrylic resin splint on this cast.

Advantages

1. The prepared teeth and tissues are spared contact with surface monomer and polymerization heat.
2. Polymerization shrinkage is minimized by leaving the resin splint on the cast throughout the procedure; distortion is minimized.

3. This extraoral procedure can be performed by an auxiliary thereby freeing the dentist for other productive procedures.

Disadvantages

1. Time consuming.
2. Extra materials, devices, and cost.

Armamentarium

- Standard dental setup (see the section on Preformed Crown and Crown Forms earlier in this chapter)
- Cord placement instrument
- No. 0 gauge retraction chord
- Impression material: irreversible hydrocolloid, silicone impression material, or reversible hydrocolloid/irreversible hydrocolloid (e.g., Duoloid Cadco) (Fig. 13–29)
- Petroleum jelly or silicone liquid

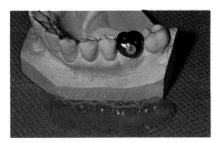

FIG. 13–21. A Ni-Chro preformed metal crown was used to "correct" the edentulous space on the diagnostic cast prior to adapting the heated plastic sheet.

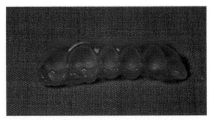

FIG. 13–22. The borders are trimmed to within 2 to 3 mm of the gingival margins.

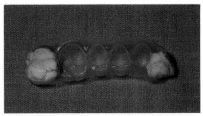

FIG. 13–23. Wet paper towel "wads" are placed into the stent adjacent to the terminal abutments.

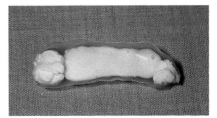

FIG. 13–24. Acrylic is placed in the stent.

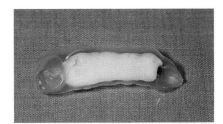

FIG. 13–25. When the surface sheen disappears the paper "wads" are removed and the stent and acrylic is carefully seated over the preparation.

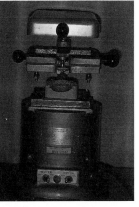

FIG. 13–26. Vacuum former (Omnivac Corp.).

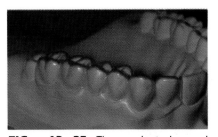

FIG. 13–27. The adapted and trimmed clear plastic matrix—facial view.

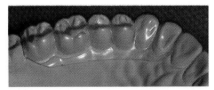

FIG. 13–28. The adapted and trimmed clear plastic matrix—palatal view.

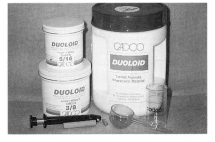

FIG. 13–29. Components of the Duoloid Impression System.

TABLE 13–8. LABORATORY PROCESSED CUSTOM PROVISIONAL SHELLS

BRAND	MANUFACTURER'S TELEPHONE NUMBER
Resista-Temps	(317) 248-2476
Den-Tek (acrylic resin with or without vitallium reinforcement	(800) 243-4722
Glidewell Laboratories (Bio-Temp)	(800) 854-7256

- Liquid releasing agent (e.g., Al-Kote (Caulk, Inc.) or Coe-Sep (Coe/ICI Dental, Inc.))
- Acrylic resin of choice (see Table 13–6).
- Acrylic bur setup (see the section on Preformed Crowns and Crown Forms earlier in the chapter)
- Acrylic finishing setup (see the section on Finishing Procedures later in the chapter)
- Shade correction setup (optional) (see the section on Color Correction and Shade Characterization later in the chapter)
- Temporary cementation setup (see the section on Cementation of Provisional Restorations later in the chapter.)

Clinical Technique

1. Prepare the teeth.
2. Place a No. 00 gauge retraction cord into the sulcus below the preparation margins.
3. Make a full arch impression using irreversible hydrocolloid.

CLINICAL TIP. To secure a more accurate impression (especially marginal detail), use a reversible hydrocolloid/irreversible hydrocolloid system (Duoloid System, Cadco Int.).

CLINICAL TIP. The hydrocolloid component may be boiled in any device that will boil water. Thus, any office without the standard hydrocolloid preparation units may still use this technique. After boiling the hydrocolloid, temper it in a standard water bath for 20 minutes at the temperature recommended by the manufacturer (usually 150° F).

---

4. The assistant mixes standard alginate with cold water and fills a stock impression tray. (Water cooled trays are not required in this technique.)
5. Using a syringe, the dentist places hydrocolloid around the prepared tooth, taking care to fill sulci, and places the tray containing the alginate over the teeth.
6. Leave the tray in place for 2 minutes.
7. Pour the impression with a fast set plaster or stone.

CLINICAL TIP. Use slurry water (water mixed with a small amount of finely ground set plaster, such as waste water from a model trimmer) to accelerate the setting of models.

---

8. Trim the cast.
9. Apply a tin foil substitute.
10. Using any of the techniques listed above, construct the provisional restoration on the model as if it was being done intraorally.
11. Reline or remarginate, if necessary. (See the section on Remargination later in the chapter.)
12. Finish and polish the restoration. (See the section on Finishing Procedures later in the chapter.)
13. Custom stain or characterize, if necessary. (See the section on Color Correction and Shade Characterization later in the chapter.)
14. Cement. (See the section on Cementation of Provisional Restorations later in the chapter.)

Laboratory Produced Shell and Reline Technique

The professional dental laboratory can assist the dentist in achieving excellence with acrylic resin provisional restorations (Table 13–8). The dentist relines a processed acrylic resin shell (provided by the laboratory) with an auto-cured resin on the prepared teeth. The shell may be auto-cured or heat processed on study casts to the dentist's prescription. Heat processing provides increased strength, durability, and stain resistance and is particularly appropriate for long-term use. Another technique uses hollow plastic denture teeth as "veneers" to which the laboratory adds resin to fill out proximal and lingual contours of the shell (Fig. 13–30). A length of 15-gauge half-round stainless steel wire may be incorporated into multiple-unit splints to add strength and rigidity.

Armamentarium

- Standard dental setup (see the section on Preformed Crowns and Crown Forms earlier in this chapter)
- Diagnostic cast
- Acrylic resin of choice (see Table 13–6)
- Acrylic bur setup (see the section on Preformed Crowns and Crown Forms earlier in the chapter)
- Acrylic finishing setup (see the section on Finishing Procedures later in the chapter)
- Shade correction setup (optional) (see the section on Color Correction and Shade Characterization later in the chapter)
- Temporary cementation setup (see the section on Cementation of Provisional Restorations later in the chapter.)

Clinical Technique

1. Provide the dental laboratory preoperative diagnostic casts, a centric occlusion and a protrusive record, shade and characterization information, and detailed instructions for the production of an acrylic resin shell.
2. The laboratory corrects anatomic contour on the study casts.
3. The laboratory under prepares the abutments on the cast (1.0 mm reduction) to provide space for resin.
4. The laboratory fabricates the splint using one of the various methods previously described.
5. Initial finishing may be performed before sending the restoration to the dental office.

6. Reline intraorally.
7. Finish and polish the restoration. (See the section on Finishing Procedures later in the chapter.)
8. Custom stain or characterize, if necessary. (See the section on Color Correction and Shade Characterization later in the chapter.)
9. Cement. (See the section on Cementation of Provisional Restorations later in the chapter.)

CLINICAL TIP. When long-term provisional splints are required, custom-cast chrome cobalt substructures, which reinforce the resin splint, offer an exceptionally strong and durable restoration (e.g., Nik-Temp, Den-Tek, Inc.). Reline the acrylic resin shells attached to the metal substructure with auto-cured acrylic resin (Figs. 13–31, 13–32).

Provisional Restorations for Coronally Debilitated Teeth

When minimal coronal dentin is available, the retention of the provisional restoration is compromised. Standard retention techniques must be altered or augmented to compensate for a lack of resistance and retentive forms.

Endodontically Treated Teeth.
If the restoration involves a dowel and core, a provisional restoration is *mandatory* (especially for anterior teeth) between the required two appointments. It is not always feasible to immediately provide a final dowel and core for endodontically treated teeth prior to temporization.

1. If the restorability of a tooth is questionable, an interim post and crown is less expensive than a restoration that will subsequently be lost.

2. During lengthy periodontal treatment periods of questionable teeth, the interim resin post core is mandatory.

When fabrication or placement of a dowel and core is delayed, an aluminum temporary post may be used to add retention to the acrylic resin provisional restoration. Accessory temporary aluminum pins are also available (Para-Post systems, Coltene/Waledent) (Fig. 13–33). These devices are incorporated into provisional restorations during reline techniques (Fig. 13–34).

The provisional aluminum postcrown must be monitored (as with any temporarily cemented provisional restoration) regularly for cement wash out and caries development.

Nonendodontically Treated Teeth.
To provisionally restore teeth that, despite having little coronal structure, do not require endodontic therapy, an interim pin-retained, light-cured composite resin "crown" may be used. This restoration can later be prepared as a pin-retained core, over which a ceramometal restoration can be fabricated (Figs. 13–35, 13–36).

Provisional Restorations for Edentulous Spaces

Interproximal contact areas are constructed wider buccolingually than the solder joint of the permanent splint to give strength to a splint. The tissue contacting surface of a pontic must be flat or convex (never concave) to permit efficient cleansing with floss and other home care devices (Fig. 13–37). (See also Pontic Design in CHAPTER 8—Ceramometal—Full Coverage Restorations.)

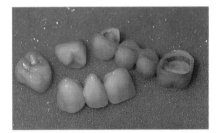

FIG. 13–30. Dental laboratory-produced shells that are to be relined with auto-cure acrylic resin and placed on the prepared abutments.

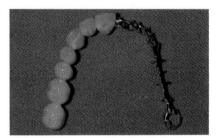

FIG. 13–31. A demonstration cast illustrating the custom-made chrome-cobalt substructure with acrylic resin crown shells (on one side).

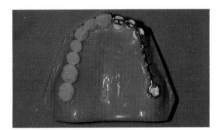

FIG. 13–32. Custom-cast chrome cobalt substructure demonstration case shown on a display model.

FIG. 13–33. Aluminum temporary posts and pins (Coltene/Whuldent) are available to add retention to acrylic resin crowns for endodontically treated teeth.

FIG. 13–34. Aluminum temporary posts and pins have been added to the provisional restoration to increase retention and resistance.

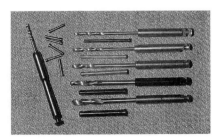

FIG. 13–33

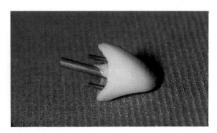

FIG 13–34

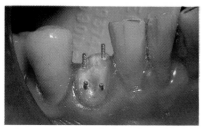

FIG. 13–35. A coronally debilitated canine with four Link-Plus Retention Pins (Coltene/Whaledent). The tooth is vital, however, limited finances do not permit elective endodontic treatment and dowel-core placement.

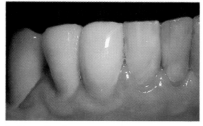

FIG. 13–36. The interim light-activated composite resin crown retained with bonding agent and retention pins.

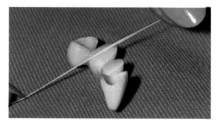

FIG. 13–37. Proper pontic contour (tissue side) is conducive to cleansing with dental floss.

FIG. 13–38. A demonstration model with the interim acrylic resin splint extending from the right maxillary second molar to the right first premolar, retained by Steri-Oss metal copings incorporated into the prosthesis attached to the implant fixture.

FIG. 13–39. The provisional splint with Steri-OSS metal copings. Also shown are plastic Steri-OSS healing caps, which may be custom-cast in metal alloy to serve as retainers for the prosthesis.

FIG. 13–40. A demonstration model with the interim acrylic resin splint on the maxillary left second premolar and first and second molars, retained by Implant Innovations' screw-retained temporary cylinders attached to the implant fixtures.

FIG. 13–41. A demonstration provisional interim acrylic resin splint retained to the implant fixture with the following temporary copings
(1) Implant Innovations #ITC30 temporary cylinder for the UCLA type abutment
(2) Implant Innovations #TC300 temporary cylinder for standard type abutment.

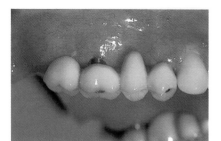

FIG. 13–38

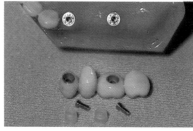

FIG. 13–39

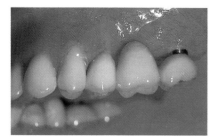

FIG. 13–40

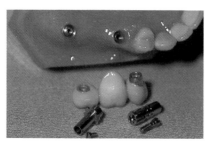

FIG. 13–41

Temporization of Implant Fixtures

Following the prescribed healing period required for osseointegration, the re-entry surgical procedure is performed. An abutment is connected to the fixture and healing caps are placed. The patient may be required to wear a modified (reline) interim removable prosthesis prior to placement of the final restoration. This may be particularly desirable when abutments are in the anterior segment.

A solution to this dilemma is the placement of an interim acrylic resin fixed prosthesis incorporating tempo rary cylinders (Figs. 13–38 to 13–41) (Table 13–9). These components may be used by the dentist in a di

rect chairside fabrication of an acrylic resin prosthesis or when prescribed for laboratory fabrication.

Whether fabricated directly (chairside) or by a dental technician, the acrylic resin incremental loading prosthesis provides many benefits to the patient. Wearing a modified fixed prosthesis, when indicated, eliminates healing caps. The patient can immediately use the osseointegrated implants, with a preview of the final prosthesis. Function and esthetics can be altered in the interim restoration until the patient and clinician are satisfied. In addition, this "fixed type" prosthesis provides an excellent training and evaluation guide for the home care regimen. It may also be retained as a back-up prosthesis in case repair or modifications are required for the final prosthesis.

TABLE 13–9. ABUTMENT AND CYLINDERS FOR SECURING PROVISIONAL CROWNS AND BRIDGES TO IMPLANT FIXTURES

TYPE	CODE	MANUFACTURER	COMMENTS
For Nobelpharma Fixtures			
Implant temporary cylinder and screw (UCLA type abutment)	#ITC30	Implant Innovations, Inc.	Attaches directly to fixture with retaining screw.
Temporary cylinder—stainless steel	#TC300	Implant Innovations, Inc.	Attaches to standard abutment. Retained with tapered abutment retaining screw. Narrow profile.
Tapered abutment temporary cylinder	#TTC30	Implant Innovations, Inc.	Attaches to standard tapered abutment.
Temporary bridge head	#TB700	Implant Innovations, Inc.	Attaches to standard abutment. Luting cement is used.
Nonrotating temporary cylinder	#NRTC3	Implant Innovations, Inc.	Single tooth replacement concept. Attaches to #NAB40 nobelpharma nonrotating abutment (4.0 mm). Retained by 3.0 mm gold screw #GS300.
For IMZ Fixtures Temporary cylinder	#IMTC3	Implant Innovations, Inc.	Must use IME. Interim crowns are screw-retained.
Abutment post	#IAH30/40 series	Implant Innovations, Inc.	Luting cement is used.
For Calcitek Fixtures Temporary cylinder	#CCC30	Implant Innovations, Inc.	Requires 4mm calcitek screw coping #830.
Gold cylinder	#CGCN3	Implant Innovations, Inc.	Nonfluted shoulder abutment.
For Steri-Oss Fixtures Healing cap (plastic)	#2119	Steri-Oss, Inc.	Screw retained. May be cast in metal alloy.
Metal copings	#2115 #2116	Steri-Oss, Inc.	Incorporate into acrylic crown.

Intraoral Technique (Direct)

This technique is a modification of the plastic matrix technique, which uses either a vacuum former unit or an Ellman Press-Form System. It requires the fabrication of a clear plastic matrix which represents the correct arch form prior to fabricating the provisional restoration.

Armamentarium. The armamentarium is the same as that listed for the vacuum former unit or Ellman Press-Form System plus:

- Periphery wax or injectable silicone
- Appropriate retention screws
- Access-Blocker (optional) (Implant Innovations, Inc.)

TABLE 13–10. FINISHING AND POLISHING MATERIALS

BRAND	MANUFACTURER
Cutting/Finishing Bur	Ellman International Mfg. Co.
Sof-Lex Discs	3M, Inc.
Fine Pumice	Kerr Manufacturing Co.
White Diamond Bar	Laboratory Products
Sulci Discs	Burlew Co.
Polier Polishing Paste	Ivoclar, International

TABLE 13–11. SHADE ALTERATION KITS

BRAND	MANUFACTURER
Stain Kit	George Taub Products
Jet Adjusters	Lang Dental Mfg. Co., Inc.
Stain-Tint Kit	Ellman International Mfg. Co.

TABLE 13–12. ACRYLIC RESIN GLAZING

BRAND	MANUFACTURER
Touchup Liquid	Lang Dental Mfg. Co., Inc.
Cyanodent (Fast/Slow)	Ellman International Mfg. Co.
Glaze	George Taub Products
Palaseal (VLC)	Kulzer International
Temp-Glaze	Ellman International Mfg. Co.

Clinical Technique

1. Secure the appropriate temporary cylinders to the abutments.
2. Inject wax or silicone into the screw access chimney to prevent resin from flowing into them.
3. Use the clear plastic matrix to carry acrylic resin intraorally.
4. Allow the resin to set to just after the rubbery stage prior to unscrewing and removing the assembly and allow complete exothermic polymerization to occur extraorally.
5. When fully set, contour the acrylic resins and refine the occlusion.
6. Finish and polish the restoration. (See the section on Finishing Procedures later in this chapter.)
7. Custom stain or characterize if necessary. (See the section on Color Correction and Shade Characterization later in this chapter.)
8. Insert and secure the restoration with retention screws. The access opening may be obturated with Access-Blocker (Implant Innovations, Inc.), cotton pellets and silicone plugs or Fermit (Vivadent, USA).

Indirect Technique

The professional dental laboratory can produce an acrylic resin interim restoration incorporating temporary cylinders following abutment connections to osseointegrated fixtures.

Armamentarium. The armamentarium is the same as that listed for the Indirect Technique, plus:

- Impression material: polyether or vinyl polysiloxane
- Irreversible hydrocolloid
- Periphery wax or injectable silicone
- Appropriate retention screws
- Access-Blocker (optional) (Implant Innovations, Inc.)

Clinical Technique

1. Fabricate a short-term removable prosthesis. This is usually a modified or relined existing denture.
2. Make a polyether or vinyl polysiloxane impression of the coping attachments.
3. Make an irreversible hydrocolloid impression of the opposing arches; make intraocclusal records and record the correct shade.
4. Connect the abutment analogs to the impression copings.
5. Pour impressions, mount the recorded case.
6. Attach temporary cylinders to abutment analogs and complete a full-contour wax-up.
7. Invest, boil out, flask, pack with resin, and process.
8. Recover and finalize the prosthesis.
9. Deliver the custom prosthesis to the patient. If the design includes natural tooth abutments in conjunction with implants, add a chairside reline procedure to convert the prosthesis to dual retention.
10. Retain the restoration to the abutment with gold screws or cement.

Remargination

If marginal discrepancies are noted, an intraoral repair procedure (remargination) is required.

Armamentarium

- Standard dental setup (see the section on Preformed Crowns and Crown Forms earlier in this chapter)
- Dappen dish
- Assorted red sable brushes—No. 00 to No. 2
- Acrylic resin of choice (see Table 13–6)
- Acrylic bur setup (see the section on Preformed Crowns and Crown Restorations earlier in this chapter)

Clinical Technique

1. Roughen the resin surrounding the defect with an acrylic cutting bur.
2. Mix a moderately fluid acrylic resin and paint it onto the dry defect area.
3. Additional mixed resin may be placed in the gingival sulcus adjacent to the defect.
4. Seat the splint is so that the fluid resin will set in the defect.
5. Remove when set; trim and finish the restoration to the correct margins.

CLINICAL TIP. Light-cured resins are an excellent, efficient material to repair marginal defects.

Finishing and Polishing Procedures

The provisional restoration must be finished so that the contour and marginal excellence equals that of the final cast restoration in order to ensure biologic compatibility. Various laboratory carbides, diamond stones, and diamond-coated discs are used to establish physiologically acceptable contours (Fig. 13−42).

Following intraoral occlusal adjustment to establish centric relation and freedom of excursive border movement, the occlusal anatomy is refined and defined with burs (see acrylic bur setup in the section on Preformed Crowns and Crown Form). Correct esthetic coronal anatomy is achieved with a series of flat planes as opposed to rounded surfaces (Fig. 13−43).

Facial textures, supplementary anatomy, and development grooves are sculpted with carbide burs. Smoothing is accomplished with a slurry of medium pumice and a wet chamois wheel on a dental laboratory lathe.

To avoid breaking the acrylic resin splint, all smoothing and polishing must be done on the *slow-speed lathe setting*. Interproximal surfaces are smoothed and polished with pumice wheels, sand paper, cuttle, and Sof-Lex (3M, Inc.) discs on a straight handpiece. High-luster polishing is accomplished with a dry rag wheel coated with a white diamond bar (Laboratory Products, Inc.) on the dental lathe or with glazing resin. However, custom staining is always performed after polishing but prior to staining (Tables 13−10 to 13−12).

Color Correction and Shade Characterization

To provide an exceptionally esthetic, life-like acrylic resin provisional restoration that will please the most demanding patient, the operator may apply surface colorants (see Table 13−11). This is readily accomplished with the Taub Minute Stain Kit (George Taub Products) (Fig. 13−44) or the Lang Jet Adjuster Kit (Lang Dental Mfg. Co., Inc.) (Fig. 13−45).

These are quick setting colored acrylic liquids that are applied by brush to modify the shades of cured acrylic provisional and permanent restorations. The stains cure and bond to all dental resins, including ethyl and methyl methacrylate, polycarbonates, vinyl methacrylate copolymers, resin crowns and laminates, denture bases, acrylic denture teeth, and composite resins. These stains can be applied intraorally or extraorally.

Armamentarium

- Standard dental setup (see the section on Preformed Crowns and Crown Forms earlier in this section)
- Assorted red sable brushes—No. 00 to No. 2
- Acrylic color correction kit: Taub Minute Stain Kit or Lang Jet Adjuster Kit

Clinical Technique

1. Finish and polish the restoration. (See the section on Finishing Procedures earlier in this chapter.)
2. Make certain the surface is clean.

CLINICAL TIP. Shake bottles *gently* to disperse pigments. Shake bottles vigorously only if intense, concentrated colors are desired.

3. Dip the brush into the bottle, wipe off excess at the bottle neck, and bleed additional excess from the brush onto the ceramic or glass mixing slab. Pigments should be evenly dispersed with a very light quick brush stroke. Additional layers may be applied following 5-second drying periods.

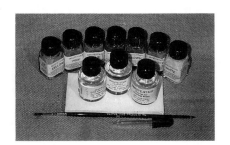

FIG. 13−42. A temporization kit containing laboratory carbide bur, diamond stone, and safe-sided disc (Brasseler).

FIG. 13−42

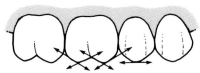

FIG. 13−43

FIG. 13−43. Subtle flat planes, meeting at gentle angles, create esthetic excellence in the provisional restoration.

FIG. 13−44. Taub Minute Stain Kit.

FIG. 13−45. Lang Jet Adjustor Kit.

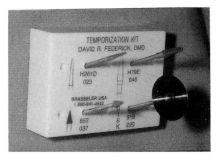

FIG. 13−44

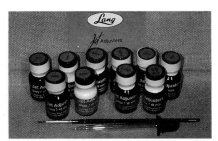

FIG. 13−45

Cementation

Cements with or without eugenol can be used for cementation of provisional restorations (Table 13–13). Cements containing eugenol are indicated for relief of pulpal sensitivity. However, the eugenol may inhibit the setting of the acrylic during subsequent reline and remargination procedures. Noneugenol formulations are easier to remove from the acrylic resin.

Armamentarium

- Standard dental setup (see the section on Preformed Crowns and Crown Forms earlier in this chapter)
- Cord placement instrument (optional)
- No. 0 gauge retraction cord (optional)
- Temporary cement: noneugenol or eugenol type
- Petroleum jelly
- Dental floss
- Dental floss threader
- Cement removal instrument: small cement spatula, 1/2 Hollenback, or red sable brushes—No. 00

Clinical Technique

1. Isolate the teeth with cotton rolls and dry them with the air syringe.

CLINICAL TIP. Lubricating the provisional splint externally with mineral oil or petroleum jelly will facilitate the removal of excess cement after setting.

CLINICAL TIP. Placing lengths of dental floss between the prepared teeth prior to cementation of the splint will facilitate dislodging interproximal excess cement.

TABLE 13–13. TEMPORARY CEMENTS

TYPE	BRAND	MANUFACTURER
Eugenol Type	ZOE Plus	Interstate Dental Equipment and Supply Co.
	ZOE	Cadco
	Flow Temp	Premier Dental Products Co.
	Temp Bond	Kerr Manufacturing Co.
	Trial Cement	Opotow Corp.
	Temrex	Interstate Dental Equipment and Supply Co.
	ZOE 2200	L.D. Caulk/Dentsply
Noneugenol Type	Zone	Cadco
	NoGenol	Coe Laboratories, Inc.
	Freegenol	GC International Corp.
	Mirage (no free eugenol)	Chameleon Central Products Co.
	Temporary Cement	Opotow Corp.
	Neotemp	Teledyne-Getz

2. Mix a eugenol or noneugenol temporary cement according to the manufacturer's instructions.
3. Deliver a thin film of cement to the restoration with a brush or small cement spatula.
4. Seat the restoration on the preparations and direct the patient to gently close the mouth into occlusion.
5. After the cement has set, gently remove the excess with an explorer or 1/2 Hollenback carver. Flossthreaders and unwaxed dental floss effectively cleanse cement from interproximal spaces.
6. Make certain no excess subgingival cement remains. This cement may contribute to gingival irritation and recession.

CLINICAL TIP. Place a section of nonimpregnated retraction cord into the sulcus prior to cementation of the provisional restoration. Retrieving this cord during excess cement removal assures that no cement remains, however, *failure to remove the cord can have adverse periodontal consequences* (Fig. 13–46).

Laboratory Prescription

A properly fabricated provisional restoration can be used as a three-dimensional laboratory prescription. A stone cast duplicate will aid the dental technician in developing crown contour, emergence profile, transitional line angles, proportion, lip and smile lines, disclusion guides, and esthetics in the subsequent restoration (Figs. 13–47, 13–48). This serves to minimize chairside adjustments and remakes. An acrylic tab accurately conveys the desired shade to the laboratory.

CLINICAL CASES
Direct Technique

A 28-year-old female patient presented with maxillary dentition in poor repair. Her medical history was noncontributory. She had some congenitally missing teeth and retained deciduous teeth (Fig. 13–49). After consultation with the patient, a maxillary porcelain-fused-to-gold prosthesis was selected as treatment. Corrected and duplicated diagnostic casts were prepared to secure clear plastic matrices for the maxillary left and right quadrants (Figs. 13–50, 13–51). The abutments were prepared for porcelain-fused-to-metal retainers, nonsalvageable teeth were extracted (Fig. 13–52), and maxillary left and right acrylic resin provisional splints were produced using the clear plastic matrix technique (Fig. 13–53).

Indirect/Direct Technique—Laboratory Processed

A 28-year-old female presented with severe gingival irritation surrounding six clinically unacceptable maxillary anterior porcelain jacket crowns (Fig. 13–54). Her medical history was noncontributory. A 6-unit laboratory processed acrylic resin shell splint was fabricated using plastic denture teeth veneers (Fig. 13–55). The existing porcelain jackets were removed, the abutments were reprepared, and the acrylic resin shell was relined

FIG. 13–46. Retrieval of the cord that was placed prior to cementation of the provisional restoration. This technique aids in debridement of excess temporary cement.

FIG. 13–47. Esthetic, well contoured acrylic resin provisional restorations.

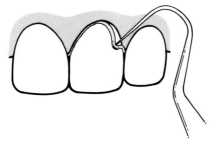

FIG. 13–46

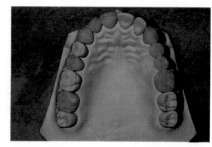

FIG. 13–47

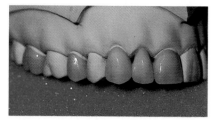

FIG. 13–48. Esthetic, well contoured acrylic resin provisional restorations.

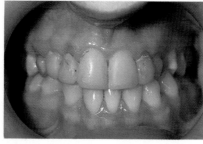

FIG. 13–49. Preoperative photograph of poorly restored maxillary dentition.

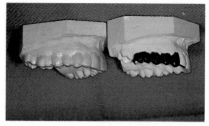

FIG. 13–50. Corrected maxillary right diagnostic cast, duplicated prior to obtaining the clear plastic matrix.

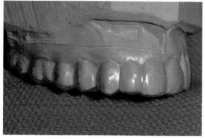

FIG. 13–51. A stone duplicate of a corrected study cast with maxillary right clear plastic matrix.

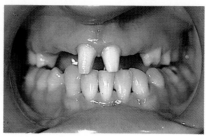

FIG. 13–52. Prepared abutments for porcelain-fused-to-gold retainers two months after extractions.

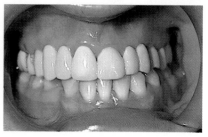

FIG. 13–53. Maxillary left and right acrylic resin provisional splints cemented to abutments.

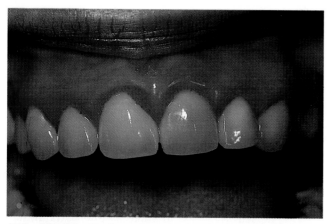

FIG. 13–54. Poorly contoured maxillary anterior porcelain jacket contributing to severe gingival inflammation and hyperplasia.

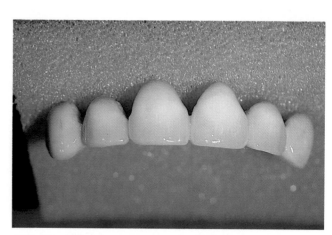

FIG. 13–55. A laboratory-produced shell splint.

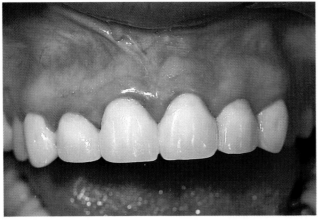

FIG. 13–56. One week postcementation photograph of the relined laboratory-produced acrylic resin shell splint. Note the favorable soft tissue response.

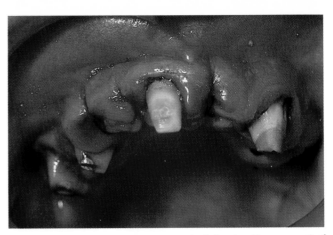

FIG. 13–57. Four abutments remain following the removal of an existing fixed prosthesis.

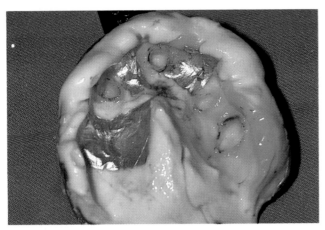

FIG. 13–58. The Duoloid (Cadco Co.) impression system used to record maxillary arch preparation.

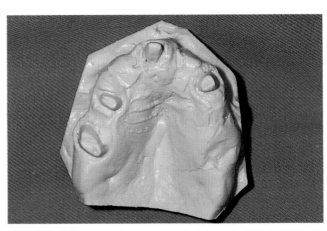

FIG. 13–59. A rapid set stone model made from the reversible hydrocolloid impression.

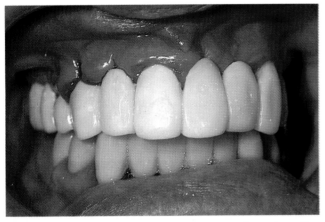

FIG. 13–60. The completed maxillary acrylic resin splint. Shade characterization and glaze will be added.

to fit the preparations. Conventional finishing techniques were employed to achieve an esthetic, biologically compatible interim splint (Fig. 13–56).

Indirect Technique

A 72-year-old male presented with a failing maxillary occlusal rehabilitation. His medical history was noncontributory. After preparatory procedures to secure a full maxillary clear plastic matrix, the patient was scheduled for preparation and temporization. Following removal of existing restorations and nonsalvageable teeth, the remaining four abutments were reprepared (Fig. 13–57). Burlew Dry Foil (J.F. Jelenko & Co.) was placed over the sutures and fresh extraction sites, retraction cord was placed apical to the preparation margins, and a Duoloid (Cadco) impression was made (Fig. 13–58). A quick set stone cast was secured from the impression (Fig. 13–59). Using the extraoral technique, a 12-unit acrylic resin splint was fabricated on the cast. The splint was cemented with a noneugenol temporary luting agent (Fig. 13–60).

FIG. 13–61. Pretreatment photograph of a complex perioprosthetic challenge.

FIG. 13–62. Postcementation photograph of ceramometal rehabilitation of the maxillary right central incisor through left first molar.

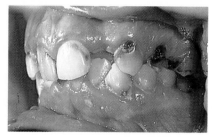

FIG. 13–61

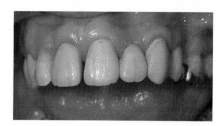

FIG. 13–62

CONCLUSION

An esthetic, biologically compatible, physiologically sound interim restoration will generate patient satisfaction, ensure tissue health, and decrease final restoration delivery and cementation time. Experience gained during this critical phase of therapy will aid the practitioner in accepting perioprosthetic challenges confidently (Figs. 13–61, 13–62).

The cosmetic dentist must never rationalize that "it is only a temporary"—a seductive invitation to abuse and potential failure in attaining treatment goals. The acrylic resin provisional restoration should be considered a permanent restoration in temporary material.[2]

REFERENCES

1. Federick, D.R. and Capilto, A.A.: Stress distribution to the supporting tissues of abutment stabilized with fixed splints. J Calf Dent Assoc 8:33, 1980.
2. Amsterdam, M., and Fox, L.: Provisional splinting: principals and techniques. Dent Clin North Am 4:73, 1959.

BIBLIOGRAPHY

Adams, W.K.: A temporary fixed partial denture. J Prosthet Dent 24:571, 1970.

Amsterdam, M. and Fox, L.: Provisional splinting: principles and techniques. Dent Clin North Am 4:73, 1959.

Antonoff S.J. and Levine, H.: Fabricating an acrylic resin fixed prosthesis for an allergic patient. J Prosthet Dent 45:678, 1981.

Barghi, N. and Simmnons, E.W.: The marginal integrity of the temporary acrylic resin crown. J Prosthet Dent 36:274, 1976.

Baumhammers, A: Temporary and Semipermanent Splinting. Springfield, IL, Thomas C Thomas, p. 99, 1971.

Bell, T.A.: Light-cured composite veneers for provisional crowns and fixed partial dentures. J Prosthet Dent 61:266, 1989.

Behrend, D.A.: Temporary protective restorations in crown and bridge work. Aust Dent J 12:411, 1967.

Berglin, G.M.: A technique for fabricating a fixed provisional prothesis on osseointegrated fixtures. J Prosthet Dent 61:347, 1989.

Binkley, C.J., et al: Reinforced heat-processed acrylic resin provisional restorations. J Prosthet Dent 57:689, 1987.

Braden, M. and Clark, R.L.: An ethyleneimine derivative as a temporary crown and bridge material. J Dent Res 50:536, 1971.

Ban, M., et al: A new temporary crown and bridge resin. Br Dent J 141:269, 1976.

Braden, L.C.: Indirect temporary acrylic restorations for fixed prosthodontics. J Am Dent Assoc 105:1026, 1982.

Brotman, I.N.: Contoured temporary aluminum shell crown. Dent Survey 28:807, 1952.

Caldwell, W.K.: A temporary fixed partial denture. J Prosthet Dent 24:571, 1970.

Campagni, W.V.: Technique for cementation of provisional restorations. J Prosthet Dent 54:13, 1985.

Campagni, W.V., et al: Provisional restorations. J Cal Dent Assoc 16:16, 1988.

Cathcart, J.: Immediate acrylic jacket crowns by the direct-indirect technique. Dent Dig 56:342, 1950.

Chalifoux, P.R.: Temporary crown and fixed partial dentures: new methods to achieve esthetics. J Prosthet Dent 61:411, 1989.

Christensen, L.C.: Color characterization of provisional restorations. J Prosthet Dent 46:631, 1981.

Cleveland, J., King, C., and Contino, S.: Custom shading for temporary-coverage restorations. J Prosthet Dent 32:425, 1974.

Cleveland, J.L. and Richardson, J.T.: Surface characterization of temporary restorations: guidelines for quality ceramics. J Prosthet Dent 37:643, 1977.

Cohn, L.A.: Staining acrylic resin restorations. J Prosthet Dent 7:400, 1957.

Cooly, R.L.: Etched-retained natural crown as a temporary fixed partial denture. Gen Dent 29:323, 1982.

Cottle, K.L.: Temporary bridge or inlay. Dent Survey 39:3541, 1963.

Crispin, B.J. and Caputo, AA: Color stability of temporary restorative materials. J Prosthet Dent 42:27, 1979.

Crispin, B.J., et al: The marginal accuracy of treatment restorations: a comparative analysis. J Prosthet Dent 44:283, 1980.

Dahl, B.L., et al: Biological tests of a temporary crown and bridge material. J Oral Rehabil 1:299, 1983.

Davidoff, J.R.: Heat-processed acrylic resin provisional restorations: an in-office procedure. J Prosthet Dent 48:673, 1982.

Deines, D.N.: Direct provisional restoration technique. J Prosthet Dent 59:395, 1988.

Dill, G., Schmidt, J., and King, C.: A technique for temporary bridge construction. South Car Dent J 27:22–24, 1969.

Doherty, M.J.: Fabrication of an acrylic and metal band provisional restoration. J Prosthet Dent 41:109, 1979.

Donaldson, D.: Gingival recession associated with temporary crowns. J Periodont 44:691, 1973.

Donaldson, D.: The etiology of gingival recession associated with temporary crowns. J Periodont 45:468, 1974.

Donovan, T.E., et al: Physical properties of acrylic resin polymerized by four different techniques. J Prosthet Dent 54:522, 1985.

Ellman, I.: Compression-formed plastic shells for temporary splints. Dent Dig 77:334, 1971.

Etkins, B.J.: Temporization. Ariz Dent J 24:17, 1978.

Federick, D.R.: The provisional fixed partial denture. J Prosthet Dent 34:520, 1975.

Federick, D.R.: The processed provisional splint in periodontal prostheses. J Prosthet Dent 33:553, 1975.

Federick, D.R.: Rationale and requirements for the provisional (treatment) restoration in fixed prosthodontics. Isr Dent Med 26:5, 1977.

Feinberg, E.: Full Mouth Restoration in Daily Practice. Philadelphia, Lippincott, p. 28, 1971.

Fiasconaro, J. and Skerman, H.: Vacuum-fired prostheses: a temporary fixed bridge or splint. J Am Dent Assoc 76:74, 1968.

Fisher, D., Dewhirst, F., and Schillingburg, H.: Indirect temporary restorations. J Am Dent Assoc 72:160, 1971.

Fox, C.W., et al.: Provisional restorations for altered occlusions. J Prosthet Dent 52:567, 1984.

Fox, C.W.: Applications for outdated composite. J Prosthet Dent 61:116, 1989.

Freese, A.S.: Impressions for temporary acrylic resin jacket crowns. J Prosthet Dent 7:99, 1957.

Fritts, K. and Thayer, K.: Fabrication of temporary crowns and fixed partial dentures. J Prosthet Dent 30:151, 1973.

Fritts, K.W.: Temporary and provisional restorations. *In* Loose Leaf Reference Services Staff: Clinical Dentistry, Vol. 4. Philadelphia, Lippincott, p. 1, 1974.

Fritts, K.W.: Temporary and Provisional Restorations. *In* Loose Leaf Reference Services Staff: Clinical Dentistry, Vol. 4. Philadelphia, Lippincott, 1983.

Gabryl, R.S., et al: Effect of a temporary cementing agent on the retention of castings for composite resin cores. J Prosthet Dent 54:183, 1985.

Garvin, D.C., et al: Fabrication of a vacuum adapter for the construction of provisional coverage splints. J Prosthet Dent 47:457, 1982.

Garvin, P.H., et al: Effect of self-curing acrylic resin treatment restorations on the crevicular fluid volume. J Prosthet Dent 47:284, 1982.

Gegauff A.G., et al: Effect of provisional luting agents on provisional resin additions. Quint Int 18:841, 1987.

Gegauff, A.G., et al: Fracture toughness of provisional resins for fixed prosthodontics. J Prosthet Dent 58:23, 1987.

Glickman, G.N.: An immediate acid-etched provisional fixed partial denture. J Prosthet Dent 49:137, 1983.

Glickman, I.: Clinical Periodontology, 3rd Ed. Philadelphia, W.B. Saunders Co., p 762, 1954.

Goldman, N.M. and Cohen, D.W.: Periodontal Therapy, 4th Ed. St. Louis, C.V. Mosby Co., p. 509, 1968.

Goteiner, D., et. al.: Temporary stabilization of periodontally questionable teeth. Gen Dent 37:52, 1989.

Grajower, R., et al: The temperature rise in pulp chamber during fabrication of temporary self-curing resin crowns. J Prosthet Dent 41:535, 1979.

Greenberg, J.R.: The metal band-acrylic provisional restoration featuring ultra-thin stainless steel bands. Comp Cont Ed Dent 2:7, 1981.

Grieder, A, and Cinnotti, W.: Periodontal Prosthesis. St. Louis, C.V. Mosby Co., p. 269, 1968.

Gross, M.D., et. al.: Transferring anterior occlusal guidance to the articulator. J Prosthet Dent 61:282, 1989.

Grossman, L.I.: Pulpal reaction to the insertion of self-curing acrylic resin filling materials. J Am Dent Assoc 46:265, 1953.

Grosso, F.P. and Sears, P.G.: Placement of temporary crown prior to root canal therapy. Dent Prac 15:31, 1977.

Guyer, S.: Recheck and retrac with the temporary. St. Louis Dent Soc Bul 35:51, 1964.

Haddix, J.E.: A technique for visible light-cured provisional restorations. J Prosthet Dent 59:512, 1988.

Haywood, V.B.: A direct temporary for a single tooth restoration. Q.I.D.D. 10:23-30, 1979.

Herlands, R., Lucca, J, and Morris, M.: Forms, contours and extensions of full coverage restorations in occlusal reconstruction. Dent Clin North Am 1962, pp 147-161.

Hudson, W.C.: Provisional coverage and splinting procedures in crown and bridge ceramics and rehabilitation. Dent Pract Dent Rec 8:198, 1958.

Hunter, R.N.: Construction of accurate acrylic resin provisional restorations. J Prosthet Dent 50:520, 1983.

Johnston, J., Phillips, R., and Dykema, R.: Modern Practice in Crown and Bridge Prosthodontics, 2nd Ed. Philadelphia, W.B. Saunders Co., p. 881, 1965.

Johnston, J.F., Mumford, G., and Dykema, R.W.: Modern Practice in Dental Ceramics. Philadelphia, W.B. Saunders Co., p. 59, 1969.

Jones, E.: Vacuformed Clear Resin Shells. J Prosthet Dent 29:46462, 1973.

Jordan, R.D., et al.: Temporization of an extensively fractured anterior tooth. J Prosthet Dent 47:182, 1982.

Jordan, R.E., Suzki, M., Sills, P.S., et al.: Temporary fixed partial dentures fabricated by means of the acid-etch resin technique. J Am Dent Assoc 96:994, 1978.

Josepheson, B.A.: Efficient acrylic temporary coverage: description of technology. NY Dent J 36:7, 1966.

Josepheson, B.: A technique for temporary acrylic resin coverage in functional occlusal relationship. J Prosthet Dent 32:339, 1974.

Kalm, J.M. and Piperno, S.: Simple reproduction of a reproducible temporary crown. Dent Survey 53:447, 1977.

Kaiser, D.A.: Accurate acrylic resin temporary restorations. J Prosthet Dent 39:158, 1978.

Kaiser, D.A. and Cavazos, E.: Temporization techniques in fixed prosthodontics. Dent Clin North Am 29:403, 1985.

Kazis, H. and Kazis A.: Complete Mouth Rehabilitation Through Crown and Bridge Prosthodontics. Lea & Febiger, p. 365, 1956.

King, C., et al.: Polycarbonate resin and its use in the matrix technique for temporary coverage. J Prosthet Dent 30:78794, 1973.

Kinsel, R.P.: Fabrication of treatment restorations using acrylic resin denture teeth. J Prosthet Dent 56:142, 1986.

Knight R.: Temporary restorations in restorative dentistry. J Tenn Dent Assoc 47:346, 1967.

Kramer, I.R.N., et al.: Response of the human pulp to self-polymerizing acrylic restorations. Br Dent J 92:155, 1952.

Krug, R.S.: Temporary resin crowns and bridges. Dent Clin North Am 19:2, 1975.

LaBarre, E.E.: Fabrication of separate adjacent provisional restorations. J Prosthet Dent 49:631, 1983.

Landsman, N.M., et al.: Provisional restorations. *In* Reisbick, M.H. (ed.): Dental Materials in Clinical Dentistry. Boston, The Wright Group, Bothell, WA, 1982.

Langeland, K., et al: Pulpal reactions to crown preparation, impression, temporary crown fixation, and permanent cementation. J Prosthet Dent 15:129, 1965.

Leff, A.: An improved temporary acrylic fixed bridge. J Prosthet Dent 3:245, 1953.

Linkow, L.: Full Arch Fixed Oral Reconstruction. New York, Sprinzer Publishing Co., p. 124, 1962.

Lockard, M.W.: Excellence in dentistry: acrylic provisional crowns. Dent Man 27:60, 1987.

Lowe, R.A.: The art and science of provisionalization. Int J Periodont Rest Dent 6:65, 1987.

Lu, D.P.: Construction of temporary fixed partial dentures with prefabricated polycarbonate temporary crowns. Gen Dent 36:400, 1988.

MacEnter, J.I., Bartlett, S.O., and Loadholt, C.B.: A histologic evaluation of tissue response to three currently used temporary acrylic resin crowns. J Prosthet Dent 39:42, 1978.

Miller, S.D.: The anterior fixed provisional restoration: a direct method. J Prosthet Dent 50:516, 1983.

Mob, E.: Why temporary restorations should be radiopaque. Cal Dent J 38:12, 1972.

Moloff R.I.: A concept and technique for fixed provisional restorations. Quint Int 9:19, 1978.

Monday, J.L.L., et al.: Marginal adaptation of provisional acrylic resin crowns. J Prosthet Dent 54:194, 1985.

Moskowitz, M.E., et al.: Using irreversible hydrocolloid to evaluate preparations and fabricate temporary immediate provisional restorations. J Prosthet Dent 51:330, 1984.

Murphy, E.: A method of protecting 3/4 and full crown restorations. Dent Dig 72:391, 1966.

Naimon, F.H.: Intraoral fabrication of temporary coverage for crown and bridge (part I). Q.I.D.D. 8:19, 1977.

Naimon, F.H.: Intraoral fabrication of temporary coverage for crown and bridge (part II). Q.I.D.D. 8:19, 1977.

Naimon, F.H.: Intraoral fabrication of temporary coverage for crown and bridge (part III). Quint Int 8:23, 1977.

Naimon, F.H.: Intraoral fabrication of temporary coverage for crown and bridge (part IV). Quint Int 8:31, 1977.

Nayyar, A. and Edwards, W.S.: Fabrication of a single anterior intermediate restoration. J Prosthet Dent 39:574, 1978.

Nayyar, A. and Edwards, W.S.: Fabrication of a single posterior intermediate restoration. J Prosthet Dent 39:688, 1978.

Oliva, R.: Custom shading of temporary acrylic resin jacket crown. J Prosthet Dent 44:154, 1980.

Pokorny, D.K. and Rofe, M.G.: Temporary resin crowns and bridges. Dent Survey 54:52, 1978.

Portera, J.J.: Immediate fixed temporization utilizing extracted natural dentition. J Prosthet Dent 45:286, 1981.

Povlich, J.: Temporary coverage in crown and bridge. J North Car Dent Soc 53:22, 1970.

Preston, J.D.: A systematic approach to the control of esthetic form. J Prosthet Dent 35:39302, 1976.

Prichard, J.F.: Advanced Periodontal Disease, 2nd Ed. Philadelphia, W.B. Saunders Co., p. 885, 1972.

Richardson, J.T., Cleveland, J.L., and Cox, W.B.: Metal shell temporization: effective and protective. Dent Sur 53:34, 1977.

Robinson, F.B., et al.: Marginal fit of direct temporary crowns. J Prosthet Dent 47:390, 1982.

Rosenstiel, S.F. and Gegauff, A.G.: Effect of provisional cementing agents on provisional resins. J Prosthet Dent 59:29, 1988.

Rubin, M.: Full coverage: the provisional and final restorations made easier. J Prosthet Dent 8:664, 1958.

Rubinstein, M.N.: Immediate acrylic temporary crown and bridge. Dent Dig 60:12, 1954.

Rudick, G.S.: Fabrication and duplication of a temporary acrylic resin splint. J Prosthet Dent 28:318, 1972.

Saklad, M.: An esthetic provisional cast gold and acrylic splint. J Prosthet Dent 4:653, 1954.

Samarni, S.I.A. and Harris, W.T.: Provisional restorations for traumatically injured teeth. J Prosthet Dent 44:36, 1980.

Schmidt, J., et al.: Anterior temporary coverage. South Car Dent J 27:5, 1969.

Schneider, D.N.: Full coverage temporization—an outline of goals, methods and uses (part I). Quint. Int. 11:27, 1980.

Schneider, D.N.: Full coverage temporization—an outline of goals, methods and uses (part II). Quint. Int. 11:35, 1980.

Schneider, D.N.: Full coverage temporization—an outline of goals, methods and uses (part III). Quint. Int. 11:31, 1980.

Segat, L: Protection of prepared abutments between appointments in crown and bridge prosthodontics. J Mich Dent Assoc 44:32, 1962.

Shavell, N.M.: Mastering the art of provisionalization. J Cal Dent Assoc 7:44, 1979.

Shillingburg, H.T., et al.: Indirect temporary restorations. J Am Dent Assoc 82:160, 1971.

Silvestri, A.R. and Gagnon, W.W.: Improved temporary restorations for onlay preparations. J Prosthet Dent 37:4327, 1977.

Smith, C.C. and McGhay, R.M.: Techniques for making a template for temporary restorations. J Prosthet Dent 47:214, 1982.

Sochat, P. and Schwartz, M.: The provisional splint—trouble shooting. J South Cal Dent Assoc 41:92, 1973.

Sotera, A.J.: Direct technique for fabricating acrylic resin temps using the omnivac. J Prosthet Dent 29:577, 1960.

Stein, R. and Glickman, I.: Prosthetic considerations essential for gingival health. Dent Clin North Am 4:177, 1960.

Stein, I.B.: The status of temporary fixed-splinting procedures in the treatment of periodontally involved teeth. J Periodont 31:217, 1960.

Talkov, L.: Temporary acrylic fired bridgework and splints. J Prosthet Dent 2:693, 1952.

Talkov, L.: The copper band splint. J Prosthet Dent 6:245, 1956.

Taylor, A.G.: Temporary protection of prepared abutment teeth. Royal Can Dent Corps Quart 2:8, 1961.

Tjan, A.H.L., et al: Marginal accuracy of temporary composite crowns. J Prosthet Dent 58:417, 1987.

Tracy, W.W.: Simplified procedure for temporary crown. NY J Dent 25:191, 1955.

Troendle, K.B., et al.: Temporary replacement of missing maxillary incisors. J Prosthet Dent 55:277, 1986.

Tylman, S.D.: Theory and practice of crown and bridge prosthodontics, 5th Ed. St. Louis, C.V. Mosby Co., p. 3315, 1965.

Utley, J.I.: Chairside fabrication of an acrylic resin temporary crown. J Prosthet Dent 54:736, 1985.

Vahidi, F.: The provisional restoration. NY Dent J 51:208, 1985.

Vahidi, F.: The provisional restoration. Dent Clin North Am 31:363, 1987.

Waerhaug, J.: Effect of rough surfaces on gingival tissue. J Dent Res 35:323, 1956.

Waerhaug, J. and Zander, N.A.: Reaction of gingival tissue to self curing acrylic restorations. J Am Dent Assoc 54:760, 1957.

Waerhaug, J.: Temporary restorations: advantages and disadvantages. Dent Clin North Am 24:305, 1980.

Weinberg, L.A.: Esthetics and the gingivae in full coverage. J Prosthet Dent 10:737, 1960.

Weinberg, L.: Atlas of crown and bridge prosthodontics. St Louis, C.V. Mosby Co., p. 26, 1965.

Weiner, S.: Fabrication of provisional acrylic resin restorations. J Prosthet Dent 50:863, 1983.

Wilkie, N.D.: The search for the practical. J Prosthet Dent 32:251, 1974.

Willis, J.: Gold temporary crowns simplified. South Cal Dent Assoc J 40:51, 1972.

Wilson. E.G., Werrin, S.R., and Groom, G.S.: Temporary coverage using the double-arch impression technique. Gen Dent 31:273, 1983.

Wood, M., et al.: Visible light-cured composite resins: an alternative for anterior provisional restorations. J Prosthet Dent 51:192, 1984.

Wright, W.E., et al.: The role of restorative dentistry in the prevention of periodontal failures. J Cal Dent Assoc 13:68, 1985.

Wright, W.E.: Provisional restoration. J Cal Dent Assoc 16:18, 1988.

Yuodelis, R.A., et al.: Provisional restorations: an integrated approach to periodontics and restorative dentistry. Dent Clin North Am 24:285, 1980.

Ziebart, G.: A modified "shell" type of temporary acrylic filled partial denture. J Prosthet Dent 27:667, 1972.

Sidney I. Silverman, D.D.S.

ACRYLIC AND OTHER RESINS—REMOVABLE PROSTHESES

14

Esthetic correction of partially and fully edentulous patients with removable prostheses requires the dentist to not only replace missing teeth but also to restore lost alveolar bone. This additional flexibility comes with added complexity. The esthetic results of a removable prosthesis thus depend not only on biologic and material factors, but also on behavioral factors. Biologic factors include the replacement of missing teeth, the number and condition of the remaining teeth, the condition of the surrounding soft tissue, and the amount of alveolar bone lost because of disease and subsequent healing. Behavioral factors include both the skills and biases of the dentist combined with the perceptions and expectations of the patient. The material factors require esthetic judgement about color and form of teeth, denture base, the design of clasp retaining devices, and the effect of porcelain, resins, and metals on reflected color. These dynamic factors make esthetic judgements and treatments challenging.

CLINICAL CONSIDERATIONS

When restoring the edentulous mouth, the practitioner must use gross guidelines of soft tissues and skeletal landmarks. These landmarks may have been severely altered by periodontal disease, surgical reduction, or mandibular displacement. Often, the guidelines for centric occlusion, vertical dimension, height and inclination of the plane of occlusion, and maxillomandibular overjet are uncertain. Obviously, the absence of natural teeth eliminates the possibility of direct comparison when determining the shape and color of replacement teeth.

The loss of these landmarks, however, removes certain limitations. Placement of a fixed prosthesis is often limited by the poor positioning of the remaining teeth as well as an abnormal condition of either the alveolar ridge or surrounding structures. Often, a removable

prothesis can esthetically rehabilitate a patient when a fixed prosthesis would fail, even after orthodontics and/or corrective surgery.

The removable partial denture lies between the fixed prothesis and the complete removable prosthesis in flexibility of treatment options. A removable partial dentures allows replacement of both missing anterior teeth and alveolar bone. In addition, denture base material can be customized for both color and contour. However, unlike a fixed prosthesis, anterior tooth and bone replacements are complicated by the muscle activity and the nature of the muscle insertions and attachments of the tongue, lips, and cheeks. The tongue and lips, which are, respectively, lingual and labial to the arch form, have no bony attachment or only one bony attachment. The subtle interaction of these muscle actions and skeletal support is critical to the recovery of esthetics. Muscles collapse from disuse and atrophy from prolonged loss of function. They subsequently recover their form and tonicity when teeth and skeleton are correctly restored. Treatment should include an incremental therapy program (see the section on Incremental Treatment Program later in this chapter) to recover form, position, and function.

The recovery of muscle position, tonus, speed of motion, and contraction strength allows retrieval of the tubercle of the upper lip, the corners of the mouth, the fullness and relatively equal height of the lips, and the philtrum. This incremental recovery, by the use of the provisional prosthesis, also reduces lip collapse and lessens the vertical grooves of the nasolabial sulcus. The lip form recovery prevails for all forms of prosthesis. Removable prostheses include complete, partial, and maxillofacial appliances as well as orthodontic and temporomandibular joint treatment appliances. The principles of tissue behavior are the same for immediate, provisional, and definitive prostheses in all types of removable appliances.

BEHAVIORAL CONSIDERATION

A removable prosthesis requires greater patient cooperation than a fixed prosthesis for both functional and esthetic success. Once a fixed bridge is cemented into place, the patient has little control over treatment outcome. On the other hand, the success of a complete removable denture depends more on a patient developing the neuromuscular skill required for proper function. In addition, a complete removable denture places greater psychologic demands on the patient by requiring the incorporation of the prosthesis into the patient's concept of "self."[1] The inability of a patient to physically and psychologically accept a complete denture may manifest as a dissatisfaction with the esthetics of the prosthesis, expressed by phrases such as "it's not me," and "they're too big, too small, too dark, or too light."[2]

Severely neurotic patients who cannot stabilize their esthetic expectations or persistent demands of unrealistic size, color and position of teeth should pay a higher fee. This group of patients usually suffers from generalized chronic anxiety and depression or postural hallucination.[3] Postural hallucination, like visual or acoustic hallucination, is a disorientation of sensory perception. When it relates to body posture, patients request unnatural posture as their normal posture. For example, patients with an obvious history of horizontal or vertical overbite in their natural teeth may desire a "tip-to-tip" occlusion of the maxillary and mandibular incisor teeth. Other patients think their occlusion is "crooked" when it is in centric balance and may want either a right or left lateral position as the restored occlusion.

These patients can be intractable and often the prosthesis must be partially mutilated to satisfy them. They consume an inordinate amount of treatment time and the dentist must place limits on treatment. Fees should reflect patient responses and attitudes about change, because one component of fees is time consumed in treatment. Fees should also be charged for additional laboratory work. When patients realize they are incurring additional costs, often they conform (if they are not too psychologically disturbed), or they leave the office in anger. However, the diagnostic signs of neuroses are present at the initial diagnosis or at least early in the treatment program. A dentist must confront the patient. The patient must agree to the ground rules for treatment, including the possibility of additional fees if the prognosis is guarded. If the patient does not agree, treatment should be discontinued in an appropriate manner. (See Chapter 28,—Esthetics and Dental Jurisprudence.) Some patients who experience postural head hallucinations constantly complain about midline dislocation or occlusal plane "tilting" and often decline to accept any horizontal overjet of the maxillary dental arch. The latter group prefers an edge-to-edge relationship of the maxillary and mandibular incisors. These patients often chronically protrude the mandibular anterior teeth, inducing occlusion disharmonies and a variety of gliding prematurities during mastication and swallowing. It is often necessary to compromise and construct an unesthetic prosthesis, as long as the treatment is biologically sound.

Patients with positional distortion usually do not allow final cementation of abutment crowns or fixed prostheses associated with removable dentures. The cases "drag on" and secondary decay and periodontal problems arise, leading to hostile dentist-patient interaction. Malpractice suits are a distinct possibility when treating these psychologically unmanageable patients.

SOFT TISSUE CONSIDERATIONS

The condition of the muscles and skin surrounding the oral cavity is an important factor in determining the extent of esthetic correction that can be achieved with a removable prosthesis. Patients with long-term collagen disorders, rigid muscles, or nonpliable skin may not respond well to efforts to restore facial form and height. In these patients, increases in height and arch form should be kept close to the existing state. In addition, proper centric and balancing occlusion is imperative because these patients require greater effort to chew and incise due to a narrow envelope of motion. Finally, these patients report more denture looseness and denture abrasion irritations over a longer period of time.

DIAGNOSTIC CONSIDERATIONS

Vertical Dimension

The need to recover lost vertical dimension is a common problem in both complete and extensive partial denture fabrication. In mandibular distal extension cases, patients usually compensate for posterior tooth loss by developing a forward mandibular position to create a rest position with maximal opposing contact of the remaining teeth. The chronic forward drift may adversely affect the temporomandibular joint structures.

In addition, loss of vertical dimension often causes "splaying" and other displacements of the anterior teeth. Prolonged anterior occlusion positions may also induce tooth abrasions. The development of a diastema may be caused by a premature closing contact associated with a protruded position and frequent, intermittent occlusion force. It may be necessary to correct these problems, when restoring proper vertical dimension with periodontal, orthodontic, and restorative therapy.

It is imperative to re-establish a provisional centric jaw posture with a vertical dimension appropriate to the most desired face height. This is readily accomplished by placing diagnostic wax bite rims over the teeth and achieving a retruded occlusion record (Figs. 14–1, 14–2). Clinical observations and measurements are obtained to evaluate how much to recover face height, lip contour, and profile relationships (Fig. 14–3). Considerations also include recovery of the length of abraded teeth, the arch position of inappropriate residual artificial crown restorations, and the existing height and inclination of the plane of occlusion (Figs. 14–4, 14–5).

Face height is a function of three dimensions of space relating to the oral cavity. The mouth, a hollow chamber (viscus), is bound superiorly by the labial and buccal vestibule and the hard and soft palate. It is bounded

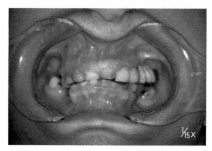

FIG. 14–1. A patient with a reduced vertical dimension of occlusion caused by a lack of posterior teeth and abrasion of the remaining anterior teeth. The mandibular position is habitually protruded in order to achieve the tooth contacts.

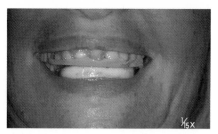

FIG. 14–2. Maxillary and mandibular occlusal rims. The maxillary occlusal rim has an acrylic base on which wax has been used to restore the length and arch form of the original teeth before they were displaced and abraded. The mandibular acrylic base is tooth-colored and has restored the lost tooth length and arch form. A centric relation record is made at this new provisional face height.

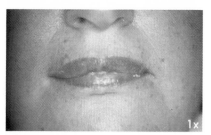

FIG. 14–3. Facial view of the patient in Figure 14–1 with teeth on wax bite rims in occlusion prior to provisional restoration of the dentition. Note that the central incisors are just visible. The lower lip shows a deep shadow in the labiogenial fold, indicating a very acute angle.

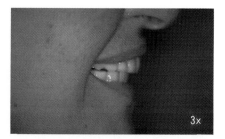

FIG. 14–4. Open lateral mouth view of the patient in Figure 14–3 with lips retracted. A horizontal overjet and equal fullness of the lips are evident.

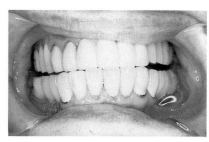

FIG. 14–5

FIG. 14–5. Five-year postoperative frontal view of the finished prosthesis with the patient in a protrusive tip to tip anterior closure. The maxillary partial denture disengages correctly and the full crown length of the mandibular teeth has been restored. There is slight evidence of gingival recession on the mandibular lateral and central incisors, but no increase in pocket depth beyond 2 mm over the period of 5 years.

inferiorly by the dorsum of the tongue, the sublingual space mucosa, the occlusal surfaces of the mandibular teeth, the lower vestibular fornix of the lips, and the cheeks; buccally by the buccinator muscles; anteriorly by the upper and lower lips; and posteriorly by the suspended soft palate and tonsilar region where the oral cavity joins the oropharynx. This space is part of the airway. It remains partially patent during quiet respiration (about 30 mm), fully opened during vowel sounds, and interrupted during consonants while air passes through the mouth. It variously opens and closes during chewing, and closes during swallowing.

Whatever function the mouth is engaged in, it always returns to the rest position or face height of rest (vertical dimension of rest). In this rest position there is a residual volume of air called "respiratory dead space." This dead space remains fairly constant for each individual because it is a function of the vital capacity of a normal patient (500 ml of air). One hundred fifty ml is dead space—the air that is always resident in the mouth, the nose, and the pharynx when a patient breathes in and out.

When patients lose all their teeth, they generally reconstitute the original dead space. This is achieved by elevating the mandible, elevating and spreading the tongue between the maxillary and mandibular ridges, and collapsing the lips and cheeks. Placing dentures in the mouth recovers the facial form by reversing the displacement after loss of teeth (Figs. 14–6, 14–7).[4]

Clinically, if a patient has collapsed facial tissues, the dentist can place wax rims over old dentures, as if on a trial base. The wax can be placed labially over the teeth to simulate an expanded arch form and occlusally on the teeth to simulate increase in height on one or both dentures. Face height and lip form will immediately change. The wax can be modified until a freeway space is created. Speech and swallowing can be tested for comfort, if not for improvement. The patient should observe, in a mirror, changes in face height. If agreement is reached, a change in tooth and flange position can be made and evaluated over a trial period.

CLINICAL TIP. Be careful to read clinical signs correctly. When a patient with collapsed face form is examined, only 2 to 3 mm of freeway space may be observed. Do not conclude that because face height is minimal it necessarily cannot be opened.

An existing 2 to 3 mm of freeway space may be a physiologic adaptation to loss of tooth and bone structure and the patient keeps this closed vertical dimension to maintain a normal "dead space." If the dead space was increased to hold the proper face form, the patient would have to correct the respiratory rate in order to obtain the necessary volume of oxygen by normal respiratory means.

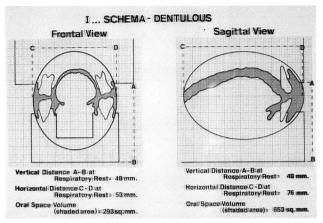

FIG. 14—6. The constancy of the oral respiratory dead space (including the intraocclusal "freeway" space) when the teeth are present. The space in the sagittal and frontal view is measured in square millimeters.

CLINICAL TIP. Using a wax rim over old dentures or a wax rim as a trial base for removable partial dentures can assist in restoring face height. Once the evaluation is made, increase vertical dimension in 2 mm increments by modifying the old complete or partial removable dentures.

One of the critical concerns in restoring face height is the level of the plane of occlusion. A simple method follows (Figs. 14—8 to 14—12).

1. Reduce the base plate in height until the lips touch at rest.
2. Place two straight pins or wooden wedges into the wax rims. (These markers on the rims approximate the distal contact point for the canine tooth position.)
3. The anterior plane of occlusion is approximately 2 mm below this point on a line parallel to the interpupillary axis of the eyes.
4. The posterior plane of occlusion is parallel to the ala-tragus line used in prosthetic cases (Fig. 14—13).
5. Contour the labial surface of the wax rim, following the catenary curve. (See the section on Catenary Curves later in this chapter.)
6. Construct the mandibular wax rim 2 mm below the canine distal contact point, as described above.
7. Construct the anterior height by joining the canines on a plane that also is 2 mm below the height of contour of the lower lip.
8. Construct the posterior plane by drawing a plane from the cuspal incisal edge to a point at least 2 mm below the top of the retromolar pad on each side.
9. Create the arch form with a hot wax spatula so that the anterior wax inclination is 10 to 15° labial from the vertical axis from the vestibular height of contour of the denture flange to the incisal plane.
10. Generate the posterior arch form with a hot spatula to be 10 to 15° lingual from the vertical axis from the flange to the occlusal plane.

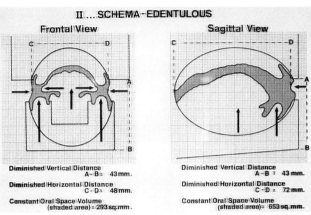

FIG. 14—7. The same schema as Figure 14—6 except the teeth have been extracted and the alveolar bone is healed. It is hypothesized that to recover the same number of square millimeters of oral space the mandible elevates; the cheeks and lips collapse medially and dorsally, respectively; the body of the tongue elevates; and the intrinsic muscles of the tongue spread into the empty interalveolar space where the teeth had been. Conversely, when a denture prosthesis is placed in the mouth the soft tissue readjusts its form and position and the mandible is displaced to recover the dead air space in the mouth. This automatically repositions and recontours the facial structures to create a new profile and frontal view of the face.

Develop these two denture bases independently using anatomic criteria to approximate the desired vertical dimension of occlusion. Minor adjustments to the rim by the addition or removal of wax after a provisional centric relation record usually results in a vertical dimension level at which the definitive centric relation record may be obtained for mounting on an articulator. The mounting is best done by face bow transfer to generate provisional tooth arrangement.

The establishment of a correct vertical dimension causes observable changes in facial contour when the dentures are in the mouth. The soft tissues are displaced by both angular and curvilinear displacement (Figs. 14—14 to 14—17).

Centric Relation

After determining vertical dimension, provisional centric occlusion should be obtained in order to mount the casts on an articulator. Ideal articulation is obtained on a semiadjustable condylar instrument with an anterior pin reaching an incisal table. This provisional centric relation position will assist in evaluating the existing intercuspal positions if teeth are present and in evaluating the available and desired arch form, the horizontal and vertical overjet, and the height and inclination of the plane of occlusion.

CLINICAL TIP. If no teeth are present, the old dentures with overlaid wax rims will assist in determining the desired centric relation and vertical dimension.

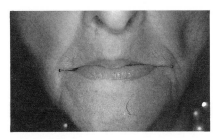

FIG. 14—8. Facial view of a patient with reduced vertical dimension of occlusion demonstrating the placement of bilaterally placed pins at the angle of her mouth to locate the plane of occlusion. The pin is 1 to 2 mm above the plane and on the distal side of the canine at the level of the contact point. The mandibular base is constructed separately so that the pin is above the wax rim by 1 or 2 mm.

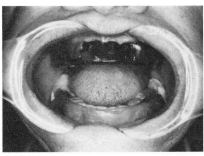

FIG. 14—9. Intraoral view of wax placed over an old mandibular complete denture to expand the mandibular arch and conform it to a catenary curve compatible with the upper curve when viewed in the mouth. The lips will reflect these arch form changes.

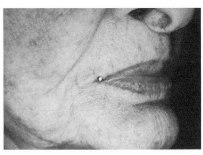

FIG. 14—10. Profile view in the absence of the mandibular wax rim demonstrates the labiogenial sulcus, which reveals an acute angle. Pins are in place.

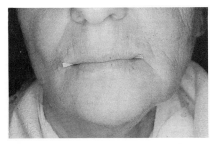

FIG. 14—11. Wooden wedges placed at the corners of the mouth at a given selected vertical dimension also may be used to mark the canine position on the trial base wax rim.

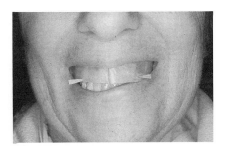

FIG. 14—12. The wedge on the bite block is located at the distal contact point of the canines.

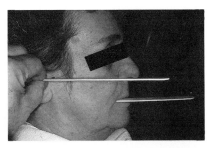

FIG. 14—13. The posterior plane of occlusion is parallel to the ala-tragus line.

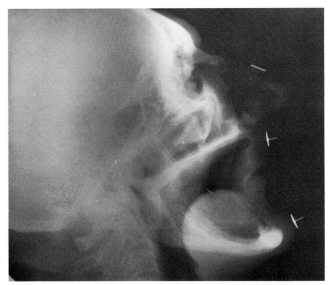

FIG. 14—14. Radiograph of an edentulous patient with thumb tacks cemented on the upper and lower lip in order to show changes in their positions. The radiograph was taken with no denture base in the mouth. Changes in pin direction with respect to parallelism reflect changes in the soft tissues of the skin. Note how the pins converge anteriorly. (From Silverman, S.I.: Prosthodontic care for the aging. Alpha Omegan 79:22, 1986.)

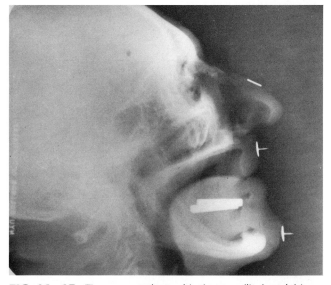

FIG. 14—15. The same patient with the mandibular trial base in the mouth. The heavy bar is a radiopaque metal used to indicate the presence of a denture base clearly. Note how the pins are almost parallel. (From Silverman, S.I.: Prosthodontic care for the aging. Alpha Omegan 79:22, 1986.)

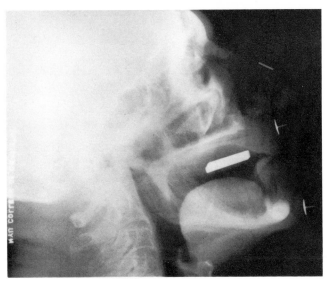

FIG. 14–16. The same patient with only the maxillary base in the mouth. Note that the pins are slightly divergent. (From Silverman, S.I.: Prosthodontic care for the aging. Alpha Omegan 79:22, 1986.)

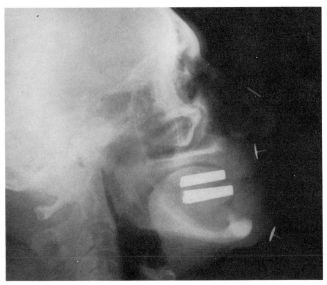

FIG. 14–17. The same patient with both maxillary and mandibular trial bases in the mouth. The pins diverge significantly. (From Silverman, S.I.: Prosthodontic care for the aging. Alpha Omegan 79:22, 1986.)

Most centric occlusion positions, (maximum intercuspal relationships) are anterior to the centric relation position.

Alteration in Vertical Dimension and Centric Occlusion

The vertical dimension of rest and centric (intercuspal) occlusion positions changes as the occlusion deteriorates by decay, periodontal disease, trauma, or alveoplasty during extraction.

These displaced relationships must first be deconditioned neurologically by modifying the occlusion with a provisional prosthesis. Then the permanent prosthesis may be modified to condition and retrain the new jaw position.

Changes in the cervical spine in some musculoskeletal disorders may cause the head and neck to maintain a state of chronic flexion with the condyle displaced anteriorly (Figs. 14–18, 14–19). Chronic obstructive pulmonary disease may induce jaw separation habituation, thus inducing changes in mandibular position. These changes may cause gliding prematurities, tooth displacement, food impactions, and occlusion trauma.

Because jaw position is readily displaced by systemic and dental disease, clinical treatment must first confirm at the diagnostic visit if change in occlusion from normal has indeed taken place. Second, it must confirm if it is possible to restore correct form and position and if the recovered occlusion positions can be maintained.

Pseudoprognathic occlusion occurs when any type of occlusion (Class I, II, or III) has one or more gliding prematurities that can drive the mandible anteriorly up to a cusp width. A gliding prematurity coupled with an overclosure of vertical height of occlusion can create a greater prognathic appearance. There may also be a lateral glide displacement in occlusion which disturbs the

midline relationship of the two jaws. Class II patients who have only anterior tooth contacts may also have pseudoprognathism. These patients develop a resting jaw posture that is displaced up to 10 mm anteriorly to accommodate opposing tooth contacts during mastication and or swallowing. They normally never retrude posteriorly to their original centric relation position unless guided there by the dentist. Jaw relationship, tooth size, and arch form arrangement depend on whether the prosthesis will conform to prevailing conformative treatment or whether rehabilitative steps will be taken (Figs. 14–20, 14–21).

Plane of Occlusion

When determining the plane of occlusion both the static centric occlusion position and the dynamic states of mastication, swallowing, speech, and respiration must be considered.

Height of Occlusion—Clinical Consideration.
The height and inclination of the plane of occlusion is esthetically critical.

CLINICAL TIP. When the plane of occlusion is too low both anteriorly and posteriorly for any given vertical dimension, the mandibular teeth will not be visible during speech and the patient will appear to be edentulous on the mandible. In addition, the maxillary teeth will appear too large and too light in color.

When the maxillary occlusion plane is too low, too much tooth structure is visible during speech. The increased reflecting surface makes the tooth surface appear lighter than it is. When the plane is elevated, the amount of reflected light is diminished and the tooth appears darker.

A poor plane of occlusion is not only unesthetic, but also can create unfavorable stress on the edentulous al-

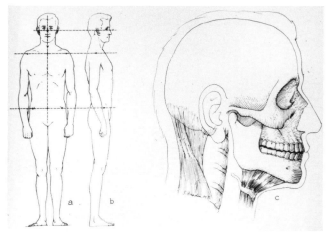

FIG. 14—18. The body has several axes of posture. Shown are the midline vertical axis when standing upright when the center of gravity is close to the center of body mass, and the horizontal axes of the eye line, the shoulder girdle, and the hip line. As disease and age progress these axes change and the effect is to change the position of the mandible and, of course, the nature of the intercuspal relationships.

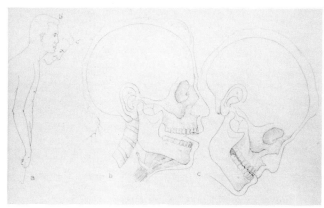

FIG. 14—19. When the neck is scoliosed, the head and neck are first extended as in (b), and there is a posterior tooth prematurity. When the scoliosis is more extreme, the head and neck are even more flexed and an anterior tooth prematurity may develop (c). The lower lip and jaw are more prognathic. A conflict of occlusion position is often created when the dentist pushes the patient's head back for occlusion record production. Sufficient horizontal overbite is required in (c) position for good esthetics.

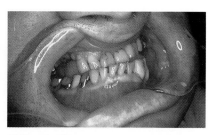

FIG. 14—20. Because this patient has lost most of his posterior teeth only his anterior teeth occlude. The mandible is deviated to the patient's right side. He exhibits loss of facial height and a chronic protruded state, and demonstrates numerous rotated or tilted teeth. The teeth are chipped and stained and have numerous defective restorations and numerous diastemata creating sites for food impaction. This patient has a myriad of esthetic problems, all of which are manifest in the soft tissue contours of the face.

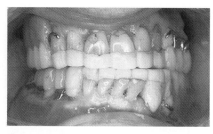

FIG. 14—21. The same patient in Figure 14—20 after bite rims have restored the vertical dimension and centric relation position. Overlay acrylic on the vitallium clasp-type partial dentures is constructed to the predetermined occlusal height and jaw relationship. The patient's vertical dimension problems have been resolved. Crowns and several kinds of partial removable dentures can be constructed to achieve an esthetic outcome.

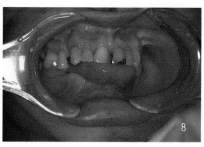

FIG. 14—22. A patient with an irregular mandibular ridge form and rotated maxillary teeth that extrude through the anticipated plane of occlusion. The mandibular ridge may require surgery to correct the asymmetric ridge form.

veolar ridge and abutment teeth (Fig. 14—22). It may result in maladaptive chewing and speaking patterns and restricted and restrained muscle function. Because facial expression is a function of comfort, pain or restrictive motion can cause limited freedom of expression. Correction of a poor plane of occlusion can be accomplished in the following manner.

1. Seat a wax rim trial base plate and the maxillary cast in a centric relation articulation.
2. Mark the teeth on the stone cast in pencil to show the desired length of the teeth for the wax rim designated plane of occlusion (Fig. 14—23).

3. Cut the teeth on the cast to the plane of the mandibular teeth that are arranged on the trial base. Reduce the corresponding maxillary teeth intraorally in the same manner. Sometimes restorations and endodontic therapy are required for a good functional and esthetic plane.

Determining the Height of Occlusion. Use the following criteria to determine the height of occlusion at rest position with the lips touching and the teeth separated 2 to 3 mm.

1. The angle of the lips is located on the distal side of the canine and about 2 mm above the canine incisal plane. (There may be a slight asymmetry in the rela-

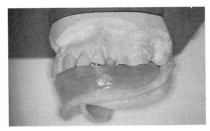

FIG. 14-23. A wax rim trial baseplate with the maxillary cast seated in centric relation articulation. Note that the teeth on the stone cast are marked in pencil to show the desired length for the wax rim-designated plane of occlusion.

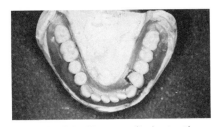

FIG. 14-24. The mandibular tooth arrangement for an Angle Class III jaw relationship. If the mandibular teeth on this removable partial denture are aligned traditionally with normal proximal contact, the protruded mandible would place heavy pressure on the posterior segment of the residual ridge during mastication. When the teeth are slightly rotated and staggered, the incisal table is widened to 3 mm, rather than the 1 mm width in the traditional tooth arrangement. Thus, in protrusive chewing positions the anterior segment retains an opposing tooth contact relationship.

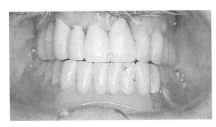

FIG. 14-25. The finished case demonstrated in Figure 14-24 several years after insertion. The wide incisal table has kept the denture and the jaw from drifting anteriorly as it might have with a narrow incisal table in a traditional incisor tooth arrangement.

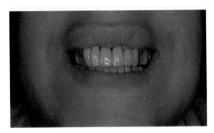

FIG. 14-26. A fixed prosthesis with a large anterior space for pontics. This unsightly restoration displays anterior teeth more than twice the length of the premolar teeth. The treatment could have had better esthetics using an overdenture with a pink acrylic removable labial stent. Judicious periodontal surgery for crown lengthening and ridge augmentation would be an alternative treatment plan if a fixed prosthesis was desired and was economically feasible.

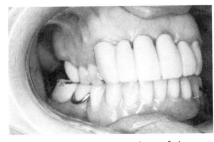

FIG. 14-27. Close-up view of the patient in Figure 14-26.

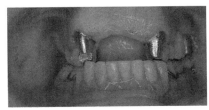

FIG. 14-28. Gold copings can be constructed for the patient in Figure 14-26 to retain a removable overdenture.

tionship of the location of the canine and the angle of the mouth.)[5]

2. The mandibular incisors are up to 2 mm below the height of contour of the vermilion border of the lower lip.
3. The mandibular plane is just below (up to 2 mm) the lateral border of the tongue and just below the buccinator muscle bulge.
4. The plane should be just below (up to 2 mm) the top of the retromolar pad on both sides, if possible.

However, because any remaining teeth may have supererupted through the occlusal plane, some posterior planes may be tilted to the right or left because of occlusal interferences. Occlusion rehabilitation may be constructed to accommodate this tilt if it does not exceed a 1 to 2 mm deviation on one side.

Two-Plane Occlusion. A more serious esthetic problems can occur when the anterior sections are in good lip approximation with a satisfactory smile line but the posterior plane is in conflict with the lateral view of the inferior border of the mandible. When the posterior

plane is too low, the maxillary posterior premolars and molars are overly visible and the prosthesis displays too much denture base.

CLINICAL TIP. Attempts to lengthen posterior teeth to avoid showing denture base may create an undesirable tooth length.

CLINICAL TIP. When the plane on the posterior teeth is too high, the premolars are not visible during speech and the patient appears edentulous in the posterior region.

In many cases of steep overbites, the 6 mandibular anterior teeth are 3 to 4 mm higher than the mandibular first premolar. In this unesthetic two-plane occlusion, the premolar length is often one-half tooth length shorter than the adjacent canine tooth. The maxillary first premolars may be severely traumatized because they, instead of the canines, act as disengagers during lateral function. Balancing-side molar prematurities are also common.

To achieve an esthetic result and to correct a two-plane occlusion:

1. Reduce the mandibular canine and the lingual cusp of the maxillary first premolar to allow the mandibular first premolar to be lengthened occlusally or
2. Perform full restorative rehabilitation treatment with a slight opening of the vertical dimension or
3. Orthodontically extrude and intrude the appropriate teeth and expand or contract the dental arch.

This action creates a more harmonious curve of Spee, as well as a canine protected occlusion. When simple conformative treatment is required, judicious grinding and simpler restorative measures can achieve remarkable improvement or recovery of esthetics.

Vertical and Horizontal Overbites

Excessive horizontal or vertical overbites are among the most difficult esthetic problems to overcome. Very steep vertical overbites that result from the loss of opposing posterior teeth are often complicated by two factors. Teeth may supererupt into the opposing plane of occlusion following the loss of the opposing dentition. This condition requires recovering lost vertical face height followed by reducing the length of the supererupted teeth to the recovered plane of occlusion. Depending on severity, treatment requires selective grinding, fabrication of a restoration (with intentional endodontic therapy, if necessary) to reduce the teeth adequately, or orthodontic therapy. In extremely severe cases, orthognathic surgery may be the only method of restoring vertical height.

A steep vertical overbite caused by loss of posterior contacts usually is accompanied by a diminished horizontal overbite, creating severe limitation in lateral excursive movements. Excess labial incisal wear on the mandibular incisors and extreme loss of lingual tooth structure on the maxillary anterior incisor teeth often occurs. An esthetic problem arises when the abraded and de-enamelized mandibular anterior teeth with variegated yellow and brown dentin and receded or calcified pulp become visible after the posterior teeth are restored to a proper vertical height of occlusion and the horizontal overbite is restored to its original position. In addition, the maxillary anterior teeth reveal a bluish or black tinged facial enamel because of increased translucency caused by their denuded lingual enamel and severely abraded dentin. The anterior teeth may be restored with crowns, laminate veneers, composite resin overlays, or removable prostheses.

Remaining Teeth

In removable partial denture treatment, the position of the replacement tooth is often limited by the remaining teeth. Sometimes existing teeth that are rotated must be recontoured or altered with restorations. A full crown restoration may not only provide more appropriate space for pontics, but also may provide more esthetic retaining devices for the removable partial denture. Laminate veneers of remaining teeth can be used to expand a tooth to an appropriate position in the arch.

Arch Form

Partially edentulous dental arches may have configurations that can create esthetic problems. Usually, the remaining natural teeth are displaced, rotated, or extruded into the opposing edentulous dental arch. These edentulous areas may be too large or too small for appropriately sized artificial teeth. It takes creativity and imagination to stagger, rotate, and modify tooth inclinations to create a harmonious tooth arrangement (Figs. 14–24, 14–25). Orthodontic, periodontic, exodontic, and restorative treatment must be considered when the remaining teeth preclude proper esthetics.

Excess Edentulous Space

When anterior teeth are lost due to advanced periodontal disease, the resultant space is often large and there is a tendency to restore the area with excessively long teeth (Figs. 14–26 to 14–30). Careful tooth contouring and color shading can be used to alter the apparent length of these teeth. (See Chapter 2—Fundamentals of Esthetics).

CLINICAL TIP. A major advantage of a removable prosthesis is that ridge augmentation is not necessary because the denture base can mask ridge loss.

Catenary Curve

The length and position of teeth can be managed by carefully separating the frontal plane of the crown portion from the long axis of the root portion of the replaced tooth (Figs. 14–31 to 14–34). This separation allows the labial height of contour of the tooth to lie on the catenary curve, a natural curve which characterizes most dental arches from the arch form in the fetal stage through adulthood.[6] The catenary curve can be demonstrated when a beaded chain is held on an axis. The apex of the curve is on a line perpendicular to the midpoint of the axis (Fig. 14–35).

Usually the heights of contour of the labial surfaces of the canines, premolars, and first and second molars lie on the catenary curve. Sixty percent of the central and lateral incisors are on the curve, 30% are 1 to 2 millimeters anterior to the curve, and 10% are 1 to 2 millimeters within the curve. These positions probably result from the muscular arrangement of the masticatory and facial muscle groups. The canines to the molars are confined between the powerful masseter and internal pterygoid muscles, which have two bony attachments, one on the mandible and the other on the craniofacial skeleton. These teeth thus have few options for displacement in the arch during the developmental and maturation stages of the dentition. The lingual and labial muscles confining the anterior teeth have fewer functional restraints and tend to generate three groups of tooth arrangement, i.e., 60% on the catenary curve, 30% exterior to the curve, and 10% interior to the curve (Figs. 14–36 to 14–38).

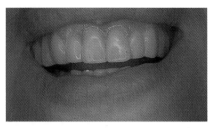

FIG. 14—29. When economics is a factor the patient in Figure 14—26 is better served by a vitallium partial denture with labial facing attached to the vitallium on the premolars.

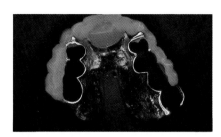

FIG. 14—30. An overdenture with a pink acrylic labial vestibular flange widens the dental arch.

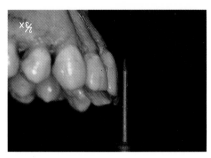

FIG. 14—31. A skeleton of the maxillary arch demonstrates that the labial facial inclination is almost vertical and the root portion inclines 30 to 40° from the vertical.

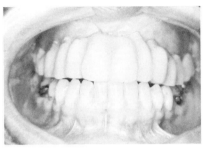

FIG. 14—32. A provisional fixed bridge for a patient with a cleft palate and a deficient premaxillary bone demonstrates the separation of the labial face of the tooth from the root portion. (From Silverman, S.I.: Prosthodontic care for the aging. Alpha Omegan 79:22, 1986.)

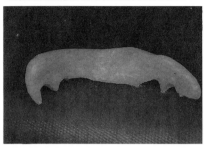

FIG. 14—33. The deficiency of bone is accommodated by an acrylic removable labial stent. (From Silverman, S.I.: Prosthodontic care for the aging. Alpha Omegan 79:22, 1986.)

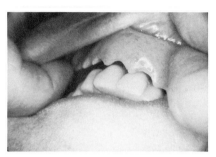

FIG. 14—34. A labial stent being placed over the root position of a fixed bridge in the patient in Figure 14—32. (From Silverman, S.I.: Prosthodontic care for the aging. Alpha Omegan 79:22, 1986.)

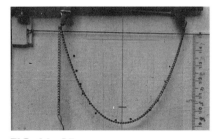

FIG. 14—35

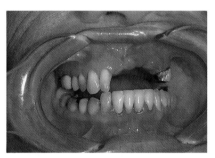

FIG. 14—36

FIG. 14—35. A catenary curve formed by a chain of metal beads superimposed in a vertical tracing from a patient's casts. The dots represent the position of the height of contour of the labial surface of the patients teeth. The chain curve corresponds to these points.

FIG. 14—36. A patient who suffered a gun shot wound to the face and maxilla. Note two planes of occlusion on the mandible, i.e., the high plane of the right canine, and the low plane of the right first premolar.

FIG. 14—37. The patient in Figure 14—36 wearing a provisional maxillary removable partial denture.

FIG. 14—38. The stone diagnostic cast with wax added to expand the arch to conform to the catenary bead chain curve.

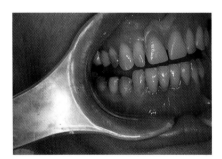

FIG. 14—37

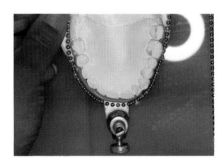

FIG. 14—38

Soft Tissue Landmarks

In completely edentulous mouths, skill and knowledge are required to locate soft tissue and bony landmarks before and after tooth replacement (see Figs. 14–22, 14–23). However, soft tissues and alveolar bone landmarks vary, and clinical judgment is required to anticipate how tissues recover their form and position (see Figs. 14–14 to 14–17).

TOOTH SELECTION

Tooth position, size, shape, color, and composition are crucial in removable denture esthetics. The esthetic outcome of the prosthesis depends eventually on a coherent mosaic of natural tissues, teeth, lips, skin, mucosa, bone, and artificial materials like porcelains, metals, and resins. The mosaic of tissue and artifacts should create the illusion of reality both during function and at rest.

However, tooth size matching and color matching are not necessarily symmetrical. Colors need to be blended harmoniously, not identically. Similarly, maxillary and mandibular teeth are usually not identical in shade. Mandibular teeth have more dominant body shades, whereas anterior maxillary teeth tend to have more dominant translucent incisal shades. Nevertheless, harmonious colors and blends, when variegated, are more likely to be accepted than strikingly different shading between the materials, and the natural colors.

In addition, genetic and familial characteristics of the skeletal face form, height and width of the facial bones, the arch form, tooth size, and contour should be considered. Examining old photographs of the patient and examining siblings or parents is often helpful in resolving acceptable composition.

CLINICAL TIP. *Often for psychologic or emotional reasons, the patient dislikes (sometimes intensely) his genetic and familial esthetics. These feelings should be noted and heeded.*

Color

In removable prosthetics, color choice is difficult for partial prosthesis selection when remaining natural teeth have stains, checks, rotations, and other malpositions that influence color matching. In complete removable dentures, choices are simpler in this regard. No less significant then the absolute hue, chroma, and value[7] is the placement of the arch in relation to lip contour and the residual alveolar ridges. When the arch is too far forward, i.e., labially and or buccally, the color appears brighter than if the arch form is contracted and arranged closer to the alveolar ridges, i.e., the tooth arrangement is more medial in the posterior arch and more dorsal in the anterior arch form. Another factor in making the arch form appear lighter or darker is the position of the incisal edges of the teeth. When the incisal line is too labial in the maxillary area or too superior on the mandibular arch the teeth appear lighter because too much tooth is revealed when the lips are elevated or contracted during speech or when smiling.

A more subtle differentiation in lighter or darker appearance of any given tooth color is created by the position of each tooth within the arch form. When a tooth is in lingual version, it appears darkened because less tooth surface is available for reflecting light. Conversely, when a tooth is in labial version, it often appears lighter because more tooth structure is available for light reflection. The light reflection is further enhanced because the curvilinear and generally convex surfaces of the proximal and buccal surfaces of the tooth reflect and scatter the reflected light. This scatter effect of light is diminished when the tooth is in lingual version and the light is not reflected from larger and convex proximal surfaces of the teeth, which are hidden by the approximating teeth.

Still another factor in individual tooth position is the inclination of the labial and buccal surface of the teeth. When the gingival half of the facial surface of the maxillary tooth is in buccal version relative to the incisal half of the tooth, light is reflected downward away from the viewer's visual field and little light is reflected outward. When the incisal half of the labial surface is buccal to the gingival half, the inclination of the tooth surface reflects the ambient light to the eye of the viewer, and accordingly the same tooth appears lighter and brighter.

The light source used during shade selection is another critical factor (see Chapter 2—Fundamentals of Esthetics). Other functional factors make successful color selection even more artistic. They are: dynamic states of the lips and jaws during speech, laughter, chewing, and breathing. A high smile line creates a "lighter, whiter, toothier" appearance. The proverbial "stiff upper lip," which displays little tooth structure, masks out reflected light and creates a grayer, darker, relatively smaller, if not edentulous, look. In both cases the vertical dimension is critical. (See the section on Vertical Dimension earlier in this chapter.)

The other major factor in color choice is related to the patient's psychological and emotional attitude regarding tooth color. The patient who is intransigent and desires only "pearly whites" is rarely satisfied with nonintrusive natural color reproduction. They have a rigid resolution to obtain "dead white" teeth and no rational analysis of tooth color or form will be accepted.

CLINICAL TIP. *A dentist's ultimate responsibility is to please the patient, no matter how irrational, as long as the treatment is not detrimental to the patient's health and function.*

Color selection is difficult, and despite the many shade guides that manufacturers provide and the color selection "tricks" that dentists concoct, color selection remains an art form, unique for each patient and dentist.

In each unique relationship between the patient and dentist, a constant psychological variable is reflected by the patient with respect to whether the patient is "field dependent" or "field independent."[8] The field independent patient is confident and has a reasonable measure of self worth; rationally assessing the options available for the choice of color and shade, making a decision jointly with the dentist, and accepting a satisfactory outcome. Such a patient is easily treated without undue incident. However, the field dependent patient cannot make a decision derived from internal intellectual and emotional expression. This patient relies on a parent, spouse, friend, or even a casual acquaintance to determine the correct shade. This type of patient wants what the last person in a series of 10 or 20 consultation wants.[9] Then, when given a choice, rejects it because the dentist didn't "get it right." In a retrospective study on more than 200 patients with burning mouth syndrome, 10% experienced crooked head syndrome (Verkrumpte Kopf Syndrome),[3] in which the patient describes that the jaw is not centered, the head tilts, or the maxillary and mandibular incisors are not edge-to-edge. The latter problem presents an insoluble behavioral phenomenon. The dentist is advised to avoid these patients if possible and, if it is necessary to treat them, to advise them by letter of the guarded outcome of treatment. In addition, firm financial arrangements for fee payment should be presented.

It is also prudent to have a third party participate in color and tooth form selection, such as a family member, a close friend, or a member of the dental office staff whom the patient trusts—a hygienist, assistant, or dental colleague.

Size and Shape

Tooth size and shape are related factors, selected partially on the basis of anthropomorphic data about skeleton size and on criteria devised by dentists[11,12] and manufacturers based on studies of the preferences of dentists and patients. Some dubious studies related psychological and emotional states.[13] Other published works by so-called physiognomists,[14] now discredited, still influence the dentist's choice of size. Notwithstanding these unreliable influences, there are some physical limitations to the choice of color and shade of teeth based on hard data. Lieb, et al.[5] located the position of the distal contact point of the maxillary canines. It varied from 1 to 3 mm of displacement from the commissure of the mouth. The incisal plane is also 2 to 3 mm below the commissure of the mouth. These findings accordingly suggest that tooth size for the six anterior teeth should not be measured as a function of the residual bony ridge form of the maxilla, but rather that a trial base plate with a well formed wax rim be contoured to provide esthetically appropriate lip contours with corresponding vertical dimension of occlusion and a centric relation position. This wax rim will provide the measurement of the curved width of the maxillary arch of the anterior six maxillary teeth.

A second factor in selecting tooth size is the distance from the resting position of the lip to the smile line and to the speaking line of the elevated and retracted upper lip.

There are, however, extreme lip patterns of elevation. For example, the "tight" upper lip, usually immobile in the taciturn, emotionally unexpressive persons or the patient with a developmentally short upper lip and rel-

CLINICAL TIP. When the vowel "e" is sounded vigorously, the upper lip is elevated to the mid or upper one-third of the anterior teeth. When a forced smile is expressed, the patient usually elevates the upper lip to almost the gingival margins (to the highest point on the labial face of the tooth). This position sometimes reveals the interproximal gingival papilla.

ative overgrowth of the labial maxillary alveolar bone, exposes not only the entire tooth on lip elevation, but also 3 to 4 mm of gingiva during laughter and speech. In the nonrevealed arch form, judgements of tooth size and shape are not critical, except for patient desires. However, in the fully exposed mouth there are often difficulties in pleasing patients resulting from the anatomic limitations.

Usually, the selection of tooth size can be determined by simple measurement of the arch width as described above. However, a complicating factor in tooth selection is the often observed contradictions between mouth, face, and head size. Because the maxillary and mandibular skeletal height, width, and length develop over 24 years, the early loss of teeth and alveolar bone does not leave enough room for a genetically determined tooth size and form. In these cases, one can effectively select the genetically sized tooth and create an arch form by rotating, lapping, or omitting some teeth. Patients often have photographs or casts of remaining teeth that offer a guide for tooth size and shape. In summary, teeth can be rotated and overlapped to accommodate small bony arch forms (see Figs. 14–24, 14–25).

The shape of teeth should conform to the size of the teeth selected as well as accommodate the available tooth space. Unfortunately, when excessive alveolar bone loss is accompanied by high lip retraction, the space available makes teeth look too long.

CLINICAL TIP. Teeth can be made to appear shorter by creating a festoon on the ridge end of the tooth so that the labial facial form is appropriate for the face size and genetic history. For example, when a central incisor crown form is genetically 14 mm long and 9 mm wide and the space to be filled is 18 mm long, the tooth should be constructed with a 14 mm labial face and the additional 4 mm of tooth length should be root length contour.

Characterization

Teeth do not have uniformly distributed color. Not only does the enamel layer vary in thickness from the gingival to the incisal edge in each millimeter segment of the vertical plane but also in each millimeter horizontal segment from the mesial to the distal surface of each tooth. These arbitrarily selected millimeter dividing planes create a millimeter square grid, which assists in color and characterization options. The normal healthy tooth usually has a gradient-like blending of not only the varied layer of enamel but also the yellower color of the dentin. Light passing through a tooth and light reflected back from a tooth surface mingle and appear to the viewer as a blend of hue, chroma, and value, commonly known as the shade. Traditionally, teeth are judged and selected by dividing the tooth into 3 major segments, gingival one-third, central body, and incisal one-third. These subdivisions usually allow satisfactory shades to be selected when the choice is made in the mouth environment where the dark recesses of the oral cavity and the lip and skin color in both the dynamic conditions of speech and smile and the static condition of rest collectively mediate the color choice.

However, a patient's age, trauma, caries, endodontic therapy, gingival recession and periodontal disease or therapy, and gold, amalgam, composite resin, porcelain, and porcelain-fused-to-metal restorations each alter the color characteristics of the teeth. In restoring prosthetic teeth in an environment where color markings are apparent on the remaining natural teeth, it is important to not be too aggressive in frank duplication of gray, white, brown, and yellow markings or striations.

CLINICAL TIP. Characterizations or exaggeration of color on natural teeth are usually subliminally accepted as natural. When placed on artificial teeth, they appear harsh and intrusive to patients. The reason may be perceptual because of the inherent characteristics of porcelain, metal, or accompanying resins, or because of psychologic or emotional reasons. Muting the character markings to barely perceptible levels may be a more prudent approach to esthetic outcomes.

A practical method of applying color and characterization markings is achieved by an induction process of slow incremental changes in color from the original natural teeth to the provisional replacements and then to the final restoration. Shade selection and characterization should be evaluated and recorded with the full participation of the patient and in the following sequence. Evaluate:

1. Before any treatment, including prophylaxis, periodontal treatment or occlusion, or caries treatment. Obtain good quality color prints with reliable reproducible light, camera distances, and lenses. (See Chapter 17—Esthetics and Oral Photography.)
2. After initial prophylaxis and scaling and curettage.
3. After periodontal surgery, if necessary.
4. When the provisional prosthesis is constructed.
5. At the final bisque bake and try-in of the fixed prosthesis or removable prosthesis.

There are, however, some patients who participate in numerous cooperative shade sessions and then deny responsibility for shade outcomes. They are few, but when encountered, the prosthesis should not be finally cemented until they agree to color and characterization. Obviously, these patients require more treatment time and the fees should reflect these extra sessions of treatment. It is thus prudent to anticipate those patients who are uncertain about color outcome. Accordingly, dentists should be guarded if during the early diagnosis and treatment phases patients talk about friends, family, and other doctors they consulted about their appearance and the shade and form of their prosthesis.

Position

The ultimate position of any tooth in a removable partial prosthesis is largely dependent upon the remaining abutment teeth. Of course, the abutment teeth may be modified. All natural or artificial teeth can be moved bodily, tilted, rotated, depressed, or extruded in some measure to create improved esthetic orientation for removable partial prostheses.

The placement of each tooth in the arch form is relative to the curvature of the arch and the height of the plane of occlusion. The curve and plane are clearly defined by the residual natural teeth when the missing teeth are not canines and second molars. These four natural teeth usually provide a reference for placement of the incisors, premolars, and first molars. However, sometimes these reference teeth may drift or extrude and a more critical assessment must be made of the desired arch form and plane. Earlier in this chapter the catenary curve was discussed as a guide for the general contour of the arch form, suggesting any given tooth should be contained within the curve. If a natural tooth abutment is in buccal or lingual version to this curve, a crown or laminate veneer restoration can help to align it. Another option is to orthodontically reposition the tooth.

The relationship of an individual tooth to the plane of occlusion is termed infraocclusion when the tooth is short of the plane and supraocclusion when the tooth extends through the plane to be closer to the opposing maxillary or mandibular bone. Orthodontic treatment may be used to extrude or depress a tooth to conform to the plane. When an abutment tooth is in infraocclusion it can alternatively be restored to proper occlusion with a restoration. When the tooth is in supraocclusion the tooth may be reduced by judicious grinding or by restoration (with endodontic therapy and periodontal crown lengthening, if necessary).

When treating the completely edentulous mouth, there are no tooth guidelines so soft tissue and skeletal guidelines are required to define the arch form and level of the occlusal plane. This is a more complex decision making process and is discussed earlier under vertical dimension of occlusion and arch form determination.

CLINICAL TIP. Once the arch form and plane of occlusion are determined for the gross position of a tooth, the inclination of the labial face of the tooth is the critical factor in tooth placement.

A review of the natural tooth form in the alveolus reveals that each tooth has a mean root vertical axis and a mean coronal axis, which are usually at some obtuse angle to each other (see Fig. 14–31). The labial face of each tooth has a vertical axis, which may or may not be parallel to the mean coronal axis. These facial planes are unique to each tooth and the facial plane at the height of contour fits the arch form curve, especially the catenary curve.

The individual tooth position can be modified easily in the artificial tooth. However, the facial plane contour of an abutment tooth requires appropriate tooth preparation for crown form restoration. For example, when a canine is prepared for a crown restoration, if insufficient tooth structure is removed on the labial incisal one-third of the tooth, the incisal one-third of the resultant crown will be outside (in labial version to) the dental curve. Thus, the crown will be too large on its labial contours and the lip form will be distorted, displaying a "peeking canine tip" when at rest. According to Roizen a useful guideline for tooth position of the labial face is:[15]

1. The molars are inclined 12 to 15° medially from the vertical
2. The premolars are inclined 4 to 8° medially from the vertical
3. The canines are inclined 0 to 4° medially from the vertical
4. The central incisors are inclined 12 to 15° labially from the vertical

Further consideration of individual tooth position relates to variations from the "ideal tooth" position. Teeth may be separated, rotated, overlapped, and slightly above the plane. All of these positions can be changed to cope with existing residual alveolar bone and natural teeth. It is at this point that the "art phenomena" inherent in dental esthetics dominates the procedure.

Composition

Material choices—resin, porcelains and metals—influence the esthetic outcome. The incompatibility of differing materials is revealed when light is transmitted through or reflected by the materials in vivo. The critical location where differences are noted is in the midline. Therefore, when two central incisors are replaced with crowns or artificial teeth, both should be of the same material. For example, if the maxillary left central is restored with a ceramometal crown it is prudent to use a porcelain tooth or even a porcelain-fused-to-metal crown on a removable partial denture to replace the right central incisor.

Metals accompanying denture bases or crown construction always create some measure of concern, if not conflict, between the patient and the dentist. Patients should always be informed that the metals may be visible during an intraoral examination but not usually by the viewer during normal functioning.

DENTURE BASE ESTHETICS

The denture base has several components that require careful management to achieve an esthetic outcome. The base is used:

1. As a labial flange to restore lost bone contours
2. As a retaining mechanism to attach teeth
3. As a retaining mechanism to attach retainers to abutment teeth (removable partial dentures)
4. As a connecting device to hold together all the elements in the prosthesis
5. As a support for the lip form and position (especially the labial and buccal flanges)

Although other factors such as color, stippling effects, and gingival contour are important, they are secondary to lip support and tooth position.

The denture base flange structure acts as a stimulus in the provisional denture to recover lip form and position. Many elderly denture wearers whose artificial teeth were placed over residual ridge crests, have a marked loss of muscle bulk and skin tone because the arch was constructed dorsally and medially to reflect the nature of maxillary bone loss. In the mandible, the method of tooth arrangement has usually expanded the arch, creating a more permanent thickened lower lip. In addition, there is often a loss of vertical height exacerbating a prognathic look.

Denture flanges generally are required to expand the upper lip, bringing the tubercle of the upper lip anteriorly and also moving the junction of the philtrum of the upper lip and the columella of the nose anteriorly. The tubercle of the upper lip can be moved anteriorly up to 23 mm from the edentulous state to the support position of a complete denture flange. The junction of the columella and the philtrum can be moved up to 8 mm anteriorly in cases of long standing edentulousness.[16]

The second aspect of the role of the denture flange relates to the size of the teeth selected. There is a "golden proportion" ratio of tooth width to tooth height that dominates most of the desired tooth sizes (see Chapter 2—Fundametals of Esthetics). The width of the six anterior teeth is about equal to the curved width of the lips at rest with natural teeth.[5] Given these guidelines for tooth selection, the extent of elevation of the high lip line (when the lips is elevated for the "e" sound or full smile elevation) will determine the effects of the denture base.

CLINICAL TIP. The most usual and desired exposure of teeth and denture base material is obtained when the high lip line reveals the full length of the teeth up to the cervical line, and usually only to the top of the resin interproximal papilla.

Many patients reveal no denture base in speech. However, some patients who have genetically or developmentally short upper lips and relatively protruded maxillary bone and teeth will display denture base material when laughing. These patients must be advised that solving this problem by reducing the vertical dimension or modifying the arch form may adversely effect the esthetics of the rest position. It requires a compromise for the dentist and patient to reach a mutually satisfactory outcome.

The secondary factors of stippling, staining, tinting, and root inclination are minor compared to the above.

1. **Stippling.** Stippling creates a textured surface that disperses reflected light. It mutes the brilliant reflection of light from a smooth polished surface. It also simulates the textured, stippled surface of the natural mucosa. Inflamed, unhealthy mucosa is smooth and glossy, therefore, stippling is always desirable unless the mucosa is very smooth on the adjacent area associated with natural teeth.
2. **Staining.** Some ethnic groups display heavy concentrations of melanin in the mucosa. It is appropriate to stain these denture flanges to match the existing distribution of melanin pigmentation. Also, some

acrylic resins have light and dark bluish tints available. The one most nearly matching the skin or mucosa should be selected.

3. **Root simulations.** Subgingival root simulations are usually critical in the canine regions where most lip collapse takes place when the canine eminence of bone is lost. Root simulations elsewhere generally are not required, but a slight contouring may be pleasant to the eyes, reinforcing an anatomic concept of natural bone contours. When too exaggerated, contours may collect food, calculus, and debris.

The denture base form, position, and color are essential elements in the esthetic composition. These considerations, however, generally should not compromise the fundamental aspects of denture retention and stability. It is a question of clinical judgement, esthetic expectation, and the patient's ability to cope with sacrificing retention and stability for esthetic improvements. Patients must share in responsibility for not only esthetic but functional factors. For example, a field dependent patient often places a finger over the lip, feeling the flange below the lip. Thinking it redundant, they desire it to be thinned to feel more "natural" despite the explanation that its removal may alter retention of the denture or induce wrinkling of the lip. Sometimes it is necessary to reduce the flange to satisfy the patient.

ATTACHMENT CONSIDERATIONS

Extracoronal clasp-retained removable partial dentures are inherently unesthetic. The I bar design reveals somewhat less metal facially and occlusally as compared to the circumferential clasp design and may in some cases be a viable esthetic design. In all cases, the functional lip line and patient desires determine the acceptability of any clasp design. Esthetic "cover-up" of the metal clasps has demonstrated only limited success. Semiprecision (mill-in) and precision attachments provide optimal esthetics as compared to the extracoronal clasp-retained partial denture.

GENERAL TREATMENT PRINCIPLES

Diagnostic Procedures

In addition to the usual radiographs, diagnostic casts, periodontal evaluation, and medical and dental history, diagnostic wax occlusal rims should be fabricated to replace missing teeth and alveolar tissues. These wax rims can be contoured over the remaining natural or restored teeth to approximate the anticipated vertical dimension, arch form, and centric relation of the articulated occlusion. They may also be used to evaluate the anticipated lip form and facial contour in both the static and dynamic states (Figs. 14–39 to 14–46). The stone teeth on the casts can be altered to approximate a more esthetic individual tooth position, contour, and alignment. These waxed up casts can be duplicated and used by the laboratory as clinical guides.

In addition, the patient should evaluate the anticipated tissue and tooth alignment and new facial form in both frontal and lateral profile view. Patient responses are important in determining the final success of the prosthesis. Because patient cooperation is crucial, it may be prudent not to treat those who cannot tolerate a change in facial appearance during this initial diagnosis.

The diagnostic wax occlusal rims also allow for evaluation of the response of the skin and muscles of the face to different approaches to treatment. The vermillion border of the lips should be increased and the prognathic lower lip associated with loss of face height should be reduced when the trial bases are in place.

Computer imaging may also be helpful in predicting treatment results (see Chapter 29—Esthetics and Advanced Technology).

The Incremental Treatment Program

The treatment indicated by the diagnostic casts and the wax occlusal rims should generally be provided through an incremental treatment program. This often involves a series of modifications to the patient's old prostheses or to a new provisional prosthesis. For example, if the vertical height is to be ultimately increased 4 mm, the first change should be 2 mm. If the plane of occlusion is to be modified, acrylic bite block additions can be made on the posterior teeth. The anterior teeth may be replaced simultaneously along with vertical height and centric relation modifications (see Figs. 14–20, 14–21). Centric relation record checks and remount procedures should be used when indicated. These alterations should simultaneously improve esthetics as well as function.

The Immediate Prosthesis

Immediate replacements of extracted teeth can be accomplished with modifications of an existing prosthesis or with an immediate prosthesis constructed before or at the time of surgery. The prosthesis permits the wound to maintain its form and prevents injury from impaction of foreign objects or food. For best results, the immediate denture must be constructed with proper prosthetic techniques. It must not create excessive occlusion forces, gliding prematurities or undue passive or dynamic stresses on teeth adjacent to the surgical sites. The tooth to be extracted is reduced out of occlusion on mounted casts and the prosthesis is equilibrated to a bilateral stable occlusal schema. If the tooth extracted is a canine, then group balance on the premolars should be established to provide a group function protected occlusion (Figs. 14–47 to 14–53).

If periodontal surgery is contemplated or performed simultaneously with the extractions, the immediate partial denture should provide room for retaining a periodontal packing. In addition, because tissue form changes rapidly during the first few days after a surgical procedure, the removable denture should be observed, adjusted, and if necessary, relined or teeth reset during this healing period.

A second objective of the immediate denture is the protection of the patient's psyche. People, when sud-

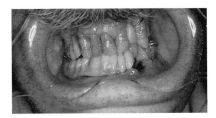

FIG. 14—39. A patient requiring maxillary and mandibular removable partial prostheses has loss of vertical height and severely decayed and periodontally compromised natural teeth. He is wearing defective partial dentures.

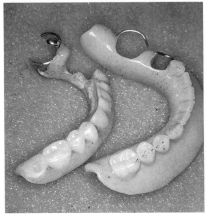

FIG. 14—40. The old and new mandibular partial denture. The old partial denture has anterior teeth inclined lingually, whereas the new partial denture has anterior teeth inclined labially and an increased vertical height of occlusion.

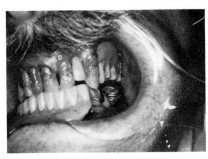

FIG. 14—41. Note the increased height of occlusion with the new provisional mandibular partial denture. The maxillary posterior teeth on the left side will be increased in length by adding quick-setting tooth-colored resin.

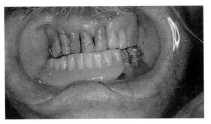

FIG. 14—42. The left canine was extracted and the partial denture maxillary teeth reset.

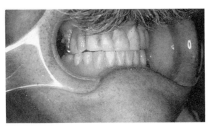

FIG. 14—43. Provisional acrylic crowns are placed on the remaining natural teeth with a reduction in stain and dark color. This slow color improvement was essential for this patient, who did not want to look different suddenly. The slow color change conditioned his psyche while the incremental change in arch form and vertical height conditioned the jaw muscles.

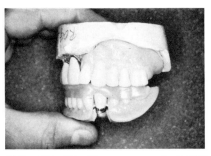

FIG. 14—44. The processed partial denture before mounting for refining the occlusion.

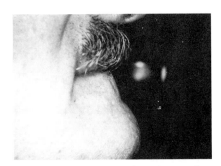

FIG. 14—45. The profile view before treatment. Note the thin lips and relatively straight 180° angle of the labiogenial sulcus. (From Silverman, S.I.: Prosthodontic care for the aging. Alpha Omegan 79:22, 1986.)

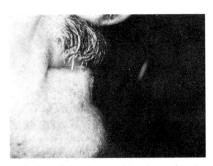

FIG. 14—46. The profile view after insertion of the new partial dentures with increased vertical dimension of occlusion and the expansion of the dental arches. The labiogenial sulcus has an obtuse angle approximating 150°. (From Silverman, S.I.: Prosthodontic care for the aging. Alpha Omegan 79:22, 1986.)

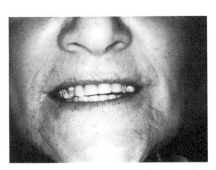

FIG. 14—47. A patient with a defective maxillary partial denture replacing the central and lateral incisors. Defective crowns are on the canines and remaining posterior teeth. She also has a defective mandibular complete denture.

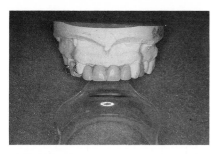

FIG. 14—48. Cast with defective maxillary partial denture. Note the absence of a denture flange, which might have supported the upper lip.

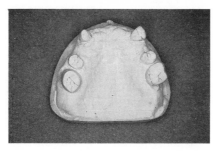

FIG. 14—49. Cast without maxillary partial denture. The maxillary left canine and molar are splayed beyond the contours of the catenary curve. These teeth have poorly contoured cast veneer crowns.

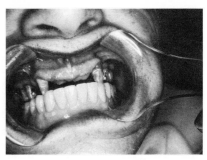

FIG. 14—50. The patient in Figure 14–47 with crowns removed and teeth prepared prior to placing the provisional fixed bridge and the new provisional mandibular complete denture. Periodontal treatment is required.

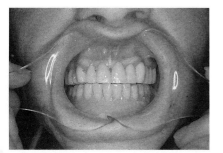

FIG. 14—51. The provisional fixed bridge placed in the mouth.

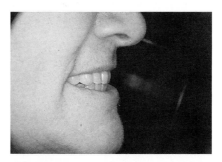

FIG. 14—52. Profile view with lips retracted and new prosthesis.

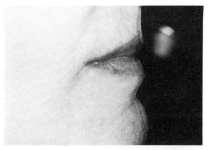

FIG. 14—53. Profile view demonstrating full lip profile and labiogenial sulcus angle of 125°.

denly partially edentulous, may become emotionally traumatized and avoid social interaction unless an immediate replacement of lost teeth is provided.

Provisional Prosthesis—Incremental Therapy

When preliminary healing is complete, the immediate prosthesis may be converted to a provisional prosthesis or a new provisional prosthesis may be constructed. The provisional prosthesis may be worn from a week to a year or more. The more extensive the surgery, the more frequent will be the change in denture form.

The prosthesis may be used to rotate, extrude, or intrude teeth or to move them buccolingually or mesiodistally. It may also be used to incrementally recover face and lip form, to increase vertical height, to expand or contract the dental arch, or to reposition the condyle in the temporomandibular joint.

The provisional prosthesis also allows patients to neurologically decondition mandibular posture and motion patterns. Newly conditioned patterns can improve consonant production and vowel differentiation for improved speech, voice, and resonance quality. Maladaptive, unesthetic chewing and swallowing patterns can be eliminated by wearing provisional dentures for several weeks.

When provisional removable partial or complete dentures are not worn, new prostheses often require multiple and prolonged adjustments because existing habituated occlusion patterns dominate during mastication and when at rest. This will cause the final prosthesis to look worn and abraded.

The provisional prosthesis also allows the patient to cope with changes in tooth color, shape, size, and arrangement. It provides the patient with time and experience in accepting changes in vertical and horizontal overbite.

CLINICAL TIP. A "trial run" with staggered and slightly irregular yet natural tooth forms and arrangements may result in an acceptance of a truly lifelike prosthesis in lieu of a preconceived notion of "perfect" teeth.

Women with provisional prostheses can learn to apply lipstick and facial foundation creams, to accept changes in reduced creasing of skin folds and to cope with new facial planes. (See Chapter 26—Esthetics and Cosmetology.) Men may require facial hair recontouring and, along with women, be encouraged to progressively reduce or eliminate tobacco and coffee, which may stain their new smile.

One of the most resisted changes is from a tip-to-tip anterior tooth position in the intercuspal and rest positions to a horizontal overbite at rest, which requires the mandible to move anteriorly to the tip-to-tip incisal position to produce the sibilant "s" sound. Usually in the old dentures the mandible moves anteriorly with the "s" sound into a protruded position. This is the characteristic position of aging patients who have lost face height or have complete or partial maxillary dentures replacing anterior teeth and labial alveolar bone loss.

The incremental program of change induces a subtle acceptance of all the stages in the recovery of esthetics of the face form and the dynamics of mastication, deglutition, and respiratory functions. Few patients resist this method of improved esthetics. In summary, the provisional prosthesis is an active appliance with a principle function of inducing change and recovery of tissue form and activity.

Definitive Prosthesis

When all dental and psychologic criteria are achieved, the patient is ready for the third stage of treatment, the definitive prosthesis.

The final removable prosthesis insertion, with or without accompanying fixed restorations, should be performed when all soft and hard tissues have been brought to optimal health. If there is a question about pulp health of an abutment tooth, about a gingival margin or sulcus depth, or about a mucosal irritation from a pontic or base, then the denture and crowns should not be permanently cemented into place until these treatment issues are resolved.

Definitive removable prostheses require a preventive maintenance program as frequently and thoroughly as natural teeth. To prevent jaw displacement (especially laterally or protrusively) and loss of face height, patients should be examined periodically.

CONCLUSION

Esthetics that satisfy the patient, the dentist, and the laboratory technician, in addition to satisfying the biomedical criteria of treatment, are the highest objective a dentist can attain in treatment.

REFERENCES

1. Silverman, S., Silverman, S.I., Silverman, B., and Garfinkel, L.: Self image and its relationship to denture acceptance. J Prosthet Dent 35:131, 1976.
2. Silverman, S.I.: Psychology of esthetics. New York, Esthetics Medcom Learning Systems, 1973.
3. Silverman, S.I.: The burning mouth syndrome. J Dent Assoc S Africa 30:163, 1976.
4. Silverman, S.I.: Vertical dimensions: a three dimension phenomenon. Part II. J Prosthet Dent 53:420, 1985.
5. Lieb, N., Silverman, S.I., and Garfinkel, L.: An analysis of soft tissue contours of the lips in relation to the maxillary cuspid. J Prosthet Dent 18:292, 1967.
6. Silverman, S.I. and Hayashi, T.: Dental arch form, alveolar bone contours and the catenary curve. Abst Dent Res 48:152, 1970.
7. Preston, J.D. and Bergen, S.F.: Color science and dental art, a self-teaching program. St. Louis, C.V. Mosby Co., 1980.
8. Silverman, S. Silverman, S.I., Silverman, B., and Garfinkel, L.: Self image and its relationship to denture acceptance. J Prosthet Dent 35:131, 1976.
9. Silverman, S.I.: The burning mouth syndrome. J Am Dent Assoc 33:459, 1967.
10. Roizen, A.: A mathematical analysis of maxillary tooth position. Master of Science Degree Thesis, New York University College Of Dentistry, 1976.
11. Hallarman, E.: A statistical survey of the shape and management of human male and female teeth. Master of Science Degree Thesis New York University College Of Dentistry, 1971.
12. Hallarman, E.: A statistical survey of skin color, natural tooth color in adult caucasians. Master of Science Degree Thesis, New York University College Of Dentistry, 1971.
13. Frush, J.P. and Fisher, R.D.: Introduction to dentogenic restorations. J Prosthet Dent 5:586, 1955.
14. Morison, A.: Physiognomy of Mental Disease, 2nd Ed. Burke, VA, American Publishing, 1976.
15. Roizen, A.: A mathematical analysis of maxillary tooth position. Master of Science Degree Thesis, New York University College Of Dentistry, 1976.
16. Silverman, S.I.: *Oral Physiology*. St Louis, Mosby, 1961.

Barry G. Dale, D.M.D.

BLEACHING AND RELATED AGENTS

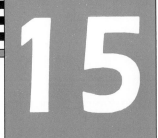

Esthetic improvement of acceptably shaped but discolored teeth by chemical means is highly desirable because of its conservative nature. The chemical agents and specific procedures used depend on a number of factors, including the type, intensity, and location of the discoloration.

HISTORY

A professional response to the unrelenting quest for whiter teeth dates back at least 2,000 years. First century Roman physicians maintained that brushing teeth with urine, in particular Portuguese urine, whitened teeth.[1] In the 1300s, the most requested dental service, other than extractions, was tooth whitening. Barbersurgeons, after abrading the enamel with coarse metal files, would apply "aquafortis," a solution of nitric acid, to whiten the teeth. This common practice continued into the eighteenth century.[1]

In the late 1800s, the combination of hydrogen peroxide, ether, and electricity was reported to be an effective method of lightening teeth.[2] Circa 1916, hydrochloric acid was used to successfully treat "Colorado brown stain" (endemic fluorosis).[3] In 1937, the combination of five parts 100% hydrogen peroxide with one part ether and heat, was reported as a treatment for this same type of discoloration.[4] Two years later, successful bleaching of fluorosis staining using 30% hydrogen peroxide, ether, and heat was described.[5] In 1966, the use of hydrochloric acid combined with hydrogen peroxide was advocated.[6] It was not until 1970 that hydrogen peroxide was demonstrated to be effective for the treatment of dentinal discoloration as well.[7]

MECHANISM AND APPEARANCE OF DISCOLORATION

Tetracycline Staining

The broad spectrum tetracycline group of antibiotics was first introduced in 1948 for use in the treatment of respiratory illnesses. However, tooth discoloration caused by incorporation of systemic tetracycline into tooth structure was not reported until 1956.[8]

Mechanism. The exact mechanism of tetracycline staining is not completely understood. It is hypothesized to occur by the joining of the tetracycline molecule with calcium through a chelation process and a subsequent incorporation into the hydroxylapatite crystal of the tooth during the mineralization stage of development.[9-12] A second theory maintains that the discoloration involves a binding of the tetracycline to tooth structure by a metal-organic matrix combination of the tetracycline complex.[13,14] Although some tetracycline accumulates within the enamel, it is primarily deposited into the dentin[15] because of the large surface area of the dentin apatite crystals compared to enamel apatite crystals.[16] Enamel hypoplasia, however, can also result.[17]

Extracted tetracycline stained rat,[18] dog,[19] and primary human teeth[20] have been shown to darken when exposed to sunlight. Interestingly, further exposure to various light sources (sunlight, incandescent, or ultraviolet lights) produces a subsequent lightening of the tetracycline stain.[11,18,20-23] It has been postulated, therefore, that tetracycline incorporated into hydroxylapatite, when oxidized by light (photo-oxidation), produces the red quinone product 4-α, 12-α anhydro-4-oxo-4-dedimethylaminotetracycline (AODTC).[24,25] Continued photo-oxidation of AODTC photolyzes, or bleaches, the red quinone.[24] Addition of diluted hydrogen peroxide yields an irreversible bleaching of the red quinone as well.[24]

Appearance. Tetracycline discoloration may be yellow, yellow-brown, brown, gray, or blue. The intensity of the staining varies widely. Distribution of discoloration is usually diffuse and severe cases may exhibit banding. Staining is usually bilateral and affects multiple teeth in both arches.

The hue and severity of tooth discoloration depends upon four factors associated with tetracycline administration:

1. **Age at time of administration.** Anterior primary teeth are susceptible to discoloration by systemic tetracycline from 4 months in utero through 9 months postpartum. Anterior permanent teeth are susceptible from 3 months postpartum through age 7 years.[26]
2. **Duration of administration.** The severity of the staining is directly proportional to the duration of administration of the medication.[27,28]
3. **Dosage.** The severity of the staining is directly proportional to the administered dosage.[26,29,30]
4. **Type of tetracycline.** Coloration has been correlated to the specific type of tetracycline administered:[31]
   A. Chlortetracycline (Aureomycin)—gray-brown stain
   B. Dimethylchlortetracycline (Ledermycin)—yellow stain
   C. Doxycycline (Vibramycin)—does not cause staining
   D. Oxytetracycline (Terramycin)—yellow stain
   E. Tetracycline (Achromycin)—yellow stain

Yellow tetracycline staining slowly darkens to brown or gray-brown when exposed to sunlight. Therefore, the anterior teeth of children often darken first, while the posterior teeth, because of reduced exposure to sunlight, darken more slowly.[32] In adults, however, natural photobleaching of the anterior teeth (see the preceding section on Tetracycline Staining—Mechanism) has been observed, particularly in individuals whose teeth are excessively exposed to sunlight because of maxillary lip insufficiency.[21] Hypocalcified white areas of varying opacity, size, and distribution may also be present.

Fluorosis

Mechanism. Endemic fluorosis, or mottling, results from the presence of excessive systemic fluoride during enamel matrix formation and calcification.[33,34] Fluorosis is actually a form of enamel hypoplasia,[33] hence the white spotting. Darker discoloration occurs through extrinsic staining of the hypoplastic enamel. Thus, the darker stains occur only after tooth eruption.[32] Studies show little clinically significant fluorosis when municipal water fluoride levels are less than 0.9 ppm. However, levels greater than 4.4 ppm cause fluorosis in more than 97.8% of the population.[35]

Appearance. Staining is usually bilateral and affects multiple teeth in both arches. Fluorosis presents as mild, intermittent white spotting, chalky or opaque areas, yellow or brown staining of varying degrees, and, in the most severe cases, surface pitting of the enamel.[34,36]

Extrinsic Environmental Stains

Mechanism. Essentially limited to enamel, extrinsic environmental staining is caused by a variety of factors including foods, beverages, and tobacco products.

Appearance. Environmental staining affects multiple teeth and appears as yellow or brown stains of varying intensities. They are diffuse in nature, however, pits and other enamel defects may be more intensely stained because of inadequate oral hygiene procedures on these concave "protected" surfaces (Figs. 15–1, 15–2).

Staining of Pulpal Etiology—Trauma or Necrosis

Mechanism. Intrinsic staining results from the deposition of hemorrhagic byproducts into the dentinal tubules after pulpal trauma[37–39] or necrosis.[39]

Appearance. Discoloration of pulpal origin can be red, yellow, yellow-brown, brown, gray, or black. Discoloration is obviously limited to the affected tooth or teeth (Fig. 15–3).

Staining Following Endodontic Therapy

Mechanism. Staining following endodontic therapy can result from excessive hemorrhaging during pulp removal or from the decomposition of pulpal tissue following incomplete extirpation.[37,40]

CLINICAL TIP. Carefully remove all tissue and debris from the sometimes elusive pulp horns and lateral extensions of the pulp chamber. This will reduce the likelihood of subsequent tooth discoloration (Fig. 15–4).

Various endodontic medicaments and sealers containing barium, iodine, or silver may also cause discoloration as can gutta percha.[37,41–43]

CLINICAL TIP. All remnants of endodontic filling materials and sealers should be carefully removed from the pulp chamber. This will reduce the likelihood of subsequent tooth discoloration.

Appearance. Discoloration of pulpal origin can appear yellow, yellow-brown, brown, gray, or black. Discoloration from endodontic medicaments and sealers ranges from orange-red to dark red, or gray to

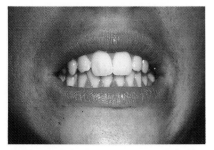

FIG. 15—1. Extrinsic environmental staining may be similar in appearance to developmental discoloration (see Figure 15—16).

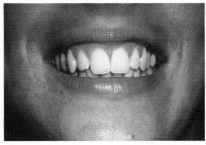

FIG. 15—2. Some extrinsic stains may be eliminated by simple prophylaxis.

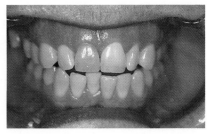

FIG. 15—3. Intrinsic staining results from the deposition of hemorrhagic byproducts and decomposition of pulpal tissue into the dentinal tubules after pulpal trauma (see also Figure 15—46).

FIG. 15—4. Elusive pulp horns and lateral extensions of the pulp chamber often remain untouched during routine endodontic access preparation. (The access preparation is highlighted in black.) Careful removal of tissue and debris from these areas may help prevent subsequent tooth discoloration.

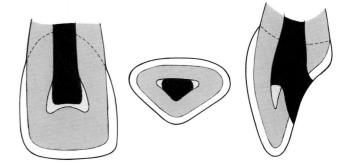

FIG. 15—5. Intrinsic staining results from the deposition of hemorrhagic byproducts as well as from endodontic medicaments deposited into the dentinal tubules.

FIG. 15—6. Congenital white spot lesions. Note that brown developmental discoloration is also present (see also Figure 15—14).

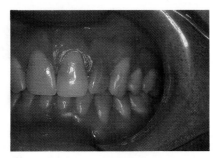

FIG. 15—5

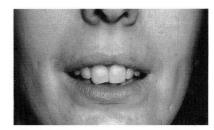

FIG. 15—6

black.[40,41] Discoloration is obviously limited to the affected tooth or teeth (Fig. 15—5).

Staining from Pre-Eruption Trauma—Direct and Indirect

Mechanism. Discoloration of a permanent tooth may occur after trauma to its primary counterpart.[44] Blood breakdown products from the traumatized site can infiltrate into the developing enamel during the calcification stage.[32]

In addition, the apex of the primary tooth may directly traumatize the ameloblasts or the enamel matrix. Discoloration of a permanent tooth may also result from jaw fractures associated with the developing dentition, periapical inflammation of a primary tooth, or other infections in the area of a developing tooth bud.[32]

Appearance. Discoloration is usually white or yellow-brown and often sharply demarcated or spotty rather than diffuse.[44] This discoloration can closely mimic that caused by endemic fluorosis or tetracycline ingestion, however, it is usually limited to the facial enamel surface of one or two teeth, usually the maxillary incisors.[45] Enamel defects may also be present if the ameloblasts or the enamel matrix was disturbed.[32]

White Spot Lesions

Mechanism. White spot enamel lesions can be developmental, acquired, or a combination of the two.

Developmental lesions result from alterations during the matrix formation or calcification stages of tooth development. Endemic fluorosis and trauma are two of the most common causes, however, developmental disturbances during this period from genetic disorders, febrile and other illnesses and from unknown causes also occur. The term "dysmineralization" has been introduced to refer to these lesions because of the difficulty often encountered in determining the precise nature of these mineralization abnormalities.[46]

Acquired white spot lesions occur after tooth eruption. One source of such lesions is localized discoloration from chronic stasis of bacterial plaque. This often results around fixed orthodontic appliances in patients with poor oral hygiene.[46]

Appearance. White spot lesions manifest as discrete areas that are lighter than the surrounding normocalcified enamel (Fig. 15–6). The intensity of the lesion varies from mildly decreased chroma to opaque chalky white. Size, distribution patterns, and penetration depth vary greatly.

Staining from Silver Amalgam

Mechanism. Tooth discoloration from silver amalgam is primarily caused by the visibility of a restoration through relatively translucent tooth structure. It may also, to varying degrees, be caused by direct staining of the tooth structure by the reaction products of intraoral sulfides and the copper or silver ions of the amalgam.

Appearance. Tooth discoloration from silver amalgam is gray to black in color.

Other Discolorations

There are numerous other types of discolorations resulting from a plethora of causes. Some chromogenic bacteria may cause yellow, orange, brown-black, or green stains.[35,47] Salivary components can cause brown stains.[36] Sulfmethemoglobin, a blood pigment breakdown product, can cause a green coloration to remnants of Nasmyth's membrane.[31,35] Chlorophyll in dental plaque may also cause green stains.[31] The deposition of porphyrin into developing dentin in patients with erythropoietic porphyria, an inborn error of metabolism, may result in a red, purplish brown, or brownish discoloration.[36,48] Phenylketonuria, another inborn error of metabolism, can produce brown discoloration.[31] Erythroblastosis fetalis, a syndrome resulting from Rh incompatibility in an infant, is characterized by the hemolysis and breakdown of the infant's blood, producing jaundice. These pigments may produce an intrinsic blue, brown, or green discoloration.[35] Thalassemia and sickle-cell anemia may cause similar discolorations.[31] Amelogenesis imperfecta may result in yellow or brown stains.[35] Dentinogenesis imperfecta can cause brownish violet, yellowish, or gray discolorations.[35] Generalized yellow or gray coloration may not result from a pathologic entity, but may simply be a variant within the normal range of tooth shade (Figs. 15–7, 15–8). Some discolorations are of unknown origin.

TREATMENT AGENTS

Solutions for treating unwanted tooth discolorations can permeate the enamel and dentin, ultimately reaching the pulp.[49–53] The exact mechanism of discoloration removal during this process depends upon the chemical agent and technique used.

Hydrochloric Acid

Although hydrochloric acid is not a true bleaching agent, its applications warrant inclusion in any discussion of tooth discoloration treatments.

Hydrochloric acid is a potent decalcification agent. Nonselective in nature, it decalcifies both the tooth structure and the accompanying stains. When hydrochloric acid is used in conjunction with abrasive agents, the affected enamel is totally removed along with the stain. Unfortunately, the preponderance of the literature only deals with the use of acid and acid/abrasion techniques for the treatment of brown fluorosis staining.[4,6,54–63] Hydrochloric acid treatment of other superficial enamel stains and hypocalcifications[64] has been suggested, but multiple source long-term evaluations

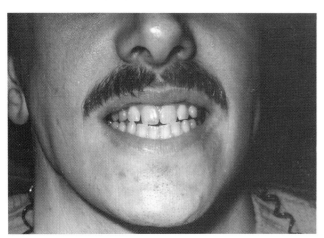

FIG. 15–7. Generalized yellow coloration of nonpathologic etiology.

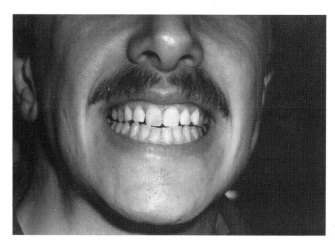

FIG. 15–8. The same patient as shown in Figure 15–7 after four vital thermo-photocatalytic bleaching treatments.

ESTHETIC DENTISTRY

Bleaching Agents

The most commonly used bleaching agents are sodium perborate, hydrogen peroxide, and carbamide peroxide. Carbamide peroxide (also known as hydrogen peroxide carbamide, carbamide urea, urea hydrogen peroxide, urea peroxide, perhydrol urea, and perhydelure) breaks down into hydrogen peroxide and urea.

The exact mechanism of discoloration removal is not entirely understood, but likely includes oxygen-releasing, mechanical cleansing actions[32] and oxidation or reduction reactions. Tetracycline staining may, more specifically, be bleached through an oxidative degradation of the quinone ring.[24] (See the section on Mechanism and Appearance of Discoloration—Tetracycline earlier in this chapter.) The mechanisms will differ according to the type of discoloration involved and the chemical and physical environment present at the time of action (i.e., pH, temperature, cocatalysts, lighting, and other conditions).[65]

Hydrogen peroxide, depending upon conditions, is capable of releasing free radicals ($H_2O_2 \rightarrow H\cdot + \cdot OOH$ or $H_2O_2 \rightarrow HO\cdot + \cdot OH$), perhydroxyl anions ($H_2O_2 \rightarrow H^+ + :OOH^-$), or a combinations of both free radicals and anions ($HOO\cdot + OH^- \rightarrow O_2^-\cdot + H_2O$ in a basic solution and $HOO\cdot \rightarrow O_2^- \cdot + H^+$ in an acidic solution).[65] These compounds tend to be attracted to electron-rich alkene (double) bonds and form epoxides that are unstable and can form alcohols

$$(C = C + O\cdot \rightarrow \overset{O}{\underset{C\text{-}C}{\wedge}} + H_2O \rightarrow \overset{OH\ OH}{\underset{C\text{-}C}{|\ \ |}}).$$ Double bonds can create discoloration; thus breaking these bonds often eliminates discoloration. In addition, more water-soluble compounds are created, which are more easily removed.[66]

Hydrogen peroxide also increases the permeability of tooth structure, thus increasing the movement of ions through the tooth.[67] This probably occurs because of the low molecular weight of hydrogen peroxide and its ability to denature proteins.[67]

UV Photo-Oxidation

Laboratory evidence that photo-oxidation is both the cause of and a "cure" for tetracycline staining (see the section on Mechanism and Appearance of Discoloration—Tetracycline earlier in this chapter) suggests that light alone is potentially a viable treatment for some tooth discolorations. In vitro ultraviolet (UV) irradiation of tetracycline stained rat dentin produced complete stain removal after 24 hours of exposure.[21] However, UV light does not penetrate enamel easily. Other sources of higher intensity UV light, such as deuterium arc sources or UV lasers, may overcome this obstacle, but problems such as high temperature generation, skin and mucosal burns, eye damage, potential carcinogenicity, and structural damage to enamel and dentin have not yet been suitably addressed, making this an unacceptable alternative at this time.[21]

TREATMENT MODALITIES

As with any therapeutic treatment, proper diagnosis should be attempted before a course of treatment is promulgated. Although the etiology of a specific tooth discoloration may be difficult to discern, an accurate history, as well as an evaluation of the factors discussed earlier (see the section on Mechanism and Appearance of Discolorations earlier in this chapter) help in establishing a differential diagnosis. The presence or absence of pulp tissue is also a treatment planning factor.

Currently, only three modalities of stain removal are available:

Acid Application Combined with Mechanical Abrasion

Acid/abrasion techniques are enticingly efficient because of the short treatment times. However, the non-selective, destructive nature of this procedure limits its application to only the most superficial discolorations and those cases in which treatment time (and subsequent cost) is a factor. Obviously, whether or not a discoloration is superficial enough to be treated in this way can only be determined through trial and error,[46] and patients should be so informed.

Bleaching Systems

Bleaching systems can also be used to treat superficial staining and are the only technique available for deeper enamel stains and for staining of the dentin. Repeated treatment applications are often necessary, especially for vital teeth.

Combination Therapy

It has been suggested that the acid/abrasion techniques can be attempted for discolorations that appear to be superficial, followed by the use of bleaching systems, if necessary.[32]

RESTORATIVE IMPLICATIONS

The return of discoloration after successful or partially successful treatment has been observed. Similar regression despite subsequently placed porcelain or composite resin laminate veneers is therefore possible. Although restorative materials may offer some protection against color changes of the underlying tooth structure, long-term multiple source investigations of this phenomena are lacking. This must be considered if discoloration removal therapy is followed by restorative treatment of any kind. The esthetic effects of such color regression depend on the amount of regression and the degree of translucency of the overlying restoration.

It has also been demonstrated that hydrogen peroxide application to tooth structure diminishes the bond strength between unfilled resin and acid etched enamel.[68-70] Presumably, oxygen inhibition of resin polymerization and the creation of voids in the resin tags may be caused by the presence of residual hydrogen peroxide or peroxide-related substances in the interprismatic enamel areas after bleaching.[69,70] This residual substance is apparently not removed by either a 1 min. water rinse or by thoroughly drying the surface.[70] However, the changes within the tooth structure which cause the diminished bond strength seem to be reversible.[68] Therefore, bonded restorations should be postponed for a minimum of 1 week[71] after bleaching with hydrogen peroxide to allow for the elimination of this residual hydrogen peroxide.

TREATMENT PLANNING AND PROGNOSIS

General Considerations

Mandibular teeth generally require fewer stain removal treatments than maxillary teeth when office-based techniques are used (e.g., thermo-photocatalytic method). This is probably because of the thinner enamel and dentin of the mandibular anterior teeth when compared to their maxillary analogs. The reverse, however, is true for the "home-use" techniques. This most likely occurs because the bleaching solution quickly empties from the mandibular tray as a result of gravity.

If both the mandibular and maxillary arches are similarly discolored, it may not be necessary to treat the discoloration of the mandibular teeth. In many cases, the lower lip completely hides the mandibular arch during normal smiling (Figs. 15–9, 15–10).

During function, the coloration of the mandibular arch is often obscured because of shadowing from the upper lip, particularly in Class I and Class II horizontal overjet relationships. In addition, the visual perception of the mandibular teeth is further reduced because of the continuous motion of the mandible during speaking, as opposed to the maxillary arch, which remains relatively stable in space during function. These factors may permit an esthetically acceptable result despite significantly contrasting shades between the maxillary and mandibular arches.

Tetracycline Staining

Tetracycline stains reside primarily in the dentin. Therefore, bleaching systems, rather than acid/abrasion techniques, are indicated. In general, the results of bleaching yellow, yellow-brown, and brown stains are more favorable than blue-gray to gray stains. When teeth exhibit any combination of yellow, brown, blue, or gray stains, the blue and gray component may remain to some degree despite a more favorable bleaching of the yellow and brown component (see Fig. 15–13). In addition, less intense stains have a better prognosis and usually require fewer treatment visits. Teeth with diffuse staining generally respond better than those with banding.

Tetracycline staining has been classified into three groups:[36]

1. **First degree stains.** First degree stains are light yellow, light brown, or light gray, and are uniform throughout the clinical crown. No banding is present. A successful result is usually accomplished in approximately three treatments (Fig. 15–11).
2. **Second degree stains.** Second degree stains are more intense than first degree stains. No banding is present. Up to six treatments usually are necessary to achieve a satisfactory result (Fig. 15–12).
3. **Third degree stains.** Third degree stains are intense and the clinical crown exhibits horizontal color banding. Ten or more treatments usually are required. Bleaching is generally contraindicated because of the time involved and the poor prognosis. However, although less than ideal results are to be expected, the outcome may be esthetically satisfactory to the patient. The yellow-brown to brown component will generally respond better than the blue to blue-gray component (Fig. 15–13).

Fluorosis

Fluorosis staining is limited to the enamel. If the staining is yellow to brown, the prognosis is favorable. Acid/abrasion techniques can be attempted first if the staining is presumed to be extremely superficial. If acid/abrasion techniques are unsuccessful (of if they are not attempted) two to four treatments with a bleaching system will usually be successful. Bleaching systems are equally effective when compared to acid/abrasion systems for treatment of superficial fluorosis stains.[72]

Extrinsic Environmental Staining

Superficial extrinsic staining can often be removed during routine prophylaxis (see Figs. 15–1, 15–2). Long

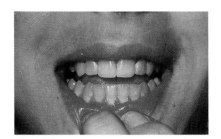

FIG. 15–9

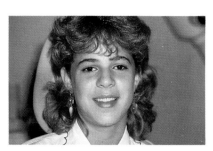

FIG. 15–10

FIG. 15–9. Patient with second degree tetracycline staining following bleaching of the maxillary teeth.

FIG. 15–10. The same patient as shown in Figure 15–9. A full lower lip hides the mandibular arch during function precluding the need for mandibular bleaching.

standing, deeper staining is usually amenable to bleaching system treatments. Two to four treatments are usually necessary, depending on the intensity of the staining. It has been suggested that acid/abrasion techniques will be successful if the staining is superficial[46] although long-term, multiple source studies are lacking.

Staining of Pulpal Etiology or from Endodontic Therapy

Only bleaching systems, rather than acid/abrasion techniques, are indicated for stains of pulpal etiology. The absence of pulp tissue allows for placement of bleaching agents directly into the pulp cavity.

Staining caused by medications, sealers, and filling materials are generally less amenable to bleaching than those resulting from biologic causes.[73] However, the bleaching of stains caused by endodontic materials can nevertheless be quite successful.[40]

Staining from Pre-Eruption Trauma

The prognosis and treatment time for discoloration resulting from pre-eruption trauma is similar to that for fluorosis. A normal response to pulp vitality testing can aid in distinguishing between staining induced by developmental trauma and that arising from pulpal etiology.

White Spot Lesions

A tooth with localized white spot lesions can, for treatment planning purposes, be considered a mosaic of light areas on a background of normocalcified tooth structure. If the background tooth structure is a desirable color, acid/abrasion techniques can be considered, although long-term, multiple source studies of treatments of white lesions are lacking. It has been estimated that between 50 and 75% of white enamel defects are sufficiently superficial to be successfully treated with acid/abrasion.[46]

However, if the background color is undesirable and the discoloration is deemed to penetrate deeper than the most superficial levels, a bleaching system should be used. In this situation, the contrasting white spot lesions are often significantly less noticeable and esthetically acceptable after a successful bleaching of the normocalcified background area. The intensity, size, and distribution of the hypocalcified areas, as well as the efficacy of the bleaching of the surrounding areas, determines whether this approach is appropriate (Figs. 15-14 to 15-18).

Staining from Silver Amalgam

Tooth discoloration from silver amalgam is not routinely amenable to bleaching. Restorative treatments are the usual solution.

Other Discolorations

The precise etiology of many stains is not always dis-

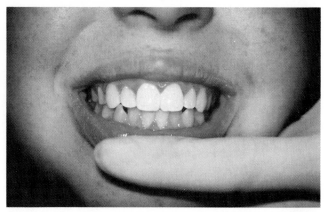

FIG. 15–11. First degree tetracycline staining after three vital thermo-photocatalytic bleaching treatments. The mandibular arch remains untreated and serves as a comparative control.

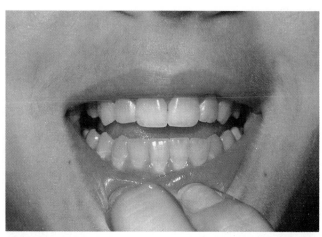

FIG. 15–12. Second degree tetracycline staining after four vital thermo-photocatalytic bleaching treatments. The mandibular arch remains untreated and serves as a comparative control.

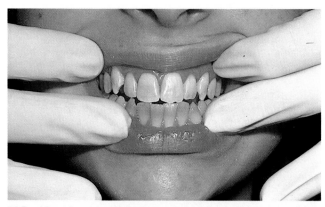

FIG. 15–13. Third degree tetracycline staining with typical banding pattern. The mandibular arch remains untreated and serves as a comparative control. Note the complete removal of the yellow-brown component and the partial removal of the more tenacious blue-gray band. Although a less than ideal result was achieved, it was esthetically satisfactory to the patient, who desired no additional treatment. Sixteen thermo-photocatalytic vital bleaching treatments were performed.

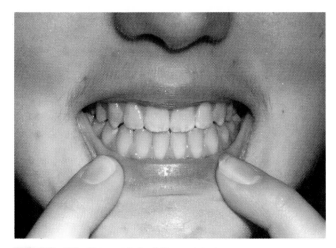

FIG. 15–14. Congenital white spot lesions.

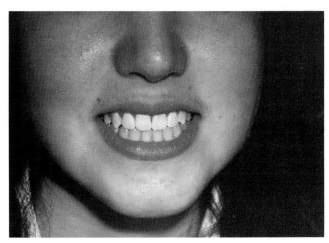

FIG. 15–15. The same patient as in Figure 15–14 after three vital thermo-photocatalytic bleaching treatments. Lightening of the "background" color eliminates the perceptual impact of the white spot lesions.

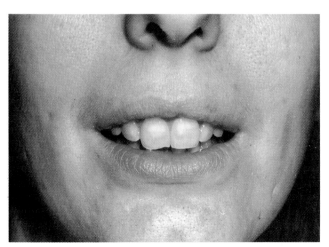

FIG. 15–16. The central incisors exhibit both brown and white developmental discolorations.

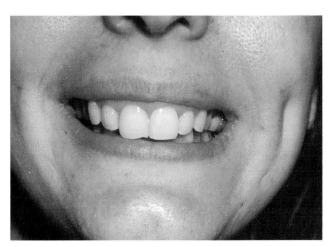

FIG. 15–17. The same patient as in Figure 15–16 following three vital thermo-photocatalytic bleaching treatments. Whitening of the "background" color and removal of the brown stain eliminates the perceptual impact of the white spot lesions, creating an esthetically pleasing result.

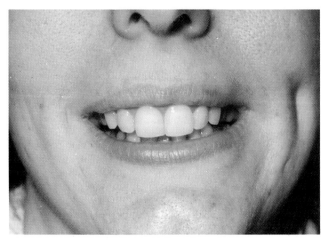

FIG. 15–18. The same patient as in Figure 15–16 after cosmetic recontouring.

cernible. This may complicate the generation of a reasonable treatment plan and prognosis.

Some discolorations may be treated with routine prophylaxis. It has been suggested that any discoloration limited to only the most superficial enamel can be eliminated with acid/abrasion.[67] Stains resulting from erythropoietic porphyria and erythroblastosis fetalis can sometimes be successfully treated with bleaching agents.[74,75] Treatment of discoloration resulting from amelogenesis imperfecta and other etiologies that interfere with normal matrix formation or calcification of enamel is often less effective.[75] In addition, treatment is often contraindicated if the current structural integrity of the tooth is sufficiently compromised.

The prognosis for the treatment of generalized coloration of nonpathologic origin is highly unpredictable.

VITAL TEETH—ACID/ABRASION

General Considerations

Acid/abrasion is a relatively simple procedure that removes both tooth structure and stain simultaneously. Techniques vary and include at least one commercially produced set of armamentarium (Figs. 15–19 to 15–22).

Safety

The acid/abrasion technique empirically appears relatively safe if performed properly. Primary safety considerations include patient cooperation, careful gingival isolation, minimal duration of exposure of the tooth structure to the acid, minimal mechanical abrasion, and meticulous protection of the patient and personnel from the acid. However, the long-term safety of the procedure has not been documented by controlled long-term studies.

Five repetitions of a 5-second acid/pumice application with a wooden stick removes 112 microns of tooth structure.[76] This results in an 11% loss of enamel thickness, assuming a permanent incisor midlabial enamel thickness of approximately 1 mm.[55] It has been reported that enamel losses of 25%[64] and 30%[55] are clinically acceptable.

It has been suggested that hydrochloric acid applied to the enamel surface does not penetrate into the pulpal tissue.[51,77] It is possible that the acid forms a calcium or phosphorous salt precipitate that limits further penetration of the acid into the dentin. These salts may, in addition, further neutralize the acid.[51]

Scanning electron microscopy performed after treatment with 18% hydrochloric acid and Italian ground pumice reveals a "smeared" enamel surface with tooth structure loss from both chemical erosion and mechanical abrasion.[78] Qualitative elemental analysis of this same enamel surface demonstrates a chemical pattern similar to unetched enamel and an absence of any foreign residue.[78]

There is no question that alterations in the enamel continue after treatment is completed. The duration of such alterations and the detrimental clinical significance, if any, is unknown at this time. The treated enamel surfaces may continue to change for at least 6 months. These changes may include a further improvement in color correction, as well as a smoother, brighter, and more lustrous surface. Color improvement has been attributed to a change in the optical characteristics of the tooth surface, which may be a function of the manner in which the acid treated enamel remineralizes.[46] The other changes have been alternately described as resulting from an anatomically smoother surface, increased plaque resistance,[46] plaque accumulation in residual defects, or continuous abrasion from dentifrices.[78]

Mechanical abrasion using rotary instrumentation alone is an alternative approach. However, this approach requires care to avoid ditching, altering labial contours, and excessive enamel reduction.

Acid Abrasion (after Croll)[79]

Armamentarium

- Protective glasses with side shields (for patient and operator)
- Heavy rubber dam
- Copal varnish (e.g., Copalite, Cooley and Cooley, Ltd.)
- 36% hydrochloric acid U.S.P. (available from chemical supply house)
- Two glass dappen dishes or two disposable plastic medicine cups (available at most local pharmacies)
- Distilled water

FIG. 15–19. Preoperative view of white spot lesions. (Courtesy of Dr. T.P. Croll.)

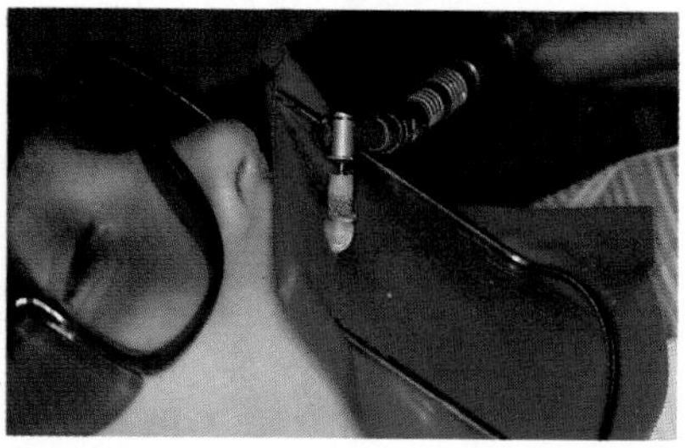

FIG. 15–20. Application of a commercially produced hydrochloric acid abrasive paste (Prema) with a specially designed low-speed handpiece and mandrel. (Courtesy of Dr. T.P. Croll.)

FIG. 15–21. The same patient as in Figure 15–19. The mandrel is used to apply commercially produced hydrochloric acid abrasive paste (Prema). (Courtesy of Dr. T.P. Croll.)

FIG. 15–22. Same patient as in Figure 15–19 after removal of what proved to be a superficial white spot lesion. (Courtesy of Dr. T.P. Croll.)

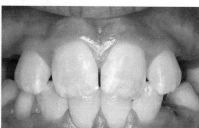

FIG. 15–19

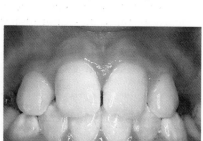

FIG. 15–20

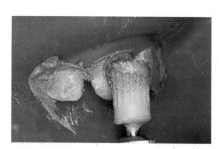

FIG. 15–21

FIG. 15–22

- Flour of pumice
- Sodium bicarbonate powder U.S.P.
- Tongue blade
- Cotton-tipped applicator
- 1.1% neutral sodium fluoride (e.g., Prevident, Colgate-Hoyt Laboratories)
- Fine fluoridated prophylaxis paste
- Superfine aluminum oxide polishing disc (e.g., Soflex, 3M, Inc.)

Clinical Technique

CLINICAL TIP. WARNING: Protective glasses with side shields must be worn by the patient, dentist, and any auxiliary personnel while working with hydrochloric acid. The dentist and auxiliary personnel should wear rubber gloves and the patient must be draped. The procedure is contraindicated if patient behavioral management problems exist or if the teeth are sensitive to temperature changes or acidic liquids.

CLINICAL TIP. This technique should not be attempted if the operatory is not equipped with a high volume evacuation system.

1. Apply a heavy rubber dam to the teeth to be bleached.
2. Seal the labial and lingual (or palatal) rubber dam margins with copal varnish.
3. Prepare an 18% hydrochloric acid solution by mixing equal volumes of 36% hydrochloric acid and distilled water in a dappen dish or disposable medicine cup.

CLINICAL TIP. Always add acid to water. Adding water to acid can cause splattering because of the exothermic reaction that occurs upon mixing.

4. Add flour of pumice to the acid solution to make a thick, wet paste.
5. Prepare a thick paste of sodium bicarbonate and water.
6. Place sodium bicarbonate paste on the rubber dam to help neutralize any splashed acid.

CLINICAL TIP. WARNING: Neither hydrochloric acid nor any mixture containing or instrument contacting hydrochloric acid should ever be held in the region of, or passed over, the patient's face.

7. Apply the acid/pumice mixture to the labial enamel with a wooden tongue blade. Simultaneously use a cotton-tipped applicator to absorb any excess solution.

CLINICAL TIP. The tongue blade can be cut or split to better adapt it to the facial surface.

CLINICAL TIP. WARNING: Rotary instrumentation of any type is strictly contraindicated because of the danger of splattering the acid.

8. With firm finger pressure on the tongue blade, grind the mixture into the enamel.

CLINICAL TIP. Total acid contact time should not exceed 5 seconds.

9. Rinse thoroughly with water for 10 seconds while carefully evacuating with high powered suction.
10. Evaluate for excessive enamel wear by viewing, with a mirror, the labial surface from an incisal direction.
11. Wet the tooth with saliva and evaluate for appropriate color change.

CLINICAL TIP. White enamel discoloration is usually more visible on dry tooth structure.[46] Color evaluation of dry teeth may, therefore, result in overtreatment and unnecessary enamel removal.

12. If color change is esthetically acceptable, skip to step 14.

CLINICAL TIP. To avoid excessive wear, limit the acid/abrasion application to a maximum of five attempts. However, if no change is observed after the third attempt, discontinue treatment and skip to step 14.

13. If color change is unacceptable, repeat steps 6 through 13. These steps should not be performed more than five times.
14. Apply a 1.1% neutral sodium fluoride gel for 3 minutes.
15. Polish with a fine fluoride prophylaxis paste and superfine aluminum oxide composite resin polishing discs.

Alternate Method

Clinical Technique. A commercially manufactured kit (Prema, Premier Dental Products Co.) uses a hydrochloric acid abrasive compound of paste-like consistency, a 10:1 gear reduction contra angle handpiece, specialized mandrel tips, and hand applicators.[46] Specific instructions are provided in the kit. The acid concentration is presumably lower than 18%,[46] however the precise concentration is unavailable proprietary information.

VITAL TEETH—OFFICE BLEACHING

Bleaching of vital teeth in the dental office involves the application of bleaching agents (usually 30 to 35% hydrogen peroxide) often in combination with heat and light.

Safety

The efficacy of bleaching teeth with heat and hydrogen peroxide is well documented.[7,36,80-84] Although histologic changes within the dental pulp are evident after heat and hydrogen peroxide application, pulpal damage appears to be reversible.[53,85-87]

Histologic changes in the enamel and dentin have also been demonstrated.[82] However, spectroscopic analysis reveals no change in surface chemistry of enamel after exposure to hydrogen peroxide.[70] The clinical significance of this in vivo has yet to be determined, however, the scarcity of any negative clinical sequelae over the long-term is well established.[74,75]

Acid Etching

The application of phosphoric acid to the enamel surface prior to bleaching is controversial. It presumably facilitates the bleaching process by creating porosities, thus increasing the penetration of the bleaching agent. Whether this truly affects the efficacy of bleaching, however, has not been determined by multiple source controlled studies. Further, if acid is applied, the precise concentration and duration of exposure is an additional uncertainty. Suggested acid application times vary from 10 to 60 seconds, with acid concentrations ranging from 37 to 50%, and rinsing times of from 30 to 60 seconds.[34,74,75,88]

Acid etching prior to bleaching results in a dull, roughened tooth surface. Subsequent polishing is necessary to immediately restore some of the original surface luster. The often repetitive nature of the bleaching process necessitates multiple exposure to these procedures. The amount of tooth structure removed by repeated etching and polishing is a function of the type and concentration of the acid, as well as the frequency and duration of exposure. It is also a function of the abrasiveness of the polishing material and the manner, frequency, and duration of application. The clinical significance, if any, of this tooth loss has not been adequately investigated. Therefore, the use of acid must be based upon clinical judgment.

Postoperative Complications

Hydrogen peroxide contact with soft tissue will cause a transient chalky white lesion. The lesion usually heals within a few hours without scarring.

CLINICAL TIP. *A burning or stinging sensation from hydrogen peroxide contact with soft tissue can be alleviated by placing Orabase Plain (Colgate-Hoyt Laboratories) on the affected tissue.*

Mild spontaneous steady postoperative pain will usually not persist for more than 24 hours and can be successfully treated with nonprescription analgesics. Transient sharp shooting pains can also occasionally occur. These usually cease within 36 hours. If the symptoms persist beyond these time frames, further bleaching should not be attempted.

CLINICAL TIP. *If any postoperative tooth pain occurs, reduce the heat intensity, treatment time, or both during subsequent visits. This usually eliminates a recurrence of the symptoms.*

Treatment Modalities

Treatment modalities generally involve the use of 35% hydrogen peroxide in either liquid or gel form. Various treatment alternatives involve the application of the bleaching agent at room temperature, in combination with heat (thermocatalytic technique), or in combination with both heat and light (thermo-photocatalytic technique).

35% Hydrogen Peroxide with Heat (Thermocatalytic Technique).
The thermocatalytic technique involves the use of a spatula- or paddle-shaped heating element, which is approximately the size of a single tooth (Fig. 15–23). After 35% hydrogen peroxide is applied to the tooth surface, the heating element is positioned over the tooth. Each tooth is treated individually and in sequence. Treatment duration, frequency of application, and temperature vary depending on the system used and the type of discoloration.

35% Hydrogen Peroxide with Heat and Light (Thermo-Photocatalytic Technique).
The thermo-photocatalytic technique is the most commonly used procedure. A rheostatically controlled heating lamp provides efficient uniform heating and lighting of an entire arch.

35% Hydrogen Peroxide Alone.
This technique eliminates the addition of both heat and light. It usually involves the use of 35% hydrogen peroxide, which is combined with a proprietary component to produce a gel.

There have been no controlled scientific studies comparing the clinical efficacy of one technique over another. However, it has been generally accepted that heat increases the rate of decomposition of hydrogen peroxide (thereby accelerating the release of the activated bleaching molecules). Light energy also accelerates the decomposition of hydrogen peroxide.[89] Acceleration of the decomposition of hydrogen peroxide by both heat and light is further implied by the storage precautions, which recommend protection from both light and heat.[90,91] The thermo-photocatalytic technique is the only treatment that incorporates both heat and light. It is also more efficient than the thermocatalytic technique when treating entire arches.

In light of these and the other factors described above (see the section on Vital Teeth—Office Bleaching—Safety earlier in this chapter), the thermo-photocatalytic technique appears to be the most reasonable approach.

Other Considerations

Bleaching should not be performed in the presence of caries, large pulps, areas of exposed labial dentin, or improperly placed or leaking restorations. Teeth with large restorations or with numerous small restorations also should not be bleached. Minimal amounts of exposed incisal dentin are not a contraindication for bleaching.

CLINICAL TIP. Composite resin restorations are not amenable to bleaching. If they are appropriately shaded prior to bleaching, they may need to be subsequently replaced if the surrounding tooth structure is successfully lightened.

CLINICAL TIP. The immediate postbleaching appearance is virtually always a lightening of the tooth surface. However, a large percentage of cases that ultimately attain a satisfactory result return to the original prebleaching shade after the initial one or two treatments. Therefore, a minimum of three bleaching treatments should be performed. If, after the third bleaching treatment, the teeth remain lighter in appearance for two weeks, bleaching should be continued until the desired appearance is obtained or until the treatments are no longer effective. If, after the third treatment, the appearance remains unchanged, lightening still may be possible, however, the prognosis is highly questionable.

CLINICAL TIP. The patient should be informed prior to beginning treatment that a minimum of three visits will be necessary before the effectiveness of bleaching can be ascertained. Explaining the conservative nature of this technique may help the patient overcome psychologic ambivalence about the uncertainties of the ultimate effectiveness of the treatment.

CLINICAL TIP. The patient should be informed prior to treatment that annual touch-up treatments may be necessary. In many cases, however, the frequency between required touch-ups is considerably longer or the treatments may be unnecessary. Explaining the conservative nature of this technique may help the patient overcome psychologic ambivalence about the uncertainties of the longevity of results.

Office Bleaching of Vital Teeth

Armamentarium

- Shade guide (e.g., Vita, Lumin, or Trubyte Bioform Extended Range Shade Guide, Dentsply International, Inc.)
- Protective sunglasses (patient and operator)
- Orabase-Plain (Colgate-Hoyt Laboratories)
- Cotton swabs
- Medium or heavy rubber dam
- Rubber dam frame
- Waxed dental floss
- Flat ended "plastic" instrument
- Scissors
- Wooden wedges or dental dam stabilizing chord (e.g., Wedjets, The Hygienic Corp.)
- Glass dappen dish
- Pumice
- 37% phosphoric acid (optional)
- 35% hydrogen peroxide liquid (e.g., Superoxol, Union Broach Corp., also available generically at some local pharmacies) or 35% hydrogen peroxide gel (optional) (e.g., Starbrite, Stardent Laboratories, Accel, Brite Smile)
- Bleaching light (e.g., New Image Bleaching Unit or Illuminator, Union Broach Corp.)
- Composite resin polishing cup (Vivadent USA, Inc.)
- Explorer or scaler

- Cotton gauze
- Toothbrush and toothpaste

Clinical Technique

1. Evaluate radiographs for caries, inappropriate restorations, and excessive pulp size. Minimally sized, properly placed small restorations are not contraindications for bleaching. (See the section on Vital Teeth—Office Bleaching—Other Considerations earlier in this chapter.)

CLINICAL TIP. As a comparative control, record in the patient's record the color of the teeth to be bleached. If the color of the opposing arch matches that of the teeth to be bleached, it can be used as a comparative control. This permits easy monitoring of the effectiveness of bleaching as treatment progresses.

2. Position the protective sunglasses over the patient's and operator's eyes.
3. Apply Orabase Plain (Colgate-Hoyt Laboratories) to labial and lingual (or palatal) gingiva with a cotton swab. Do not attempt at this time to keep Orabase Plain off the enamel surfaces because this may result in the placement of an insufficient quantity of material (Fig. 15—24).

CLINICAL TIP. The actual bleaching process must be completely painless without the use of anesthetic. Therefore, use only Orabase Plain (Colgate-Hoyt Laboratories). Orabase with Benzocaine may cause an unwanted partial anesthesia of the gingiva or teeth which may mask any symptoms (Fig. 15—25).

4. Place the rubber dam around each tooth to be bleached.
5. Position the rubber dam frame.

CLINICAL TIP. Do not place rubber dam clamps for retention of the rubber dam. They are cumbersome, may be painful to the patient, and will be subjected to heating by the bleaching lamp. Layers of dental floss, a strip of rubber dam, wooden wedges, or rubber dam clamp substitutes are effective and efficient retention aids and should be placed only *after* floss ligation is completed.

6. Ligate each tooth with a waxed floss slip knot. (Create a loop with the first half of a one-hand tie surgeon's square knot *before placing the floss on the tooth* is an efficient way to accomplish this.)

CLINICAL TIP. Unwaxed dental floss should not be used because it will absorb the 35% hydrogen peroxide, which can subsequently leak beneath the ligation and contact the soft tissue.

7. Gently position the floss below the lingual (or palatal) height of contour of the tooth. While the dental assistant secures the floss in position apical to the height of contour with a plastic instrument, alternate tightening the knot (Fig. 15—26) and pushing the floss apically with one index finger (Fig. 15—27) in order to secure a tight seal.

CLINICAL TIP. Place the dental floss loosely around the retention projections of the rubber dam. At this point, do not cut any of the remaining dental floss. The resulting small "ends" of the floss may partially cover the enamel and thereby impede proper contact between the tooth structure, acid etchant, and bleaching solution (Figs. 15–28, 15–29).

8. Stabilize the rubber dam bilaterally at the distal contact area of the distal-most teeth with a strip of rubber dam (Figs. 15–30 to 15–33), wooden wedges (Fig. 15–34), layers of dental floss (Fig. 15–35), or commercially produced rubber dam stabilizing material (Fig. 15–36).
9. Clean the labial enamel surfaces with pumice. Remove all of the Orabase Plain (Colgate-Hoyt Laboratories) from the labial tooth surface at this time (Fig. 15–37). Carefully determine that no soft tissue will be exposed.
10. Acid etch, rinse, and dry (optional). If only a section of the tooth surface is to be bleached because of banding or other staining, apply acid only to this section. A gel form of acid provides optimum control in this case. (See the section on Acid Etching earlier in this chapter.)

11. *Liberally* apply Orabase Plain (Colgate-Hoyt Laboratories) to the lingual (or palatal) tooth surface and the adjacent section of the rubber dam (Fig. 15–38).
12. Using the wooden end of the cotton-tipped applicator, apply Orabase Plain (Colgate-Hoyt Laboratories) to any exposed incisal dentin.

CLINICAL TIP. If only a section of the tooth surface is to be bleached because of banding or other staining, Orabase Plain (Colgate-Hoyt Laboratories) should be carefully applied to the remaining section of the tooth with a toothpick or the wooden end of a broken cotton-tipped applicator. This will prevent the bleaching solution from contacting that section of tooth structure.

13. Adjust the dental chair so the patient is seated in a comfortable upright position.

CLINICAL TIP. Stereo headphones playing the patient's choice of music often help the patient to pass the time pleasantly.

14. If the thermo-photocatalytic technique is used, po-

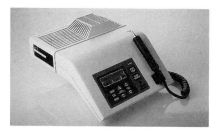

FIG. 15–23. Bleaching unit with paddle shaped heating attachment (Union Broach).

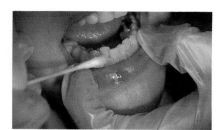

FIG. 15–24. Liberal application of Orabase-Plain is essential to protect the gingiva from contact with the bleaching agent.

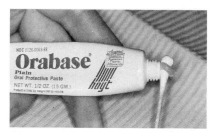

FIG. 15–25. Orabase-Plain should be used to protect the tissue. The use of any form of topical anesthetic is contraindicated during office bleaching procedures.

FIG. 15–26 and 15–27. Alternately tightening and apically positioning the knot efficiently positions the floss ligature.

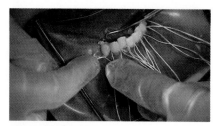

FIG. 15–26

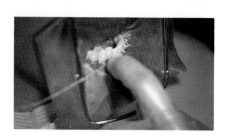

FIG. 15–27

FIG. 15–28. The free ends of the dental floss are loosely wrapped around the retention points of the rubber dam frame.

FIG. 15–29. Repositioning the rubber dam secures the free ends of the dental floss.

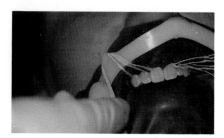

FIG. 15–28

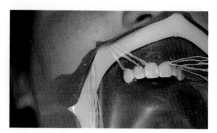

FIG. 15–29

sition the heat lamp so that it is 13 in. from the labial surface of the central incisors.

CLINICAL TIP. If the New Image Bleaching Unit (Union Broach Corp.) is used, cover one-half of the front of the light source with a piece of cardboard. (Cover the lower half when bleaching maxillary teeth and the upper half when bleaching mandibular teeth.) This significantly lessens the amount of heat transmitted to the lip areas opposite the arch being bleached (i.e., mandibular lip when the maxillary arch is bleached and the maxillary lip when the mandibular arch is bleached). This will usually eliminate the need for placement of wet cotton gauze on these lip areas, which would be necessary if the entire circumference of the light source was exposed (Figs. 15–39 to 15–41).

15. If the gel technique is used, apply the 35% hydro-

gen peroxide gel onto the teeth according to the manufacturer's instructions and skip to step 19.

If the thermo-photocatalytic technique is used, place a small amount of 35% hydrogen peroxide into a dappen dish. Apply the hydrogen peroxide liquid onto the teeth with a cotton-tipped applicator (Fig. 15–42).

CLINICAL TIP. It is not necessary to use cotton gauze or other retention mechanism for the liquid hydrogen peroxide.

16. Turn on the bleaching unit. The warmest portion of the projected light is a zone approximately three-

FIG. 15–30. A small strip of rubber dam (approximately one-eighth to one-quarter in. wide and three-quarters to 1 in. long) is a preferable substitute for metal rubber dam clamps.

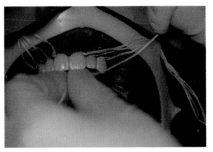

FIG. 15–31. The rubber dam strip is stretched until it approximates the thickness of dental floss.

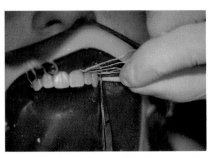

FIG. 15–32. After positioning the rubber dam strip below the contact area, the labial portion is stretched and cut at a point near the tooth.

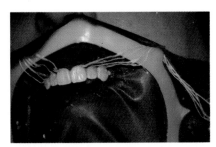

FIG. 15–33. A properly positioned and cut rubber dam strip.

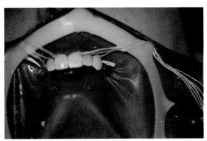

FIG. 15–34. A wooden wedge may be used in lieu of metal rubber dam clamps.

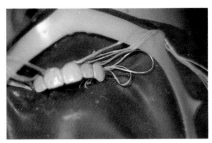

FIG. 15–35. Multiple folds of dental floss are an additional alternative to metal rubber dam clamps.

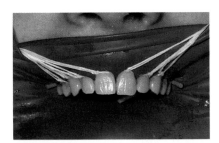

FIG. 15–36. Commercially prepared rubber dam "wedges" are used in a manner similar to the rubber dam strip (see Figures 15–30 to 15–33).

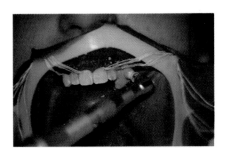

FIG. 15–37. The labial enamel surfaces are pumiced to remove plaque, debris, and remaining Orabase-Plain.

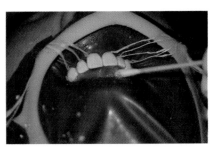

FIG. 15–38. Orabase-Plain is applied liberally to the palatal (or lingual) tooth surface and rubber dam.

quarters of an inch wide, beginning approximately three-eighths of an inch in from the periphery of the projected light beam.[92] Direct this area of the light source on the teeth to be bleached. Adjust the heating lamp so that the patient has no sensation in the teeth. The patient may, however, experience a slight warming of the lips.

CLINICAL TIP. Do not adjust the heating lamp to just below the pain threshold because this may result in postoperative sensitivity. The lamp should be adjusted to just below the "sensation threshold." This usually eliminates the need for placement of wet cotton gauze over the lip areas of the bleached arch.

17. Re-wet the enamel surface with 35% hydrogen peroxide as needed to prevent the drying of the tooth surface.

CLINICAL TIP. Discontinue the bleaching process immediately if any untoward symptoms occur.

18. After 30 minutes, recline the dental chair.
19. Gently and thoroughly rinse the patient's teeth of any remaining hydrogen peroxide with warm water. Avoid splattering. The patient's eyes should be closed.

CLINICAL TIP. Do not rinse with cold water. The sudden change in temperature may be detrimental to the pulp. If the air water syringe does not have a heat control gauge, a cup filled with warm tap water may be used. Avoid splattering.

20. Dry the teeth and gently polish them with a composite resin polishing cup using intermittent light pressure. This will partially restore an enamel-like luster. The patient's eyes should be closed during the polishing procedure. When the teeth are subsequently wet with saliva, they will appear to have a normal luster.

21. Cut the dental floss ligations as close to the knot as possible.
22. Untie the slip knot by sliding an explorer or scaler underneath the knot and pulling in a labial direction. Note that the knot will remain on one end of the floss.
23. Remove the floss using college pliers.

CLINICAL TIP. The knot that remains on the floss generally will not pass through the embrasure space. It is, therefore, necessary to grasp the knot with the college pliers and pull in a labiogingival direction. Do not attempt to remove the floss in an incisal direction through the contact area of the teeth.

24. Carefully remove the rubber dam and wipe the bulk of the Orabase Plain (Colgate-Hoyt Laboratories) from the labial and palatal (or lingual) gingiva with cotton gauze.

CLINICAL TIP. If an appropriate amount of Orabase Plain (Colgate-Hoyt Laboratories) was used, patients often find the sensation after the rubber dam is removed to be quite unpleasant. Provide a toothbrush and toothpaste in the operatory or the lavatory for immediate post-treatment use.

25. Advise the patient to avoid or severely limit the use of any substance that may stain the teeth (e.g., tobacco, tea, cola, coffee), especially for 2 weeks following the bleaching treatment.

CLINICAL TIP. If patients will not comply with food and beverage precautions, advise them to use a straw to prevent any potentially staining liquid from contacting the labial tooth surfaces.

FIG. 15–39. The bleaching lamp projects a focused circular light.

FIG. 15–40. A semicircular piece of cardboard is affixed to the front surface of the lower one-half of the bleaching lamp.

FIG. 15–41. Covering one-half of the light source significantly lessens the amount of heat transmitted to the lip areas opposite the arch being bleached. This usually eliminates the need for placement of wet gauze on these lip areas.

FIG. 15–42. Hydrogen peroxide is applied directly to the labial enamel. It is not necessary to use cotton gauze or any other mechanism to retain the bleaching agent.

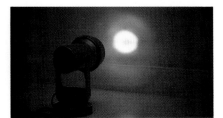

FIG. 15–39

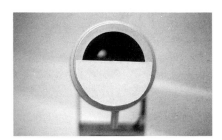

FIG. 15–40

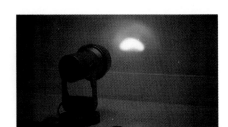

FIG. 15–41

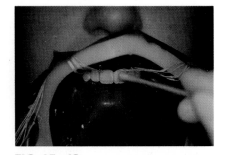

FIG. 15–42

26. Schedule another appointment in 3 weeks, if necessary.

Home Bleaching of Vital Teeth

General Considerations. Patient self-application of bleaching agents performed outside of the dental office is a recent variant of the office bleaching technique described above. Carbamide peroxide or dilute hydrogen peroxide are the bleaching agents most often used, usually in a liquid or gel form. The bleaching agent is held in close proximity to the teeth by means of a custom fabricated tray (Fig. 15–43). Techniques vary widely as to the design of the custom tray, the materials used, the use of spacers on the working model, the use of foam liners, the exact formulation of the bleaching agent, and the frequency and duration of application of the materials.

This lack of consensus concerning treatment techniques and the absence of multiple source long-term studies precludes the inclusion of any specific step by step instructions based on purely scientific evidence.

Safety. Within 1 hour, over one-half of the bleaching agent is ingested by the patient.[93] The total amount of systemic exposure, therefore, depends on the frequency of replenishment. Controlled long-term studies of the effects of systemic ingestion and mucosal contact with bleaching agents used in this manner are lacking. The effects of hydrogen peroxide on tooth structure and the dental pulp when used in office bleaching techniques have been discussed above. (See the section on Vital Teeth—Office Bleaching—Safety earlier in this chapter.) It may be inappropriate to infer that these effects hold true for the same or similar bleaching agents used in the home technique because of the urea component of the carbamide peroxide used in some systems and because the exposure times are longer and the recovery times are less frequent and of shorter duration than the parameters investigated in these studies.

Soft tissue sloughing, nausea, sore throat, tooth hypersensitivity, and temporomandibular disorder secondary to tray usage have been reported,[93] although long-term effects, if any, have not been adequately investigated.

Other possible side effects include periodontal tissue damage with prolonged use, delayed wound healing, an alteration of the normal oral flora leading to hypertrophy of the tongue papillae, chronic oral infection from opportunistic organisms such as candida albicans, and inhibition of some pulpal enzymes.[94]

The mutagenic potential[94] of the free radicals released by hydrogen peroxide, as well as their ability to potentiate the effects of known carcinogens, have also been reported.[95] Therefore, smoking,[94] or the use of any known carcinogen, while performing home bleaching is contraindicated. In addition, this technique should not be used by pregnant women.

Proper informed consent and caution is appropriate because many factors involved in home bleaching are unknown. In 1991, the Food and Drug Administration

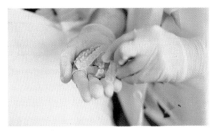

FIG. 15–43. Home bleaching tray (White and Brite).

questioned the safety of these techniques. The practitioner should, therefore, determine whether any prohibitions or restrictions are currently applicable.

NONVITAL TEETH

General Considerations

Discoloration of endodontically treated teeth has been treated with acid/abrasion (if the staining is superficial and therefore not related to the devitalization), bleaching agents (with or without heat), or a combination of both. Treatment is expedited by the absence of pulpal tissue concerns. Bleaching agents can be applied both internally (directly into the empty pulp chamber) and externally. Techniques in which bleaching solutions remain in the pulp cavity for limited periods of time (the so-called "walking" bleach) also have been advocated.

Safety

External resorption is a possible sequela of internal bleaching. It is likely that resorption occurs as a result of one or more of the following:

1. In 10% of all teeth, the cementoenamel junction is defective or absent, resulting in a portion of the tooth being devoid of cementum coverage.[96] Thirty-five percent hydrogen peroxide may denature the dentin, invoking a foreign body response by elements in the approximating gingival tissue, ultimately causing cervical resorption.[97]

2. Internally applied 35% hydrogen peroxide may directly contact the periodontal membrane or the gingival sulcus by passing through patent dentinal tubules[98,99] or through lateral root canals or accessory foramina.[100] This may elicit an inflammatory reaction, ultimately resulting in cervical resorption.

3. Hydrogen peroxide may inadvertently directly contact the periodontal membrane tissues during the bleaching procedure, causing cervical resorption.[99]

4. Bleaching agents may infiltrate between the gutta percha and the root canal walls. They could then communicate with the periodontal membrane through the dentinal tubules, lateral canals, or apex. This may invoke a resorptive process anywhere along the root area, including the apical regions.

5. Heat application during treatment may invoke a resorptive process.[99]

6. Thirty-five percent hydrogen peroxide mixed with sodium perborate can lower the pH in the periodontal membrane area, which may induce cervical re-sorption.[100]

It has also been demonstrated in vitro that when heat is combined with 35% hydrogen peroxide-sodium perborate paste during an internal bleaching technique, not only is the crown bleached, but also the entire root surface. Significantly less of the root surface is bleached when the heat is omitted.[101] This suggests that heat facilitates the permeation of bleaching agent, in all directions, thus increasing the likelihood of external resorption through any of the above mechanisms.

Tooth discoloration is often the result of a traumatic injury to the tooth. Resorption also may be a sequela of the original trauma.

Other Considerations

The walking technique primarily involves the use of hydrogen peroxide, sodium perborate, or a combination of the two. The combination apparently enhances the effectiveness of the treatment.[38] It has been demonstrated, however, that a large percentage of cases can be successfully bleached using sodium perborate alone.[38,102] Therefore, the use of the more caustic 35% hydrogen peroxide may be unnecessary for the successful treatment of some cases.

A comparison of thermocatalytic bleaching using 35% hydrogen peroxide, walking bleaching using a mixture of sodium perborate and 35% hydrogen peroxide, and a combination of the two showed all to be equally effective in bleaching the crowns of extracted pulpless teeth which were experimentally stained with hemolyzed red blood cells. However, the roots of the teeth that were exposed to heat were also bleached.[101] This suggests that heat may potentiate the penetration of the bleaching process through the tooth. Therefore the use of heat, with its potential risks, may be unnecessary for successful treatment of some cases, however, it may be helpful in unresponsive cases.

Polymorphonuclear leukocytic and osteoclastic activity is enhanced in an acidic environment.[103] An in vitro study[100] demonstrated that a mixture of sodium perborate powder and 35% hydrogen peroxide placed in the pulp chamber resulted in an increased acidity of the external tooth structure. The subsequent placement of calcium hydroxide paste into the pulp chamber caused a significant elevation to an alkaline pH. Presumably, similar pH changes in vivo would cause comparable pH changes in the approximating periodontal membrane. An alkaline environment is antagonistic to osteoclastic activity.[100]

Treatment Considerations

The available information suggests the following procedures and treatment sequence should provide the best chance of reducing postoperative sequelae when bleaching nonvital teeth:

Proper Endodontic Treatment. A properly sealed endodontic filling is a prerequisite before attempting

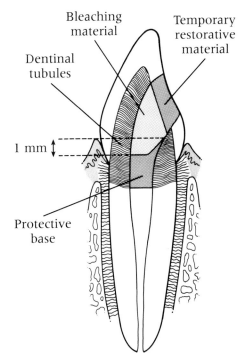

FIG. 15–44. The "walking" bleach technique. The direction of the dentinal tubules requires that the bleaching material extend 1 mm apical to the level of desired bleaching. The lingual portion of the protective base (and the proximal extensions which are not shown in this cross-sectional representation) extends incisally to a supragingival level when possible. The temporary restorative material extends into undercut areas to prevent dislodgement.

bleaching. Silver points may be dislodged during the preparatory stages and, therefore, must be replaced with gutta percha prior to bleaching.

Protective Base. A protective base of zinc phosphate or polycarboxylate cement at least 2 mm thick should be placed between the bleaching agent and the gutta percha.

CLINICAL TIP. The cervical dentinal tubules are obliquely oriented and tilt in an incisal direction from the pulp chamber toward the tooth surface (see Fig. 15–44). To compensate for this, the incisal termination of the base should be 1 mm below the height of the free gingival margin if the entire clinical crown is visible during maximum smiling or functioning (see Chapter 11—Porcelain—Laminate Veneer and Other Partial Coverage Restorations.)

CLINICAL TIP. If the gingival portion of the clinical crown is not visible during function or maximum smiling, the incisal termination of the base should be appropriately positioned to further reduce the chance of cervical resorption. Explaining this advantage may help the patient overcome psychologic ambivalence about leaving a segment of the tooth unbleached.

CLINICAL TIP. *The position of the lip during maximum smiling may be deceptive. Patients with unattractive smiles often habitually adapt a high smile line lip position, which is significantly lower than anatomically possible. After successful bleaching, this smile line may significantly change because the psychologic barriers inhibiting full smiling have been removed. Therefore, this crucial lip position must be critically evaluated before the final height of the base is determined.*

Limited Treatment Duration and Frequency.

Treatment time should be limited as much as possible. As soon as a successful result is achieved, bleaching material should be removed. A successful result is the attainment of an appropriate shade or possibly a shade slightly lighter than desired to allow for possible regression.

CLINICAL TIP. *If a slightly lighter shade is considered, it should not be so light as to be cosmetically unacceptable to the patient in the event color regression does not occur.*

Avoid Heat and Hydrogen Peroxide if Possible.

A "walking" bleach therapy should be used. Only a mixture of sodium perborate and water should be used for the first two treatments. (Sodium perborate mixed with water is alkaline, whereas 35% hydrogen peroxide alone or mixed with sodium perborate is more acidic.)[104] If this is unsuccessful, a mixture of sodium perborate and 35% hydrogen peroxide should be attempted for one more treatment. If this also is unsuccessful, a final thermocatalytic treatment should be attempted.

Calcium Hydroxide Application.

The final visit should involve the removal of all bleaching agents and the application of a thick paste of calcium hydroxide mixed with sterile water. This should be left in the canal for 4 days. Although a mixture of sodium perborate and water is not acidic, calcium hydroxide and water is more alkaline.

Treatment Protocol and Rationale

The above considerations suggest the following protocol for bleaching nonvital teeth (Fig. 15–45).

First bleaching treatment: sodium perborate alone, without heat.

Second bleaching treatment (if necessary): repeat of first treatment.

Third bleaching treatment (if necessary): sodium perborate and 35% hydrogen peroxide without heat.

Fourth bleaching treatment (if necessary): sodium perborate and 35% hydrogen peroxide with heat followed immediately by calcium hydroxide therapy (see Final treatment).

Final treatment: calcium hydroxide paste therapy for 4 days. The calcium hydroxide is placed after completion of the "walking" bleach treatments or immediately after the thermocatalytic treatment.

The time between each bleaching treatment is 2 to 3 days. This limits the exposure to the bleaching agents to a maximum of 2 weeks or less. Each successive step is only performed if the previous step is unsuccessful. Only a maximum of 4 bleaching treatments are attempted. The chance of a successful result from further bleaching is slight and does not warrant increasing the risk of external resorption.

This protocol limits the chance of postoperative sequelae by:

1. Limiting the duration of exposure to resorptive stimuli
2. Limiting the frequency of exposure to resorptive stimuli
3. Providing a treatment sequence that begins with the least potential for negative postoperative sequelae
4. Sequentially progressing to treatments with higher postoperative sequelae potential only when necessary
5. Including calcium hydroxide therapy after bleaching to raise the pH in the periodontal area.

Nevertheless, the possibility of resorption still exists, and the patient should be so informed. It has been shown that resorption can occur up to 7 years after bleaching has been performed.[99]

Nonvital Bleaching

Armamentarium

- Orabase Plain (Colgate-Hoyt Laboratories)
- Protective glasses for the patient
- Protective clear glasses for the operator
- Cotton swabs
- Medium or heavy rubber dam
- Rubber dam frame
- Rubber dam clamps
- Waxed dental floss
- Flat ended "plastic" instrument
- Scissors
- Wooden wedges
- Sodium perborate powder U.S.P. (Sultan, Inc.; also available at some local pharmacies)
- Glass slab
- Cement spatula
- Explorer or scaler
- 35% hydrogen peroxide (e.g., Superoxol, Union Broach Corp.; also available generically at some local pharmacies)
- Pumice
- 37% phosphoric acid
- Placement instrument (e.g., instrument provided in Delton Pit and Fissure Sealant Kit, Johnson & Johnson Dental Care Co.) (see text below)
- Bleaching unit (heating type) with paddle and probe attachments (e.g., Illuminator, Union Broach Corp.)
- Temporary restorative material (e.g., Cavit, ESPE-Premier Sales Corp.; Provit, Svedia, USA)
- Cotton gauze
- Composite resin polishing cup (Vivadent USA, Inc.)
- Toothbrush and toothpaste
- Calcium hydroxide powder U.S.P. (Eli Lilly and Co.)
- Sterile water (Abbott Laboratories)

Clinical Technique

1. Evaluate the high smile line.

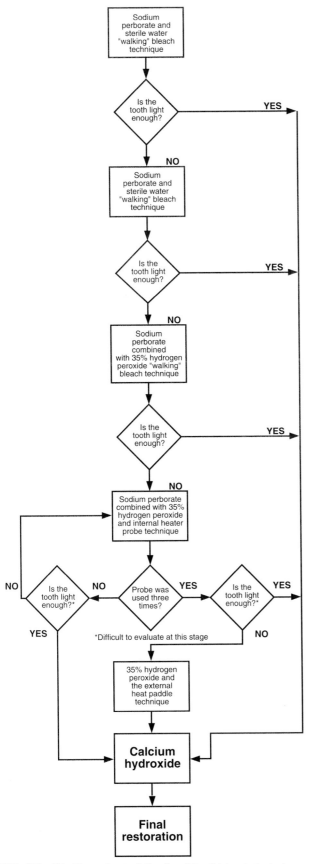

FIG. 15−45. Flow chart of the "walking" bleach technique.

The following text accompanies the flow chart:

- Sodium perborate and sterile water "walking" bleach technique
- Is the tooth light enough? — YES
- NO
- Sodium perborate and sterile water "walking" bleach technique
- Is the tooth light enough? — YES
- NO
- Sodium perborate combined with 35% hydrogen peroxide "walking" bleach technique
- Is the tooth light enough? — YES
- NO
- Sodium perborate combined with 35% hydrogen peroxide and internal heater probe technique
- Is the tooth light enough?* — NO / YES
- Probe was used three times? — YES
- Is the tooth light enough?* — YES / NO
- *Difficult to evaluate at this stage
- 35% hydrogen peroxide and the external heat paddle technique
- **Calcium hydroxide**
- **Final restoration**

CLINICAL TIP. Be certain of the precise position of the lip during maximum smiling because it may change following therapy. (See the Clinical Tip in the section on Treatment Considerations.)

2. If the cervical area of the tooth remains hidden by the lip during maximum smiling and functioning, consult with the patient about bleaching only the visible portions of the crown.

CLINICAL TIP. Leaving a gingival segment of the tooth unbleached lessens the chance of cervical resorption. (See the Clinical Tip in the section on Treatment Considerations.) Explaining this advantage may help the patient overcome psychologic ambivalence about this alternative.

3. Position protective glasses over the patient's eyes.
4. Apply Orabase Plain (Colgate-Hoyt Laboratories) to the labial and lingual (or palatal) gingiva.
5. Isolate the tooth with a rubber dam (Figs. 15−46, 15−47).
  A. If the endodontic access opening is distant from the palatal or lingual gingival tissues, only the tooth to be bleached needs to be isolated.
  B. If the endodontic access opening or existing restorations are close to the gingival tissues, thereby impeding proper rubber dam clamp placement, isolate one additional tooth on each side of the discolored tooth and ligate the discolored tooth with waxed dental floss. (See Office Bleaching of Vital Teeth—Clinical Technique—Step 7.)
6. Apply additional Orabase Plain (Colgate-Hoyt Laboratories) to the rubber dam and the tooth (Fig. 15−47).
7. Remove the access restoration and any remaining pulp tissue from the crown (Fig. 15−48). Leave a slight undercut in the access opening to retain the temporary restorative material that will be placed later (Fig. 15−44).

CLINICAL TIP. When performing initial endodontic therapy, carefully remove all tissue, debris, endodontic sealers, and filling materials from the sometimes elusive pulp horns and lateral extensions of the pulp chamber. This will help prevent subsequent tooth discoloration (see Fig. 15−4).

8. Remove excess gutta percha and endodontic sealer.
  A. If the entire crown is visible during function (see steps 1 and 2) remove gutta percha to 3 mm subgingival to the free marginal gingiva.
  B. If more than 2 mm of the gingival portion of the clinical crown is not visible during function (see steps 1 and 2), remove gutta percha to 5 mm below the high smile line. This will allow for a 2 mm base and a 3 mm margin of error.

CLINICAL TIP. Measure the length of the labial portion of the tooth to be bleached with a periodontal probe using the incisal edge as a reference point. Then use this measurement and reference point palatally (or lingually) and within the pulp chamber to determine the precise amount of gutta percha to remove.

CLINICAL TIP. The cervical dentinal tubules tilt in a slightly incisal direction. Therefore, the base should be placed to a level approximately 1 mm below the level of desired bleaching (Fig. 15–44).

9. Place a 2 mm thick base of zinc phosphate or polycarboxylate cement.

CLINICAL TIP. Because only the labial portion of the tooth must be bleached, extend the lingual and proximal portions of the base as incisally as possible in order to help prevent infiltration of the bleaching solution through the lingual and proximal wall dentinal tubules (Fig. 15–44). This will further reduce the chance of cervical resorption.

10. Mix a thick paste of sodium perborate and sterile water on a glass slab and place the mixture into the tooth.

CLINICAL TIP. The mixture can be easily manipulated with the placement instrument provided with the Delton Pit and Fissure Sealant Kit (Johnson & Johnson Dental Care Co.) (Fig. 15-49). The sodium perborate must be thoroughly crushed to produce a homogenous paste, otherwise an excess of liquid will be drawn into the applicator tube.

11. Tamp the mixture into place with a wet cotton pellet so that appropriate space is provided for the temporary restorative material.

CLINICAL TIP. Be certain that the walls of the access opening are cleared of bleaching material in order to ensure an intimate seal of the temporary restorative material.

12. Seal the access with temporary restorative material.
13. Schedule the next appointment for the patient for 2 to 3 days later.
14. If a successful result is achieved after 2 to 3 days, skip to step 32.
15. If a successful result has not been achieved after 2 to 3 days, isolate the tooth with rubber dam, remove the temporary filling, carefully wash the internal tooth chamber with water and repeat steps 10 through 13 one additional time.
16. If a successful result is achieved after 2 to 3 days, skip to step 32.
17. If, after two attempts with sodium perborate paste, a successful result has not been achieved, mix a thick paste of sodium perborate and 35% hydrogen peroxide on a glass slab and place the mixture into the tooth.

CLINICAL TIP. Place the mixture with the placement instrument provided with the Delton Pit and Fissure Sealant Kit (Johnson & Johnson Dental Care Co.). (See the Clinical Tip between steps 10 and 11.)

18. Tamp the mixture into place with a wet cotton pellet so that appropriate space is provided for the temporary restorative material.

CLINICAL TIP. Be certain that the walls of the access opening are cleared of bleaching material in order to ensure an intimate seal of the temporary restorative material.

19. Seal the access with temporary restorative material.
20. Schedule the next appointment for the patient for 2 to 3 days later.
21. If a successful result is achieved after 2 to 3 days, skip to step 32.
22. If two attempts with sodium perborate paste and one attempt with sodium perborate combined with hydrogen peroxide have not produced a successful result, thermocatalytic bleaching may be attempted.
23. Isolate, protect, and clean the teeth. Use the same technique described for Vital Teeth Office Bleaching, steps 2 through 9.
24. Acid etch, rinse, and dry (optional). (See the section on Acid Etching earlier in this chapter.)
25. Mix a thick paste of 35% hydrogen peroxide and sodium perborate and place the mixture into the tooth.

CLINICAL TIP. Place the mixture with the placement instrument provided with the Delton Pit and Fissure Sealant Kit (Johnson & Johnson Dental Care Co.). (See the Clinical Tip between steps 10 and 11.)

26. Insert the probe attachment of the heating instrument for 2 to 5 minutes.
27. Carefully flush out the bleaching solution with water and high-speed suction. Be careful to avoid splattering the caustic bleaching solution.

CLINICAL TIP. It is difficult to periodically assess the adequacy of bleaching at this stage. Teeth may appear transiently lighter because of desiccation and visual contrast with the rubber dam.

28. Repeat the application of sodium perborate, hydrogen peroxide, and heat (steps 25 through 27) for a maximum of three attempts, if needed. If a successful result is achieved, skip to step 32.
29. Apply a single layer of unfilled gauze saturated with 35% hydrogen peroxide to the labial surface.
30. Place the paddle shaped heating attachment onto the labial surface.
31. Re-wet the gauze as it dries. Check frequently for sufficient color change. Apply heat for a maximum of 10 to 15 minutes. Then carefully rinse the labial surface with water, evacuating with high-speed suction.

CLINICAL TIP. No additional bleaching treatments should be attempted. The chances of a successful result after further bleaching is slight and does not warrant increasing the risk of possible cervical resorption.

32. Carefully wash the internal tooth chamber with water.
33. Mix a thick paste of calcium hydroxide powder and sterile water and place the mixture into the tooth.

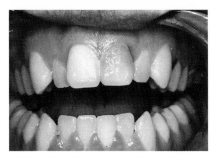

FIG. 15–46. Preoperative view of staining caused by the deposition of hemorrhagic byproducts into the dentinal tubules following pulpal trauma (courtesy of Dr. Kenneth W. Aschheim).

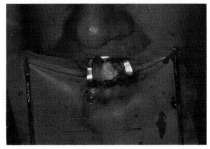

FIG. 15–47. Tooth following rubber dam isolation and placement of Ora-base-Plain (courtesy of Dr. Kenneth W. Aschheim).

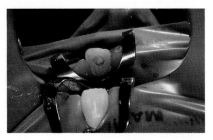

FIG. 15–48. Occlusal view of access opening with gutta-percha in place. The appropriate amount of gutta-percha must be removed prior to the placement of the bleaching agent into the chamber (courtesy of Dr. Kenneth W. Aschheim).

FIG. 15–49. A thick paste of sodium perborate and sterile water is placed into the pulp chamber. The mixture can be easily manipulated with the Delton Pit and Fissure Sealant Kit placement instrument (Johnson and Johnson) (courtesy of Dr. Kenneth W. Aschheim).

FIG. 15–50. Six-month postoperative view following treatment (courtesy of Dr. Kenneth W. Aschheim).

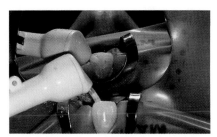

FIG. 15–49

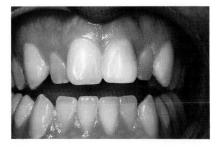

FIG. 15–50

34. Tamp the paste into place with a wet cotton pellet so that appropriate space is provided for the temporary restorative material.
35. Seal the access with temporary restorative material.
36. Schedule the next appointment for the patient for 4 days later.
37. After 4 days, remove the calcium hydroxide paste and restore the tooth (Fig. 15–50).

POSTOPERATIVE COMPLICATIONS

It has been shown that resorption can occur up to 7 years after bleaching has been performed.[99] Periodic follow up radiographs, therefore, are necessary. Cervical resorption can be treated with tooth extrusion, surgical curettage, and calcium hydroxide treatment.[38]

CONCLUSION

The use of bleaching agents or acid/abrasion techniques provides an effective and conservative approach to the removal of unesthetic discolorations from vital and nonvital teeth. As with all therapeutic modalities, proper diagnosis and treatment planning is essential.

REFERENCES

1. Panati, C.: Panati's Extraordinary Origins of Everyday Things. New York, Harper and Row, p. 210, 1987.
2. Westlake, A: Bleaching teeth by electricity. Am J Dent Sci 29:101, 1895.
3. Adams, T.C: Enamel color modifications by controlled hydrochloric acid pumice abrasion. A review with case summaries. Indiana Dent Assoc J 66:23, 1987.
4. Ames, J.W.: Removing stains from mottled enamel. J Am Dent Assoc 24:1674, 1937.
5. Younger, H.B.: Bleaching fluorine stain from mottled enamel. Texas Dent J 57:380, 1939.
6. McInnes, J.: Removing brown stain from teeth. Ariz Dent J 12:13, 1966.
7. Cohen, B.A. and Parkins, F.M.: Bleaching tetracycline-stained teeth. Oral Surg Oral Med Oral Pathol 19:465, 1970.
8. Schwachman, H. and Schuster, A.: The tetracyclines applied pharmacology. Pediatr Clin North Am 3:295, 1956.
9. Albert, A. and Rees, C.W.: Avidity of the tetracyclines for the cations of metals. Nature 177:433, 1956.
10. Finerman, G.A.M. and Milch, R.A.: In vitro binding of tetracyclines to calcium. Nature 198:486, 1963.
11. Stewart, D.J.: The effects of tetracyclines upon the dentition. Br J Dermatol 76:374, 1964.
12. Weinstein, L.: Antimicrobial agents. In Goodman L.S., Gilman A. (eds.): The Pharmacologic Basis Of Therapeutics. New York, MacMillan Publishing Co., p. 1183, 1975.
13. Sayegh, F.S. and Gassner, E.: Sites of tetracycline deposition in rat dentin. J Dent Res 46:1474, 1967.
14. Sayegh, F.S.: H3-proline and tetracycline as marking agents in the study of reparative dentine formation. Oral Surg 23:221, 1967.
15. Milch, R.A., et al.: Bone localization of the tetracycline. J Natl Cancer Inst 18:87, 1957.
16. Urist, M. and Ibsen, K.: Chemical reactivity of mineralized tissue with oxytetracycline. Arch Pathol 76:484, 1963.
17. Martin, N.O. and Barnard, P.D.: The prevalence of tetracycline staining in erupted teeth. Med J Aust 1:1286, 1969.

18. Bridges, J.B., Owens, P.D.A., and Stewart, D.J.: Tetracycline and teeth—an experimental investigation into five types in the rat. Br Dent J 1:306, 1969.

19. Walton, R.E., et al.: External bleaching of tetracycline stained teeth in dogs. J Endodont 8:536, 1982.

20. Stewart, D.J.: Teeth discolored by tetracycline bleaching following exposure to daylight. Dent Practitioner 20:309, 1969.

21. Lin, L.C., Pitts, D.L., and Burgess L.W.: An investigation into the feasibility of photobleaching tetracycline-stained teeth. J Endodont 14:293, 1988.

22. Ibsen, K.H., Urist, M.R., and Sognnaes, R.F.: Differences among tetracyclines with respect to the staining of teeth. J Pediatr 67:459, 1965.

23. Wallman, I.S., and Hilton, H.B.: Teeth pigmented by tetracycline. Lancet 1:827, 1962.

24. Davies, A.K., McKellar, J.F., Phillips, G.D., and Reid, A.G.: Photochemical oxidation of tetracycline in aqueous solution. J Chem Soc Perkin Trans II 1979;369–375.

25. Davies, A.K., Cundall, R.B., Dandiker, Y., and Slifkin, M.A.: Photo-oxidation of tetracycline adsorbed on hydroxyapatite in relation to the light-induced staining of teeth. J Dent Res 65:936, 1985.

26. Moffitt, J.M., Cooley, R.O., Olsen, N.H., and Hefferren, J.J.: Prediction of tetracycline-induced tooth discoloration. J Am Dent Assoc 88:547, 1974.

27. Genet, M.T.: Effects of administration of tetracycline in pregnancy on the primary dentition of the offspring. J Oral Med 25:75, 1970.

28. Swallow, J.N.: Discoloration of primary dentition after maternal tetracycline ingestion in pregnancy. Lancet 2:611, 1964.

29. Grossman, E.R., Walchek, A., and Freeman, H.: Tetracycline and permanent teeth: the relation between dose and tooth color. Pediatrics 47:567, 1971.

30. Wehman, J., and Porteous, J.R.: Tetracycline staining of teeth: a report of clinical material. J Dent Res 42:1111, 1963.

31. Eisenberg, E. and Bernick, S.M.: Anomalies of the teeth with stains and discolorations. J Prevent Dent 2:7, 1975.

32. McEvoy, S.A.: Chemical agents for removing intrinsic stains from vital teeth. II. Current techniques and their clinical application. Quint Int 20:379, 1989.

33. Stewart, R.E., et al: Pediatric Dentistry. St Louis, C.V. Mosby Co., p. 87, 1982.

34. Swift E.J.: A method for bleaching discolored vital teeth. Quint Int 19:607, 1988.

35. Shafer, W.G., Hine, M.K., and Levy, B.L.: A Textbook of Oral Pathology, 3rd Ed. Philadelphia, Saunders, 1974.

36. Jordan, R.E. and Boksman, L.: Conservative vital bleaching treatment of discolored dentition. Compend Contin Ed Dent 5:803, 1984.

37. Grossman, L.I., Oliet, S., and del Rio, C.E.: Endodontic Practice, 11th Ed. Philadelphia, Lea & Febiger, p. 436, 1988.

38. Ho, S. and Goerig, A.C.: An in vitro comparison of different bleaching agents in the discolored tooth. J Endodont 15:106, 1989.

39. Imber, S., and Gorfil C.: A one visit bleaching technique for the endodontically treated tooth. Refuat Hoshinayim 4:7, 1986.

40. Van der Burgt, T.P. and Plasschaert, A.J.M.: Bleaching of tooth discoloration caused by endodontic sealers. J Endodont 12:231, 1986.

41. Crane, D.L.: The walking bleach technique for endodontically treated teeth. Chi Dent Soc Rev 1984; January-February 77:49–51.

42. Gutierrez, J., and Guzman, M.: Tooth discoloration in endodontic procedures. Oral Surg 26:706, 1968.

43. Nutting, E.B. and Poe, G.S.: Chemical bleaching of discolored endodontically treated teeth. Dent Clin North Am 11:655, 1967.

44. Andreasen, J.O., et al: The effect of traumatic injuries to the primary teeth on their permanent successors: a clinical and histologic study of 117 injured permanent teeth. Scand J Dent Res 79:219, 1971.

45. McEvoy, S.A.: Bleaching stains related to trauma or periapical inflammation. Compend Contin Ed Dent 7:420, 1986.

46. Croll, T.P.: Enamel microabrasion for removal of superficial dysmineralization and decalcification defects. J Am Dent Assoc 120:411, 1990.

47. Finn, S.B.: Clinical Pedodontics, 4th Ed. Philadelphia, Saunders, p. 301, 1973.

48. Faunce, F.: Management of discolored teeth. Dent Clin North Am 27:657, 1983; 27:657–670.

49. Atkinson, H.F.: An investigation into the permeability of human enamel using osmotic methods. Br Dent J 83:205, 1947.

50. Bartlestone, H.J.: Radioiodine penetration through intake with uptake by bloodstream and thyroid gland. J Dent Res 30:728, 1951.

51. Griffen, R.E., et al.: Effects of solutions used to treat dental fluorosis on permeability of teeth. J Endodont 3:139, 1977.

52. Hardwick, J.L. and Fremlin, J.G.: Isotope studies on the permeability of the dental enamel to small particles and ions. Proc Royal Soc Med 52:752, 1959.

53. Seale, N.S., McIntosh, J.E., and Taylor, A.N.: Pulpal reaction to bleaching of teeth in dogs. J Dent Res 60:948, 1981.

54. Bailey, R.W. and Christen, A.G.: Bleaching of vital teeth stained with endemic dental fluorosis. Oral Surg 26:871, 1968.

55. Bailey, R.W. and Christen, A.G.: Effects of a bleaching technique on the labial enamel of human teeth stained with endemic dental fluorosis. J Dent Res 49:168, 1970.

56. Colon, P.G.: Improving the appearance of severely fluorosed teeth. J Am Dent Assoc 86:1329, 1973.

57. Colon, P.G.: Removing fluorosis stain from teeth. Quint Int 2:89, 1971.

58. Douglas, W.A.: A history of dentistry in Colorado 1859–1959 (book review). J Col State Dent Assoc 38:19, 1960.

59. McCloskey, R.J.: A technique for removal of fluorosis stains. J Am Dent Assoc 109:63, 1984.

60. McMurray, C.A.: Removal of stains from mottled enamel of teeth. Texas Dent J 59:293, 1941.

61. Raper, H.R., and Manser, J.G.: Removal of brown stain from fluorine mottled teeth. Dent Digest 47:390, 1941.

62. Smith, H.V. and McInnes, J.W.: Further studies on methods of removing brown stain from mottled teeth. J Am Dent Assoc 29:571, 1942.

63. Wayman, B.E. and Cooley, R.L.: Vital bleaching technique for treatment of endemic fluorosis. Gen Dent 29:424, 1981.

64. Croll T.P. and Cavanaugh R.R.: Enamel color modification by controlled hydrochloric acid-pumice abrasion. II. Further examples. Quint Int 17:157, 1986.

65. Feinman, R.A., Madray, G., and Yarborough, D.: Chemical optical and physiologic mechanisms of bleaching products: a review. Pract Periodont Aesthetics 3:32, 1991.

66. Loudon, G.M.: Organic Chemistry Today. Reading, MA, Addison-Wesley Publishing, p. 661, 1984.

67. Arwill, T., et al: Penetration of radioactive isotopes through the enamel and dentine. II Transfer of 22 Na in fresh and chemically treated dental tissues. Odontol Rev 20:47, 1969.

68. Titley, K.C., Torneck, C.D., Smith, D.C., and Adibfar, A.: Adhesion of composite resin to bleached and unbleached bovine enamel. J Dent Res 67:1523, 1988.

69. Titley, K.C., Torneck, C.D., and Smith, D.C., et al: Scanning electron microscopy observations on the penetration and structure of resin tags in bleached and unbleached bovine enamel. J Endodont 17:72, 1991.

70. Torneck, C.D., Titley, K.C., Smith, D.C., and Adibfar, A.: The influence of time of hydrogen peroxide exposure on the adhesion

of composite resin to bleached bovine enamel. J Endodon 16:123, 1990.

71. Titley, K.C.: Personal communication, March 1, 1991.

72. McEvoy, S.A.: Chemical agents for removing intrinsic stains from vital teeth. I. Technique development. Quint Int 20:323, 1989.

73. Sommer, F.S., Ostrander, F.D., and Crowley, M.L.: Clinical Endodontics, 3rd Ed. Philadelphia, Saunders, p. 489, 1966.

74. Feinman, R.A., Goldstein, R.E., and Garber, D.A.: Bleaching Teeth. Chicago, Quintessence Publishing Co., Inc., p. 12, 1987.

75. Goldstein, R.E.: Bleaching teeth, new materials—new role. J Am Dent Assoc 115:44E, 1987.

76. Waggonner, W.F., Johnston, W.M., Schumann, S., and Schikowski, E.: Microabrasion of human enamel in vitro using hydrochloric acid and pumice. Pediatr Dent 11:319, 1989.

77. Baumgartner, J.C., Reid, D.E., and Pkett, A.B.: Human pulpal reaction to the modified McInnes bleaching technique. J Endodont 9:527, 1983.

78. Olin, P.S., Lehner, C.R., and Hilton, J.A.: Enamel surface modification in vitro using hydrochloric acid pumice: an investigation. Quint Int 19:733, 1988.

79. Croll, T.P. and Cavanaugh, R.R.: Enamel color modification by controlled hydrochloric acid-pumice abrasion. I. Technique and examples. Quint Int 17:81, 1986.

80. Christensen, G.J.: Bleaching vital tetracycline-stained teeth. Quint Int 9:13, 1978.

81. Ingle, J.I. and Taintor, J.F.: Endodontics, 3rd Ed. Philadelphia, Lea & Febiger, p. 607, 1965.

82. Ledoux, W.R., et al.: Structural effects of bleaching on tetracycline-stained vital rat teeth. J Prosthet Dent 54:55, 1985.

83. Reid, J.S., and Newman, P.: A suggested method of bleaching tetracycline-stained vital teeth. Br Dent J 142:261, 1977.

84. Wilson, C.F., and Seale, N.S.: Color change following vital bleaching of tetracycline-stained teeth. Pediatr Dent 7:205, 1985.

85. Cohen, S.C.: Human pulpal response to bleaching procedure on vital teeth. J Endodont 5:134, 1979.

86. Robertson, W.D. and Melfi, R.C.: Pulpal response to vital bleaching procedures. J Endodont 6:645, 1980.

87. Seale, N.S., Wilson, C.F.: Pulpal response to bleaching of teeth in dogs. Pediatr Dent 7:209, 1985.

88. Nathanson, D. and Parra, B.: Bleaching vital teeth: a review and clinical study. Compend Ed Dent 8:490, 1987.

89. Hardman, P.K., Moore, D.L., and Petteway, G.H.: Stability of hydrogen peroxide as a bleaching agent. Gen Dent 33:121, 1985.

90. Budavari, S. (ed.): The Merck Index, 11th Ed. Rahway, NJ, Merck & Co, Inc., p. 760, 1989.

91. Martindale, W., Reynolds, J.E. (ed): Martindale's, The Extra Pharmacopoeia. London, The Pharmaceutical Press, 1989.

92. Union Broach technical reference material for New Image Bleaching Unit.

93. Tooth bleaching, home use products. Update report. Clinical Research Associates Newsletter. 13(12):1, 1989.

94. Berry J.H.: What about whiteners? Safety concerns explored. J Am Dent Assoc 121:223, 1990.

95. Weitzman, S.A., et al.: Effects of hydrogen peroxide on oral carcinogenesis in hamsters. J Periodontol 57:685, 1986.

96. Bhaskar, S.N. (ed.): Orban's oral histology and embryology, 8th Ed. St Louis, C.V. Mosby, 1976.

97. Lado, E.A., Standley, H.R., and Weisman, M.I.: Cervical resorption in bleached teeth. Oral Surg 55:78, 1983.

98. Taylor, G.N., Madonia, J.V., Wood, N.K., and Heuer, M.A.: In vivo autoradiographic study of relative penetrating abilities of aqueous 2% parachlorophenol and camphorated 35% parachlorophenol. J Endodont 2:81, 1976.

99. Harrington, G.M. and Natkin, E.: External resorption associated with bleaching of pulpless teeth. J Endodont 5:344, 1979.

100. Kehoe J.C.: pH reversal following in vitro bleaching of pulpless teeth. 13:6, 1987.

101. Freccia, W., Peters, D., Lorton, L., and Bernier, W.: An in vitro comparison on nonvital bleaching techniques in the discolored tooth. J Endodont 8:70, 1982.

102. Holmstrup, G., Palm, A.M., and Lambjerg-Hansen, H.: Bleaching of discolored root-filled teeth. Endodont Dent Traumatol 4:197, 1988.

103. McCormick, J.E., Weine, F.S., and Maggio, J.D.: Tissue pH of developing periapical lesions in dogs. J Endodont 9:47, 1983.

104. Kaplan, A., Aschheim, K.W., and Dale, B.G.; Unpublished data.

Fred B. Abbott, D.D.S., M.D.S.
Nellie Abbott, Ph.D., R.N.

ESTHETICS AND PSYCHOLOGY

16

Recent advances in dental materials and procedures have greatly increased the ability to provide esthetic treatment. The wide array of available options increases the need for understanding the patient as a person and places greater emphasis on effective communication. Personality, motivations, desires, expectations, self esteem, an ability to accept change and willingness to cooperate are important factors for successful treatment.[1,2] An awareness of self theory and a broad application of psychologic and sociologic principles can greatly enhance a dental practice that emphasizes esthetics.

HISTORY OF PSYCHOLOGY AND DENTAL ESTHETICS

Early History

As early as 1872 White reminded the dental profession of the need to relate esthetic appearance to the laws of nature, i.e., facial contours, age, and temperament.[3] White later attempted to apply this theory to tooth selection; temperamental forms of teeth were produced as "named sets."[4] Named sets refers to the categorization of maxillary anterior teeth.

The search for teeth that would enhance personality and appearance continued. In 1895, a prominent American dentist and artist, J. Leon Williams, expressed his concern about the unlifelike nature of teeth available for dentures. He carried out extensive research on teeth shape and size. He picked up on White's "named sets" and classified anterior maxillary teeth as square, ovoid, tapering, or a combination of these types. A newly emerging company (now called Dentsply International, Inc.) used his research to create a mold guide system and techniques that made it possible for the first time for the dentist to select the size and form of teeth that would look best on the patient.[5] It was believed that Williams had discovered nature's law of the face-form-tooth-form harmony.[6]

House refined and expanded upon the work of Williams to include form and color harmony into denture esthetics.[7] The theories of Williams and House still serve as the frame of reference for tooth selection as taught in many dental schools today. A study by Brown failed to support Williams' and House's face-form-tooth-form theory.[8]

In 1937, House classified patients into four types based upon psychologic assessment.[9] According to House,

1. The philosophical patient accepts his lot in life, copes with frustration, and is well organized with respect to time and habits.
2. The exacting individual is very methodical, accurate, demanding, and extremely precise in life's activities.
3. The indifferent patient is unconcerned and apathetic, and lacks motivation.
4. The hysterical patient is emotionally unstable, highly excitable, and extremely apprehensive.

Although House's classification furnishes guidelines for diagnosing patients, the psychologic assessment of a patient goes beyond simple categorization.

"Dentogenic" Movement

In the 1950s, the "dentogenic" movement became popular. Dentogenics was defined as the convergence of art, practice, and techniques that enabled a denture to add to a person's charm, character, dignity, and beauty in a fully expressive smile.[10] As proponents of dentogenics, Frush and Fisher placed great emphasis on projecting a denture wearer's personality, sex, and age. In collaboration with the Swissedent Foundation they stressed the need to avoid the "denture look." They added to face-form and tooth-form the SPA factor—sex, personality, and age.[11]

They hypothesized a personality spectrum ranging from vigorous to medium pleasing to delicate. Based on their experience, Frush and Fisher believed that about 15% of the population is the vigorous type. These individuals tend to be male. About 5% is delicate, and they tended to be female. The remaining 80% is the medium pleasing type, composed of both sexes. Tooth selections and characterizations for prostheses were partially guided by the perceived personality type.[11] Frush and Fisher placed great emphasis on the need for sculpting the tooth and for selecting the color and position, in order to enhance the masculinity or femininity of the patient. They stressed the use of characterization to enhance age and sex.[12] Enhancing age means to make someone appear more youthful; enhancing sex means to make a "rugged" masculine type appear more ruggedly masculine or a "delicate" feminine type appear more delicately feminine, for example. Recent studies, however, do not support the belief that tooth shape and size have identifiable masculine or feminine characteristics.[8,13] In a study of 300 diagnostic casts (equal numbers of male and female) judgements of sex were made by a layman, dental students, and dental faculty. The results showed an inverse relationship between correct judgement of the sex of the patient and the level of dental knowledge and experience of the judge.[13] However, from an artistic perspective, the consummate delicacy of femininity and the ruggedness of masculinity remain as accepted guidelines reinforcing the dentogenic theory. The SwisseDent Corporation still strongly adheres to incorporating personality, age, sex, and physiologic characteristics in the design of teeth (Fig. 16–1).

THE CONCEPT OF SELF

Evolution of Self Theory

Humankind has long sought to understand the causes of behavior and to create a sense of identity. The term "self-concept" has a twentieth century origin. Most pretwentieth century discussions of self were embedded in philosophic and religious dogma.

A precursor to self theory goes back to antiquity. Synthesizing ideas from classical Greek medicine and astronomy, a theory of temperaments evolved, which prevailed for many centuries. In essence, it stated that an individual's personality type was predetermined by physiology. In the mid 1800s the temperament theory of personality was still in vogue, although it had been modified somewhat. Three classifications of temperaments were believed to exist:[14]

1. **Sanguine.** This type of personality radiates good humor and enthusiasm for life. It was believed to result from a predominance of blood over other body humors (fluids).
2. **Choleric.** This type of personality is irritable and finds it difficult to establish a positive relationship. It was believed to result from a predominance of bile over other humors.
3. **Phlegmatic.** This type of personality is characterized by torpor and apathy. It was believed to result from a predominance of phlegm over other humors.

In the clinical situation it is common to find patients whose personalities fall into these categories. The sanguine personality is certainly easier to relate to; the other two may pose a challenge. The choleric type usually is harder to satisfy; and it may be difficult to obtain active involvement on the part of the phlegmatic type. The dentist must develop skill in recognizing personality types early in the data collection stage.

Near the turn of the century, William James postulated that the empirical self includes four components, which he classified in descending order of impact on self esteem.

1. **Spiritual self.** By spiritual self James meant thinking and feeling. This is the center around which all other aspects of the empirical self are clustered. He perceived it to be the source of interest, effort, attention, will, and choice. In other words, the spiritual self is a composite of intellectual, religious, and moral aspirations from which a sense of either moral superiority or inferiority or guilt could arise.
2. **Material self.** The material self refers to the clothing and material possessions that an individual views as an important part of himself. Many people define themselves by what they own rather than by what they do.
3. **Social self.** The social self refers to the various aspects of personality that are reflected in the individuals and groups to which one relates. These aspects are designed to serve social ends, such as gaining love and admiration or obtaining influence and power.
4. **Bodily self.** The bodily self was placed last in importance by James; others question this placement. This aspect refers to body image. Achieving an awareness of the self begins with experiencing one's body and feelings, often via the reactions of significant individuals. An individual who has a high degree of self awareness is often perceived to be "more alive."

These four components interrelate in unique ways to constitute each person's view of his empirical self.[15]

The development of self theory was temporarily sidetracked by the ascendancy of behaviorism and its emphasis on the scientific method. During this period, psychology was directed to a rigorous study of only those aspects of behavior that were observable and measurable. However, by about 1930 there was a retreat from this hard line and the importance of internal events was reintroduced into research and therapy. By the mid twentieth century the self concept was firmly established as an important construct in the study of human behavior.[16-18] Since then a massive amount of theorizing and experimenting has occurred in all components of self theory.

Self Theory: Relevant Constructs

Self theory might be defined as that evolving constellation of self-referent constructs that are used to attain a more plausible and complete theoretical account of hu-

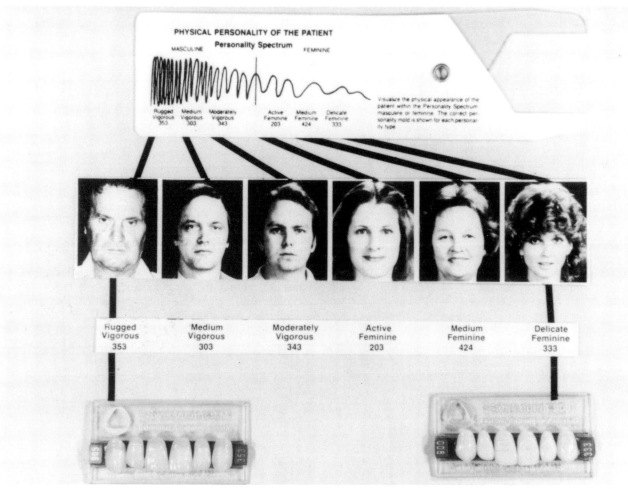

FIG. 16–1. *Two of the sex and personality attributes (SPA) that influence, from an artistic perspective, the mold and shade selection of teeth. The two extremes are shown (Copyright 1989 PTC).*

man conduct. Some of the relevant constructs of self theory are:

1. **Self awareness.** Self awareness has been defined as knowledge of one's own traits or qualities; insight into, and understanding of one's own behavior and motives.

2. **Self concept.** Many contemporary psychologists ascribe a key role to the self concept as a factor in integrating personality, motivating behavior, and achieving mental health. Volumes have been written on this subject.[19-22] Basically, self concept is a person's view of himself, which includes not only the person as an object of self-knowledge, but also the feelings about what the person conceives himself to be.

3. **Self image.** Self image is the self that one thinks oneself to be. It is not a directly observed self-object but rather a complex concept of personality, character, status, body, and bodily appearance. It may differ greatly from objective fact.[14] A concept closely related to self image is body image.

4. **Self esteem or self evaluation.** Self evaluation is the process by which an individual examines his performance, capabilities, and attributes according to his personal standards and values, which have been internalized from society and significant others. These evaluations promote behavior consistent with self knowledge. For example, an individual who firmly believes that he has unattractive or ugly teeth may develop speaking patterns or behavioral mannerisms that keep the teeth concealed. He may avoid pursuing certain lines of work which, in his opinion, require a certain degree of attractiveness because of face to face contact with the public. The image a person has of himself may or may not coincide with reality. A person may be more or less attractive than conceptualized.

5. **Self actualization.** The most recent development in self theory stresses the importance of a drive labeled "self actualization." Abraham Maslow proposed that self actualization results in a striving to develop one's capacities, self understanding, and self acceptance in accord with one's "inner nature."[23,24] Maslow looked to a more positive side of nature than many of his contemporaries. He believed that human nature was essentially good. He further believed that as personality unfolded through maturation, the creative powers manifested themselves ever

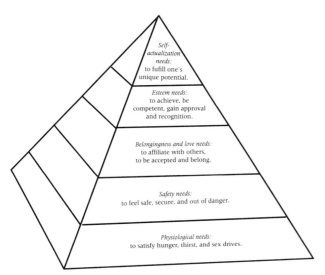

FIG. 16–2. Abraham Maslow's hierarchy of human needs. (Adapted from Rubin, Z. and McNeil, E.B.: Psychology of Being Human, 4th Ed. New York, Harper & Row, 1985.)

more clearly. If people became neurotic or miserable, he felt that was caused by the environment. Humans became destructive or violent only when their inner nature was twisted or frustrated. Maslow assumed that basic needs, such as physiologic needs, safety, love, belonging, and esteem must be satisfied before self actualization can be achieved (Fig. 16–2). Although it is well established that people who have not satisfied their basic physiologic needs are not likely to be interested in much else, the relative order of some of the other needs may vary from person to person. Also, several different needs may motivate our behavior at any given time.[25]

PHYSICAL AND PHYSIOLOGIC INFLUENCES

Facial Appearance

A study in 1921 highlighted the importance of facial appearance by proposing that the physical characteristics of individuals exert a profound influence over their associates.[26] However, researchers did not quickly pick up on this observation. Some speculate that our society's emphasis upon egalitarianism may have contributed to this omission. In other words, the belief that a person's appearance ought not to make a difference in opportunities for development and success may have produced an "ostrich effect."[27]

It was not until the 1960s that studies of facial appearance began appearing in the literature. In the 1970s, research on the social psychology of facial appearance became more frequent. A vast number of studies have been reported, but the quality of most of these studies is questionable.[28] A growing body of information is now accumulating on facial appearance.

Facial attractiveness has an important impact upon an individual's life,[29] a fact increasingly recognized by personal injury lawyers, physicians, and dentists.

Few studies of facial appearance have investigated in a scientific manner those dimensions of the face and teeth that are responsible for a pleasant or an unpleasant face. In general, individuals in our society tend to reject the open bite facial types (either Class II or Class III) but more readily accept the deep bite facial type (Fig. 16–3).[30,31]

Regardless of the results of studies relating facial attractiveness to success in academics, careers, or interpersonal relationships, the personal testimonies of patients are suggestive that improved appearance is a goal worth pursuing as the following case clearly demonstrates.

Mr. Z is a 49-year-old real estate agent. He originally presented with a dour, morose appearance and was somewhat argumentative. Over the years he had abraded his teeth through bruxism until they were no longer visible when he talked or smiled. Eating was no longer enjoyable because of the significant loss of vertical occluding dimension, which led to facial distortion when he chewed. He was embarrassed at his image. He hoped for a "quick fix" to his problem.

A transitional diagnostic acrylic splint was placed to determine his tolerance for a restored vertical occlusion. The attractive splint dramatically changed his appearance. Composite resin veneers further enhanced the esthetics (Figs. 16–4 to 16–6).

Over the next few weeks Mr. Z's personality gradually changed. He began to smile and appeared more relaxed. When questioned about this perceived change he stated, "You're absolutely right. You can't believe how good I feel inside. I want to smile at everybody. I can't pass a mirror without stopping to look at my new teeth. I can hardly wait to get my permanent restorations. Already I've started on a self improvement program, losing a few pounds and toning up. Business has become a pleasure, and I feel more confident in social situations."

The Mouth and Oral Cavity

The mouth has long played a prominent role in psychologic theories (e.g., Freud incorporated the "oral" stage of development into psychoanalytic theory). Throughout life the mouth assumes a prominent role in our link with the outside world—nutritionally, sexually, and through verbal communication.[32] When individuals first meet, the mouth is often the first body part to be noticed. Given the prominence of the mouth, it is surprising that more people do not show sufficient concern for the appearance of their teeth and mouth.

Sex and Age

Many stereotypes regarding sex have changed over the years. Still, the sexes have major differences that must be considered in a dental practice. The dentist needs to be aware of how a patient views his or her own sexual-

ESTHETIC DENTISTRY

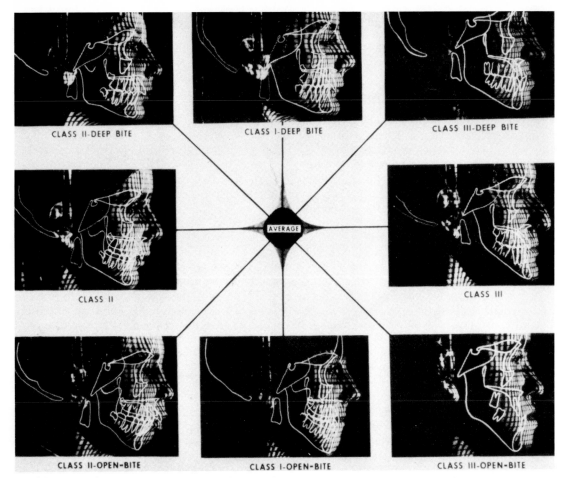

FIG. 16—3. Composite of four basic facial types and their combinations (From Sassouni, V.: A classification of skeletal facial types. Am J Orthod 55:120, 1969.)

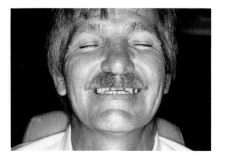

FIG. 16—4. Mr. Z prior to treatment.

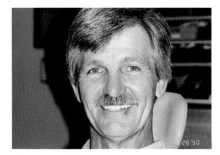

FIG. 16—5. Mr. Z following restorations.

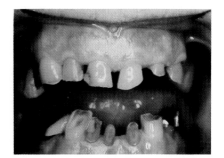

FIG. 16—6. Pretreatment photograph that convinced a patient of the need for treatment.

ity and the degree to which he or she wishes to have masculinity or femininity emphasized.

The dentist also must consider a person's age. Psychologic age and chronologic age must be determined. Through the use of veneers and bleaching, a more youthful appearance may be created. Although many people wish to appear more youthful, this is not universally true. As one woman so emphatically stated, "I am a little old lady and I want to look like one."

PSYCHOLOGIC INFLUENCES

Personality

An individual's personality is the result of many factors. The degree to which facial, and specifically oral, appearance contribute to personality is difficult to ascertain. We have referred to just a few of the many attempts to broadly classify personality. The individual dentist must choose an approach for determining personality. Because personality is the filter through which relationships take place, an accurate assessment of a patient's personality can be critical to the successful outcome of dental treatment.

Measurement and Evaluation

A number of studies in the dental literature include personality variables in the assessment of patient satisfaction with their current dental condition,[33] as well as with treatments involving complete dentures,[34-37] partial dentures,[38] temporomandibular disorders and chronic pain,[39] orthognathic surgery,[40] preprosthetic surgery,[41] and orthodontics and prosthodontics.[42]

Many of these studies dealt with captive audiences (e.g., veterans or patients at dental school clinics). Therefore, the results were not extensively generalizable. Findings from one study sometimes conflicted with findings from another. No clear picture emerges. Very few studies have been done relating personality characteristics to esthetics, per se.

A wide variety of tools and techniques have been used to obtain information from patients. They include self designed questionnaires, focused interviews, projective figure drawing, and standardized tests. Some specific tests that have been recommended include: the Cattell 16 PF questionnaire (Form C)[35] and the Cornell Medical Index.[34] Dentists considering using standardized psychologic tests should seek the assistance of a psychologist trained in measurement and evaluation.

A decision must be made regarding how psychologic information will be obtained and recorded.[43] Will it be an informal process based on an interview and observation of the patient? Or will it be more formal? Will special forms be used to collect specific information? If so, how do you present this idea to patients and gain their cooperation? Who will interpret this information? How will this information be used?

Motivations, Desires, and Expectations

A host of factors may bring a patient to a dental office initially, as well as cause him to return. A partial listing of motivations include:

1. The desire to be better able to eat and enjoy food
2. The desire to improve speech patterns
3. The fear of losing teeth through decay or fracture
4. The desire to be free of pain and discomfort
5. The desire to have fresh breath
6. The desire to enhance appearance or self image to compete more effectively for attention or advancement.

Not all patients are motivated by self actualization; however, some may be moved in that direction.

In some instances the patient's expectations are unachievable. They may have personality problems or interpersonal problems that they believe will be corrected or improved by the desired dental treatment. The dentist must be on guard for this problem and avoid getting into an unresolvable situation. The dentist should not promise more than can be delivered. The dentist should be sensitive to cues that the patient or those accompanying the patient reveal during the initial examination and interview process. The quintessential question that the practitioner must seek to answer is: What motivated this person to seek dental treatment? If the patient is primarily concerned about appearance, what is the underlying motivation? If a particular problem has existed for a long time, what change in the person's life caused him to initiate possible treatment at this time.

Once the patient has been able to articulate his motivation or concerns, the dentist has a starting point from which to begin moving the patient in the direction of a proper treatment plan. When the patient realizes that the dentist is truly listening to his concerns, he will be more able to listen to the dentist's concerns. For example, if the patient's primary concern is the ability to eat, the most appropriate treatment to improve mastication should be addressed first. In order to achieve that objective, a complete or partial denture may be required. Once that need is addressed, improved esthetics can be incorporated later in connection with the design.

Determining motivation, coupled with a fairly accurate personality assessment, is crucial to successful treatment planning and ultimately to patient satisfaction with the treatment.

CLINICAL TIP. Often it is input from sensitive staff members that provides insight into the patient's needs and desires. Patients often perceive the dentist as an authority figure and have difficulty expressing themselves to someone in that role.

Basic information should be obtained from the patient upon entry into the office. This usually is obtained by means of a form. Auxiliary personnel set the tone in the manner in which they request this information from the patient. Much can be learned by observing how the person studies the form, from unanswered questions, and from conversations with significant others while filling out the form. Seeking clarification or using information from this form to initiate conversation may elicit valuable information that can illuminate the patient's personality and motivations. This can also help to determine whether the patient is able to articulate his expectations in a clear manner.

Developing a Trusting Relationship

CLINICAL TIP. A judgment must be made regarding whether the patient can form a trusting relationship. When an individual is suspicious of every suggestion and asks an inordinate number of questions, it may indicate an inability to form a positive relationship.

At times, it is difficult for a patient to reveal all the relevant aspects of his life. The dentist may need to gain the trust of the patient to enable that individual to open up and be forthright and honest. Borrowing heavily from Roger's client centered therapy,[18] three qualities that help to engender trust have been identified:[44]

1. **Accurate empathy** involves the dentist's sensitivity to his patient's feelings and his ability to communicate this awareness and acceptance of him as a unique individual.
2. **Nonpossessive warmth** refers to the dentist's nonjudgmental acceptance of the patient regardless of behavior. The patient should not be criticized for allowing his oral health to deteriorate.
3. **Genuineness** implies an openness and spontaneity on the part of the dentist.

Decision Making Ability

Efforts should be made very early to engage the patient in decision making activities. To the extent possible, the patient should be an active participant in his treatment.

CLINICAL TIP. When the patient cannot make decisions, it is important to identify a "significant other" in the patient's life and include that person in the process.

Cooperation and Follow Through

Optimal oral health and a beautiful smile require cooperation from the patient, as well as persistence in maintenance activities. Some people are "starters" but not "finishers." Prior to initiating treatment the patient must be adequately informed of the need for followup care. Some reconstruction patients, for example, fail to accept responsibility for maintenance, and end up losing all benefit of their extensive treatment.

Abnormalities and Problem Patients

Occasionally, "troubled" or "difficult" patients with irrational perceptions of self seek treatment or esthetic alterations that are unrealistic. They may be narcissistic, depressed, paranoid, or have labile or hysterical personalities. Often, these individuals are skillful at masking their condition, especially during the interview process.

Only by careful listening over a period of time can the patients' problems be identified. The patient may have unrealistic expectations, or may be unable to internalize information provided by the dentist. These patients may be obsessed with perceived or minor flaws or may be unable to develop a trusting relationship.

Once a relationship has been established between a patient and a dentist, termination of that relationship must be handled very carefully to avoid a possible charge of abandonment. (See Chapter 28—Esthetics and Dental Jurisprudence.) Once treatment has been undertaken, it must be completed at least to the point where the patient is not left in a precarious position. Prior to terminating a relationship, efforts must be made to correct the problem, improve communication, and gain cooperation. These efforts may not be successful.

If the patient's psychologic problems are severe, the dentist may determine that professional help is needed. He should not attempt psychologic therapy unless he has training and certification in this field. However, the dentist must appreciate the delicate nature of making a referral to a mental health professional; the referral should be made with care, empathy, and tact.

Not all problems can be anticipated and prevented. The dentist must think about the type of problems which will be faced in an esthetic dental practice and consider an approach to dealing with these problems. It is logical to believe that the following problems are likely to occur:

1. The patient has an unrealistic esthetic expectation that cannot be satisfied.
2. The patient expects that an esthetic improvement will remove or correct deep-seated psychologic problems in his life.
3. The patient is not satisfied with results that are technically and esthetically correct. In other words, the "it's not me" phenomenon.
4. The patient is satisfied with the results but family and friends are not.
5. The patient does not wish to have esthetics enhanced and the dentist does.

In dealing with these problems the dentist must be explicit in what the proposed treatment can and cannot do. He should actively involve the patient and his family in the treatment phase to increase the chance of acceptance (e.g., have them select shades and shapes of teeth). Multiple joint esthetic evaluations may be required. At some point the dentist may have to accept the fact that he and the patient do not agree on what is perceived as appropriate.

CLINICAL TIP. As long as no physiologic or ethical principles are violated, the patient should be permitted to make the final esthetic determination.

If the patient wants to remain homely, let him. This may be a defense mechanism that has been built up over time and served the patient well.

CULTURAL INFLUENCES

Anthropologists have shown us that standards of beauty vary widely not only from society to society, but also locally. Even in societies where it is fashionable to go naked, the face is extremely important. Malinowski has pointed out that the naked Trobiand Islanders of the Western Pacific devoted tremendous energy to the decoration and elaboration of the face.[33]

The desire to alter the face is universal. In many primitive societies painful elaborations were undertaken not only in pursuit of beauty, but also for ritual significance. In Australia and New Guinea the native peoples celebrated the achievement of adulthood and maturity by having their two maxillary anterior teeth removed. This custom also prevailed in South Africa, where adults who still had all their teeth were considered ugly. In Borneo, teeth were blackened and holes were drilled through the labial surfaces of the six maxillary anterior teeth. Plugs of brass with outer ends shaped like stars, were inserted. In the East Indies, the mesial, distal, and incisal aspects of the teeth were filed off and shaped into points as part of the ceremony of marriage, puberty, or mourning. This custom prevails today among the pygmies of central Africa, specifically the Efe group.[45]

Within the United States today many cultures exist. The practicing dentist should become aware of the various cultural groups that may be in his care. In each community there are pockets of racial or ethnic groups that have developed traditions of eating and self care that have implications for dentistry. The dentist can become aware of these groups by subscribing to a local newspaper, becoming involved in community affairs, such as health fairs, and communicating with other health professionals who may be a part of the racial or ethnic groups. It may be necessary to use or develop teaching materials geared specifically toward the customs and traditions of these groups.

Mores and Values

Our mores and values have changed a great deal from those in vogue when the country was founded. Then plainness and austerity were the norm. Individuals who stressed beauty often were ostracized.

Gradually, a broad acceptance has come about in our society that health and beauty occur simultaneously. Religious and psychologic barriers have been lowered. Today, people are admonished to achieve the "natural look" and to "become all you can be." Styles have been modified to expose more of the body. We no longer feel guilty about seeking products and treatments to enhance beauty (or image). Feeling good about oneself now is acceptable behavior. In fact, the pendulum has almost swung too far in the opposite direction. When we see people who pay little attention to their personal appearance, we often wonder, "What's wrong with them?"

SOCIOLOGIC INFLUENCES

A number of sociologic trends in our society are believed to contribute to the ability and willingness of individuals to seek out esthetic dentistry.

Affluence

An increasing number of individuals are obtaining more discretionary income. Available funds, coupled with the newer emphasis on self actualization and the freedom to spend money on self, has led to an increase in the demand for self improvement, including esthetic dentistry.

CLINICAL TIP. The patient's socioeconomic status can be misleading. Some patients who appear to be able to afford treatment may not value oral health or appearance enough to incur the expense. Other patients with limited resources are able to rearrange their priorities and mobilize resources. Therefore, the dentist should not initially consider the patient's socioeconomic status, but rather should present the ideal treatment as well as acceptable alternatives.

Emphasis on Health, Wellness, and Fitness

After decades, and perhaps even centuries, of basing health care on a sickness model, the changes in recent years have been dramatic. Escalating health care costs, coupled with a national effort to curtail these increasing costs, has resulted in more emphasis on the prevention of illness, physical fitness, and health maintenance.

The dental profession has been at the forefront of this wellness movement. In the 1960s scientific evidence supported the efficacy of fluoridation. Dental disease was perceived to be preventable. Dentists were asked to change their clinical perspective from disease orientation to health orientation and many did. As newer concepts have been accepted, chair time has increasingly been used for maintenance of health and esthetic dentistry.

Media Influence

Possibly the greatest single factor responsible for increased esthetic awareness among the public is the media. We have been virtually bombarded by television, radio, and magazine reports and advertisements regarding the newest advances in bleaching, bonding, veneering, crowns, implants, orthodontic therapy, and surgery.[46]

Changed Attitudes Toward Medical and Dental Treatment

No longer willing to allow the physician or dentist to solely determine their needs and how to address those needs, many patients expect to be active participants in the analysis and planning phases of their care. They want to know what options are available and the pros and the cons of each option.

Attitudes toward the cost of treatment are also slowly changing. Just as the expense of a college education is considered an investment, so is esthetic dentistry viewed as an investment by some individuals who are convinced that their success in life depends on appearance. Quality of life is becoming a value for the elderly.[47]

CLINICAL PRACTICE
Dentist-Patient Interaction

To some extent, psychologic bonding occurs between the patient and dentist. Early in the relationship it is important to determine that a positive relationship can exist. The personalities of the patient and dentist must be compatible. The patient must have confidence in the dentist and believe that the dentist not only understands what the patient desires or needs, but also that the dentist has the creativity, knowledge, skill, and state of the art equipment and materials to meet these needs. One dentist who had gone to great pains to design a modern office where all extraneous items were kept out of sight was surprised to learn that a patient believed he was not fully equipped. Her previous experience had been with traditional offices where the counters were filled with instruments and materials.

Following the diagnostic workup, the clinical information is integrated with the psychologic and sociologic information relevant to the patient. A detailed, written treatment plan is formulated. The plan sets forth the optimum treatment, as well as possible acceptable options. In other words, usually there is more than one way to achieve the treatment objectives. Choices must be made. Economics, as well as personality factors, influence which specific plan is selected.

CLINICAL TIP. The presentation of treatment options should be carefully structured. If possible, schedule it at the close of the day when time is available for discussing and exploring alternatives. By giving the patient specific treatment options along with the rationale for each, the patient is made to recognize his active role in the treatment planning process.

The dentist should be prepared for some negative reactions to the comprehensive treatment plan. In some instances the plan can be overwhelming and even devastating. Patients who have ignored their oral health for years often have such great needs that they may say, "Why don't you just pull them all out and make me some dentures." They see that as the solution to their problem, not realizing that they are opening the door to a host of other problems. The dentist must be frank with the patient, explaining the many problems that they could face with dentures (e.g., problems with stability, pressure, potential inability to eat certain foods, and the need for relines). In addition, the dentist must point out the ethical and legal problem related to the extraction of teeth with adequate root structure.

Other patients can be more philosophical. They might say, "Well, this didn't happen over night. Let's get on with the treatment." Sometimes their treatment can be extended over time.

Still others may not wish to be too involved. They may claim to be "confused" by the various options. They say, "Just tell me what I need to have done." When the patient places the dentist in the decision making role, he must be guided by his conscience and the Golden Rule. He should consider the options and arrive at the most permanent, most physiologic, and most esthetic treatment to address the need. The rationale should be explained to the patient and recorded in the chart. This approach assumes that the dentist is knowledgeable of state of the art dentistry. (See also the Clinical Tip in the section on Decision Making Ability earlier in this chapter.)

Cheney suggests that the dentist avoid standardized treatment plans. In order to obtain greater patient acceptance, he believes that each treatment plan should be customized, based on an assessment of the patient's personality, needs, wants, and desires.[48] He utilizes the psychologic construct known as locus of control, to help determine the individualized treatment plan for a given patient. To the degree possible, the patient's needs, wants, and desires are incorporated into the treatment plan; however, both dental and physiologic limitations may prevent the dentist from fulfilling the patient's esthetic demands. For example, the patient may have a diastema that he wants closed. Treatment options include orthodontic treatment, crowns, composite resin restorations, or porcelain veneers. The treatment of choice is orthodontic treatment. The patient does not want this treatment, yet he insists that he does not want the anterior teeth to be larger than they are now. The dentist is faced with a dilemma. A provisional restoration could be placed to allow the patient to see whether he could accept it. Once the treatment plan has been agreed upon, the treatment phase should proceed as expeditiously as possible in order to reinforce the patient's motivation and to achieve the desired results. On the other hand, efforts by the patient to expedite the treatment should be resisted if this will compromise the desired results. This can be accomplished by explaining to the patient the specific steps required to achieve a plan of treatment, e.g., if a transitional removable partial denture is indicated, immediately placing a cast removable partial denture can result in poor function and esthetics.

CLINICAL TIP. The dentist should not allow himself to be pressured into shortcuts that will affect quality.

Dentist-Dental Laboratory Technician Interaction

The relationship between the dentist and the technician is crucial to success. In addition to the knowledge and skill that each possesses, psychologic factors enter into this relationship. Mutual respect for each other as individuals should exist, as well as a clear understanding of the role that each plays in patient treatment. The dentist must seek out a technician with whom he can communicate, must set the tone for collaboration, and must provide for a two-way evaluation process that will foster progressive excellence. Both oral and written lines of communication must be kept open. Work authorization forms may need to be redesigned.

CLINICAL TIP. Whenever possible, the dentist should visit the laboratory. It is helpful to know the key personnel and be personally reassured of the quality of their work.

When the dentist and the technician collaborate on a difficult case and the results are pleasing, each gains satisfaction and the relationship is strengthened.

Photographs give visual feedback to the technician, especially "before" and "after" views. They show color and texture dimensions that cannot be seen on the stone casts alone. When the dentist thinks of staff appreciation, he should not overlook laboratory technicians even though they may not be on the premises.

CLINICAL TIP. The technician is usually delighted to receive photographs of a completed case. This type of evaluation serves as a motivator. Providing pictures also may provide status to the technician in the eyes of his coworkers.

Prior to deciding to launch full scale into esthetic dentistry, the dentist should make an effort to determine on a small scale whether he has the personality characteristics needed for this arena. The success of esthetic dentistry depends to a high degree upon discipline and consistent adherence to procedures. Many newer esthetic materials are very technique-sensitive.

PRACTICE MANAGEMENT

The entire dental practice should take into consideration psychologic and sociologic principles. It should function as a well integrated system.

Physical Environment

An esthetic dental practice should operate in an attractive, neat, clean environment. The patient should be surrounded by pleasing colors and textures that complement each other and suggest that the treatment provided in this setting will be competent and esthetic. Colors, however, should be carefully selected and placed so that they do not interfere with tooth shade selection (muted colors are most desirable). Employing an interior decorator may be a worthwhile investment in creating the proper physical environment. If background music is played, it should be carefully selected to help create the mood for the office. Odors should be carefully monitored and controlled.

Care should be given to the selection and arrangement of furniture. Adequate space should be available in the reception area to provide a display area for teaching materials that highlight the esthetic nature of the practice (e.g., photographs, videotapes).

Psychologic Environment

The greater the use of technology in the practice, the greater the need for the human touch. A sincere caring and concern should emanate from each member of the office staff toward the patient. Patients should be made to feel important. They should be treated with dignity and respect. Staff members should radiate concern for their comfort, privacy, and time. This is manifested in how patients are addressed, where conversations take place, and the scheduling process.

Scheduling appointments presupposes that the proper amount of time is budgeted and that necessary laboratory work has been completed. The patient should know what to expect and approximately how long it will take. Verifying appointments in advance and alerting a patient to possible delays, reinforce the value of the time that has been set aside specifically for him. Coordinating treatment between various specialties is another way to reduce stress for the patient and to ensure a more successful outcome.

Personnel as an Extension of the Dentist

Although members of the dentist's staff have their own unique characteristics, a conscious effort should be made to select individuals who complement the dentist and reinforce his practice philosophy when they fulfill their specific roles. Just as the physical environment of the office is important, so is the appearance of each member of the team. Attention to small details such as hair, nails, uniforms, shoes, weight, and smoking will reap rewards. Above all, the staff members should have good oral health. Educating by example yields rewarding results.

Careful planning should go into patient communication. The burden of education must not rest entirely upon the dentist but rather should be shared, when appropriate, with other members of the team. Resources to facilitate understanding must be carefully selected. For example, there should be a wide variety of teaching materials, ranging from three dimensional models, to photographic displays, to brochures, booklets, and videotapes. Informed consent implies patient understanding.

Critical points for communication are: at consultation, diagnostic work-up, presentation of the treatment plan, and initiation of treatment. Although technical terminology may be used, it should be translated into the layman's language.

Communication

Specific terms may need to be clarified prior to the implementation of treatment, e.g., "white teeth." If the dentist has a bias against restorations that lie outside the parameters of the natural color of teeth, this must be made clear. There may be a significant difference between patient's expectations and the dentist's philosophy or attitude. This point was illustrated when a dentist interacted with a patient who desired "white teeth." The patient was not swayed when the dentist explained that the shade the patient wanted was not "natural." She replied, "I bleach my hair blond, put rouge on my cheeks, and mascara on my eyelids; I paint my lips red. These are not natural. So give me white teeth!"[49] If the request or desire of the patient does not conflict with ethical codes and does not cause physiologic harm to the oral environment, then the dentist has great freedom to cooperate. (See also the section on Abnormalities and Patient Problems earlier in this chapter.)

CLINICAL TIP. When treatment is initiated, the dentist should verify with the patient the treatment that is planned. Any misconceptions that have arisen between the time of the treatment conference and initiation of treatment should be clarified.

Styles of communication vary widely. Some people communicate directly and honestly; others play games with their communication.[50,51] They may or may not be aware of this game playing. An understanding of transactional analysis therapy may facilitate true communication. This is not to say that the dentist should be a therapist, however. The objective is to get the patient to communicate as an adult and for the dentist not to be trapped into a "child" or "parent" communication style, but rather to also be able to communicate as an adult.

FINANCIAL CONSIDERATIONS

Clinical treatment should be separated from the business aspects of the practice. In other health related disciplines treatment is not determined by the patient's ability to pay. By avoiding a discussion of fees at the time of treatment planning, the dentist can be more objective in his discussion of options. Other than helping to decide the fee structure, the dentist should avoid getting involved in this aspect of the practice. This is not to say that the patient's decision won't be largely influenced by cost. However, cost may not be the most crucial consideration. Patients may be willing to invest more time and money than dentists have previously assumed. (See also the section on Affluence earlier in this chapter.)

The team member responsible for the financial dealings must be psychologically strong and able to help the patient to view esthetic dentistry as an investment. Money and time will be expended upon self improvement which has potential payoff in meeting some of the patient's goals and dreams, e.g., to help get an advancement or better sell a proposal and win a contract. In order to accomplish this, the business manager must be aware of the patient's personality and socioeconomic status and relate to each patient in a manner consistent with the philosophy of the practice.[52]

Photography and Computer Technology

Some patients who have become complacent about their deteriorating oral health are shocked when they see a photograph.[53-55] (See Chapter 17—Esthetics and Oral Photography.) For example, Mrs. X exclaimed, "Is that me?" when she saw a picture (Fig. 16–6) of her mouth; this helped to motivate her to pursue treatment. A fairly recent breakthrough in dental photography is the color video intraoral camera, which has the capacity to store images as well as to alter them to present different treatment options.[55] (See Chapter 29—Esthetics and Advanced Technology.)

Ethics, Quality Assurance, and Risk Management

Clinical dental ethics focuses on decisions, both the decision making process and the outcome, as they are reached in everyday practice.[56-58] Dentists are legally and morally obligated to:

1. Benefit the patient's health
2. Do no harm to the patient
3. Help the patient weigh the risks or harms of treatment against the anticipated end result.

Responsible treatment decisions must be made weighing the costs of the care against the anticipated benefits.

Although it is important to discern what a patient desires as a treatment outcome, desires may not always be consistent with treatment goals. For example, a patient may desire esthetic restorative dentistry for the maxillary anterior teeth without replacing mandibular posterior teeth. To provide the desired treatment would be unethical because it is doomed to failure. Continuous occlusal trauma of the mandibular anterior teeth will result. When a patient's cosmetic preferences compromise professional standards, the dentist faces a moral dilemma. Even if the patient is willing to take calculated risks, inappropriate treatment should not be undertaken. The dentist is not legally protected from charges of inappropriate treatment, even when the patient signs a release. (See Chapter 28—Esthetics and Dental Jurisprudence.)

CONCLUSION

The patient and the dentist each bring to the relationship unique personalities, values, expectations, and motivations, which have been shaped by their respective backgrounds. The dentist has the educational responsibility to learn about psychologic and sociologic concepts and to incorporate them into his practice. If he assumes this responsibility, the practice will be enriched immensely.

Quality esthetic dentistry rendered to appreciative patients has lasting psychologic rewards for all involved.

The authors wish to recognize editorial assistance of Marc B. Applelbaum, DDS, Morristown, NJ.

REFERENCES

1. Abbott, F.B.: Psychological assessment of the prosthodontic patient before treatment. Dent Clin North Am 28:361, 1984.
2. Murrell, G.A.: Esthetics and the edentulous patient. J Am Dent Assoc Spec No. 58E, 1987.
3. White, J.W.: Aesthetic dentistry. Dent Cosmos 14:144, 1872.
4. White, J.W.: Editorial. Temperament in relation to teeth. Dent Cosmos 22:113, 1884.
5. Williams, J.L.: A new classification of tooth forms with special reference to a new system of artificial teeth. Dent Cosmos 56:627, 1914.
6. Clapp, G.W.: How the science of tooth form selection was made easy. J Prosthet Dent 5:596, 1955.
7. House, M.M.: Full denture techniques. Unpublished notes of Study Club No. 1, 1937.
8. Brown, F.: Doctoral dissertation. Washington, D.C., Howard University, 1975.
9. House, M.M. and Loop, F.L.: Form and color harmony in the dental art. Monograph. Whittier, CA, 1939.
10. Frush, J.P. and Fisher, R.D.: Introduction to dentogenic restorations. J Prosthet Dent 5:586, 1955.
11. Frush, J.P. and Fisher, R.D.: How dentogenics interprets the personality factor. J Prosthet Dent 6:441, 1956.
12. Frush, J.P. and Fisher, R.D.: How dentogenic restorations interpret the sex factor. J Prosthet Dent 6:160, 1956.
13. Abbott, F.B.: Unpublished study. Philadelphia, Temple University, 1986.
14. English, H.B. and English, A.C.: A Comprehensive Dictionary of Psychological and Psychoanalytical Terms. New York, David McKay Company, Inc., 1958.
15. James, W.: Principles of Psychology. New York, Holt, 1890.
16. Lewin, K.: Field Theory in Social Sciences. New York, Harper, 1951.

17. Combs, A. and Snygg, D.: Individual Behavior: A Perceptual Approach. New York, Harpers, 1959.
18. Rogers, C.R.: Client Centered Therapy. Boston, Houghton Mifflin, 1951.
19. Burns, R.B.: The Self Concept: Theory, Measurement, Development and Behavior. New York, Longman, 1979.
20. Fitts, W., et al.: The Self Concept and Self Actualization: Studies on the Self Concept and Rehabilitation. Nashville, Dade Wallace Center, 1971.
21. Wegner, D. and Vallacher, R.R.: The Self in Social Psychology. New York, Oxford University Press, 1980.
22. Wylie, R.: The Self Concept: A Critical Survey of Pertinent Research Literature. Lincoln, NE, University of Nebraska Press, 1961.
23. Maslow, A.H.: Motivation and Personality. New York, Harper & Row, 1954.
24. Maslow, A.H.: Toward a Psychology of Being. Princeton, Van Nostrand, 1968.
25. Rubin, Z. and McNeil, E.B.: Psychology: Being Human, 4th Ed. New York, Harper & Row, 1985.
26. Perrin, F.: Physical attractiveness and repulsiveness. J Exp Psychol 4:203, 1921.
27. Hatfield, E. and Sprecher, S.: Mirror, Mirror . . . The Importance of Looks in Everyday Life. Albany, N.Y., State University of New York Press, 1986.
28. Bull, R. and Rumsey, N.: The Social Psychology of Facial Appearance. New York, Springer Verlag, 1988.
29. Bersheid, E. and Gangestad, S.: The social psychological implications of facial physical attractiveness. Clin Plast Surg 9:289, 1982.
30. Sassouni, V.: A classification of skeletal facial types. Am J Orthodont 55:109, 1969.
31. Sassouni, V. and Sotereanos, G.C.: Diagnosis and Treatment of Dento-Facial Abnormalities. Springfield, IL, Charles C Thomas Publishers, 1974.
32. Ruel-Kellermann, M.: What are the psychosocial factors involved in motivating individuals to retain their teeth? Int Dent J 34:105, 1984.
33. Liggett, J.: The Human Face. New York, Stein & Day Publishing Co., 1974.
34. Bolender, C.L., Swoope, C.C., and Smith, D.E.: The Cornell Medical Index as a prognostic aid for complete denture patients. J Prosthet Dent 22:20, 1969.
35. Reeve, P., Watson, C.J., and Stafford, F.D.: The role of personality in the management of complete denture patients. Br Dent J 156:356, 1984.
36. Smith, M.: Measurement of personality traits and their relation to patient satisfaction with complete dentures. J Prosthet Dent 35:492, 1976.
37. Silverman, S., Silverman, S.I., Silverman, B., and Garfinkel, L.: Self-image and its relation to denture acceptance. J Prosthet Dent 35:131, 1976.
38. Watson, C.L., et al.: The role of personality in the management of partial dentures. J Oral Rehabil 13:83, 1986.
39. Oakley, M.E., et al.: Dentists' ability to detect psychological problems in patients with temporomandibular disorders and chronic pain. J Am Dent Assoc 118:727, 1989.
40. Kiyak, H.A., et al.: Predicting psychologic response to orthognathic surgery. J Oral Maxillofac Surg 40:150, 1982.
41. Reeve, P., Stafford, G.D., and Hopkins, R.: The use of Cattell's personality profile in patients who have had preprosthetic surgery. J Dent 10:121, 1982.
42. Albino, J.E., Tedesco, L.A., and Conny, D.J.: Patient perceptions of dental-facial esthetics: shared concerns in orthodontics and prosthodontics. J Prosthet Dent 52:9, 1984.
43. Warman, E.: Psychological aspects of the patient's history. NY J Dent 46:52, 1976.
44. Mittelman, J.S.: Getting through to your patients: psychological motivation. Dent Clin North Am 32:29, 1988.
45. Bailey, R.C.: The Efe: archers of the rain forest. National Geographic, 176:683, 1989.
46. Sheets, C.G.: Modern dentistry and the esthetically aware patient. J Am Dent Assoc Spec No. 103E, 1987.
47. Giddon, D.B.: Psychologic aspects of prosthodontic treatment for geriatric patients. J Prosthet Dent 43:374, 1980.
48. Cheney, H.G.: Effect of patient behavior and personality on treatment planning. Dent Clin North Am 21:531, 1977.
49. Ibsen, R.: Advances in conservative porcelain bonded restorations. Washington, Cerinate Laboratories Seminar, September 21, 1989.
50. Berne, W.: Games People Play. New York, Grove Press, 1964.
51. Kotwal, K.R.: Beyond classification of behavior types. J Prosthet Dent 52:874, 1984.
52. Goldstein, R.E.: Survey of patient attitudes toward current esthetic procedures. J Prosthet Dent 52:775, 1984.
53. King, M.: Photos reinforce change in smile. Dentist, 67:27, 1989.
54. Leinfelder, K.F., Isenberg, B.P., and Essig, M.E.: A new method for generating ceramic restorations: a CAD-CAM system. J Am Dent Assoc 118:703, 1989.
55. McCane, D. and Fisch, S.: Dental technology: knocking at high tech's door. J Am Dent Assoc 118:285, 1989.
56. Nash, D.A.: Professional ethics and esthetic dentistry. J Am Dent Assoc 117(4):7E, 1988.
57. Siegler, M., Bresnahan, J.F., Schiedermayer, D.L., and Roberson, P.: Exploring the future of clinical dental ethics: a summary of the Odontographic Society of Chicago Centennial Symposium. J Am Coll Dent 56:13, 1989.
58. Simpson, R., Hall, D., and Crabb, L.: Decision-making in dental practice. J Am Coll Dent 48:238, 1981.

Mark King, D.D.S., M.S.

ESTHETICS AND ORAL PHOTOGRAPHY

17

Dental photography has always been an important potential adjunct to dental records. However, prior to the advent of recent esthetic procedures, the dental camera could have been considered a dispensable item. With today's technological advances and the proliferation of new procedures, yesterday's luxury item, the 35 mm dental camera, is part of today's indispensable armamentarium.

HISTORY

In the early half of the twentieth century, dental photography had to be limited to the professional photographer's studio. Prior to the early 1960s, dental photography for the clinician was impractical because of a lack of proper through-the-lens viewing, lighting complications, exposure difficulties, and affordability.

The first 35 mm single lens reflex (SLR) camera was available just prior to World War II. These cameras, which incorporate a mirror and a prism, allow the photographer to see the same image the lens is "viewing" (Figs. 17–1, 17–2). Non-SLR cameras (called range finder cameras) use a viewing window located 3 to 4 inches above the film plane. This means that the image the viewer sees and the image the film exposes are not identical. This problem is referred to as parallax, and it makes accurate close-up dental photography impossible (Fig. 17–3).

For a camera system to be practical in dentistry, it must be fairly lightweight, have adequate lighting mounted on the end of the lens barrel, be automatic enough to factor out most of the technical problems for the user, have a high degree of image-accuracy, and be affordable. Most of these problems were not solved until the advent of the bellows system in the early 1960s. This camera has a short-mount lens attached to an ac-

cordion-like tube that expands and contracts to achieve the desired magnification. The automatic macro lens was soon developed as a more practical approach than the racking system of the bellows.

Today, the basic high quality close-up camera system is composed of a 35 mm SLR camera body, a macro lens (or short-mount lens for the bellows system) in the 100 mm range, a ring light or point source flash mounted on the end of the lens barrel, and a power source, either separate or encased in the light unit. Modern through-the-lens metering systems automatically determine the proper setting for a given film type and lighting condition. Electronic cameras remove almost all manual control of the parameters of photography. The operator has only to focus and shoot to produce good, accurate dental photographs.

Most recently, automatic focus 35 mm SLR cameras have become available, but the combination of automatic camera cost coupled with automatic lens cost makes these units expensive by comparison to most manual focus systems. If the clinician desires a unit that requires minimal manual input, manual focus cameras give extremely satisfying results at an affordable price.

USES OF DENTAL PHOTOGRAPHY

Quality Control. Dental photography can be an effective quality control measure. The magnified image in a dental photograph often highlights imperfections that the clinician may have overlooked. Such feedback is an excellent learning device.

Patient Records. Photographs are an effective treatment planning adjunct. With a thorough medical history, intraoral charting, study models, radiographs, and intraoral and extraoral photographs, the treatment

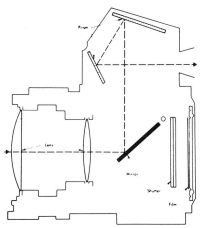

FIG. 17–1. A single-lens reflex (SLR) camera with the mirror in the view-finding position. In this position the mirror and prism mechanism allows the SLR camera to see the exact same image as the viewer's eye.

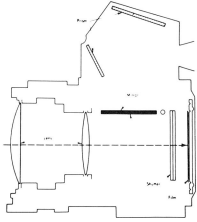

FIG. 17–2. An SLR camera with the mirror in the "exposing" position. In this position the mirror is lifted out in order to allow light to expose the film.

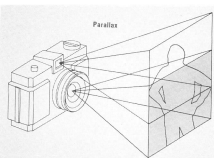

FIG. 17–3. The parallax problem of range finder (any non SLR) cameras.

planning may be accomplished almost as if the patient were present. In addition, attaching a photograph to the outside of the patient record facilitates instant recall of that patient by all staff members.

Case Presentation. Photographs of the patient's current condition enhance the patient's understanding of a proposed treatment plan, especially when accompanied by a portfolio of before and after photographs of similar, successfully treated cases. In addition the acceptance of treatment plans may increase through this approach.

Treatment Documentation. Before and after photographs provide accurate visual documentation. The dentist should obtain a release from the patient in order to display these photographs (especially full face photographs) for any other purpose (see Appendix D).

Laboratory Communication. A color photograph or slide of the restorative case facilitates communication with the laboratory. Photographing the shade tab adjacent to the teeth to be restored makes the chances of success higher. A good camera and Kodachrome 64 film will not capture the subtle differences between shades with 100% accuracy, however, the relative shade of the tab to the shade of the tooth is the important parameter. When the laboratory technician compares the actual tab to the photograph, appropriate adjustment can be made.

Insurance. Submitting color prints for insurance claims may increase the chances of treatment plan acceptance. Often, the condition in question is not radiographically evident, although a color photograph presents the situation clearly. A claim can also be made for reimbursement for the photographs just as one does for radiographs (ADA Code 00471).

Education. Photography can be used for conferring with a colleague or for lecturing at dental meetings, study clubs, or in table clinics. It can be used in publications or, as mentioned above, in patient consultation. Once again, a signed release is necessary before any such use of photographs.

Community Service. Presentations to local organizations raises the dental health consciousness of the community, improves the image of the profession, and expands the dentist's future patient base by creating a greater awareness of advances in dentistry.

Marketing. Photography has a tremendous capacity to help any dental practice grow more effectively through internal and external marketing. Just being photographed may make a patient feel more important. After treatment has been completed, before and after color prints can be sent in attractive and inexpensive frames. Before and after photographs of some dramatic esthetic cases can be included in a patient newsletter. Representative esthetic cases can be illustrated in a three panel brochure format fairly inexpensively and purchased in small quantities. These can then be mailed to individuals in the community, as well as given to patients who visit the office.

Children in the practice can be rewarded for good oral hygiene by having their pictures placed on a bulletin board in the waiting room. Displays of representative cases can be placed throughout the office to be seen by other patients.

Presentations to civic clubs and other organizations are greatly enhanced when slides and photographs are used.

If the practitioner involves the staff in this particular area of the practice, the collective creative capacity of the group can be tapped.

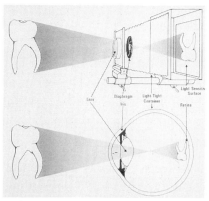

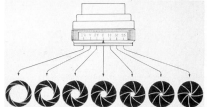

FIG. 17–5. F-stop numbers have an inverse relationship to the size of the aperture. A smaller number means a larger opening.

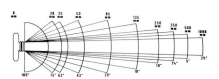

FIG. 17–6. A representative range of focal lengths of various lenses used in photography.

FIG. 17–4. An SLR camera mechanism "sees" in a manner similar to the human eye.

Medicolegal. Any and every form of record keeping is vital for defense litigation. Color photographs can be critical in esthetic treatments because the quality of the end result is subjective.

BASIC PRINCIPLES
Terminology

It is possible to use equipment that is so automated that the operator needs no particular knowledge in order to achieve the desired results, other than minimum focusing skills. However, knowledge of the workings of the camera is advantageous (Fig. 17–4).

Shutter

The shutter is a device inside the camera body that opens and closes, allowing light to strike the film for a selected period of time. This predetermined period of time is referred to as shutter speed. The various shutter speeds are indicated on a dial located on the camera body. Each shutter speed is exactly one-half the speed of the next highest one on the dial. In dental photography, a flash is used to produce the necessary light. In flash photography, only a single, predetermined synchronized shutter speed is used for proper exposures. This is usually indicated by either a different color on the dial or a broken arrow. This speed is usually $1/125$ or $1/60$ of one second and is indicated on a dial or readout located on the camera body. This eliminates one of the variables that the operator must control in order to achieve the desired quality of the resulting image. In close-up photography, most of these variables are preset and, therefore, little manipulation of the camera system is necessary to achieve quality in the finished product.

Aperture

The aperture is an opening inside the lens that controls the amount of light striking the film. The terms "aperture setting," "aperture size" and "f-stop" are synonymous. These terms refer to the size of the opening of the aperture selected by the operator (or by the camera in a fully automated system) (Fig. 17–5). The various aperture settings are indicated on a dial on the lens or on a display on the camera body. Each change in the aperture settings allows exactly one-half the amount of light to reach the film as the next larger size aperture on the dial. However, the larger the aperture; the smaller the corresponding f-stop number, which indicates the amount of opening. This is because the f-stop number is a ratio of the focal length of the lens to the diameter of the opening at a particular f-stop. In dental photography, the usual images are close-up or full face, therefore, only two aperture settings are necessary, again factoring out most of the variables. Fully automated systems set these openings for the operator and, therefore, require the operator to have no knowledge whatsoever of this function.

The sometimes confusing relationship between f-stop number and shutter speed is easily clarified by using the analogy of a water faucet. If the handle controlling the length of time the faucet remains on is likened to the shutter in the camera, and the size of the opening of the faucet through which the water runs is likened to the aperture size, it is immediately apparent that the amount of water that exits the system is a result of two variables. When the circular opening of the faucet is left open for 2 seconds, a specific volume of water is collected. If the opening is reduced to one-half that size, the faucet would have to remain on for twice as long, (i.e., 4 seconds) to collect the same volume of water. Therefore, the total volume of water collected is controlled by the total area of the size of the opening and the length of time the orifice is allowed to remain open. This is exactly how the camera and lens system works to control the amount of light that reaches the film. Because the shutter speeds are related by increments of two when traveling up or down the dial and the aperture settings are also related by increments of two, several combinations of shutter speed and aperture size result in exactly the same amount of light reaching the film.

Focus

Focus refers to the degree of clarity of the image on the film. This clarity is controlled in one of two ways. If the operator wishes to have a uniform magnification of all of the photographs in a series, then the magnification is chosen and the focus is adjusted by moving the camera away from or closer to the subject until the image is in focus. The chosen magnification remains unchanged. If this uniformity is not important, focus is achieved by rotating the lens barrel.

Lens

The lens refers to the barrel mounted on the camera body, which houses the lens optics that control the focus of the image on the film. Dental photography requires a macro lens in order to achieve close-up images. The term macro lens refers to a close-up lens. (See the section on Macro Lens later in this chapter.)

Focal Length

The focal length of a lens is the distance from the film to the optical center of the lens, measured in millimeters (Fig. 17–6). For all practical purposes, this optical center coincides with a point located at the center of the aperture. For the most accurate images in dental close-up photography, the appropriate focal lengths are between 90-120 mm.

Film Speed

Film speed refers to the relative sensitivity of the film to the available light. The higher the film speed, the more sensitive the film is to the light. For example, a film speed of 64 requires less light for the desired exposure than one of 25. Lower film speed renders less graininess in the finished photo, therefore, the lowest film speed that will render the desired result is preferred. Flash photography is best used with film speeds that are made to simulate daylight situations. The appropriate film speeds are ASA 100 or less. Film speed is indicated on the film by either ASA, ISO, or DIN. These abbreviations refer to the international organizations that control these parameters of film production. (See the section on Film later in this chapter.)

Exposure

Exposure refers to the amount of light that must reach the film in order to get a proper photograph. This single most important principle of photography is controlled by four factors and will determine the success of the end results. These four factors are: shutter speed, aperture size, light source, and film speed.

As previously discussed, several combinations of aperture settings and shutter speeds can result in the same amount of light entering the camera. When photographing in natural lighting this is important; however, in flash photography shutter speed is fixed because it must be synchronized with the camera flash. Therefore, only the aperture can be varied. A full face photograph requires more light than a close-up because the film is farther away from the subject. This means a larger aperture size (smaller f-stop number) is required for the full face photograph than for the close-up. An average range is f22 for the close-up and f5.6 for the full face. The f-stop for any particular camera can be one f-stop on either side of these numbers, depending on the cam-

era, film, film speed, type of macro lens, light source, and possible use of filters.

Light Source

The third factor affecting exposure is the light source. In close-up photography, the usual light source is either a point source or a ring light (Fig. 17–7). The point source is mounted on a rotating bracket on the end of the lens. It is rotated around the lens to achieve the most advantageous lighting for each photograph. Generally, this type of flash creates a visual environment, that is similar to natural light, producing more shadows, with greater depth, contrast, and texture. Absolute familiarization with the proper position for the point light must be gained or an entire series of photographs can be ruined. This can be very disconcerting because the practitioner does not always have a second chance.

The other type of flash lighting used in close-up photography is the ring light. The ring light completely encircles the end of the lens barrel and gives more even lighting, resulting in a flatter surface with less depth, contrast, and texture. The major advantage of the ring light is that its position remains unchanged, resulting in one less variable for the operator to control.

No consensus has been reached regarding the light source to choose for dental use. The operator should make an informed choice and please only himself. Fortunately, there are suppliers who offer both light sources with their standard systems because in some clinical situations one is preferred over the other.

At least one company, Nikon, offers a a graded ring flash unit. One side of the ring flash produces more light than the other, resulting in an image with all the elements of even lighting, depth, contrast, and texture. Minolta's Maxxum ring flash has switches that individually control the left, right, top, and bottom tubes. The Maxxum automatically increases the total light output to compensate for any tubes that are turned off. If only a single tube is left on, the system acts as a point flash. This unit is discussed in a subsequent section. Altering any of the above variables can achieve any combination of results, from completely natural appearing photographs to surrealistic images. In flash photography, the only variable that can be changed is aperture setting. The single shutter speed is determined by the manufacturer and is never changed. The flash unit produces a set amount of light and the film speed setting, on the camera should never differ from the speed indicated on the film itself.

Depth of Field

Depth of field is the range of distance from the lens within which objects will appear in focus (Figs. 17–8, 17–9). In dental photography, the more depth of field achieved, the sharper the image in front of and behind the specific object being focused on. In flash photography, the two variables controlling depth of field are aperture size and distance from the focused image. The smaller the aperture (larger f-stop) and the farther the distance from the focused image, the more depth of

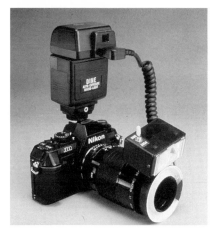

FIG. 17—7. A camera with both a point source and a ring light (Lester Dine Unit C).

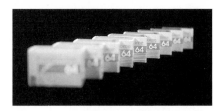

FIG. 17—8. Small depth of field, large aperture size (f/2.8).

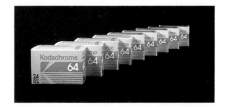

FIG. 17—9. Large depth of field, small aperture size (f/32).

field. Because close-ups require the least amount of light, smaller openings can be used. This results in the maximum depth of field appearing on the photographs where it is desired. As the operator moves farther from the subject for full face photographs, the lighting requirements demand a larger aperture size, but the greater distance from the image helps compensate for this larger opening, thus maintaining good depth of field. In order to achieve the maximum depth of field, the photographer should focus on an object that is one-third the distance into the desired depth of field.

Magnification

Magnification indicates the relationship between the size of the image on the film and the size of the actual image. These relationships are expressed in ratios. If the size of the photographed image on the film is exactly the same as the actual image, the magnification is 1:1. A magnification of 1:2 means the image on the film is one-half the actual size of the object. Most close-ups are taken at approximately 1:1.2 or 1:1.5, and full faces are usually in the 1:8 to 1:10 range. Proper use of magnification produces a series of photographs of the same dental case with uniform magnification over a period of time. This makes viewing these photographs much easier. Magnification indicator markings appear on most cameras.

Composition

Composition simply refers to the content of the photograph. The image should contain only those items intended for view. Many times, magnification is the only variable that needs to be changed to achieve proper composition. Superfluous objects in slides or prints are very distracting.

Summary

Good photographs combine proper exposure, depth of field, and composition. The use of a flash as a light source significantly simplifies the process because when using a flash, most other variables cannot be altered: exposure is controlled only by the aperture setting; depth of field is automatically determined by the chosen focused point, and composition and magnification are determined by what the operator wants in the photograph. Attention to these few easily controlled variables makes dental photography simple and satisfying.

BASIC ARMAMENTARIUM

The basic equipment required for proper dental photography is a 35 mm SLR camera body, a macro lens, a flash unit, accessories such as mirrors and lip retractors, and the appropriate film.

35 mm SLR Camera Body

The 35 mm camera body is the part of the system that has the least requirements for use in dentistry. The camera body's only function is to hold and advance the film and to trip the shutter for the proper timing. The shutter speed for flash photography is predetermined by the manufacturer, therefore, the camera body's function is greatly simplified when compared to other, nondental photographic situations. For these reasons, the operator need not make a large expenditure on this part of the system. The main consideration is that the camera body is compatible with the macro lens chosen. Most manufacturers make bodies with interchangeable mounts, in order to achieve this compatibility. Novices should purchase camera bodies produced by major manufacturers.

Bellows Systems

The bellows system is unsurpassed for image quality, but many clinicians find the modern 90 to 120 mm macro lenses more practical and less time consuming. The slight increase in image accuracy when compared to the macro lenses is not a practical consequence to most clinicians.

Macro Lens

The term macro refers to the close-up capability of the focusing range of macro lenses. There are several reliable macro lenses on the market, which function well for dental use. For the most distortion-free images, the focal length should be in the 90 to 120 mm range. These lenses provide less distortion and more comfortable working lengths than lenses with shorter or longer focal lengths. At least one manufacturer sells a 55 mm lens. This focal length functions fairly well for dental purposes, except the working distance for the close-ups is short and the distortion on the full-face is evident. The other important factor in choosing a lens is the magnification capabilities. Many good macro lenses achieve a 1:1 magnification without additional converters or extenders to expand the magnification range. Some older models only achieved 1:2 magnification and required extenders for 1:1 magnification, which added expense.

Flash

In order to obtain the proper lighting effects in intraoral photographs, the light must be mounted on the end of the lens barrel, otherwise the lips will cause harsh shadows. The choice for proper lighting is either a point or a ring flash (see Fig. 17–7). There are legitimate applications for both, depending on the needs and preferences of the operator. (See the section on Light Source earlier in this chapter.) The operator can have both units in the same system, allowing for personal preference in each situation; the added expense of having both types of flashunits is minimal.

Data Backs

Many cameras offer an optional data back. This device replaces the back of the camera and is capable of permanently imprinting the time and date the picture was taken on the film. Some units can imprint exposure information (e.g., shutter speed and aperture setting) in order to permanently record the optimal camera setting required for different lighting conditions. Although the data back can be switched off, once the data is imprinted on the film it cannot be removed. In some situations printed information may detract from the esthetics of the photograph.

Retractors and Mirrors

Proper lip (cheek) retractors are made of double-ended clear plastic (Fig. 17–10). The clear plastic allows the tissue to be seen through the retractor (lessening distraction), and the double-end allows for versatility because the two ends can be different sizes. These plastic retractors can be reshaped with an acrylic bur to any size the operator finds useful. Sometimes metal retractors can be used in combination with buccal mirrors (the long slender mirrors that reflect buccal views and fit between the zygomatic arch and the lower border of the mandible).

The best mirrors available are front surface glass mirrors. Just as in dental mirrors, front surface mirrors give a clearer single image view, instead of the sometimes double (shadowed) view of back surface mirrors.

Chrome-plated mirrors work well, except they require a larger aperture setting for proper exposure. The light does not reflect as brightly off them as compared to glass mirrors.

Two differently shaped mirrors are required, one for

CLINICAL TIP. To determine mirror type, place an explorer directly onto the mirror surface. On a front surface mirror the "tips" will meet. On a back surface mirror, there will be a space between the tips which represents the distance between the glass and the reflecting surface on the back.

full occlusal views and one for buccal and lingual views (Fig. 17–11). The clinician with a varied practice of all age groups will probably need at least two sizes of each of these mirrors.

CLINICAL TIP. A commonly encountered problem is mirror fogging caused by the patient's breath. This can be eliminated by either soaking the mirrors in warm water, or by having the assistant gently blow air from the syringe onto the mirror while it is in use.

CLINICAL TIP. If saliva splatters on the mirror, the mirror must be removed and cleaned because this causes a significant distraction on the finished photograph.

Film

Several companies produce good film for dental purposes. Some of these companies, however, have not been manufacturing film long enough to guarantee archival (longevity) quality. Kodak produces a wide range of film that is ideally suited for dental purposes (Fig. 17–12). The proper film for flash photography is daylight film of 100 ASA or lower, such as Kodacolor 100 for prints and Kodachrome 64 or 25 for slides. The difference in grain between 64 and 25 is undetectable, but the tooth and tissue tones are more correct with Kodachrome 64. Kodachrome 64 is unsurpassed for photographing the human body because of its correct red coloration and unequaled worldwide consistency of manufacturing and developing. When speed of processing is the top priority, Ektachrome 100 is useful, however, the tooth and tissue tones are not correct without the use of filters, and it has inferior archival quality compared to other films.

If the practitioner wants prints only for use in the office, Kodacolor 100 is the only film needed. However, if slides are necessary for either office use or seminar purposes, Kodachrome 64 can be used exclusively because a good custom color laboratory can render an extremely high quality print from a properly exposed slide.

There are several types of instant Polaroid films for different cameras and needs. The Dental Pro (Trojan Clinical Camera Systems) and the Dine Instant Model 4 (Lester Dine, Inc.) cameras use type 600+ and 779 film. For dental use, the 779 produces more consistent color at the same price.

The DPX (Lester A Dine, Inc.) and CU-5 (Trojan Camera Systems, Inc.) cameras use type 669 film, which is a higher quality film that is color balanced for skin tones and can be purchased at large retail stores and professional stores.

Type 691 film can be purchased for instant 3¼ × 4¼ transparencies. Polaroid Polachrome is an instant slide

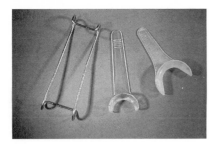

FIG. 17–10. Plastic and metal retractors.

FIG. 17–11. Various dental mirrors.

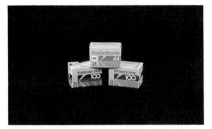

FIG. 17–12. Recommended Kodak film for slides and prints.

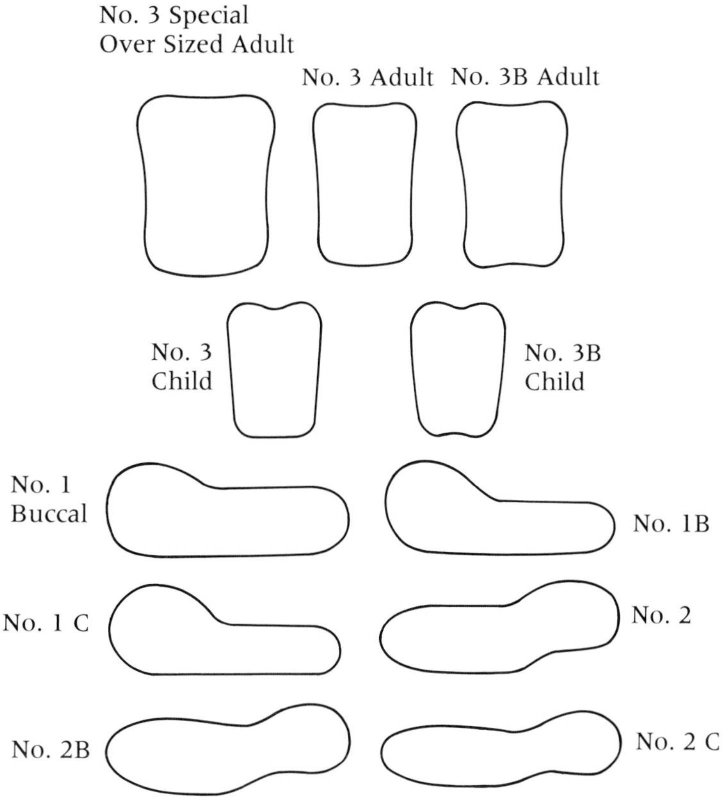

No. 3 Special
Over Sized Adult

No. 3 Adult   No. 3B Adult

No. 3
Child

No. 3B
Child

No. 1
Buccal

No. 1B

No. 1 C

No. 2

No. 2B

No. 2 C

FIG. 17–11

film used in 35 mm cameras, which requires some additional hardware for instant self-developing. The quality is sharp but grainy and lacks color brilliance.

Summary

The critical elements of the necessary dental photography equipment are the macro lens, the flash unit, and the film. The mirrors, retractors, and camera body are important, however the specific selection from among the available choices is less critical.

AVAILABLE EQUIPMENT

The choice of system can have a lot to do with who will be taking the photographs, as well as the particular needs of the office. If the dentist finds employee turnover to be high, a simple system may be a good choice. If the clinician will be taking most of the photographs, a higher quality and more complex camera will present no problem.

This discussion does not cover every detail of every available unit, but it includes the important major differences. The units are listed in order of expense, with the most expensive first. Any combination of cameras, macro lenses, and flash units can be used in dentistry, but companies which exclusively serve dentistry simplify the choices. Some of the listed equipment can be obtained wholesale through mail order, and will require some investigation on the part of the purchaser. It is important to check with the manufacturer prior to pur-

chase to ensure that the options are still available, if enhancements have been made to the cameras, and if noted limitations still exist.

Nikon 120 mm Medical Nikkor

This unit is unsurpassed for ease of use and quality (Fig. 17–13). It provides full automation of every aspect of close-up photography, except focus. A manual or automatic Nikon camera body can be used with the 120 mm Medical Nikkor lens. The extreme high quality of the ring light is this unit's biggest advantage. The ring light is built into the lens, and was specifically designed for extremely accurate lighting for close-ups. The ring flash is graded so that one side of the flash emits more light than the other. This creates an image which is more three dimensional than those obtained with conventional ring lights while simultaneously producing more even distribution than available with point lights. This lens can only be used for close-up photography at magnifications from 2:1 to 1:11 and has a minimum aperture of f32, which allows for maximum depth of field. The f-stops are harnessed to the magnification, so the operator must only select the desired magnification, move toward or away from the subject for focus, and engage the shutter. This unit can be used with either AC or DC power. The lens has a mottling light that illuminates the field for preview prior to exposure. A data button is also provided which will print the magnification on the film. An optional data back will print additional characters. This unit can be obtained through mail order if the purchaser does not want the personalized attention obtained from local retail camera stores.

Minolta Maxxum

The Minolta Maxxum is available in several different models. The 7000i is the most popular for dental use, but it must be purchased with a 100 mm macro lens and a special ring flash (Fig. 17–14). It has a focal range of 1:1 to infinity. Unlike the other cameras mentioned, the Maxxum is capable of autofocusing, however, some very close subjects require manual focus. The ring light consists of four individually controlled tubes. When only a single tube is used, the camera automatically increases the light output to simulate a point flash. An optional, inexpensive, computer chip modifies the camera for close-up photography. Many other options are available, including a data back. The camera is available through mail order or from local retail camera stores.

Yashica Dental Eye II

The Yashica Dental Eye II (Fig. 17–15) is the new edition of the earlier Yashica Dental Eye and the Yashica Medical, which are no longer being manufactured. This system employs a 100 mm lens with a built-in ring flash, power winder, data back, and battery source. The 100 mm lens offers magnifications from 1:1 to 1:15. Because the lens does not focus outside this range it cannot be used for recreational photography. The camera offers automatic film loading, automatic film advance, and automatic film speed setting when used with DX film. Options include a 2× teleconverter lens for increased magnification and an AC power adaptor. This camera, lens, and power source are compact and easy for the beginner to use. Because the f-stop selections are automatically set by the magnification choices, this unit has the least amount of potential operator induced errors. In fact, the only user selectable function is the ASA selector, which must be used on non-DX encoded films. This system is manufactured by Kyocera International and is available through selected retail and mail order outlets.

Yashica Medical

This unit is similar to the Medical Nikkor except the lens barrel is much more cumbersome and the ring light cannot be graded (Fig. 17–16). The ring light is also built into the lens and is charged by a DC power source. The lens for the Medical Yashica is 100 mm, and can be used with either manual or automated camera bodies. The f-stops are harnessed to the magnifications (2:1 to 1:15), so again all the operator must do is select the desired magnification. A data back is provided, which imprints up to ten characters. The Medical Yashica and the Medical Nikkor are similar; the difference is in the Medical Nikkor's more streamlined design and more sophisticated technical in-workings of the ring light. The Yashica Medical was recently discontinued and replaced with the Yashica Dental Eye II, however it may still be available from selected retailers or mail order houses.

Lester Dine

Lester Dine has been involved with dental close-up equipment for many years (Fig. 17–17). They provide quality equipment, while keeping choices simple. One unit uses a Nikon N2000 body with a modified Kiron 105 mm lens and either a ring light, a point light, or both. Unlike the Medical Nikkor and the Medical Yashica, the Lester Dine unit focuses from 1:1 to infinity. This lens has a minimum aperture of f32 for maximum depth of field. The proper magnification for each photograph is conveniently marked on the lens barrel. This unit requires the user to change the f-stop for different exposures. This is an excellent choice for the user who wants both dental and recreational use from the camera. The N2000 camera body has a built-in motor drive, automatic film loading, and automatic ASA setting. An optional data back is also available. Lester Dine offers less expensive Kodak 35 mm cameras of significantly lower quality and a Polaroid for instant photos. They offer a complete line of dental photography accessories and a "how to" guide for the beginner or those desiring to improve their techniques. Lester Dine is located at 351 Hiatt Drive, Palm Beach Gardens, FL, 33418, 407-624-9100.

Trojan Clinical Camera Systems

Trojan provides a full range of camera units from fully automated to fully manual (Fig. 17–18). The cost of each unit varies with the amount of automation. All Trojan systems utilize an Elicar 90 mm lens, with ring light, point light, or both. The proper magnification is conveniently printed on the lens barrel. Their most popular unit is the Canon T50. There are no settings to adjust on this camera body. It loads, advances, and sets the shutter speed automatically. The 90 mm Elicar lens is manually set at the desired magnification, the proper f-stop is selected, the frame composed, and the photograph taken. This unit functions in a manner similar to the Lester Dine and can be used as a recreational camera because it can focus from 1:1 to infinity. The Trojan T50 and the standard Lester Dine unit are the two most comparable and popular units available to the dental profession. Trojan also has an Elicar MS-1 system that is fully automated. It reads the light off the front of the lens and sets the f-stop automatically. The only drawback of this system is that it only uses film of certain ASA readings. Trojan has several other 35 mm SLR units with varying degrees of automation. They also market three different Polaroid cameras. Trojan provides a full range of dental photography accessories. Trojan Clinical Camera Systems is located at 3540 S. Figueroa St., Los Angeles, CA, 90007.

Bellows System, Washington Scientific Camera

Prior to the introduction of the macro lens, the bellows system was the only high quality clinical camera system (Fig. 17–19). There are still no units that surpass the quality of the finished photograph from a bellows unit, but many nonbellows units are more convenient to ma-

FIG. 17–13. 120 mm medical Nikkor C lens with a Nikon F2 body.

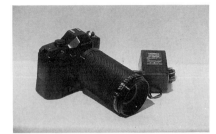

FIG. 17–13

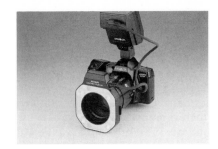

FIG. 17–14. Minolta 7000i with a 100 mm macro lens and a special ring flash.

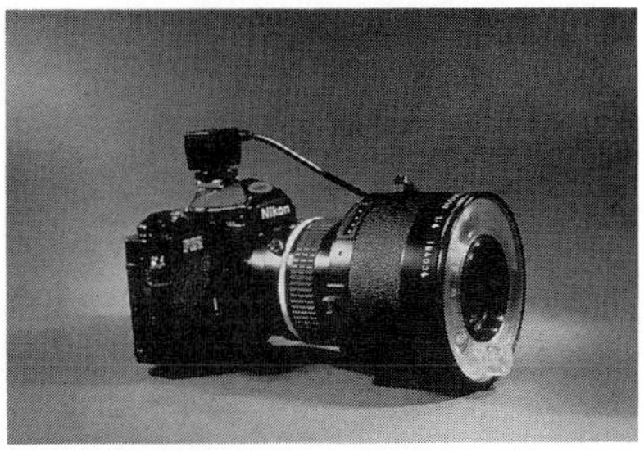

FIG. 17–14

FIG. 17–15. Yashica Dental Eye II.

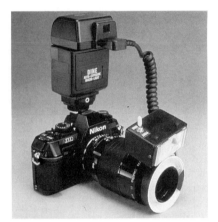

FIG. 17–16. Yashica medical camera.

FIG. 17–15

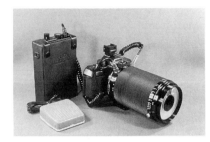

FIG. 17–16

FIG. 17–17. Lester Dine Unit C.

FIG. 17–18. Trojan cameras.

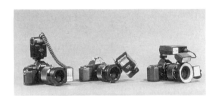

FIG. 17–18

FIG. 17–19. Bellows System (Washington Scientific Camera).

FIG. 17–17

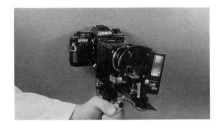

FIG. 17–19

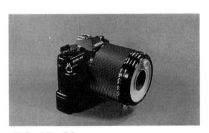

FIG. 17–20. Yashica Dental Eye.

FIG. 17–20

nipulate. This system uses a short-mount lens that is focused by moving the bellows along a tracking assembly. It provides an electronic system for maintaining the automatic diaphragm required to provide enough light for proper focusing. The aperture is manually set. Focusing ranges from 1:1 to infinity. A pistol grip is used to help support this somewhat cumbersome unit. The shutter is released by a trigger release located in the pistol grip. The components on this system have more recently been made lighter for more comfortable handling. Washington Scientific Camera is located at 615 Wood Ave., Sumner, WA, 98390.

Yashica Dental Eye

The Yashica Dental Eye has become one of the most popular clinical cameras because it is easy for the beginner to use (Fig. 17–20). This system has a compact 55 mm lens that requires very close focusing ranges. This unit has the least chances of potential operator induced errors because the camera only has one adjustable function, the ASA selector. The Yashica Dental Eye focuses from 1:1 to 1:10, and the f-stops are harnessed to the magnification, so no selections must be made by the user. The dental eye also has a built-in power pack, which eliminates cords and plugs. This feature, along with the 55 mm lens makes the Yashica Dental Eye the most compact unit available for 35 mm SLR dental photography. The drawbacks of this system are the close focusing ranges and the distortion of the image, especially on the full face. Therefore, this unit may be inappropriate for certain office situations. The Yashica Dental Eye (manufactured by Kyocera International) was recently discontinued and replaced with the Yashica Dental Eye II. It may, however, still be available from selected retailers or mail order houses.

Adolph Gasser

Adolph Gasser offers a range of clinical camera systems that use various 35 mm SLR camera bodies, coupled with either 100 or 105 mm macro lenses, and a point source light. These systems all have a focusing range from 1:1 to infinity. They are all excellent choices for the user who wishes to use the camera recreationally as well as clinically. These units require the user to set the f-stop, and they do not offer a ring flash as an option. Adolph Gasser is located at 5733 Geary Boulevard, San Francisco, CA, 94121.

Others

For the user who does not want to make the necessary investment for the excellent results achieved by 35 mm SLR units, Kodak makes a simple 35 mm camera that can be used to produce slides or prints of fair to poor quality (Fig. 17−21). This camera uses the fixed focus photographic technique. Fixed brackets with preselected magnifications are used to frame the photograph. The brackets usually come in three different focus ranges, which greatly limits the uses of this system. The three focus ranges are head and shoulder view, full view smile, and quadrant view. This is a very inexpensive and easy system suited to the beginner. These advantages must be weighed against the disadvantages of fixed focus range and poor to fair quality. This Kodak unit can be purchased through Lester Dine at 100 Milbar Boulevard, P.O. Drawer F, Farmingdale, NY, 11735.

Instant Photos

There are four units available for instant dental photographs: the Dental Pro II (Fig. 17−22) and the Dine Instant Model 4 (two different versions of the same unit); the DPX; and the CU-5 (Fig. 17−23). The basic units are all made by Polaroid and are altered for dental close-up use. The Dental Pro and the Dine are the least expensive and produce the lowest quality photographs. The most expensive, the CU-5, produces the best quality photographs. The Dental Pro, Dine, and DPX take close-up and full face standard views, whereas the CU-5 requires an added, and expensive, attachment to produce full face photographs. The DPX and the CU-5 use the same higher quality instant film. The DPX is a good choice because it frames both full face and close-up views and it uses the higher quality Polaroid film. Instant photographs are immediately available to supplement the laboratory prescription and also serve as an excellent patient education tool. Such is not the case with 35 mm film, which must be developed. The Dine Instant Model 4 is sold by Lester Dine and the Dental Pro II, DPX, and CU-5 are sold by Trojan. However, some of the same components can be purchased at other dealers throughout the United States.

Summary

Many cameras and lenses for dental use can be purchased at a local camera store, but the necessary ring light may or may not be available, and the point light will surely not be available because it is a customized component made specifically for close-up use. Companies familiar with the specific requirements of good dental photography provide the necessary equipment. It is discouraging to purchase equipment and later find that it is unsuitable for good close-up dental photography.

INTRAORAL TECHNIQUE

The post-treatment photograph can be repeated at any time, but the pretreatment photograph can never be reproduced. A good photograph is the result of proper equipment, organization, a procedural check list, and good technique. It is important that the procedure be organized and simplified so that new employees can work into the team easily.

CLINICAL TIP. The dental camera should be readily available, stored either in a wall-mounted bracket or on a counter near the work area. If the camera is not readily available it will not be used. It is not advisable for the dental camera to double as a recreational camera because it will probably be at home when needed.

CLINICAL TIP. The camera should be stored at room temperature because excessive heat can adversely affect the film.

A simplified check list will prevent error.

1. Load the film and set the proper ASA.
2. Turn on the power unit.
3. Check the film advance and shutter speed for flash synchronization.
4. Set the f-stop.
5. Position the subject, flash, retractors, and mirrors.
6. Choose the desired magnification.
7. Focus and release the shutter.

(Note: Many automatic cameras eliminate some of these steps).

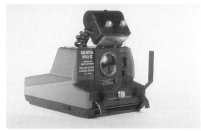

FIG. 17—22. Polaroid Dental Pro II.

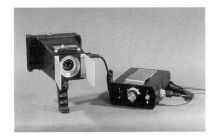

FIG. 17—23. Polaroid CU-5.

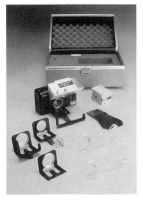

FIG. 17—21. Kodak 35 mm (non-SLR).

CLINICAL TIP. The most common single error committed by the beginner is incorrect magnification choice. A typical magnification error is including the nose and chin in a frontal view of the oral cavity. This extraneous information is distracting for the viewer. The photographer must decide what the desired photograph should contain, and then choose the magnification that will eliminate everything else.

CLINICAL TIP. Good intraoral photographs should appear as if the camera was aimed directly at the desired subject whether or not mirrors were used. The photographs should be devoid of mirror edges, fingers or thumbs, fog, saliva, lip retractors, or any elements other than the desired aspect of the oral cavity.

CLINICAL TIP. Lip retractors are not always easily eliminated, but clear retractors are an excellent compromise. Some photographs may require only the patient's assistance, whereas others require assistance from the patient, the photographer, and one or even two auxiliary staff members.

Anterior (Frontal) View

The anterior or frontal view is the most common view used in dental photography (Fig. 17—24). It ranges from a single tooth to a full face view.

Clinical Technique

1. Seat the patient semi-upright with the head turned toward the photographer.
2. Place retractors at the corners of the mouth and pull gently outward and forward so the buccal tissue is away from the teeth.
3. If a point light is used, it should be at the 9 o'clock position in order to create a sense of depth with shadows.
4. Set the f-stop.
5. Hold the camera so the occlusal plane is perpendicular and centered horizontally to the plane of the film.
6. Align the patient's midline with the center of the frame. Compose the photograph to include all relevant teeth and soft tissue. Adjust the magnification (usually 1:2).
7. Focus the camera.

CLINICAL TIP. In order to achieve maximum sharpness of the image, focus the camera on the canines, not on the central incisors.

Maxillary Occlusal View

The maxillary occlusal view is the most difficult view to obtain and requires patience (Fig. 17—25). This photograph usually requires assistance from two staff members.

Clinical Technique

1. Seat the patient in a semi-upright position with the head turned toward the photographer.
2. Instruct assistant 1 to gently rotate the retractors upward and outward.

CLINICAL TIP. A standard set of retractors can be modified by removing the flange on one side of the retractor (Fig. 17—26) such that when the retractor is rotated toward the desired arch, there is no interference between the mirror and the retractor.

3. Instruct assistant 2 to rest a full arch mirror on the maxillary tuberosity, not on the teeth. The mirror should diverge from the occlusal plane as much as possible so the camera can be held 90° to the plane of the mirror.
4. If a point light is used it should be at the 9 o'clock or 3 o'clock position.
5. Set the f-stop.
6. Hold the camera so the plane of the film is parallel to the full arch in view.
7. Align the midline of the palate with the center of the frame. Compose the photograph to include all relevant teeth and soft tissue. Adjust the magnification (usually 1:2).
8. Focus on the premolar area.

Mandibular Occlusal View

The mandibular occlusal view is the reverse of the maxillary occlusal view (Fig. 17—27).

Clinical Technique

1. Seat the patient in the supine position, parallel to the floor.
2. Tip the patient's head slightly back, turned toward

the photographer so the occlusal plane is parallel to the floor.

3. Rotate the retractors gently downward toward the mandible and outward.

CLINICAL TIP. *When photographing the mandibular occlusal view, use the same altered lip retractors that were described for the maxillary view. (See the preceding Clinical Tip.)*

---

4. Rest a full arch mirror on the retromolar pad, not on the teeth.
5. The mirror should diverge from the occlusal plane as much as possible so the camera can be held 90° off the plane of the mirror.
6. If a point light is used it should be at the 9 o'clock or 3 o'clock position.
7. Set the f-stop.
8. Hold the camera so the plane of the film is parallel to the full arch in view.
9. Align the midline of the tongue with the center of the frame. Compose the photograph to include all relevant teeth and soft tissues. Adjust the magnification (usually 1:2).
10. Focus on the premolar area.

Buccal View

Buccal views are ideal for photographing the patient's centric occlusion (Figs. 17–28, 17–29).

Clinical Technique

1. Seat the patient in a semi-upright position with his head facing straight for left buccal views and toward the photographer for right buccal views. (Reverse for left-handed dental units.)
2. Place a buccal mirror distal to the last tooth in the arch. Move it as laterally as possible while retracting the lip at the same time. The mirror also serves as a retractor.

CLINICAL TIP. *Buccal views can be taken without mirrors if a view of the distal end of the terminal molar is not required.*

---

3. If a mirror is used, place a single retractor on the side opposite the mirror.
4. If no mirror is used, pull the retractor on the side being photographed as distally as comfortably possible for the patient. Passively hold the retractor on the side that is not being photographed.
5. If a point source light is used, place it on the same side of the camera as the mirror.
6. Set the f-stop.
7. Hold the camera so the plane of the film is as perpendicular to the mirror as possible.
8. Compose the photograph to include from the distal area of the canine to the most posterior tooth, with the plane of occlusion parallel to the film plane and in the middle of the frame. Set the magnification (usually 1:1.5 to 1:2).
9. Focus the camera on the premolar area.

Lingual View

Lingual views of the maxilla (Figs. 17–30, 17–31) or the mandible are obtained similarly (Figs. 17–32, 17–33).

Clinical Technique

1. Position the patient semi-upright with his head facing straight for right views and toward the photographer for left views. (Reverse for left-handed dental units.)
2. Place retractors at the corners of the mouth, rotated toward the photographed arch, and passive on the opposite side.
3. For a mandibular photograph, place a mirror between the tongue and the quadrant being photographed, distal to the terminal tooth, parallel to the long axis of the teeth, and pushed laterally as much as possible. For a maxillary photograph, place the mirror against the palate in the midline, distal to the terminal tooth, parallel to the long axis of the teeth, and as lateral as possible.
4. If a point source light is used, place it on the same side of the camera as the mirror.
5. Set the f-stop.
6. Hold the camera so the plane of the film is as perpendicular to the mirror as is possible.
7. Compose the photograph to include from the distal area of the canine to the most posterior tooth, with the plane of occlusion parallel with the film plane and in the middle of the frame. Set the magnification (usually 1:1.5 to 1:1.2).
8. Focus the camera be on the distal of the canine.

Others

Any of the above views can be modified to meet the needs of the user. Usually, only a change in magnification is necessary to suit the specific needs. For example, if only an occlusal view of a quadrant is necessary, the buccal or lingual mirror can be used in a similar manner as described for the full arch occlusal view, along with a modification in the magnification. For a view of only the premaxilla, only the necessary portion of a full arch mirror is used and the magnification is adjusted (1:1.2). The creativity of the photographer will allow for any other specific views that are needed (Figs. 17–34 to 17–36).

EXTRAORAL TECHNIQUE

Good, finished full face and profile photographs require a pleasant colored background. An art store can furnish art paper in a number of suitable colors. The best is usually a pastel color that contrasts with normal hair color and skin tones. A soft blue is the best overall. This paper can be taped to the wall in the operatory and removed as needed.

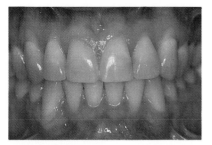

FIG. 17–24. Anterior (frontal) view (1:2 magnification).

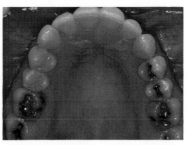

FIG. 17–25. Maxillary occlusal view (1:2 magnification).

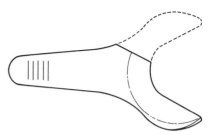

FIG. 17–26. A standard cheek retractor can be modified by removing a flange from one of its sides. This provides increased working space and allows for better visualization of the dental arch.

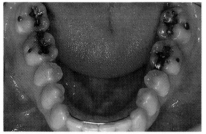

FIG. 17–27. Mandibular occlusal view (1:2 magnification).

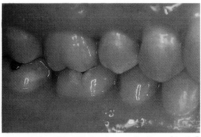

FIG. 17–28. Right buccal view (1:1.2 to 1:1.5 magnification).

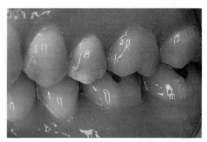

FIG. 17–29. Left buccal view (1:1.2 to 1:1.5 magnification).

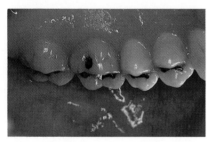

FIG. 17–30. Maxillary left lingual view (1:1.2 to 1:1.5 magnification).

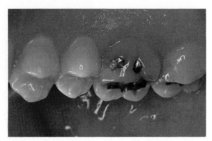

FIG. 17–31. Maxillary right lingual view (1:1.2 to 1:1.5 magnification).

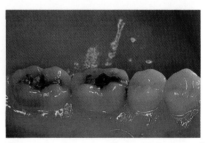

FIG. 17–32. Mandibular left lingual view (1:1.2 to 1:1.5 magnification).

FIG. 17–33. Mandibular right lingual view (1:1.2 to 1:1.5 magnification).

FIG. 17–34. Lateral view.

FIG. 17–35. Occlusal quadrant view.

FIG. 17–36. Incisal quadrant view.

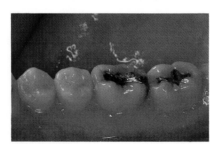

FIG. 17–33

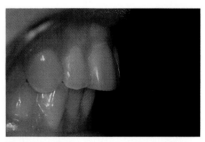

FIG. 17–34

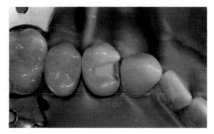

FIG. 17–35

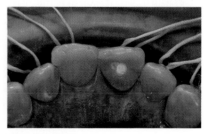

FIG. 17–36

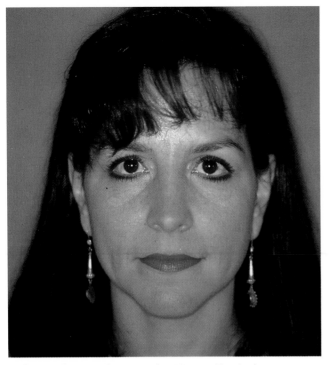

FIG. 17–37. Full face view (1:10 magnification).

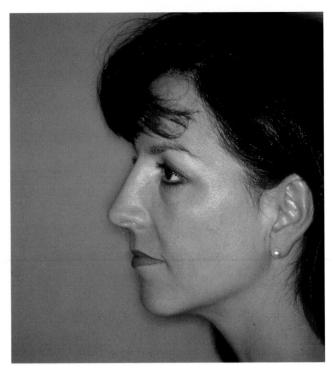

FIG. 17–38. Profile view (1:10 magnification).

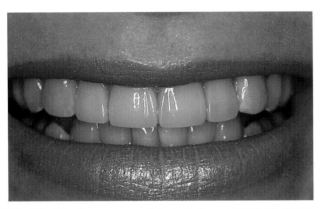

FIG. 17–39. Relaxed, casual buccal view without lip retractors.

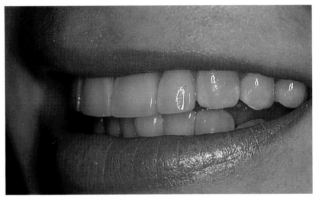

FIG. 17–40. Relaxed, casual three-quarter view without lip retractors.

Full Face (Fig. 17–37)

Clinical Technique

1. Position the patient approximately 18 to 24 inches in front of the background to help minimize shadows.
2. Position the head such that a line from the ala of the nose to the tragus of the ear is parallel to the floor.
3. If a point source is used, place it at the 12 o'clock position.
4. Set the f-stop.
5. Position the camera vertically at the level of the patient's eyes.
6. Compose the photograph to include from the infe-rior border of the hyoid to above the top of the head. Set the magnification (usually 1:10).
7. Focus the camera on the patient's eyes.
8. Take a photograph with the teeth in occlusion.
9. Take a second photograph with the patient smiling.

Profile (Fig. 17–38)

Clinical Technique

1. Position the patient approximately 18 to 24 inches in front of the background to help minimize shadows.
2. Position the head such that a line from the ala of the nose to the tragus of the ear is parallel to the floor. The teeth should be in occlusion.

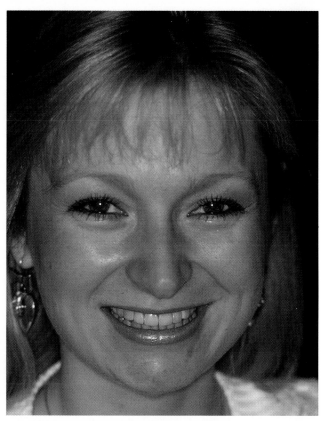

FIG. 17–41. Relaxed, casual full face view without lip retractors.

CLINICAL TIP. The head should be turned slightly toward the photographer so that the off-side eyelash is just visible. This prevents the appearance of the patient looking away from the camera.

3. If a point source is used, place it on the side of the camera that the patient is facing. The camera should be in a vertical position at the level of the patient's eyes.
4. Set the f-stop.
5. Compose the photograph so the profile dominates the center of the frame, with the area just behind the ear visible. Set the magnification (usually 1:10).
6. Focus the camera on the patient's eyes.

CLINICAL TIP. A more relaxed or casual view without lip retractors is useful and appropriate for esthetic dentistry, especially when designed for patient viewing (Figs 17–39 to 17–41). Never show patient's with lips retracted when illustrating esthetic dentistry.

TABLE 17–1. COMMON PHOTOGRAPHIC PROBLEMS AND POSSIBLE CAUSES

PROBLEM	POSSIBLE CAUSES
Incomplete image	Improperly loaded film Improper shutter speed for flash synchronization
Black image	Improperly loaded film Inadequate initial film advance Improperly connected flash Broken flash
Shadows	Improperly positioned point flash Extraneous overhead lighting reflected into mirrors disrupting the flash
Improper exposure	Weak flash batteries Improperly set flash Incorrect f-stop Improperly set ASA
Out of focus image	Improperly focused Fog on the mirror Camera movement Patient movement

TECHNICAL ERRORS

Some of the common problems encountered in the finished photograph can be caused by technical errors. Table 17–1 lists some of the major mistakes committed when using the camera and lens system, however, it is not meant to be an exhaustive list.

CONCLUSION

The clinical use of photography in dentistry has many practical, profitable, and satisfying applications. The clinician should analyze how the camera will be used and select a system accordingly. Through photography, the rewards of dentistry will be experienced at a higher level of quality for everyone.

BIBLIOGRAPHY

1. Swift, E.J., Jr., Quiroz, L., and Hall, S.A.: An introduction to clinical photography. Quint Int 18:859, 1987.
2. Freehe, C.L.: Symposium on dental photography. Dent Clin North Am 27:3, 1983.
3. Gehrman, R.E.: Dental Photography. Tulsa, OK, Penn Well Publishing, 1982.
4. Hook, S.: The camera is a practice builder. Dent Econ 77:71, 1987.
5. Freedman, G.: Standardization in dental photography. Compend Contin Educ Dent 10:682, 1989.
6. Goodlin, R.M.: The Complete Guide to Dental Photography. Montreal, Michael Publishing Co., 1987.

Mark King, D.D.S., M.S.

ESTHETICS AND ELECTROSURGERY

18

Esthetic evaluation of the oral cavity often concentrates on the color, spacing, and arrangement of the teeth without considering the architecture of the soft tissue. The gingival architecture is just as important as other parameters to good overall esthetics.

CONCEPTIONS AND MISCONCEPTIONS

Electrosurgery allows for easy, quick, safe alteration or removal of living tissue of the oral cavity with little or no bleeding. The esthetic results can be remarkable. It can also be used for gingivoplasty, hyperplastic tissue removal, mucoperiosteal surgery, overhanging tissue excision in Class I, II, III, IV, and V lesions, frenuli removal, sulcus expansion, hemorrhage control, endodontic procedures, bleaching, root sensitivity, and biopsy excisions. Yet electrosurgery is one of the least used techniques in the contemporary dental armamentarium because of misconceptions caused by fear, and misunderstanding.

BASIC CONCEPTS

Electrosurgery is the surgical application of fully controlled, partially self-limiting, high frequency, electrically generated heat energy to living tissue to alter or remove it for therapeutic purposes, while permitting and promoting desirable tissue repair.[1]

Brief History

Prior to 1891, the instruments used for heat generated surgical alteration or removal of organic tissue were crude, uncontrollable flame-heated cautery instruments.[1] In 1891, D'Arsonval discovered that alternating current oscillating at frequencies higher than 10,000 cycles per second produced no potentially lethal neuro-muscular pain or shock.[1] D'Arsonval's experiments led to the development of the spark-gap generator, which eventually evolved into electrosurgery. Doyen, et al., in 1907 were the first to use extremely high frequency current (3 million cycles per second) in combination with an active and passive electrode to achieve suitable surgical cutting ability. This cutting current, utilizing spark-gap generators, proved to be of poor quality. In 1908, DeForrest created the first radio tube high frequency apparatus. This led, in 1920, to a more refined apparatus, which used three electrode vacuum tubes to produce a much finer cutting current than those that had been available previously.[2] Dr. George A. Wyeth used this latest technology to develop the endotherm knife, which was the prototype electronic scalpel capable of delivering true surgical cutting energy. In the 1960s William Coles, an engineer, converted these vacuum tubes into solid state transistors, and the first pure continuous cutting current became available to dentistry.[1] This fully rectified filtered current has revolutionized electrosurgical cutting because of its ability to produce very low levels of heat energy. Modern technology has ushered in an era of potentially problem-free electrosurgical cutting procedures.

Mechanism of Action

A major misconception about electrosurgical cutting energy is that it is simple household electrical current. Everyday electricity is an alternating current, which cycles or oscillates from positive to negative 60 times per second (60 Hz). Applied to living tissue, it causes cell membrane polarization to change 60 times per second. This repeated polarization of the cell membrane results in contraction of muscle tissue and can be painful and potentially lethal. This reaction occurs at frequencies of up to 10,000 cycles per second (10 Khz).[1] Electrosurgical units convert household current into an electromagnetic radio frequency (RF) wave, which oscillates at a rate of 2 to 4 million cycles per second (2 to 4 Mhz). Because it is impossible for a cell to depolarize at this rate, the resistance of the tissue produces localized intracellular heating without the accompanying muscle contraction.[3]

As the RF wave leaves the unit, it travels from the active electrode (the handpiece), through the tissue, to the passive electrode in contact with the patient, and then back to the unit. Both electrodes remain at room temperature throughout the process. The passive electrode is often incorrectly referred to as the ground. The dental chair is grounded and no additional grounding is necessary. The passive electrode simply allows for a smoother and more efficient passage of current through the patient. At the proper current setting, the RF wave passes through the tissue and produces a slight rise in temperature, which causes the volatilization of one cell layer and leaves adjacent cell layers intact.[4] If the current is set too low it will result in drag; if it is set too high it will create sparking and result in excessive heat at the tissue site.[4] Absolute familiarization with the unit is crucial in order to achieve optimum results.

Current Types

With alternating current (including RF current) electric flow changes direction during each cycle. The amplitude of the current also changes continuously, exhibiting a classic sine wave pattern on an oscilloscope. Because this type of current causes excessive tissue damage it is not suitable for dental purposes and must be modified by the electrosurgical unit. At present, there are four basic types of current used in dentistry, each for a specific application.

1. **Sparking current.** This type of alternating current is a disorganized high frequency wave that causes localized but superficial destruction of cells (fulguration) (Fig. 18–1). It is used in the removal of fistulas and cystic growths.

2. **Partially rectified current.** Unlike alternating current, partially rectified current pulses but does not change direction (Fig. 18–2). During the first half of the cycle, partially rectified current flows in one direction while continuously changing amplitude. During the second half of the cycle there is no current flow. This type of current coagulates tissue.

3. **Fully rectified current.** During the first half of the cycle, fully rectified current is identical to partially rectified current. However, unlike partially rectified current, this flow is repeated again during the second half of the cycle (Fig. 18–3). Because this current incises and coagulates at the same time, it is used to cut edematous tissue.

4. **Fully rectified filtered current.** This current exhibits the same properties as fully rectified current, except that the change in amplitude is reduced (Fig. 18–4). On an oscilloscope the "peaks of the hills" have been eliminated, forming a more continuous flow in one direction. It is the current of choice for esthetic gingival recontouring because it provides the cleanest incision.

Lateral Heat

During an electrosurgical procedure, it is possible to cause inadvertent heating of tissue adjacent to the surgical site. This lateral heating results from the resistance of the adjacent cells to RF wave current flow. By controlling the electrode size, the time it contacts the tissue, and the type and intensity of the current, and by keeping the tissue moist, this heating can be minimized. The electrode should contact the tissue for a maximum of 1 to 2 seconds with 5 to 10 seconds between each application.

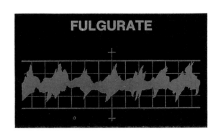

FIG. 18–1

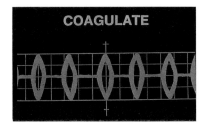

FIG. 18–2

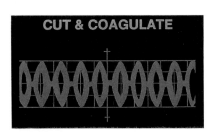

FIG. 18–3

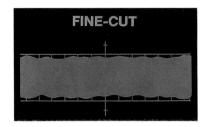

FIG. 18–4

FIG. 18–1. Sparking current. (Ellman International Manufacturing Co.).

FIG. 18–2. Partially rectified current. (Ellman International Manufacturing Co.)

FIG. 18–3. Fully rectified current. (Ellman International Manufacturing Co.)

FIG. 18–4. Fully rectified filtered current. (Ellman International Manufacturing Co.)

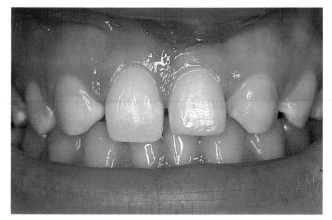

FIG. 18—5. Preoperative view of unesthetic gingival margins.

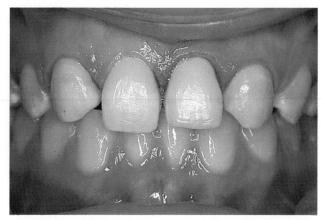

FIG. 18—6. Postoperative view immediately following surgery.

CLINICAL TIP. To dissipate excess heat and cool the adjacent tissue, moisten it with water, saliva, or saline solution prior to beginning the procedure.

The power should be set at the lowest level that still allows the electrode to move through the tissue smoothly. Use thin straight, bendable needle electrodes with fully rectified filtered cutting current.[4]

Applicable Research

One source of misconceptions about electrosurgery is found in the literature. Several investigators[5-8] have reported adverse postoperative effects of electrosurgery. Notably missing from many of these studies were descriptions of waveform, machine type, size and shape of electrode, and the speed of the electrode movement through the tissue. These variables must be properly controlled and their omission leaves these studies flawed.[9]

Many more investigators have reported overwhelmingly positive postoperative responses to electrosurgery.[10-19] When the electrode briefly contacted the oral cavity in a conventional manner, regardless of the current level, no conduction changes were detected in the heart during monitoring[1] and no damage was seen histologically in the dental pulps of animals.[20,21] When the therapist is equally competent in the use of both electrosurgery and the scalpel surgery, postoperative healing is comparable.[22-24] However, in deep resection procedures with approximation to bone, electrosurgery is contraindicated because of delayed wound healing.[24]

The overwhelming conclusion in evaluation of the literature is that when the variables in electrosurgery are properly controlled, uneventful postoperative healing is the end-result (Figs. 18—5 to 18—7).

Basic Equipment

Electrosurgery units deliver various surgical modalities, depending on the currents they produce. It is advisable to choose a unit that delivers all four current types. There are several modern, multiple-circuit, fully recti-

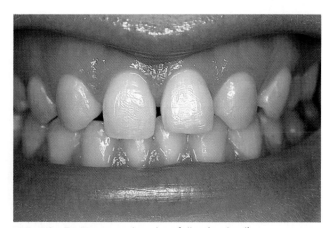

FIG. 18—7. Postoperative view following healing.

fied units available which utilize vacuum-tube power generators and solid state transistorized components to deliver these currents (Fig. 18—8). A proper unit should provide:

1. **A current selector switch** which has definitive "clicks" to indicate the type of current being used.
2. **A separate current intensity switch** that allows for continuous, linear adjustments in power.
3. **An insulated passive electrode** to create the most efficient cutting, as well as the least eventful postoperative healing. These can be incorporated into the dental chair to create less patient apprehension.
4. **A foot pedal control** for activation, rather than a handpiece control. Handpiece control requires the fingers to flex for activation, which may interfere with proper hand positioning.
5. **Thin, straight, bendable needle electrodes** (Fig. 18—9).

DIAGNOSIS AND TREATMENT PLANNING

Indications

Electrosurgery can be used to recontour any gingival architecture that is not conducive to good esthetics or

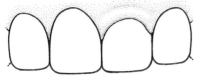

FIG. 18-8

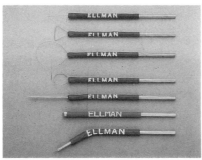

FIG. 18-9

FIG. 18-8. Electrosurgical unit. (Ellman International Manufacturing Co.)

FIG. 18-9. Electrodes are available in a multitude of shapes. For esthetic dental work a thin, straight, bendable needle electrode is used. (Ellman International Manufacturing Co.)

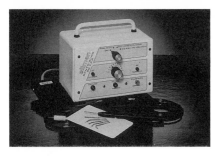

FIG. 18-10. Excess tissue caused by ectopic eruption of the maxillary left central incisor.

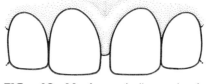

FIG. 18-11. An apically malpositioned papilla between the maxillary central incisors makes diastema closure difficult.

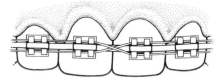

FIG. 18-12. Inflamed, hypertrophied gingiva during orthodontic treatment.

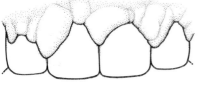

FIG. 18-13

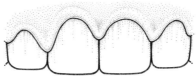

FIG. 18-14

FIG. 18-13. Hypertrophied gingival tissue during Dilantin drug therapy.

FIG. 18-14. Hypertrophied tissue caused by poor oral hygiene.

periodontal health, if attention is paid to *proper probing* and *respect for the biologic width.* The biologic width extends from the alveolar crest and includes 2 mm of gingival attachment and 1 to 2 mm of gingival sulcus. This biologic width must not be violated. Electrosurgery can be performed only on gingiva with a sulcus depth exceeding this amount.

Electrosurgery is indicated when improper contours result from any of the following causes and when the biologic width will not be violated:

1. Excess tissue caused by ectopic eruption or incomplete passive eruption of one or more teeth (Fig. 18-10).
2. Hypertrophied or malpositioned papilla (Fig. 18-11).
3. Inflamed, hypertrophied gingiva during or after orthodontic treatment (Fig. 18-12).
4. Any hypertrophied tissue from drug therapy such as Dilantin (Fig. 18-13).
5. Any hypertrophied tissue of pathologic origin, including poor oral hygiene (Fig. 18-14).

Excess Tissue Caused by Ectopic Eruption or Incomplete Passive Eruption. One of the most overlooked dental problems is excess tissue caused by ectopic eruption or incomplete passive eruption of one

or more teeth (Fig 18-15). If the eruptive force of the tooth is either misdirected or dissipates before the height of contour emerges, the gingival crest remains incisal to this height of contour. The result is inadequate crown length for proper esthetics. In the classic case, all maxillary anterior teeth are involved and the patient displays excess gingiva. Treatment of this situation depends on the cause of the excess gingiva. This excess can result from incomplete passive eruption of the teeth, insufficient lip height, overgrowth of the maxilla, or a combination of these factors. If probing reveals a sulcus of 1.5 mm or less or the radiographs reveal that the alveolar bone is in an inappropriate position, electrosurgery is contraindicated. Orthognathic or periodontal surgery involving bone removal should be considered as an alternative. If probing reveals an excess gingival sulcus and the crestal bone is in the correct position, electrosurgery alone may solve the problem, or a combination of electrosurgery and periodontal or orthognathic surgery may be required (Fig. 18-16). (See also Chapter 21—Esthetics and Periodontics.)

When teeth have improper gingival height because of ectopic eruption, orthodontic repositioning of these teeth usually will not correct this defect. Surgical recontouring is normally required after orthodontic treatment is completed.

ESTHETIC DENTISTRY

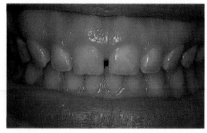

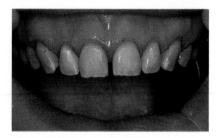

FIG. 18–15. Excess tissue caused by incomplete passive eruption.

FIG. 18–16. Postoperative view following electrosurgical procedure.

FIG. 18–15

FIG. 18–16

Hypertrophied or Malpositioned Papilla. Proper restorative diastema closure requires access to the most gingival and interproximal areas of the involved teeth. If the papilla is positioned either too far incisally or too far facially, this enamel is inaccessible and the restored teeth will have an imbalance between the mesiodistal width at the cervical as compared to the incisal: Electrosurgery can quickly make this enamel available.

Inflamed, Hypertrophied Gingiva During or After Orthodontic Treatment. This is treated in the same manner as other redundant tissue.

Hypertrophied Tissue from Drug Therapy, such as Dilantin. This is treated in the same manner as other redundant tissue.

Hypertrophied Tissue from Pathologic Origin or Poor Oral Hygiene. This is treated in the same manner as other redundant tissue.

Electrosurgery can be used to change gingival contours in any of the above conditions for esthetic purposes alone, for periodontal treatment alone, or for periodontal treatment as a precursor to esthetic treatment. Any periodontal treatment required for improved gingival health should precede esthetic treatment.

CLINICAL TIP. Treatment planning is important if electrosurgery is used in combination with esthetic restorative treatment. Although it may be possible to complete both electrosurgical and restorative procedures at the same appointment, best results are achieved with a 1 to 2 week healing period prior to the initiation of restorative treatment.

Contraindications

Electrosurgery should not be used in the following situations:

1. Within 16 feet of a pacemaker of unknown frequency (coaxially shielded pacemakers allow for safe use). The RF wave of the electrosurgery unit can interfere with the frequency of the unshielded pacemaker; this includes both patient and operator.[1]
2. When the patient has undergone radiation therapy of the head and neck. Because of the decrease in vascularization that follows radiation therapy this procedure as well as all oral surgery, carries an increased risk of osteoradionecrosis.
3. In the presence of certain chemicals, such as ethanol and chloroform, because of the danger of explosion.[1]

Advantages

The many advantages of electrosurgery include:

1. No pressure is needed for tissue separation.
2. The incision is smooth.
3. Access to remote regions of the oral cavity is easier than with other surgical modalities.
4. Tissue separation occurs with less coagulation. Scalpel incisions result in much coagulation because of trauma to the tissue, resulting in a large wound, more shrinkage, and resulting scar tissue postoperatively. Electrosurgery lessens the effects of all these healing steps because of less initial trauma upon incision and, thus, less tissue coagulation.
5. Coagulation control provides for better visibility.
6. Little or no scar tissue results.
7. Sterility is more easily controlled. All bacteria in the line of the incision are volatilized at the electrode in a similar manner as the cell (tissue) layer.
8. Electroplaning (the ability of the electrode to be placed just tangent to the tissue and plane off, i.e., remove, a minimal layer of tissue, in the manner of a carpenter's plane) of tissue is possible.
9. Allows for the planned restorative procedures to be completed in the same appointment if it is *absolutely* necessary. (See the preceding Clinical Tip.)

Nitrous Oxide Analgesia

Simple precautions allow for the confident, safe, and consistent use of nitrous oxide in conjunction with electrosurgery.[1] This should be performed with great caution. The oropharynx should be draped with slightly moist gauze to avoid accumulation of oxygen in the oral cavity. Coat any metal restorations in the surgical area with petrolatum and avoid contact with them because of the potential for excessive sparks to ignite any accumulated oxygen.

CLINICAL APPLICATIONS

In an ideal gingival architecture of the maxillary anterior teeth, the gingival heights of the central incisors and canines are equal and the gingival height of the lateral incisor is just slightly incisal to the central incisor or canine height. If the first premolar is included in the recontouring, the gingival height should be approximately 1 to 2 mm incisal to that of the canine. Precise application of instrumentation and technique cannot be over emphasized. Consistent success will follow with strict adherence to a few simple concepts.

Armamentarium:

- Standard dental setup
  cotton rolls
  explorer
  alcohol sponges
  plastic mouth mirror
  periodontal probe
  2 × 2 gauze
- Appropriate electrosurgical unit
- Thin straight bendable needle electrodes
- Passive electrode
- Extra small bite block
- Plastic high volume suction tip
- Topical anesthetic
- Local anesthetic
- Straight edge
- Hydrogen peroxide
- Tincture of benzoin and myrrh
- Aromatic oil (various flavors of fruit or flowers)

Clinical Technique:

1. Administer topical anesthetic followed by local anesthetic. Profound anesthesia is critical for a completely pain-free procedure.
2. Select a thin, straight, bendable needle electrode. Ensure that the needle electrode is completely seated into the handle of the handpiece in order to avoid contacting the metal of the shaft with the soft tissues of the lips and cheeks. Place the insulated passive plate under patient's thigh. Be certain that the patient has no metal in his pockets or on his undergarments because if the plate contacts these metal objects it can cause a burn. (The thigh is preferred because in extremely thin individuals with very sharp scapula or vertebral eminence the very thin layer of tissue may be burned if the plate is placed under the shoulder.)[1] If the plate is insulated and properly placed there is no chance of untoward occurrences.[1]

CLINICAL TIP. *The operator must be in a comfortable position to ensure a steady hand motion. The patient's head must be low enough to allow the operator's upper arms to hang comfortably at his sides with the elbows bent at 90° or more. This keeps tension off the muscles, and relaxes the upper arm.*

3. Stabilize the dentition with an extra small bite block to ensure that the mandible does not move during the procedure.
4. Place moist cotton rolls on either side of the maxillary labial frenum to retract the upper lip away from the operating area. Keep everything (tissue, cotton rolls, etc.) moist to minimize the temperature of the tissues. Also, moist cotton rolls will not stick to soft tissue during *any* procedure, thus preventing tearing of the tissue.
5. Probe the sulcular area of the appropriate teeth to determine the orientation of the gingival attachment and the depth of the sulcus (Fig. 18–17).
6. As a guide for the surgically repositioned gingival height of the involved teeth, use a maxillary anterior tooth which is not included in the surgical procedure and which has an appropriately esthetic crown length.
7. Hold a straight-edge tangent to the gingival height of the guide tooth and parallel to the pupils of the patient's eyes to determine the necessary amount of gingiva to be removed on the other teeth in order to achieve symmetry (Fig. 18–18).

CLINICAL TIP. *In orienting for the incision, disregard the occlusal plane because many patients have worn their teeth at uneven angles. Orientation with this uneven angle would result in subsequent uneven gingival orientation.*

8. Probe the affected teeth to determine if there is sufficient gingiva to perform electrosurgery and leave proper sulcular depth. Do not remove gingiva apical to the cemento-enamel junction.
9. If absolute symmetry cannot be realized, then remove as much gingiva as possible while leaving at least 1 mm of sulcus. This will result in the optimum possible esthetics in these cases.

CLINICAL TIP. *If all the maxillary anterior teeth are to be included in the surgical procedure, the tooth with the most incisally positioned gingival attachment becomes the guide for the surgically repositioned gingival height. This eliminates the possibility of violating the biologic zone on any of the teeth, and at the same time ensures the most esthetic crown length and symmetrical architecture on all teeth.*

CLINICAL TIP. *In anterior teeth, the height of the curvature of the incision is slightly toward the distal area of the tooth. The exception to this rule occurs in very square teeth, where the gingival curvature is symmetric from mesial to distal.*

10. After orienting with the pupils and determining the amount of tissue to remove, penetrate the gingival thickness at the desired height with an explorer at a right angle to the long axis of the teeth. With a periodontal probe, confirm that surgery to this new gingival height will not violate the biologic zone, while leaving the sulcus at least 1 mm deep. (Fig. 18–19).

CLINICAL TIP. *Care should be taken not to make the teeth too long. The mesiodistal width of central incisors averages 80% of their gingivoincisal height. During electrosurgery, be sure to account for any planned widening of the central incisors by bonding or laminating techniques.*

11. These gingival penetrations will bleed slightly.
12. Reorient with the pupils and confirm that surgery at the height of these penetrations will result in the desired symmetry (Fig. 18–20). If the penetrations are asymmetrical, repeat the orientation procedure until the desired balance is achieved.
13. Activate the electrosurgical unit and allow it to

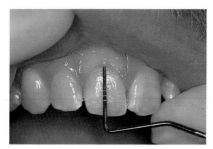

FIG. 18–17. The sulcular area is probed to determine the orientation of the gingival attachment and the depth of the sulcus.

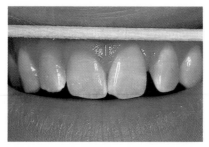

FIG. 18–18. Holding a straight edge tangent to the gingival height and parallel to the pupils of the patient's eyes, helps to determine the amount of gingiva to be removed in order to create symmetry.

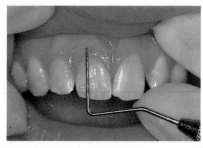

FIG. 18–19. The gingiva is penetrated at the predetermined position with an explorer at a right angle to the long axis of the tooth.

FIG. 18–20. Confirm that the height of the marks will result in the desired symmetry.

FIG. 18–21. With the handpiece held at a 45° angle toward the incisal aspect of the tooth, a smooth, pressureless hand motion should begin the incision.

FIG. 18–22. The new gingival height is confirmed for accuracy using the straightedge.

FIG. 18–23. Under normal conditions, the tissues involved in electrosurgery should heal in 7 to 14 days.

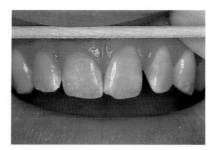

FIG. 18–20

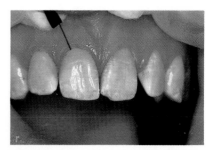

FIG. 18–21

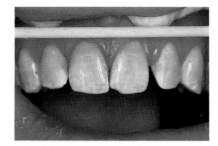

FIG. 18–22

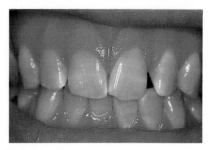

FIG. 18–23

warm up for a short period of time. Set the current selector switch on fully rectified filtered current. The separate current intensity switch should be set to maximize cutting efficiency. (Sufficient practice sessions on a cut of beef or a calf mandible will determine this setting.) Perform electrosurgery only when completely familiar with all aspects of the surgical equipment and the procedure.

CLINICAL TIP. *Reanesthetize the papilla just prior to making the incision. This assures complete anesthesia of any collateral innervation, as well as hydrates the tissue, which allows for better cutting conditions.*

CLINICAL TIP. *Keep the tissue and the surrounding areas slightly moist with saliva, water, or saline (see step 4). A dry field creates more heat and possible tissue damage.*

14. Prior to the initial incision, make a few practice cutting motions to help visualize the desired gingival contour.

CLINICAL TIP. *The odor from electrosurgical cutting of organic tissue can be strong. To mask this odor, place a 2 × 2 gauze impregnated with a pleasant smelling aromatic oil just under the nose. Many patients, however, do not find these strong smelling aromatic oils pleasant, therefore, it is best to consult the patient just prior to surgery regarding preferences.*

15. When properly oriented for the incision, activate the foot rheostat.
16. Wait momentarily for the current surge to pass and then begin the incision.
17. With the handpiece held at a 45° angle toward the incisal area of the tooth, begin the incision with a smooth, pressureless hand motion. (Fig. 18–21).

ESTHETICS AND ELECTROSURGERY

Hold the electrode tip extremely close to the tooth, but not touching it. Contacting the unevenly textured tooth surface with the electrode tip will cause drag and lead to an uneven incision. The spark-gap completes the current connection, thus initiating the incision.

CLINICAL TIP. The intensity level of the electrical current must be at a level which neither creates drag (too low) nor sparking (too high).

18. The depth of the incision should be reached on each individual pass of the electrode. However, the length of the incision does not have to be completed in one motion. Three to four short connected incisions will complete the procedure. To prevent overheating, the needle electrode should contact the tissue for not more than 1 to 2 seconds at a time while constantly in motion. Always allow 5 to 10 seconds between reapplication of the electrode at the same tissue site to prevent overheating.

CLINICAL TIP. Particular attention should always be paid to the speed and time of electrode contact with the tissue, as these are the most important aspects of the entire procedure.

CLINICAL TIP. Remove any accumulation of tissue on the electrode with an alcohol sponge. Never allow tissue remnants to remain on the electrode while cutting.

19. Care should always be taken not to over-incise the tissue; it cannot be replaced. After completion of the initial incision, use the straight edge to confirm the new gingival height for accuracy (Fig. 18–22). If needed, make necessary adjustments to achieve desired end results.
20. Surgery is incomplete without adequately cleansing the site. This includes removing all tissue tags with the electrode, curette, scaler, explorer, or any sharp sterile instrument; thorough cleansing with water, saline, or alcohol preparation; and placement of surgical dressing of 4 to 5 separate air-dried layers of tincture of benzoin and myrrh if needed. If the patient has good gingival health, as well as good overall physical health, this dressing is not required.
21. Under normal conditions, the tissues involved in electrosurgery should heal in 7 to 14 days (Fig. 18–23).
22. If the tissues were overheated during the procedure, adverse tissue reactions, such as pain, swelling, excessive inflammation or infection can occur; however, these reactions are rare. Also, overheating the tissues results in grossly delayed healing, thus, a periodontal pack may be considered to enhance healing. Smoking and drinking are contraindicated because they can delay healing.
23. Postoperative instructions include cleansing with 3% hydrogen peroxide, mixed on a cotton swab with a small amount of regular toothpaste and rinsing with warm saline solution two to three times daily for the first week. The patient should maintain a bland diet for a few days.

CLINICAL TIP. Direct toothbrush application to the surgical site is contraindicated until healing is completed.

24. If the patient experiences postoperative pain, prescribe an appropriate analgesic. Infections can be controlled with antibiotics.

CLINICAL CASES

A 45-year-old female presented with previously fractured maxillary left and right central incisors and maxillary left lateral incisor. Her medical history was noncontributory. These teeth had subsequently over-erupted, creating an imbalance in the gingival architecture of her maxillary anterior teeth (Fig. 18–24). The patient requested cosmetic bonding. Probing revealed 4 mm sulci around the central incisors and a 3 mm sulcus around the left lateral incisor. Electrosurgery was indicated on all three teeth in order to achieve a more balanced gingival architecture prior to a bonding procedure (Fig. 18–25).

A 22-year-old female presented with tetracycline stains of all teeth and a gingival imbalance of all maxillary anterior teeth (Fig. 18–26). The patient requested cosmetic bonding. Probing revealed 4 mm sulci around the right and left lateral incisors and 3 mm sulci around the right and left canine and right central incisor. Electrosurgery was indicated on all involved teeth to achieve a more balanced gingival architecture prior to cosmetic bonding (Fig. 18–27).

CONCLUSION

The architecture of the gingiva must be included in the assessment of the patient undergoing esthetic procedures. Electrosurgery allows for dramatic soft tissue changes with a great degree of confidence.[25]

The clinician can gain skill rapidly with adequate practice. Proper familiarization with the equipment, along with adherence to precise rules for application of this equipment, will allow the operator to approach each surgical case in a confident and relaxed manner. As the operator's use of and proficiency with electrosurgery increases, the recognition of unesthetic gingival defects will become intuitive.

REFERENCES

1. Oringer, M.J.: Electrosurgery in Dentistry, 2nd Ed. Philadelphia, Saunders, 1975.
2. Malone, W.F.: Electrosurgery in Dentistry. Springfield, IL, Charles C Thomas, 1974.
3. Pollack, B.F.: Understanding dental electrosurgery. NY State Dent J 50:340, 1984.
4. Krause-Hohenstein, U.: Electrosurgery: fundamental requirements for successful use. Quint Int 14:1, 1983.
5. Nixon, K.C., Adkins, K.F., and Keys, D.W. Histological evaluation of effects produced in alveolar bone following gingival incision with an electrosurgical scalpel. J Periodontol 46:40, 1975.

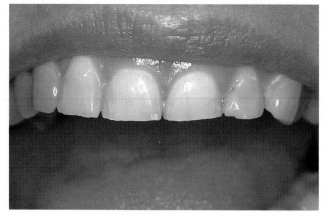

FIG. 18—24. A 45-year-old female with poor gingival architecture.

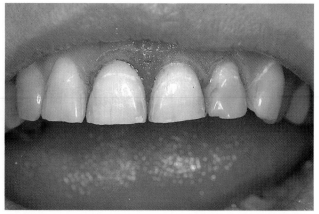

FIG. 18—25. Postoperative view immediately following surgery.

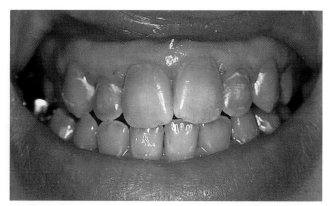

FIG. 18—26. A 22-year-old female presented with tetracycline staining of all teeth and a gingival imbalance of all maxillary anterior teeth.

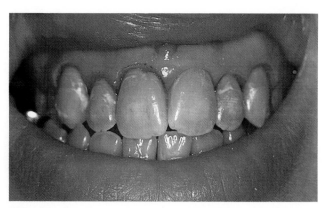

FIG. 18—27. Postoperative view immediately following surgery.

6. Simon, B.I., et al.: The destructive potential of electrosurgery on the periodontium. J. Periodontol 47:342, 1976.
7. Robertson, P.B., et al.: Pulpal and periodontal effects of electrosurgery involving cervical metallic restorations. Oral Surg 46:702, 1978.
8. Pope, J.W., et al.: Effects of electrosurgery on wound healing in dogs. Periodontics 6:30, 1968.
9. Williams, V.D.: Electrosurgery and wound healing: a review of the literature. J Am Dent Assoc 108:220, 1984.
10. Coelho, D.H., Cavallaro, J., Rothchild, E.A.: Gingival recession with electrosurgery for impression making. J Prosthet Dent 33:422, 1975.
11. Malone, W.F. and Manning, J.L.: Electrosurgery in restorative dentistry. J Prosthet Dent 20:417, 1968.
12. Armstrong, S.R., et al.: The clinical response of the gingival tissues to electrosurgical displacement procedures. Tenn Dent Assoc J 48:271, 1968.
13. Klug, R.G.: Gingival tissue regeneration following electrical retraction. J Prosthet Dent 16:955, 1966.
14. Schieda, J.D., DeMarco, J.J., and Johnson, L.E.: Alveolar bone response to the electrosurgical scalpel. J Periodontol 43:225, 1972.
15. Fisher, D.W.: Conservative management of the gingival tissue for crowns. Dent Clin North Am 29:273, 1976.
16. Stark, M.M., et al.: The effects of retraction cords and electrosurgery upon blood pressure and tissue regeneration in rhesus monkeys. J Dent Res 56:881, 1977.
17. Aremband, D. and Wade, A.B.: A comparative wound healing study following gingivectomy by electrosurgery and knives. J Periodont Res 8:42, 1973.
18. Kalkwarf, K.L., Krejci, R.F., Wentz, F.M.: Healing of electrosurgical incisions in gingiva: early histologic observations in adult men. J Prosthet Dent 46:662, 1981.
19. Schneider, A.R. and Zaki, A.E.: Gingival wound healing following experimental electrosurgery: an electron microscope investigation. J Periodontol 45:685, 1974.
20. Beube, F.E.: Periodontology. New York, MacMillan, 1953, pp. 605-607.
21. Agnew, R.G. and Kaiser, W.F.: Effects upon the dental pulp of the macacus rhesus of externally applied high frequency electrosurgical currents. Dental Research Abstract #105, 30th meeting, Colorado Springs, 1952.
22. Malone, W.F., Eisenmann, D., and Kusek, J.: Interceptive periodontics with electrosurgery. J Prosthet Dent 22:555, 1969.
23. Eisenmann, D., Malone, W.F., and Kusek, J.: Electron microscopic evaluation of electrosurgery. Oral Surg, Oral Med, Oral Pathol, 29:660, 1970.
24. Glickman, I. and Imber, L.R.: Comparison of gingival resection with electrosurgery and periodontal knife—a biometric and histologic study. J Periodont 41:142, 1970.
25. Strong, D.: Esthetics enhanced with electrosurgery. NY State Dent J 50:358, 1984.

Richard Lazzara, D.M.D., M.Sc.D.

ESTHETICS AND IMPLANT PROSTHETICS

19

Long-term success rates for osseointegrated dental implants have been well documented.[1-3] However, the esthetic restoration of the dental implant has lagged behind its biologic counterpart.

The Branëmark restorative protocol requires that several millimeters of titanium be exposed above the soft tissue. However, these early Swedish implants were originally placed into totally edentulous, severely resorbed ridges. The borders of the subsequent restoration were apical to the lip and smile line and did not present an esthetic problem. Acrylic denture flanges and acrylic teeth were used to replace the lost natural teeth and alveoli. Interpore's IMZ type restoration also requires at least 1 mm of plastic and a small amount of titanium to be exposed supragingivally. Ridge-lapping is a way of covering these exposed elements, but this creates difficulties in oral hygiene.

Because of the exposed metal or plastic elements, both the Branëmark and the IMZ technique result in restorations with flat, apical contours and crowns that are shorter than the adjacent teeth which further compromises esthetics (Fig. 19–1).

Implant surgery is divided into two stages. Stage I involves implant placement. This is followed by a healing period, with the implants submerged, while osseointegration occurs.

Following Stage I surgery, the denture can be replaced immediately as long as adequate relief is provided in the denture at the surgical site. The denture should then be relined with a soft material. The patient thereby leaves the office esthetically comfortable. In the maxillary arch particularly, the denture that is placed immediately following Stage I surgery acts as a healing stent to provide an appropriate amount of pressure on the surgical site. In the mandibular arch, some incision designs produce increased swelling and make function difficult. In these cases, the denture serves a purely cosmetic purpose.

In Stage II surgery, the implants are exposed and, after the soft tissue is allowed to heal, the prosthesis is fabricated. During Stage II surgery, an abutment or temporary abutment is connected to the implant. If an abutment is placed, a temporary screw should be used to cover the abutment until the final prosthesis can be constructed. The temporary screw will prevent tissue hyperplasia over the abutment, as well as prevent debris accumulation in the area of the retaining screw. A temporary retention cylinder can be used in place of a temporary screw. This provides additional retention for the removable appliance by creating an O-ring effect in the soft reline and adds stability to the transitional appliance.

ACCEPTANCE

Implantology and implant prosthetics are exciting and rapidly evolving fields. A number of organizations, including the Food and Drug Administration (FDA) and the American Dental Association (ADA), are currently involved with evaluation and acceptance (both provi-

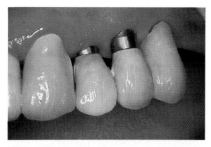

FIG. 19–1. The implant restorations using standard techniques exhibit flat apical contours as well as crowns that are shorter than the adjacent teeth. Also, exposed metal creates an unesthetic result.

sional and full) of these devices. However, it is the responsibility of the dentist to be adequately trained and experienced in the placement and use of these implants, to exercise proper judgement in case selection, and to provide the patient with appropriate information for informed consent. (See Chapter 28—Esthetics and Dental Jurisprudence.)

Currently, the number of manufacturers receiving provisional and complete ADA acceptance is limited. As more long-term clinical studies become available, more manufacturers are expected to receive acceptance for a wider array of applications. The exact type and extent of acceptance for each device is available from the ADA.

TERMINOLOGY

An implant restoration consists of three stages. The first stage is the *implant* itself, which is placed in the bone and becomes osseointegrated. Once this osseointegration has taken place there must be a mechanism to extend the implant through the soft tissues. This transmucosal extension is called an *abutment.* Abutments come in a variety of different types, each designed to manage the particular clinical situation at that location. The abutment generally consists of an abutment and an abutment screw. The abutment screw maintains the abutment in place and provides an area of retention for the prosthetic retaining screw. The third stage, or restoration, is based on the use of a *gold cylinder.* The premachined gold cylinder becomes incorporated into the final restoration and provides a premachined surface contact where the final prosthesis will meet the abutment or second stage. The use of a machined cylinder reduces potential laboratory error. The final restoration is held by a prosthetic retaining screw. These are generally constructed of gold or titanium and are recessed internally in the crown, seating at the coronal aspect of the gold cylinder and holding the final restoration in place on the second stage or abutment. There are situations when a custom post is constructed on the abutment or at the implant level and the final prosthesis is then placed on this custom post. The final prosthesis or superstructure can be cemented to the custom post or screw retained.

MATERIALS

In order to provide successful osseointegration, the implant materials must be biocompatible. The most popular biocompatible material used in implant construction today is titanium, either commercially pure titanium or titanium alloy. Generally, pure titanium is used. Titanium has proved to be biocompatible in long-term documentation of successful implant longevity.[4,5] It is light and noncorrosive and seems to be the most predictable material for implant construction. Pure titanium can also be plasma sprayed on the surface thereby maintaining the titanium surface for osseointegration as well as greatly increasing the surface area for attachment of bone to the implant. These implants are generally cylindrical, and are now available with a coronal hexagon elevation to provide maximum prosthetic options and stability.

Hydroxyapatite has also been used for the last several years as a surface coating on osseointegrated dental implants. Long-term documentation of results with this material is not available, but it appears that hydroxyapatite may resorb from the surface of the implant and, therefore, may not provide long-term benefit.

Generally, the screw type implant has been well documented for use in dense bone or where stability at the time of placement is critical. The use of a screw type of implant provides engagement of cortical bone to provide maximum stability and the most predictable precise placement. The cylindrical plasma-sprayed implant, which has a larger surface area may have some advantage in the maxillary arch where most of the foundation bone is cancellous in nature. Long-term studies are necessary in this area in order to make accurate scientific statements about what is best in each location.

TYPES OF IMPLANT RESTORATIONS
Denture Type

The denture type of implant restoration is a cost effective method. In addition, it provides the best lip support and speech control. Denture implant restorations are generally constructed by connecting the implant abutments with a gingival bar and using an overdenture clip for retention.

Indications

1. **Lip support requirements.** Especially in the maxillary arch, a fixed prosthesis may be inadequate to provide sufficient lip support in the anterior regions because of resorption of the maxillary ridges. The use of an overdenture provides the option of extending the labial flange to properly support the lip. This will maximize esthetics and facial contours.
2. **Psychologic concerns.** Patients who have worn removable appliances for many years sometimes feel that a removable appliance allows them to better cleanse their mouth. Psychologically, they are used to removing their appliance for adequate oral hygiene. These patients feel more comfortable having a removable prosthesis and are primarily concerned about appliance stability.
3. **Financial concerns.** The overdenture usually is the least expensive alternative for the restoration of multiple osseointegrated implants in an edentulous arch. Because the bar requires fewer laboratory procedures, laboratory costs can be reduced considerably. Retentive abutments, such as O-ring or Dal-Ro (Implant Innovations, Inc.), eliminate the need for a laboratory constructed substructure and, therefore, a conventional denture may be constructed for the patient and the attachments cold-cured intraorally.

Contraindications

1. **Psychologic concerns.** Many patients have a psychologic aversion to wearing a removable appliance. This aversion can be extremely strong and these patients may try to avoid removable prostheses at all costs.

2. **Hyperactive gag reflexes.** The overdenture requires extension onto the tuberosity area of the maxillary arch and onto the posterior mandible. Placement into these areas may activate the patient's gag reflexes.
3. **Unilaterally edentulous areas.** When a patient presents with a unilaterally edentulous area, an overdenture is not indicated because it is not possible to adequately stabilize the appliance. Therefore, in these instances, only a fixed restoration should be considered.
4. **Poor supporting bone.** As with any implant, adequate bone type and configuration must be available.

Crown and Bridge Type—Single Tooth

The single tooth replacement is one of the most challenging esthetic restorations. An antirotational mechanism must be present for stability. An implant with a built-in antirotational mechanism eliminates the need for external stabilization appendages and is essential if the maintenance of a diastema is desired.

Indications

1. **Conservation of tooth structure requirements.** The usual alternative to a single tooth replacement is either a conventional or acid-etch retained bridge. These require the removal of tooth structure.
2. **Diastema maintenance.** If adjacent diastemas can be maintained, over-contouring contact areas or placing a palatal bar can be avoided.
3. **Existing clinically acceptable adjacent bridgework.** There are instances when a single tooth must be removed and the adjacent multiple unit bridgework is clinically acceptable. Conventionally, this would require replacement of the adjacent fixed bridge in order to replace this single tooth. Generally, this also includes extending the bridgework one tooth beyond the edentulous area. Placement of a single implant allows the maintenance of the clinically acceptable fixed bridge as well as avoids the preparation of an additional tooth adjacent to the new edentulous area.

Contraindications

1. **Poor supporting bone.** As with any implant, adequate bone type and configuration must be available.
2. **Restoration of adjacent teeth is necessary for other reasons.** If adjacent teeth require extensive rehabilitation, a fixed bridge should be considered.

Crown and Bridge Type—Small Span Bridge

Small span, unilateral fixed bridges eliminate the need for removable partial dentures and provide stable abutments for fixed bridgework. This includes bridges solely supported by implants or by a combination of implants and the natural teeth connected by some type of retrievable mechanism.

Indications

1. **Unilateral edentulous posterior or anterior areas.** A unilateral fixed prosthesis can be placed in edentulous posterior or anterior areas of the dentition to avoid the use of removable partial dentures. If the adjacent natural dentition is in need of preparation and is stable, several implants can be placed to support a fixed prosthesis in addition to the natural dentition. However, the appropriateness of splinting natural teeth to implant borne restorations still requires further research.
2. **Large edentulous area with unprepared adjacent natural teeth.** In this situation an independent implant-borne bridge can be constructed using an adequate number of implants to provide maximum stability. It is especially important to provide an appropriate number of implant abutments to resist lateral occlusal forces.

Contraindications

1. **Poor supporting bone.** An adequate number of implants must be placed to support a fixed prosthesis. As with any implant, adequate bone type and configuration must be available.
2. **Inadequate interarch space.** There must be an adequate amount of interarch distance between the residual ridge and the opposing occlusion to provide room for the restorative components. This is especially important in the posterior regions where implants are placed in the tuberosity area and mandibular posterior areas.

Crown and Bridge Type—Full Arch Bridge

Full arch crown and bridge type restorations can be constructed on osseointegrated implants, provided there is adequate supporting structure and that an acceptable esthetic result can be realized. Under ideal circumstances a patient can convert from a complete denture to a totally fixed restoration.

Indication

1. **Adequate ridge height.** Full arch crown and bridge type restoration can only be considered for totally edentulous patients when there is adequate ridge height to produce a normally sized and shaped final restoration. Minimal resorption of the residual ridge permits the final restoration to be tooth-like in size and shape. This is the ideal situation for using a conventional crown and bridge type restoration supported by osseointegrated dental implants.

Contraindications

1. **Moderate to severe ridge resorption.** When there has been moderate to severe bone resorption, a fixed restoration requires replacement of more than just tooth crowns. Root dimension and alveolus height must be replaced in a fixed restoration. This is difficult to achieve using a conventional crown and bridge type restoration because of framework con-

siderations. In addition, because the ridges generally recede in a lingual or palatal direction, as well as in an apical direction, unusual contours would be required in the final restoration or in the final fixed bridge. This is difficult to restore with conventional metal and porcelain type restorations.

2. **The need for extensive cantilevering.** In totally edentulous patients, implants are generally placed anterior to both the mental foramen and the maxillary sinus. This requires extensive distal cantilevering to provide some posterior occlusion. Fixed restoration using conventional crown and bridge type procedures with porcelain and metal have no shock absorbing affect when in occlusion and the extensive cantilevering may affect the stability of the porcelain surface.

3. **Inadequate lip support.** The prosthesis may not adequately support the lip in the vestibular area and may produce a soft tissue crease under the nose.

Hybrid Type

The hybrid restoration of osseointegrated dental implants involves components of both the complete removable denture and the traditional fixed restoration. It consists of a metal framework supporting denture teeth. Denture acrylic is processed around the denture teeth, connecting them to the metal framework. This allows replacement for the lost alveolar structures as well as root structures in the edentulous patient with moderate to severe bone resorption. Generally, these restorations are associated with extensive cantilevering at the distal aspects of the restoration.

Indications

1. **Totally edentulous arches with moderate to severe resorption.** The hybrid prosthesis is used in moderately to severely resorbed edentulous patients because it provides maximum flexibility when positioning the teeth, despite the location of the implants. The denture teeth can be placed in the proper position to provide lip support and occlusal function; this position may not be directly over the implants themselves.

2. **Cantilever and shock absorption requirements.** Acrylic occlusion provides some shock absorption which is particularly necessary in extensive cantilevers (10 to 15 mm) situations.

3. **Lip support, speech, and air control requirements.** The hybrid prosthesis provides sufficient bulk to the restoration to adequately seal areas that otherwise may potentially cause disturbances in air control and speech. The hybrid prosthesis can provide adequate bulk for lip support, especially in severely resorbed areas of the anterior maxilla.

Contraindication

1. **Minimal ridge resorption.** When there is minimal ridge resorption, the hybrid prosthesis is contraindicated because the open apical surface of the hybrid prosthesis will be displayed during function.

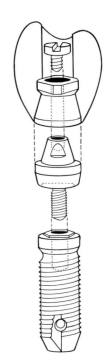

FIG. 19–2. Screw-retained prosthesis.

TYPES OF ABUTMENTS

Screw Retained Prosthesis

The screw retained final prosthesis uses a screw to attach the abutment to the implant. A second screw attaches the prosthesis to the abutment. All components are easily removed and, thus, readily retrievable (Fig. 19–2).

Indication

1. **Retrievability requirements.** A screw retained final prosthesis is indicated when retrievability of the implant prosthesis is desired.

Contraindications

1. **Inadequate arch space.** When there is inadequate room for placement of a gold cylinder, an alternative type of prosthesis must be considered, combining the abutment and crown.

2. **Occlusal esthetic requirements.** When maximum esthetics of the occlusal surface of the final restoration are indicated, a screw retained prosthesis should not be used because the screw access opening must be filled with a composite resin type material. This can partially compromise the final esthetics of the occlusal portion of the restoration.

Cement Retained Prosthesis

The cement retained prosthesis can be used on osseointegrated dental implants. However, it is important to maintain retrievability of the entire system and, therefore, the prosthesis should be cemented with a transitional type cement. The second stage, or abutment,

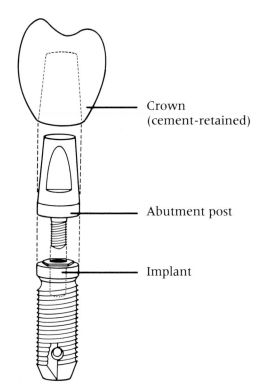

Crown
(cement-retained)

Abutment post

Implant

FIG. 19—3. Cement-retained UCLA-type prosthesis.

should be screwed into the implant and not cemented in order to maintain adequate retrievability. These second stage abutments can be custom-made using UCLA-type abutments or preconstructed abutment posts (see below).

Indications

1. **Accessibility.** The cement retained prosthesis should be utilized in posterior areas where accessibility with screwdrivers may be difficult. The cement retained prosthesis is easier to seat and to impression than other types of abutments.
2. **Simplicity requirements.** The cement retained prosthesis more clearly parallels conventional crown and bridge technique. Impressions, laboratory technology, and final restoration seating are similar to conventional procedures. In addition, there is no need for impression copings, analogs, gold cylinders, and screws.

Contraindication

1. **Inadequate interarch distance.** There must be an adequate amount of interarch distance in order to provide sufficient retention when using the cement retained prosthesis. There should be a minimum of 5 to 7 mm of abutment exposed supragingivally in order to provide adequate retention for the final restoration. When a reduced amount of interarch distance is available a screw retained prosthesis should be utilized.

UCLA-type Retained Prosthesis

The UCLA-type prosthesis, first developed at UCLA, (e.g. Unique Castable Long Abutment, Implant Innovations; or UCLA Abutment, Implant Support Systems) reduces the three stage system by combining the final restoration and abutment phase (Fig. 19—3). It consists of a castable abutment with a large retaining screw that screws directly into the implant for most implant types. For implant systems with a coronal hexagonal elevation this type abutment should be used for single tooth replacement and custom post construction.

Indications

1. **Single tooth replacement.** The UCLA-type abutment should be used for single tooth abutment restorations where there is less than 4 mm of tissue height above the implant. This will allow adequate stability of impression copings and provide ease of prosthetic procedures.
2. **Improper implant angulation.** This abutment can be used when the angulation of the implant is inappropriate and when there is less than 4 mm of tissue height. This can ideally position the abutment for construction of the most esthetic and optimally positioned final restoration.
3. **Minimal tissue height.** When there is minimal tissue height, the UCLA-type abutment is indicated because it allows porcelain to be carried to within less than 1 mm of the coronal aspect of the implant surface. This will maximize esthetics by bringing restorative material below the level of the soft tissue.

Contraindication

1. **When there is greater than 4 mm of tissue height** the UCLA-type abutment should not be utilized for single tooth or custom post construction. Most available impression copings are designed to be used when there is less than 4 mm of tissue height above the coronal aspect of the implant. When tissue height exceeds 4 mm, it limits the ability of the impression material to properly engage the impression coping.

Overdenture Retained Prosthesis

These abutments screw directly into the implant and provide a basis for the retention of the overdenture. They do not require laboratory construction of bars and connections, but rather provide immediate connection to the denture. They are usually in the form of an O-ring or ball and socket type attachment (Dal-Ro, Implant Innovations, Inc. or Overdenture Kit, Nobelpharma Inc.). These abutments screw directly into the implant and provide stable retention of a mandibular overdenture.

Indications

1. **Simplicity requirements.** The overdenture abutments provide a more simplistic approach to the retention of overdentures because they do not require impressions or laboratory procedures and construction of gingival bars.

2. **Excessive space between or inappropriate arrangement of implants.** When there is too much space between implant locations or if a gingival bar would have to be constructed in a circular fashion, individual retentive abutments are indicated. These allow retention of the overdenture without construction of oversized or poorly designed bars.

Contraindications

1. **Maintenance requirements.** O-rings must be changed periodically because they tend to wear during extended usage.
2. **Nonparallel implant orientation.** Because these abutments have male posts extending above the implant they must be relatively parallel in order to prevent damage to the retaining rings and to allow proper seating.
3. **Immobility requirements.** O-rings and ball and socket attachments allow some movement of the overdenture. If the patient requires absolute immobility to the overdenture, multiple implants and bars should be used to provide a greater area of support for stabilizing the denture.

PREOPERATIVE PLANNING

To obtain ideal esthetic results it is critical that the restorative dentist, in conjunction with the surgeon, formulate a preoperative plan. This plan culminates in the fabrication of a surgical guide stent. However, a number of factors must be considered first.

Mounted Model Analysis

Mounted models will facilitate the evaluation of interarch distance and location of opposing occlusion. In the fully edentulous patient, preoperative models mounted with occlusal rims indicate the desired lip support and occlusal requirements of the final prosthesis. This influences the shape and angle of the final restoration. For example, the rims will clinically demonstrate the amount of facial inclination of the mandibular restoration necessary for proper lip support and a functional occlusion.

Preoperative mounted models can influence decisions concerning the type of final restoration to be used. For example, if the final tooth position will be facial to the residual mandibular ridge, a hybrid-type prosthesis may be considered, as opposed to a conventional crown and bridge restoration.

In the maxillary arch, an occlusal rim (Fig. 19–4) will demonstrate the amount of facial positioning required of the replacement tooth in order to properly support the maxillary lip relative to the residual ridge. In this way, it will help determine whether a conventional crown and bridge prosthesis, a hybrid prosthesis, or an overdenture should be constructed to best support the lip.

In the fully edentulous patient, it may be necessary to construct a trial tooth set-up to precisely determine final tooth position. This is especially true when the location of the teeth is changed both in the arch to be reconstructed with the osseointegrated dental implant and in the opposing arch, which may be restored conventionally. Because tooth position in the maxillary arch will affect the mandibular teeth, the location must be determined precisely before constructing the mandibular guide stent. In those cases, a wax try-in of the maxillary and mandibular teeth should be constructed as part of a diagnostic workup prior to constructing a stent and placing implants (Fig. 19–5, 19–6).

The guidelines for selection of conventional crown and bridge prosthesis, hybrid prosthesis, or overdenture prosthesis after study model analysis follow.

1. **Patient's desire for fixed restoration.** To many patients, the avoidance of a removable appliance is paramount.
2. **The size of the framework involved.** This may eliminate the possibility of using a conventional crown and bridge type prosthesis because of the amount of metal necessary.
3. **Amount of interarch distance.** The amount of interarch distance is important because moderate to severe resorption requires a hybrid prosthesis or overdenture. If providing adequate lip support is critical, an overdenture is generally necessary, especially when there has been severe resorption. This is especially true in the maxillary anterior region where proper support of the maxillary lip and the area under the nose is critical.
4. **Number and location of implants.** For construction of a conventional crown and bridge type prosthesis, implants must be positioned in tooth locations. In addition, the implants must be adequately spaced in the anterior and posterior regions to provide adequate stabilization.

CLINICAL TIP. A conventional crown and bridge type procedure cannot be used when six implants are placed anterior to the mental foramen because of the stress created by the cantilever upon both the implants and the prosthesis.

---

5. **Strength and dimension of supporting bone.** When severe resorption has taken place, especially in the mandibular posterior region of totally edentulous patients, it is best to place an overdenture. An anterior fixed appliance can develop significant functional forces that may overstress the mandible, which thins posteriorly. This may cause fracture due to an overload of the anterior region with a fixed restoration.

Radiographic Analysis

Proper radiographic analysis is needed to evaluate the amount of bone available in the area. CT scans (Fig. 19–7) disclose bone dimension and the contours of the residual ridge and guide proper angling of an implant at a given edentulous site. The sectional portion of the CT scan is especially important because it gives an indication of buccal-lingual bone dimension, bone quality, and the location of vital structures.

FIG. 19–4. Mounted models and an occlusal rim should be used during the preoperative phase for patients undergoing osseointegrated dental implant therapy. This will give an indication of the final tooth position relative to the residual ridge.

FIG. 19–5. The maxillary tooth position of the patient shown in Figure 19–4 will be changed. This will, in turn, affect the final position of the mandibular teeth.

FIG. 19–6. A tooth setup is important in the preoperative evaluation of the final tooth position, especially when changing the position of both the maxillary and mandibular teeth.

FIG. 19–7. The precise dimension can be determined by computerized tomography scan showing the coronal evaluation and the sectional portion illustrating 1 mm slices.

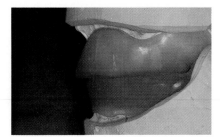
FIG. 19–4

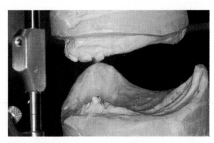
FIG. 19–5

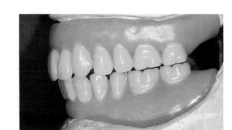
FIG. 19–6

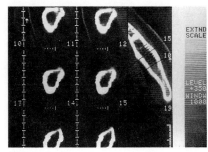
FIG. 19–7

The radiographic information, along with mounted models, allows coordination of implant position and angle.

Psychologic Considerations

The issue of patient expectation must be addressed before implant placement.

CLINICAL TIP. Some patients have unusually high expectations about the esthetics and configurations of the final restoration. If this is not considered, patients may not be satisfied with the final restoration despite its biologic success.

A patient, for example, may expect a conventional crown and bridge prosthesis with no exposed metal in a clinical situation that is best managed with a hybrid prosthesis. In this case, it may be impossible to hide all the metal and totally eliminate spaces. Patients must be informed that there may be some limitations in our ability to satisfy their concerns. If unrealistic expectations remain, alternate treatment plans should be considered.

Abutment Selection

The choice of abutment types is based on various requirements: visibility, accessibility, tissue architecture, angulation of the implant, interarch distance, tissue height, and tissue thickness.

Visibility. In areas of high visibility with thin tissue buccolingually, an abutment that allows porcelain to extend well below the soft tissue to the implant should be used (Fig. 19–8). This not only produces the best esthetic results, but also compensates for future soft tissue recession.

Accessibility. The cement retained prosthesis should be used in posterior areas where accessibility with screwdrivers when inserting and retrieving the final prosthesis may be difficult.

Tissue Architecture. If the tissue contours or levels are healthy but uneven and visible during function, the crown should follow the contours of the gingival tissue. Generally, this requires a preparable abutment or abutment post. This also helps preserve interproximal papilla, especially those adjacent to a natural tooth. Poor esthetic results occur when the unalterable flat margins of a prefabricated abutment do not conform with the gingival architecture (Fig. 19–9). Better esthetics can be obtained by using a post type abutment that can follow the gingival tissues (Fig. 19–10). Because this is a cement retained prosthesis, the occlusal surface is covered entirely with porcelain (Fig. 19–11) producing a better esthetic result. Temporary cement allows retrievability of the restoration and access to the implant.

Angle of the Implant. Precise preplanning and the construction of surgical guide stents suggest the proper positioning of the implant. However, the clinical acceptability of this predetermined position is determined by the available bone. In the maxillary premolar regions, and sometimes in the maxillary anterior region, implants must be placed with a labial flare in order to be within the supporting bone. This, however, creates an unesthetic screw access opening in the facial aspect of the final restoration.

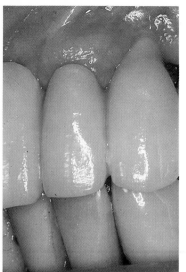

FIG. 19–8. When very thin buccal tissues are displayed, as over this maxillary canine location, a castable abutment is utilized. If recession takes place, no metal will be displayed. Also, this type of abutment allows maximum control of the emergence profile.

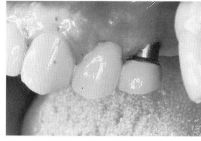

FIG. 19–9. A poor esthetic restoration is the result of an abutment that cannot be adjusted to follow precise contours of the soft tissue.

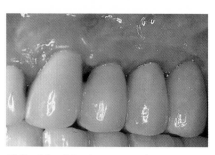

FIG. 19–10. A preparable abutment allows the final restoration to follow the contours of the gingiva.

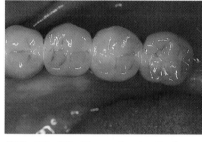

FIG. 19–11. The occlusal esthetics are preserved when using an abutment post because the prosthesis is cemented, eliminating the screw access opening.

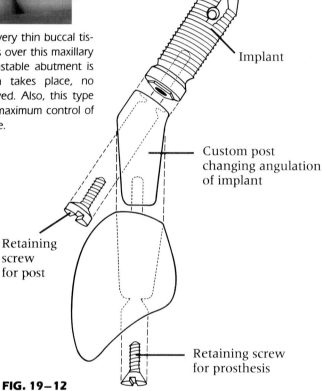

Implant

Custom post changing angulation of implant

Retaining screw for post

Retaining screw for prosthesis

FIG. 19–12

FIG. 19–12. A custom castable post is used to change angulation and create an esthetic prosthesis.

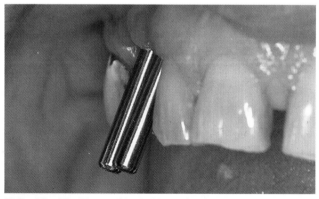

FIG. 19–13. The residual ridge of this patient necessitated positioning implants with a buccal inclination.

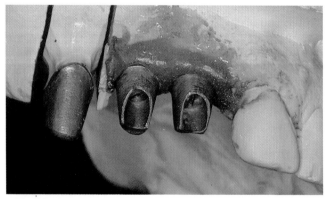

FIG. 19–14. A custom post was fabricated to realign the buccally placed implants in a more palatal direction.

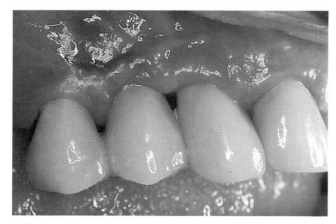

FIG. 19–15. A final restoration over a custom post with the restorative material extending below the gingival margin.

To compensate, a custom castable abutment can change the implant's angle (Fig. 19–12) so that it emerges from the soft tissue in the correct position (Figs. 19–13, 19–14). A prosthesis can be cemented over these castable abutments and extended below the soft tissue for an esthetic result (Fig. 19–15). Another option is the use of a preangled type abutment.

Interarch Distance and Tissue Height.

When there is minimal gingival height occlusal to the implant and the area is visible during function, the restoration must extend to the implant level by eliminating the second stage abutment and using a castable abutment.[6,7] This allows successful esthetic management when as little as 2 mm of soft tissue height exists above the implant (Figs. 19–16 to 19–18).

A comparison of the conventional abutment with that of the castable abutment (Figs. 19–19, 19–20) shows that in this type of case the conventional design exhibits metal supragingivally. A comparison at the metal framework stage (Figs. 19–21, 19–22) shows that the conventional design exhibits a flat apical contour of the final restoration where the abutment and metal framework meet. A more natural flow develops when the castable abutment is used. On the master cast, a conventional abutment demonstrates restorations that are shorter than the adjacent teeth, with a flat apical contour and metal exposed above the soft tissue (Fig. 19–23). The UCLA-type abutment, however, permits porcelain extension below the soft tissue for a more natural tooth-like form (Fig. 19–24). The final case exhibits the significant esthetic difference between the two systems (Figs. 19–25, 19–26).

Implant Position and Alignment

Osseointegrated implants are ideally positioned in the site previously occupied by the natural tooth. Implants placed in an interproximal position can cause considerable restorative difficulties in final crown contour and esthetics when crown and bridge type restorations are planned.

Considerations of the Interproximal Papilla.

Implant position affects interproximal tissue esthetics between the natural tooth and the implant restoration. The implant should be positioned so that a proper dimension of the interproximal papilla is maintained (Fig. 19–27), avoiding the dark, triangular space created when the soft tissue is lost.

The mesiodistal position of an implant is critical in the single tooth replacement case. Often, the implant should be placed more mesially in order to preserve the interproximal papilla at the distal aspect of the natural tooth and to create a more natural soft tissue slope between the natural tooth and the restoration (Fig. 19–28). If the implant is placed centrally in the edentulous site, the esthetics can be compromised because the papilla at the mesial aspect of the implant would be flattened leaving a visible black triangular space anterior to the implant restoration.

The exact buccolingual position for the single tooth replacement is also critical. The restorative dentist and surgeon should predetermine whether a restoration will be screw or cement retained because of the ramifications upon the optimum positioning of the implant. The implant should be placed as buccally as possible in order to manage the emergence profile of the final restoration without creating a lip on the facial area of the crown (ridge-lapping) and, if a post-like construction is used in the final restoration, this can be better accomplished (Figs. 19–29, 19–30).

However, a screw-retained prosthesis requires a more lingually placed implant so the screw access opening will be in the cingulum area. If such a prosthesis is indicated and the patient has been edentulous for some time, rebuilding of the buccal aspect of the ridge with soft tissue augmentation may be necessary to create better facial esthetics. However, the final restoration in this case will generally have a buccal ridge-lapping extension in order to esthetically manage the crown at the gingival margin (Fig. 19–31).

Anterior Diastema.

Tooth size and position are especially crucial in the maxillary anterior region. Ideally, the final restoration will simulate the natural tooth. The restored tooth should be normal sized with no component of the implant visible. Single tooth replacement can easily maintain pre-existing diastemata. However, this restoration requires an implant with a built-in antirotational mechanism, such as a coronal hexagon elevation, to prevent rotation of the final crown.

Clinical Case.

A 34-year-old female patient presented with a defective maxillary removable partial denture and maxillary anterior region diastemata (Fig. 19–32). The edentulous space was larger than the adjacent teeth. The patient's medical history was noncontributory. A single implant was precisely positioned in the edentulous space (Fig. 19–33). The correct buccolingual inclination ensures that the screw access will be confined to the cingulum area of the final restoration (Fig. 19–34).

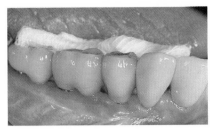

FIG. 19–16. This patient presented with minimal tissue height above the first premolar implant. Porcelain was extended down to the implant surface for maximum esthetics.

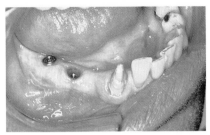

FIG. 19–17. A minimal amount of soft tissue over the facial aspect at the first premolar implant site is noted.

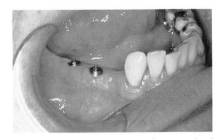

FIG. 19–18. Placement of a standard type abutment, which is approximately at tissue height at the lingual aspect, will show metal at the facial.

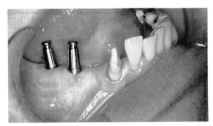

FIG. 19–19. An impression on the conventional abutment is made with a standard impression coping.

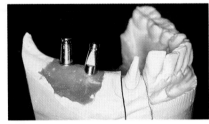

FIG. 19–20. On the side to be restored with a castable type abutment, an implant impression is made and a soft tissue model is constructed.

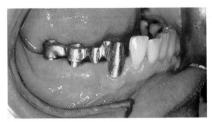

FIG. 19–21. The metal framework on the conventional abutment is beginning to illustrate a flat contour at the apical portion of the casting.

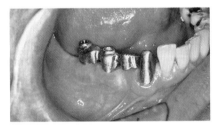

FIG. 19–22. The casting made with the castable abutment is developing more tooth-like contours.

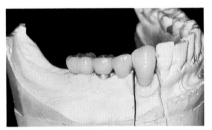

FIG. 19–23. On the master cast the final restoration on the standard abutment has a flat apical contour, is shorter than the adjacent teeth, and displays metal.

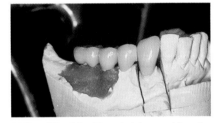

FIG. 19–24. The bridge with the castable abutment permits more natural toothlike form in the final restoration supported by the implant.

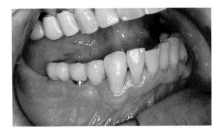

FIG. 19–25. As seen intraorally, the standard abutment is exposed supragingivally with a poor esthetic result.

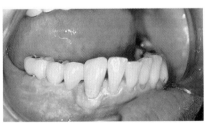

FIG. 19–26. This bridge constructed with a castable abutment exhibits porcelain extending subgingivally for a more esthetic and harmonious restoration.

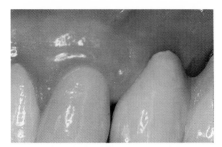

FIG. 19—27. The implant was placed in such a manner as to support the papilla at the distal aspect of the canine.

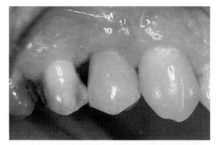

FIG. 19—28. An implant placed in an extraction site led to preservation of the interproximal contours and gingival level at the canine-first premolar site.

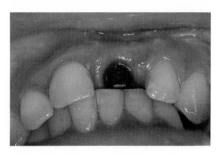

FIG. 19—29. The implant in this case was restored with a custom post for precise final crown location.

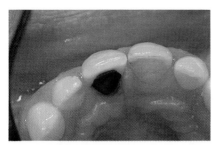

FIG. 19—30. The final crown cemented on the custom post.

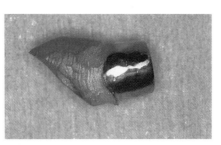

FIG. 19—31. Because of the implant position, overcontouring of the facial aspect of the crown is necessary in order to provide maximum esthetics.

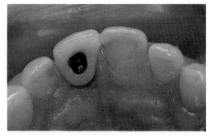

FIG. 19—34. Palatal view of Figure 19–33. An appropriate buccolingual positioning of this implant was chosen so that a screw-retained prosthesis could be constructed. Note that the screw access chamber is in the cingulum area of the tooth and the distal diastema is clearly evident.

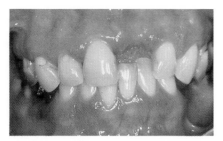

FIG. 19—32. This patient presents with an existing maxillary removable partial denture. The edentulous space is larger than the adjacent central incisor and conventional restoration of this area will be difficult with a conventional fixed bridge.

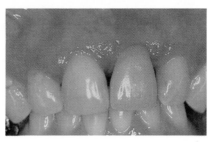

FIG. 19—33. Restoration of this maxillary central incisor area with a single implant allowed maintenance of a distal diastema and an esthetic result.

Clinical Case. A 41-year-old female patient presented with an over-retained primary canine in need of extraction (Fig 19–35). The patient's medical history was noncontributory. Restorative options included an oversized tooth to completely fill the space or a normal sized tooth with symmetrical mesial and distal diastemata. However, replacement with a normal sized tooth in mesial contact with the adjacent lateral incisor is esthetically preferable. In addition, this allows maintenance of an interproximal papilla between the natural tooth and the replacement canine. A distal diastema was created, which is not visible in normal function (Fig. 19–36). Precise positioning of the implant is especially crucial to an esthetic result in this type of case.

Small Edentulous Space with Limited Bone.
When replacement tooth size or limited bone availability prevents placement of a standard sized implant, an implant of smaller diameter may be indicated. This type of implant can be used for replacing a single mandibular incisor tooth (Fig. 19–37) or a maxillary lateral incisor.

Partially Edentulous Ridge. Implant positioning in the posterior regions often effects the esthetic outcome. When the patient presents with only a natural canine in a quadrant, strategic implant placement in the second premolar location will allow the more visible and esthetically important first premolar to be a pontic with an intact occlusal surface (Fig. 19–38). The screw access chamber and resultant occlusal restoration will now occur in the less visible second premolar. In addition, this allows the option of placing an interlock between the restoration and the natural tooth to provide retrievability of the restoration.

Totally Edentulous Maxilla. In the maxillary arch, implants should be placed in the canine locations or posteriorly, if possible (Fig. 19–39). This also allows the restorative dentist flexibility in properly placing pontics for optimal lip support, phonetics, and esthetics. This is particularly necessary when there has been considerable resorption of the maxillary anterior region. In this case, the final restoration can be placed near the anterior border of the residual maxillary ridge in order to provide proper lip support and optimal esthetics (Fig. 19–40).

Esthetically, implant retained restorations in the maxillary anterior region may be complicated by the space needed for the restorative hardware and for proper oral hygiene. These considerations may affect speech, as well as esthetics, especially in severely resorbed ridges. (See the section on Soft Tissue Management later in this chapter.)

Totally Edentulous Mandible. In the mandibular arch, the type of prosthesis influences implant location. If severe ridge resorption has taken place and a hybrid type prosthesis has been chosen, an implant must be placed in the symphysis area to properly support the final prosthesis. Because the restoration will have denture teeth and acrylic, precise control of the location of the implant is not critical as long as the implant is angled properly so that the screw access opening is within the lingual aspect of the mandibular incisors.

However, if a conventional crown and bridge type restoration is to be placed and there has been only minimal ridge resorption, it is imperative to place the implant precisely in a tooth location. If bone dimension allows, the implant should be placed in a canine or posterior tooth position rather than in a narrow lateral incisor location, which is difficult to restore with standard abutments (Fig. 19–41).

Angle of the Implant. Limited bone availability often results in implant placement with a facial or buccal inclination (Fig. 19–42). If a screw retained final prosthesis is placed, the screw access opening will emerge through the facial or buccal aspect. The closeness of the metal of the screw access chamber to the occlusal surface may limit the technician's ability to esthetically manage the porcelain in this area. Composite resin coverings of the screw access openings are subject to marginal breakdown and staining. However, a custom telescopic post can change the angle of the implant so that it is confluent with the adjacent dentition. This permits placement of an esthetic restoration (Fig. 19–43).

Occlusal Height. If the top of the implant is coronal to the cementoenamel junction of the adjacent teeth, the final restoration will be shorter than normal (Fig. 19–44). Osseous surgery can reduce bone height so that the top of the implant can be several millimeters apical to the cementoenamel junction of the adjacent teeth (Fig. 19–45). This allows the gingival margin of the abutment restoration to be level with the adjacent natural tooth. The apical-occlusal height of the implant should be determined prior to surgery because after osseointegration implant position obviously cannot be altered.

Porcelain vs. Acrylic Resin

The choice of restorative material is influenced by the type of restoration needed. For example, a full arch hy-

FIG. 19–35. A retained primary canine is to be extracted and replaced with an implant. Selecting the optimal location within the edentulous space is critical in order to obtain an esthetic final result.

FIG. 19–36. The implant is placed in the mesial portion of the edentulous area in order to create a papilla between the canine and lateral incisor. A normally sized tooth was constructed and a distal diastema maintained.

FIG. 19–37. In order to properly restore this mandibular right lateral incisor, a small diameter implant (Mini-Plant, Implant Innovations, Inc.) was placed so that proper dimension of the final restoration could be achieved.

FIG. 19–38. If possible, implants should not be placed in the first premolar region to allow maximum esthetics of this more visible area. In addition, this allows the technician more flexibility in constructing interlocks, if necessary, between the canine and first premolar position.

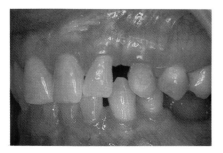

FIG. 19–35

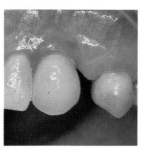

FIG. 19–36

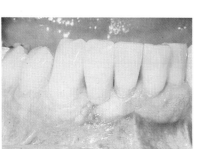

FIG. 19–37

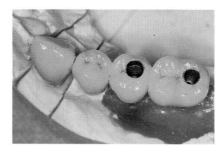

FIG. 19–38

ESTHETIC DENTISTRY

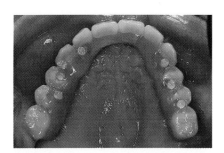

FIG. 19–39. If possible, implants are not placed in the maxillary central and lateral incisor areas in order to provide maximum flexibility for positioning pontics and for best esthetics.

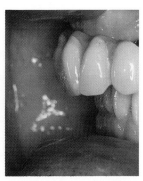

FIG. 19–40. Note the placement of pontics anterior to the existing ridge. This allows proper lip support, but would make restoration difficult if implants were placed in this area.

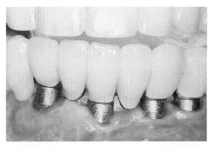

FIG. 19–41. Note the esthetic difficulty in restoring mandibular anterior teeth with crowns and standard implant abutments. The standard abutments are larger than the diameter of the mandibular incisors and therefore result in an unesthetic outcome.

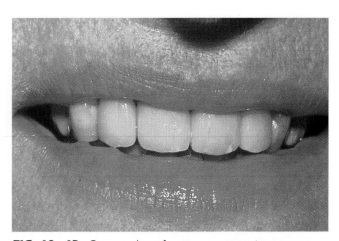

FIG. 19–43. Construction of custom posts and a superstructure that is cemented in place allows a very esthetic restoration of this difficult angulation problem.

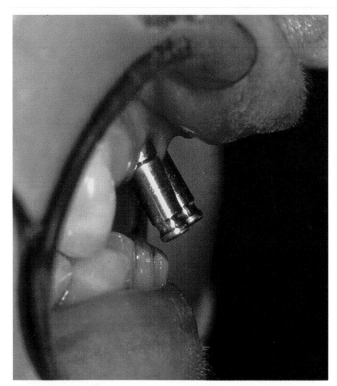

FIG. 19–42. Implants are placed with a labial flare in this maxillary anterior region due to the concavity of the facial aspect of the premaxilla.

brid type restoration over a considerably resorbed residual ridge may require long span cantilevers, possible facial overcontouring to provide lip support, and large crown to root ratios. Because the implants are positioned in the anterior region, the length of the cantilever (as long as 10 to 20 mm) may create framework flexing. The stress relief of an acrylic resin occlusion would be advantageous in this case. However, in partially or fully edentulous patients with normal sized crowns and multiple implants placed in a widely distributed pattern without long cantilevers, porcelain is the material of choice. Porcelain, when compared to acrylic resin, provides greater color stability, and imparts a more natural translucency to the final restoration. It is more wear resistent than acrylic resin and more stable under heavy masticatory function (Fig. 19–46).

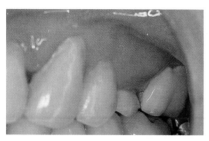

FIG. 19–44. Because the implant and abutment were placed lower than the adjacent teeth, it is more difficult to esthetically restore this area. Implants should be placed apical to the cemento-enamel junction of the adjacent teeth.

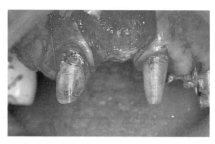

FIG. 19–45. The bone at the implant site should be adjusted in a case such as this so that the coronal aspect of the implant is several millimeters apical to the cemento-enamel junction of the adjacent teeth.

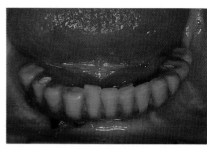

FIG. 19–46. This patient presents with severe wear of the occlusal aspect of the acrylic restoration.

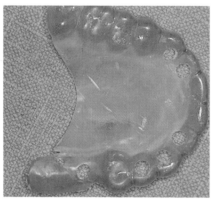

FIG. 19–47. This stent illustrates the use of the palate as a stabilizing base for the surgical stent during placement procedures.

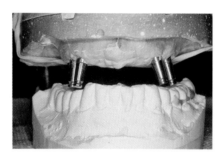

FIG. 19–48. Because of resorption of the maxillary ridge, implants had to be placed with a labial flare.

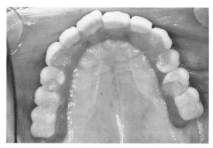

FIG. 19–49. Use of a surgical guide stent allows the final position of the screw access opening to be within the confines of the occlusal surface of the replacement teeth.

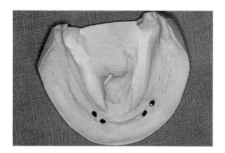

FIG. 19–50. Desired implant locations are marked on the cast after radiographic and clinical evaluation.

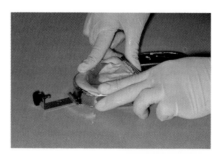

FIG. 19–51. Replication of the patient's existing denture in a denture replicating flask simplifies construction of a surgical guide stent.

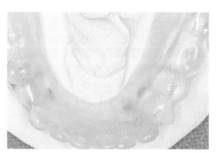

FIG. 19–52. One can determine from the replicated denture the desired implant location. Holes will be drilled from the occlusal position of the tooth to the predetermined location on the ridge.

STENT CONSTRUCTION

After the diagnostic work-up has been completed and the ideal implant type, implant location, and abutment and restoration type determined, a surgical stent is constructed to provide the surgeon with a guide during implant placement. The stent ensures proper positioning and angulation of the osseointegrated dental implants, thus coordinating radiographic analysis, clinical analysis, and model evaluation.

CLINICAL TIP. The key to an accurate surgical guide stent is a positive seat. This involves engaging the adjacent natural dentition or using the palate for positive seating of a maxillary surgical stent (Fig. 19–47). In the mandible, stent stabilization in the totally edentulous arch is more difficult and the stent usually is stabilized in the posterior areas because the implants are often placed anterior to the mental foramen.

CLINICAL TIP. Both the position and angle of the implant must be carefully evaluated. Often, the residual ridge is more lingual or palatal than the final teeth. To compensate for this in the maxilla, the implants are angled bucally (Fig. 19–48). This allows the screw access opening to emerge from the occlusal aspect of the final restoration (Fig. 19–49). The predetermined angle may produce over-angulation in the maxillary bone, which may cause the implant to be too close to the palatal crest or, in the mandible, may cause it to perforate through the lingual border. Therefore, compromises between implant placement and ideal esthetics must be reached. Custom posts or preangled abutments may be necessary to compensate for less than ideal implant position.

Stents can be classified as either *restricted* position or *variable* position.

Restricted Position Stent

If the surgeon and the restorative dentist, after clinical radiographic evaluation, are sure of the amount of bone at the implant location, a definitive stent that precisely indicates both location and angulation can be constructed.

Generally, these stents will guide implant location and angle because of the thickness of the acrylic resin or through the use of pindex tubes. In many of these appliances, the palate serves as a definite stop for the stability of the guide stent and a buccally placed flap is used to allow access to the bone.

Stent from a Pre-Existing Removable Full Denture

When existing denture tooth position is adequate in the fully edentulous patient, the existing maxillary or mandibular dentures can be replicated in order to construct a guide stent.

Armamentarium

- Basic dental setup
  explorer
  mouth mirror
  periodontal probe
  high-speed handpiece
  low-speed handpiece
  irreversible hydrocolloid impression material
  impression trays
- Denture duplicator (Lang Dental Manufacturing Co., Inc.) (optional)
- No. 10 round bur
- 2 mm twist drill

Clinical Technique

1. Make an irreversible hydrocolloid impression and pour a study model.
2. Mark the desired implant locations on the model (Fig. 19–50).
3. Duplicate the denture in *clear* acrylic resin, either in the laboratory or chairside using a denture replicating flask (Fig. 19–51).

CLINICAL TIP. Clear acrylic resin permits visualization of the implant location as marked on the study model. This expedites precise positioning of the guide holes in the replicated denture stent.

4. Drill openings in the stent from the desired tooth position to the location marked on the model (Fig. 19–52). Place the holes with a No. 10 round bur to allow for the use of a 2 mm twist drill. This provides a location guide, as well as an angulation guide, since the thickness of the replicated denture will guide the angulation of the surgeons bur.

Stent from Inadequate or Nonexistent Removable Full Denture

If the patient does not have an existing denture, or the prosthesis does not have desirable tooth position, an occlusal rim must be fabricated first.

Armamentarium

- Basic dental setup (see the section on Stent from a Pre-Existing Removable Full Denture)

Clinical Technique

1. Make an irreversible hydrocolloid impression and pour a study model.
2. Construct an occlusal rim with a preliminary tooth setup.
3. After the patient approves the esthetics of the tooth placement, duplicate the wax setup with a denture replicating flask in order to construct the guide stent.
4. Mark the model and drill holes in the stent in the same manner as for a pre-existing denture. (See the section on Stent from a Pre-Existing Removable Full Denture.)

Stent from a Removable Partial Denture

Partial dentures can be replicated in the same manner as pre-existing dentures. (See the section on Stent from a Pre-Existing Removable Full Denture.)

CLINICAL TIP. If possible, try to capture the impression of any existing precision attachments in the surgical stent to provide for a positive seat (Fig. 19–53).

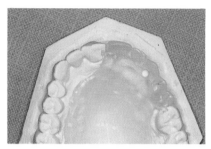

FIG. 19–53. The existing removable partial denture attachments provide a positive seat for precise placement of the stent at the time of surgery.

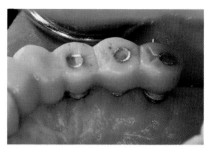

FIG. 19–54. In the transitional bridge phase it is evident that exact positioning was achieved by the use of the surgical guide stent.

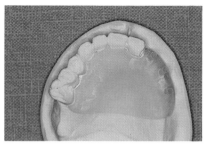

FIG. 19–55. This surgical guide stent is fabricated with a palate and pindex tubes to provide angulation guides during implant placement.

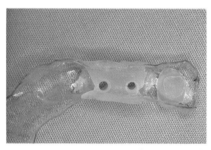

FIG. 19–56. A vacuum formed surgical stent is used in combination with tubes to guide implant location between adjacent teeth.

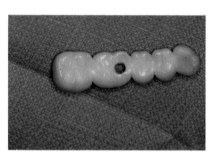

FIG. 19–57. Temporary bridges are used as surgical guide stents, especially when maintaining hopeless or questionable teeth, during the osseointegration phase.

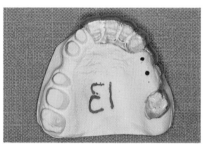

FIG. 19–58. Including the facial aspect of the teeth in the guide stent allows the surgeon flexibility in moving the location of the implant, while still remaining within the confines of a desired tooth location.

Acrylic Buildup Technique

This type of stent is especially useful when the patient is partially or fully edentulous and the screw access openings must be placed in a specific location within the occlusal aspect of the final restoration (Fig. 19–54).

Armamentarium

- Basic dental setup (see the section on Stent from a Pre-Existing Removable Full Denture.)
- Irreversible hydrocolloid
- 2 mm Pindex tubes (Whaledent)
- Clear orthodontic acrylic resin
- Cyanoacrylate cement

Clinical Technique

1. Make an irreversible hydrocolloid impression and pour a study model.
2. Lute Pindex tubes to the model at the predetermined location and angle.

CLINICAL TIP. Hold the tubes in place by luting them to the model with cyanoacrylate.

---

3. Construct a stent using a salt and pepper technique of placing liquid acrylic monomer and sprinkling clear acrylic polymer powder (Fig. 19–55).

Vacuum Form Technique

Vacuum form guide stents can be used if the patient has teeth both mesial and distal to the edentulous area.

Armamentarium

- Basic dental setup (see the section on Stent from a Pre-Existing Removable Full Denture)
- Irreversible hydrocolloid
- Vacuum forming unit (Buffalo Dental Mfg. Co., Inc.)
- Clear tray material (0.60 or 0.80 in.) (Buffalo Dental Mfg. Co., Inc.)
- 2 mm Pindex tubes
- Clear orthodontic acrylic resin
- Cyanoacrylate cement

Clinical Technique

1. Make an irreversible hydrocolloid impression and pour a study model.

2. Place denture teeth in the edentulous area of the model.

3. Vacuum form a stent in the usual manner. (See Chapter 13—Acrylic and Other Resins—Provisional Restorations.)

4. Mark the implant locations on the model.

5. Using the markings as a guide, place holes in the occlusal aspect of the vacuum-formed stent with the 2 mm twist drill.

6. Place the Pindex tubes (Whaldent) in the openings drilled in the occlusal aspect of the vacuum-formed stent.

7. Angle the tubes in the stent to the predetermined position on the cast. Lute the tubes to the stent material with cyanoacrylate and reinforce with a clear acrylic resin (Fig. 19–56).

Provisional Fixed Bridge Technique

Provisional fixed bridges may be used as surgical guide stents. This requires that teeth adjacent to the implant site are treatment planned for a fixed prosthesis (Fig. 19–57).

Armamentarium

- Basic dental setup (see the section on Stent from a Pre-Existing Removable Full Denture)
- Tooth-colored acrylic resin

Clinical Technique

1. Prepare the abutment teeth and fabricate a provisional bridge to span the edentulous area where the implants will be placed.

CLINICAL TIP. Hopeless teeth may be maintained during the osseointegration phase of treatment if they will not effect implant location or the esthetic success of the final prosthesis. They can serve as abutments to stabilize the provisional bridge, which can be used as a surgical stent during implant placement. They can also function as abutments for the provisional restoration during the integration phase of treatment.

2. With a No. 10 bur, place an opening in the pontic areas of the provisional bridge to act as a guide stent.

3. Following surgery, seal these holes with acrylic resin.

Variable Position Stent

If the clinicians are unsure about the exact dimension, quality, and configuration of the bone, or if the surgeon feels there may be some reason for deviating from the predetermined location, the stent should be relieved. This gives the surgeon a choice of acceptable implant locations while still remaining within the dimension of the replacement tooth in the final restoration. However, it can only be accomplished with a removable type stent. The variable position stent can be constructed from a replica of a pre-existing full denture, an inadequate full denture, a nonexistent denture, or a partial denture can be modified to become a variable position stent.

Maxilla

Armamentarium

- Basic dental setup (see the section on Stent from a Pre-Existing Removable Full Denture)

Clinical Technique

1. Partially construct the appropriate restricted position stent.
  A. See the section on Stent from a Pre-Existing Removable Full Denture, steps 1 to 3.
  B. See the section on Stent from Inadequate or Nonexistent Removable Full Denture, steps 1 to 3.
  C. See the section on Stent from a Removable Partial Denture, steps 1 to 3.
  D. See the section on Vacuum Form Technique, steps 1 to 3.

2. Cut away the occlusal and lingual aspect of the teeth in the surgical area opening in the stent. This allows the surgeon to place all sizes of drills, perform tapping procedures, and possibly place the implant, with the surgical stent in place (Fig. 19–58).

3. In the maxillary arch, elevate the surgical flap buccally to allow maximum access and maneuverability within the palatal aspect of the stent where the implants will be placed.

CLINICAL TIP. The facial aspect of the teeth in the stent serves as a guide to tooth location.

CLINICAL TIP. Radiographic marking balls (Implant Innovations, Inc.) can be placed in the stent to determine its intraoral position on preoperative radiographs. This allows the surgeon to take advantage of the upward extensions of bone in the floor of the maxillary sinus, allowing placement of a longer implant (Fig. 19–59). The surgeon can take advantage of areas of foundation bone under the floor of the maxillary sinus.

Mandible

Armamentarium

- Basic dental setup (see the section on Stent from a Pre-Existing Removable Full Denture)

Clinical Technique

1. Make an irreversible hydrocolloid impression and pour a study model.

2. If teeth remain, replicate an existing partial denture or wax-up in a denture replicating flask. If the arch is edentulous construct a clear occlusal rim or replicate a wax-up.

3. Cut away the entire lingual or facial portion of the mandibular teeth, leaving the facial or lingual outlines of the premolars and anterior teeth.

CLINICAL TIP. The facial or lingual aspect of the teeth in the stent serves as a guide to tooth location (Fig. 19–60).

ESTHETIC MANAGEMENT OF THE PATIENT IN TRANSITIONAL PHASES

Stage I

Following Stage I surgery, patients often object to the esthetics of not wearing their removable appliance for the initial healing period, as prescribed by some implant techniques. In the maxillary arch, it may be advantageous to place the denture immediately following surgery. Usually, a palatal incision is used and the tissue reflected bucally. The relined denture can act as a surgical compression stent to control bleeding and stabilize the flap postoperatively. The full denture should be adequately relieved in all surgical areas and soft-relined immediately following suturing to assure a pressure fit. A soft reline material provides the most comfort and avoids loading the implants through the soft tissue (Fig. 19–61).

In the mandibular arch, a similar procedure can be used, especially for vestibular deepening procedures (Fig. 19–62). Extension of soft reline material in the labial flange area provides a surface guide for tissue healing. However, when using either of these procedures, it is important that the implants are placed below the osseous crest so they bear no load through the tissue during this phase.[4]

For single tooth replacements, a transitional acrylic resin removable denture can be placed. If implant placement is performed at the time of tooth extraction, there must be adequate space over the extraction site so as to not load the implant (Fig. 19–63).[8] A transitional fixed restoration may also be bonded to the adjacent natural dentition or the replacement tooth may be luted or.ɔ orthodontic bands during the integration phase (Fig. 19–64).

Finally, wherever possible, hopeless teeth can be maintained to serve as transitional abutments during the integration phase of treatment, allowing the patient to have a fixed restoration during this time.

Stage II

Provisional fixed bridgework has many advantages when used after Stage II surgical procedures. It allows the restorative dentist to evaluate the esthetics, tooth position, lip support, pontic location, vertical dimension, and control of the gingival margin prior to constructing the final restoration. A provisional fixed bridge allows full maturation of the gingival tissues without the pressure of a removable appliance during healing. It provides the patient a degree of psychologic confidence by having an esthetically acceptable fixed appliance during the 2 months of soft tissue maturation following Stage II surgery. In addition, oral hygiene procedures can be reinitiated at an earlier stage.

Following Stage II Healing

There can be considerable recession of the soft tissue around the abutments in the Stage II postoperative period (Fig. 19–65). When healing is complete, the determination of abutment type and size is finalized. At this point, additional procedures can be performed, such as tissue recontouring or augmentation (see the section on Soft Tissue Management later in this chapter), evaluation of vertical dimension, placement of additional implants, or evaluation of tissue maturation following the extraction of hopeless teeth.

Provisional bridges at this time can either be cement retained, using temporary bridge heads on the standard abutments, or they can be screw retained with Temporary Cylinders (Implant Innovations Inc.), which provide long-term stability to the provisional prosthesis.

SOFT TISSUE MANAGEMENT

Tissue must not be inflamed, bleeding, or hyperplastic. In addition, an adequate zone of healthy attached gingiva is necessary to maintain the level of the marginal tissue around the final restoration. This is particularly critical when subgingival margins are anticipated. Proper tissue type and health also prevents irritation from oral hygiene procedures and decreases the likelihood of marginal recession. Gingival grafting for tissue augmentation or to provide vestibular extension can be done either at the time of Stage II surgery (Fig. 19–66) or after the tissue heals around the transitional healing abutments.

CLINICAL TIP. During Stage I and II surgical procedures, the surgeon must avoid incision lines and reflection of papillary tissue around the natural dentition adjacent to an implant site (Fig. 19–67). This may interfere with surgical access, however, the resultant implant will appear more natural and will blend with the adjacent tooth form and contour. If the papilla next to a natural tooth is destroyed, the loss may be irretrievable.

Papilla can be surgically created by removing the tissue directly over the facial aspect of the implant while leaving the mesial and distal tissues intact. In this procedure, implant placement must be deep enough in bone to maintain adequate tissue height above the implant for recontouring procedures. Unless sufficient facial tissue is present, the resultant gingival margin may be at a different level than the adjacent natural teeth.

Gingival Papilla

The key to successful tissue management in the partially edentulous patient is to maintain the interproximal profile of the papilla and to create a tissue flow that is similar to the natural dentition. The shape of the gingival tissues is particularly important in high smile line situations because of gingival display in the maxillary anterior and premolar regions.

Gingival Recontouring

The level and contour of the tissue in the implant area can differ from that of adjacent natural dentition (Fig. 19–68). The gingiva can be coronally positioned and without parabolic flow. Surgical correction is indicated.

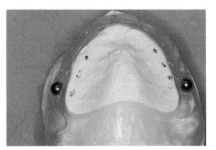

FIG. 19—59. This maxillary stent with marking indicators has two functions: to provide a guide to exact placement of the implants at the time of surgery and to help the surgeon locate areas of maximum bone support as revealed on the radiograph.

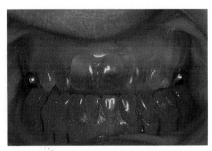

FIG. 19—60. Maxillary and mandibular guide stents for this totally edentulous patient will permit precise positioning of the implants.

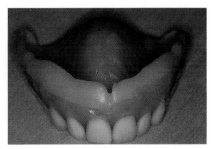

FIG. 19—61. The maxillary denture which was relined for the patient, will be placed immediately at the time of Stage I surgery. Note the thickness of the soft relining material to provide good cushioning and tissue adaptation.

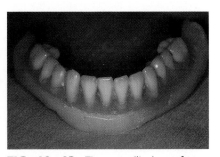

FIG. 19—62. The mandibular soft relining material is extended in the anterior area, where the vestibule has been extended.

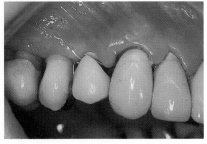

FIG. 19—63. A transitional removable partial denture was placed immediately at the time of implant placement in the first premolar location.

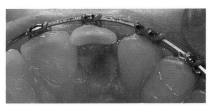

FIG. 19—64. A single tooth implant in a patient undergoing orthodontic therapy allows the replacement tooth to be bonded to the orthodontic bands.

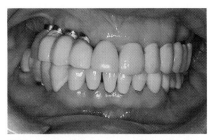

FIG. 19—65. A transitional fixed bridge fabricated following Stage II surgery.

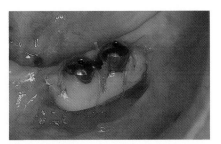

FIG. 19—66. Increasing the zone of attached gingiva around implants can be achieved by placing a gingival graft around transitional healing abutments at the time of Stage II surgery.

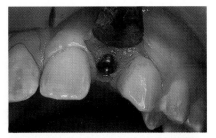

FIG. 19—67. Incisions in the papilla areas during Stage I and Stage II surgery should be avoided in order to preserve the dimension of the interproximal papillae.

Armamentarium

- Basic dental setup (see the section on Stent from a Pre-Existing Removable Full Denture)
- Alcohol pen (Masel Orthodontics, Inc.)
- No. 15 scalpel blade

Clinical Technique

1. Mark the desired gingival contour with an alcohol pen (Fig. 19–69).
2. Make a surgical incision with a No. 15 scalpel blade in order to create an even flow and blend of the soft tissue from the natural dentition through and including the implant site.
3. Healing occurs in 4 weeks. A natural flow of soft tissue should result and the interproximal papilla should remain intact (Fig. 19–70).
4. Fabricate the final restoration (Fig. 19–71).

Gingival Augmentation

The buccal dimension of tissue over an implant site is an important aspect of the esthetic restoration, especially in the maxillary anterior and premolar regions.

Armamentarium

- Peridontal surgical setup

Clinical Technique

1. Gingival augmentation procedures to enhance the dimension of the soft tissues can be performed at or following Stage II surgery.
2. An ideal donor site is connective tissue from under a palatal flap.
3. Place this tissue over the facial aspect of a temporary abutment (Fig. 19–72). This procedure will not only add tissue bulk but also provides good gingival stability, prevents recession, and allows for any necessary soft tissue recontouring.
4. Healing occurs in 6 weeks.

CLINICAL TIP. Considerable height changes occur in gingival tissue for at least 3 to 6 months following Stage II surgery.[9] The placement of a fixed provisional appliance is advisable during this period of continued tissue shrinkage (Fig. 19–73). After stabilization of the soft tissue level, the proper prosthesis should be fabricated.

Treatment of Severely Resorbed Edentulous Ridge

Severe tissue defects often create difficulties in proper positioning of the final restoration. This can result in limited support of the maxillary lip and improper contouring at the gingival margin of the final restoration. In addition, speech problems may accompany severely resorbed tissue and tissue height discrepancies. If there has been severe resorption in the region, or if there is a thin ridge, the emergence angle of the implant may not be ideal. This can result in unesthetic contours on the facial aspect of the restoration.

When an implant must be placed on a severely re-sorbed edentulous ridge next to the natural dentition, it is difficult to manage the tissue height discrepancy. Therefore, to adequately restore this region it may be necessary to use a conventional crown and bridge type restoration on the natural teeth and a hybrid type appliance on the edentulous area (Fig. 19–74). Replacing teeth and lost alveolus ensures proper lip support, esthetics, and speech management. The restorative dentist must evaluate these possibilities in the preliminary workup phase. This allows esthetic restoration of the area, some type of facial cantilevering and ridge-lapping, and provides access for oral hygiene procedures.

Coordination of Abutment Height to Soft Tissue Level

Esthetically, the ideal margin of the final restoration should be placed approximately 1 mm subgingivally. An appropriately sized abutment must be chosen to accomplish this. After maturation following Stage II surgery, the soft tissue height must be measured. For example, if the clinician measures 4 mm of tissue height at the direct facial aspect, a 3 mm abutment would be chosen (Fig 19–75). This allows the porcelain to extend approximately 1 mm subgingivally.

CLINICAL TIP. Concern with soft tissue height coordination remains when custom posts are selected to correct angle discrepancies. A castable abutment can be used to construct the custom post (Fig. 19–76). The superstructure, or telescopic crown, should extend over the custom post and below the gingival margin in the area (Fig. 19–77).

Adjustment of Abutment Post and Impressioning to Achieve Subgingival Margins

Armamentarium

- Basic dental setup (see the section on Stent from Pre-Existing Removable Full Dentures)
- Retraction cord (optional)
- Firm impression material (e.g., polyether or polyvinyl siloxane types)

Clinical Technique

1. After judging the amount of restorative material required at the occlusal level and after making determinations about angulation, mark the abutment to show where adjustments will be made.

CLINICAL TIP. A minimum of 5 mm of post must be maintained to provide adequate retention for the final restoration.

2. Because extensive preparation in the mouth may create heat damage to the implant, remove the abutment post from the mouth to make adjustments.
3. Return the abutment post to the mouth and, using copious irrigation, prepare a subgingival finish line that follows the gingival tissue (Fig. 19–78).
4. Place retraction chord, if necessary.

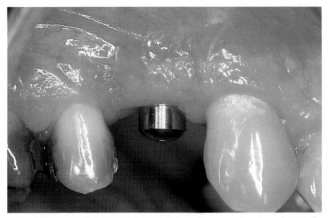

FIG. 19—68. Although successful and properly placed, the final esthetics of this implant will be compromised by the flat contour of the gingival tissues at the implant site as well as by the height of the soft tissue relative to the adjacent natural tooth.

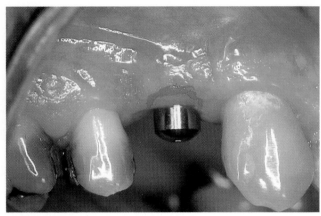

FIG. 19—69. Using an alcohol pen, the location and the amount of planned tissue scalloping is marked.

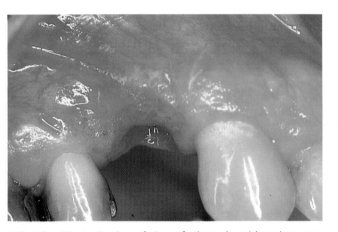

FIG. 19—70. Scalloping of the soft tissue is achieved to provide an esthetic contour.

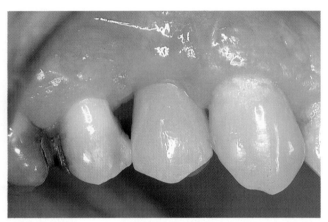

FIG. 19—71. Restoration illustrating the parabolic flow of the gingival contours. This cast ceramic crown is supported by an STR abutment (Implant Innovations, Inc.).

CLINICAL TIP. Retraction cord is usually not necessary when impressing the abutments because of the flexibility of the peri-implant tissue.

5. At this point, treat the abutment as if it were a natural tooth, both in the impression and laboratory procedures.

FABRICATION OF PROSTHESIS

It is beyond the scope of this chapter to discuss prosthesis fabrication in detail. The clinician must be well trained in implant techniques before attempting any clinical procedures. However, for the sake of simplicity, implant restorations can be grouped into three broad categories.

Denture Type

Overdenture construction is similar to conventional full denture construction over natural teeth.

Armamentarium

- Basic dental setup (see the section on Stent from a Pre-Existing Removable Full Denture)
- Irreversible hydrocolloid
- Tray acrylic for custom trays
- Border molding material
- Impression material

Clinical Technique

1. Following Stage II surgery and healing, construct a denture in the usual manner, providing adequate relief over the overdenture abutment.
2. After approximately 2 to 3 weeks, the patient should be comfortable with the denture and the overdenture attachments can be cold-cured into the denture.
3. When placing O-ring attachments be sure to provide adequate relief in the corresponding internal aspect of the denture so that the denture only contacts the O-ring.

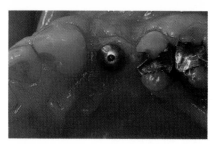

FIG. 19–72. Augmentation of the buccal tissues at the facial aspect of the temporary abutment allows construction of a normally shaped final restoration.

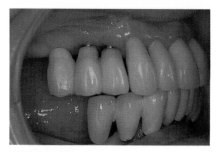

FIG. 19–73. A provisional fixed bridge in the maxillary right quadrant is supported by osseointegrated dental implants and temporary cylinders. Shrinkage in the soft tissues has taken place following Stage II surgery. Now that the tissues are mature, the proper size abutment will be placed so that the margin of the final restoration can be brought to tissue level.

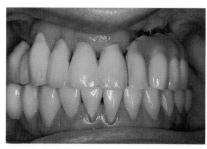

FIG. 19–74. This patient has a unilateral hybrid prosthesis in the maxillary left quadrant to replace a large alveolar defect. It provides proper lip support, good esthetics, and speech control.

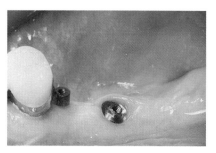

FIG. 19–75

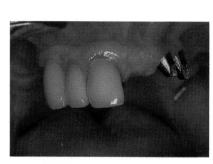

FIG. 19–76

FIG. 19–75. Placing an abutment so that the coronal aspect is approximately 1 mm below the soft tissue level is ideal for an esthetic restoration.

FIG. 19–76. The buccal inclination of these maxillary implants is corrected with custom posts.

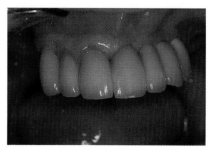

FIG. 19–77

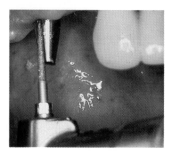

FIG. 19–78

FIG. 19–77. The superstructure over the custom post extends subgingivally for proper esthetics.

FIG. 19–78. The abutment post finishing line should be prepared intraorally, creating a finishing line that follows the gingival contours.

Cemented Type

The fabrication of a prosthesis over a cemented type abutment is similar to that of a conventional fixed prosthesis.

Armamentarium

- Basic dental setup (see the section on Stent from a Pre-Existing Removable Full Denture)

Clinical Technique

1. After judging the amount of restorative material required at the occlusal level and after making determinations about angulation, mark the abutment to show where adjustments will be made.

CLINICAL TIP. A minimum of 5 mm of post must be maintained to provide adequate retention for the final restoration.

2. Because extensive preparation in the mouth may create heat damage to the implant, remove the abutment post from the mouth to make adjustments.
3. Return the abutment post to the mouth and, using copious irrigation, prepare a subgingival finish line that follows the gingival tissue.
4. Make impressions and fabricate the prosthesis.

Screw Type

The fabrication of a prosthesis over a screw type abutment is unique to implants.

Armamentarium

- Basic dental setup (see the section on Stent from a Pre-Existing Removable Full Denture)
- Stock metallic trays
- Firm impression material (e.g., polyether or polyvinyl siloxane types)
- Impression copings
- Brass analogs

Clinical Technique

1. Remove the temporary screw from the abutments.
2. Verify the tightness of the abutments with an abutment driver.
3. Screw impression copings onto the abutments and verify that seating is complete.
4. Make an impression with firm impression material.
5. Remove the impression from the mouth.
6. Unscrew the impression copings from the abutments and attach them to the corresponding laboratory analog.
7. Reinsert the impression coping in the analog back into the appropriate position in the impression.
8. Paint stone in the area of the impression copings without using a vibrator and allow the stone to set prior to pouring the remainder of model.
9. After the initial pour has set, pour the remainder of the impression in the usual manner using a vibrator.
10. Fabricate the prosthesis.

CONCLUSION

Close coordination between the surgeon and the restorative dentist in the preoperative phase will improve the quality of the final restoration. An esthetic approach to implant placement and restoration provides patients with stable, predictable fixed appliances that enhance the patient's quality of life both functionally and esthetically.

REFERENCES

1. Branëmark, P.-I., Hanson, B.O., Adell, R., et al: Osseointegrated implants in the treatment of the edentulous jaw. Experience from a 10-year period. Scand J Plast Reconstr Surg 1977; 11(suppl15):1, 1977.
2. Adell, R., Lekholm, U., Rockler, B., et al.: A 15-year study of osseointegrated implants in the treatment of the edentulous jaw. J Oral Surg 10:387, 1981.
3. Branëmark, P.-I., Hansson, B.O., Adel, R., et al.: Osseointegrated implants in the treatment of the edentulous jaw. Experience from a 10-year period. Scand J Plast Reconstr Surg 11(suppl16):1, 1977.
4. Branëmark, P.-I., Zarb, G.A., Albrektsson, T.: Tissue-integrated prosthesis. Chicago, Quintessence Publishing Co., Inc., 1985.
5. Adell, R.: Clinical results of osseointegrated implants supporting fixed prosthesis in edentulous jaws. J Prosthet Dent 50(2):251, 1983.
6. Lewis, S., Beumer, J., Hornburg, W., and Moy, P.: The UCLA abutment. Int J Oral Maxillofac Implants 3:183, 1988.
7. Lewis, S., Beumer, J., Hornburg, W., and Perri, G.: Single tooth implant supported restorations. Int J Oral Maxillofac Implants 3:25, 1988.
8. Lazzara, R., Immediate implant placement into extraction sites: surgical and restorative advantages. Int J Periodont Rest Dent 9:333, 1989.
9. Adell, R., Lekholm, U., Rockler, B., et al.: Marginal tissue reactions at osseointegrated titanium fixtures: Int J Oral Maxillofac Surg 15:39, 1986.

Charles Citron, D.D.S., M.S.D.

ESTHETICS AND PEDODONTICS

20

The majority of adults would not consider stainless steel crowns for their anterior teeth, nor accept a partially edentulous smile for a period of 5 to 6 years. Dentistry should no longer subject children in their formative years to this fate.

The early loss of primary teeth may delay eruption of the permanent teeth if less than one-half the root structure is formed on the succedaneous tooth.[1] If a child's central or lateral incisor is extracted at 3 years of age, the permanent teeth may not erupt until age 8 or 9.

Physical appearance and superficial attributes influence a child's impression of and reaction to others. In addition, an attractive child is considered more socially adept than an unattractive child. This is perceived by both acquainted and unacquainted preschool children.[2] Children as young as 3 years old are able to distinguish between attractive and unattractive peers. Children between the ages of 3.5 and 6 preferred attractive children for friends. Their judgments are similar to those of adults.[3]

Prematurely lost or congenitally missing teeth affect speech patterns. A child learning correct production of tongue tip sounds (t, d, s, sh, and ch), as well as the labial sounds of f and v, may be aided by an appliance that restores the maxillary anterior teeth.[4,5]

The primary dentition usually has interdental spacing in the anterior portion of the dental arch; a small percentage of the population has no spacing or exhibits crowding. It is imperative that the space in the anterior portion of the dental arch is preserved in children in order to ensure correct alignment of their permanent teeth.[6]

The need for restoration of the anterior primary dentition can be caused by two main factors: traumatic injuries or caries and developmental problems.

TRAUMATIC INJURIES

The anterior primary teeth erupt between 6 and 9 months of age and exfoliate at about age 7. Treatment goals for injuries to primary teeth include:

1. Protecting the forming succedaneous tooth.
2. Avoiding infection.
3. Restoring normal form and function.

Attainment of these goals often is not possible, and these goals do not always complement each other. Although it is possible to replant an avulsed primary tooth and restore normal function, this is contraindicated because the pressure of manipulation may damage the succedaneous tooth bud.[7] It may be possible to restore a fractured primary tooth, but a child of 2 years old may not cooperate sufficiently to complete the treatment. Any form of trauma to the primary tooth can directly affect the succedaneous tooth.

Maxillary central incisors are the most frequently traumatized tooth; accidents often occurring when the child is between .5 and 2.5 years of age. Children in this age group are gaining mobility and independence while lacking coordination and motor skills.[8] Traumatic injuries to primary teeth can be classified in a manner similar to the Ellis classifications of traumatic injuries to permanent teeth (Table 20–1).[9]

It is easier to treat a child when the parent's fears are first allayed.[7] The parent can help with the treatment by providing emotional support to the child. If the parent is too distraught, it is better to exclude him or her from the operatory.

After obtaining a thorough history of trauma,[10] medical history, and neurological examination,[11] the traumatized area is cleaned and debrided so the extent of the injury can be ascertained.

TABLE 20–1. CLASSIFICATION OF TRAUMATIC INJURIES

CLASS	PROBLEM
I	Fracture of the crown into the enamel with little or no dentin involvement
II	Fracture of the crown into the dentin, but no dental pulp involvement
III	Fracture of the crown with exposed dental pulp
IV	Displacement of the tooth without fracture of the crown or root
V	Root fracture without loss of crown structure
VI	Traumatized tooth (vital or nonvital) that may or may not discolor

Class I Traumatic Injuries

Class I injuries involve the enamel of the crown with little or no dentin involvement (Fig. 20–1). When the primary tooth is chipped or slightly fractured it can be left untreated or smoothed and recontoured to prevent irritation to the soft tissue (Fig. 20–2). This will also create a more pleasing esthetic appearance (Fig. 20–3). A periapical radiograph should be taken to evaluate any changes, such as a root fracture.

Class II Traumatic Injuries

Class II injuries involve both the enamel and dentin of the crown, but not the pulp (Fig. 20–4). These injuries should be evaluated and restored by the dentist. The injured tooth may be examined clinically and radiographically to determine the extent of the damage.

Armamentarium:

- Standard dental setup
  explorer
  mouth mirror
  periodontal probe
  suitable anesthesia
  rubber dam setup
  high-speed handpiece
  burs, including a 12-fluted carbide bur
- Calcium hydroxide (e.g., Dycal, L.D. Caulk, Co.)
- Metacresylacetate (e.g., Cresatin, Schein, Inc.)
- Acid etch gel
- Bonding agent of choice (see Chapter 3—Dentin Bonding Agents)
- Composite resin of choice (see Chapter 5—Composite Resin—Fundamentals and Direct Technique Restorations)
- Teflon coated composite resin placement instrument (e.g., Fleck's Instrument, Healthco, Inc.)
- Clear plastic crown forms (e.g., Crownforms, Caulk, Inc.)

Clinical Technique:

1. Obtain a thorough medical history, neurological evaluation, and history of trauma.
2. Perform a clinical examination, including a periapical radiograph.
3. Administer local anesthesia.
4. Place a rubber dam.
5. If the fracture is deep and close to the pulp chamber there may be a microscopic exposure. Place metacresylacetate, a mild germicide and anodyne,[12] on the dentin for 5 minutes. If the fracture is small (about 1 mm or less) and does not appear to be near the pulp as seen on the radiograph, this step can be eliminated.
6. Apply calcium hydroxide to the dentin (Fig. 20–5) to promote the formation of secondary dentin.[13]
7. Acid etch the enamel for 30 to 45 seconds, rinse and dry.
8. Apply bonding agent (Fig. 20–6). (See Chapter 3— Dentin Bonding Agents.)
9. Apply an acid-etch retained composite resin to the fractured portion of the tooth.
10. Place the composite resin with a teflon-coated instrument in a manner similar to that of a Class II fracture of a permanent tooth (Fig. 20–7), but do not bevel the enamel. (See Chapter 5—Composite Resin—Fundamentals and Direct Technique Restorations.)
11. Use a crown form to hold the composite resin in place. Cure the resin both buccally (Fig. 20–8) and lingually (Fig. 20–9). For very large fractures, full coverage may be placed on the tooth. (See the section on Crowns for Primary Teeth later in this chapter.)
12. Shape and polish the restoration (Figs. 20–10, 20–11).

Class III Traumatic Injuries

Class III injuries include the enamel, dentin, and pulp of the tooth. These injuries should be examined and treated as soon as possible because the chance of a successful result decreases the longer the tooth is exposed to the oral environment.

If the pulp has been exposed for less than 24 hours and if the exposure is minimal, a pulpotomy should be performed. The roof of the pulp chamber is removed and the coronal pulp is extirpated with a spoon excavator. A vital healthy pulp will exhibit hemorrhage that can be controlled with pressure from a cotton pellet. If a tooth has been exposed for more than 24 hours, or if the exposure is large or if it is bleeding uncontrollably and can not be stopped with pressure, pulpal inflammation and degeneration are likely and a pulpectomy should be performed.

A complete pulpectomy should be performed if the pulp chamber is devoid of healthy tissue; this is evidenced by no hemorrhage from the root canal. Never perform a pulpotomy on a nonvital tooth.[14]

Vital Primary Teeth—Pulpotomy
Armamentarium:

- Standard dental setup (see the section on Class II Traumatic Injuries)

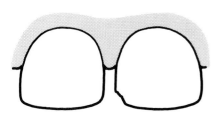

FIG. 20–1. Class I fracture of the enamel of a primary incisor.

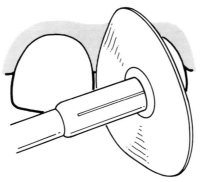

FIG. 20–2. The tooth can be smoothed and recontoured with a sandpaper disc or a fine diamond stone.

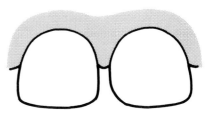

FIG. 20–3. The recontoured tooth.

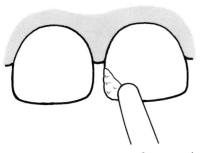

FIG. 20–4. A fracture involving the enamel and dentin of a primary incisor.

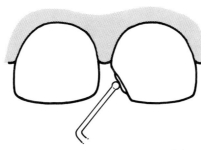

FIG. 20–5. Calcium hydroxide lining is placed on the dentin.

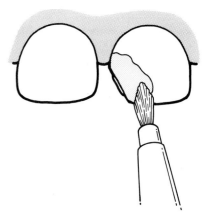

FIG. 20–6. The etched tooth with a layer of bonding agent applied.

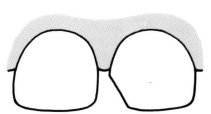

FIG. 20–7. Placement of composite resin material.

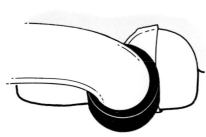

FIG. 20–8. A fitted crown form is filled with composite resin, is placed, and is cured from the buccal direction.

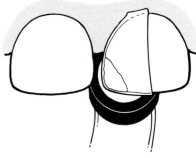

FIG. 20–9. The tooth is then cured from the lingual direction.

FIG. 20–10. The restoration is contoured and polished.

FIG. 20–11. The final restoration.

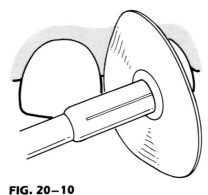

FIG. 20–10

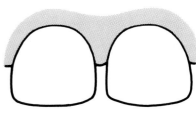

FIG. 20–11

- Buckley's formocresol (19% formaldehyde, 35% creosol, and 46% glycerine (Sultan Chemists, Inc.)
- Zinc oxide and eugenol paste
- Suitable restorative cement, such as polycarboxylate cement (e.g., Duralon ESPE-Premier Sales Corp.) or glass ionomer cement (Keta-Cem, ESPE-Premier Sales Corp.)
- Acid etch gel
- Bonding agent of choice (see Chapter 3—Dentin Bonding Agents)
- Composite resin of choice (see Chapter 5—Composite Resin—Fundamentals and Direct Technique Restorations)

Clinical Technique:

1. Obtain a thorough medical history, neurological evaluation, and history of trauma.
2. Perform a clinical examination, including a periapical radiograph.
3. Administer local anesthesia.
4. Place a rubber dam.
5. If the tooth is vital, perform a pulpotomy. Remove the coronal portion of the pulp tissue with a spoon excavator. Pulp capping for a primary tooth is contraindicated.[14]
6. Control hemorrhage with a cotton pellet.
7. Place Buckley's formocresol on the pulp tissue for 5 minutes. This will fix the pulp in the coronal portion of the tooth, but vital tissue will remain in the apical one-third.
8. Place a layer of zinc oxide and eugenol paste over the fixed pulp.
9. Place a base of polycarboxylate cement (Duralon) or glass ionomer cement.
10. Apply an acid-etch retained composite resin to the fractured portion of the tooth in a manner similar to that of a Class II fracture of a permanent tooth, but do not place a bevel (see Chapter 5—Composite Resin—Fundamentals and Direct Technique Restorations) or place full coverage on the tooth (see the section on Crowns for Primary Teeth later in this chapter).

Nonvital Primary Teeth—Pulpectomy. A pulp that is exposed to the oral environment for any length of time may lose its vitality. A pulpectomy should be initiated in these cases. Endodontic therapy for a primary anterior tooth is not as exacting a procedure as for a permanent tooth.

Armamentarium:

- Standard dental setup (see the section on Class II Traumatic Injuries)
- Paper points
- Cotton pellets
- Irrigating solution, such as chlorinated soda (Sultan Chemists, Inc.) or saline (Sultan Chemists, Inc.)
- Germicidal agent, such as Buckley's formocresol (19% formaldehyde, 35% creosol, 46% glycerine (Sul-

tan Chemists, Inc.) metacresylacetate (e.g., Cresatin, Henry)
- Endodontic files, reamers, headstroms and broaches
- Zinc oxide
- Eugenol paste

Clinical Technique

1. Obtain a thorough medical history, neurological evaluation, and history of trauma.
2. Perform a clinical examination, including a periapical radiograph.
3. Administer local anesthesia.
4. Place a rubber dam.
5. Because it is difficult to obtain exact measurements, estimate the pulp length by:
   A. Measuring the radiographic image.
   B. Ascertaining a tactile change in resistance during instrumentation.

CLINICAL TIP. Do not use an electronic apex finder on primary teeth. They are unreliable because the canals cannot always be completely dried.

---

6. It is only necessary to debride the canals of necrotic material. Unlike the permanent dentition it is not necessary to shape the canals to accept a filling (Fig. 20–12).
7. Clean the canals with a suitable irrigant.
8. Dry the canals with paper points and cotton pellets.
9. Place a germicidal agent in the canal. The medicament is not as important as the actual debridement and irrigation.
10. Seal the access opening with a zinc oxide and eugenol type cement until the next visit (4 to 7 days).[14]
11. At the next visit, open the tooth.

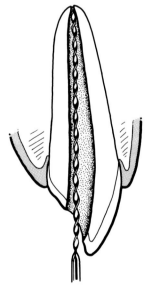

FIG. 20–12. A primary tooth with an endodontic instrument in place.

12. Pass a lentulo spiral into the canal just short of the apex to fill the canal with a resorbable zinc oxide and eugenol paste. Alternatively, a pressure syringe can be used.

CLINICAL TIP. Avoid nonresorbable types of zinc oxide and eugenol (i.e., Intermediate Restorative Material [IRM], L.D. Caulk/Dentsply) with acrylic fibers).

CLINICAL TIP. An alternate approach involves a pressure syringe (Temp-Canal Kit, Pulpdent Corp.), which uses 18- to 30-gauge needles. Insert a special dense mixture of zinc oxide powder and eugenol (provided with the kit) into the needle hub and attach it to the syringe. Insert the needle to the appropriate length in the canal and inject the material.[16] Overfills act as a foreign substance, but are usually resorbed (Fig. 20–13).[14]

---

13. Place a full coverage restoration on the tooth (see the section on Crowns for Primary Teeth later in this chapter).

Class IV Traumatic Injuries

Class IV injuries involve displacement of the tooth without fracture of the crown or root. They include intrusion injuries and buccolingual displacement of teeth.

Intruded Teeth. Intruded anterior teeth are one of the more common results of injuries to the primary dentition of the preschool child. The child's bone is soft, thus the force of a blow often can push the tooth into the maxilla. However, mandibular intrusions are rare because of the angle of blow required to cause them. The less severe the intrusion, the better the prognosis. If one-half or less of the clinical crown is intruded, and there is no clinical or radiographic evidence of fracture, the tooth is left in place. It will probably re-erupt within 3 to 4 weeks.[7]

CLINICAL TIP. Because a tooth may be totally intruded, it is common for the parent or dentist to assume the primary tooth has been avulsed. A diagnosis can only be made by examining a clear radiograph. Soft tissue swelling can also make a tooth appear more intruded than it actually is.

The primary concern involving intruded teeth is the proximity of the deciduous tooth to its successor. Only a thin layer of bone surrounds the crypt of the succedaneous tooth. If clinical judgement predicts that the intruded primary tooth will adversely affect the permanent tooth, the primary tooth should be extracted. This is determined by a radiograph that shows the primary tooth to be in direct proximity to its successor. The extent of damage to the permanent tooth depends on its stage of matrix formation and calcification at the time of injury. Trauma before the age of 3 (during matrix formation), often results in enamel hypoplasia (crater-like defects in the enamel). After the age of 3, the tooth is undergoing calcification and injury results in localized hypocalcification (chalky opaque spots).[17]

Most intruded teeth also have pulpal damage. However, pulp vitality testing is not dependable for a young

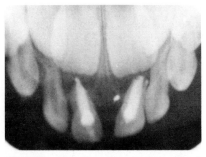

FIG. 20–13. Completed x-rays of primary incisors that were nonvital because of trauma and required pulpectomies.

child or a primary tooth, rather radiographs should be taken at 6-month intervals. Endodontic therapy should be instituted if periapical pathology is noted. Involved teeth must be followed carefully. If the intruded tooth does not begin to re-erupt within 2 months, it should be extracted. Ankylosis may have resulted, which will effect the eruption pattern of the permanent incisor.

Labially or Buccally Displaced Teeth. Because the alveolar bone is soft, injury can result in labial or lingual displacement of the primary anterior tooth. If there is no radiographic evidence of root or bone fracture, the tooth can be slowly and carefully digitally moved to its normal position. The primary concern with a lingually displaced maxillary tooth is that occlusal interference is not created. It is imperative that occlusal interference is corrected or constant trauma to the teeth will result.

If primary anterior teeth are only slightly displaced, incidental muscle pressure from the tongue and lip will restore them to their correct position in the arch. They usually do not have to be splinted in place. If there is more than 2 mm of mobility in any direction, a splint is necessary. The teeth can be etched and a thin layer of composite resin placed or a periodontal pack can be used. The splint is removed in 7 to 10 days.[10]

Splinting—Composite Resin

Armamentarium:

- Standard dental setup (see the section on Class II Traumatic Injuries)
- Acid etch gel
- 0.018 orthodontic wire (Unitek/3M, Inc.)
- Hollow jawed pliers
- Wire cutters
- Bonding agent of choice (see Chapter 3—Dentin Bonding Agents)
- Composite resin of choice (see Chapter 5—Composite Resin—Fundamentals and Direct Technique Restoration)

Clinical Technique:

1. Obtain a thorough medical history, neurological evaluation, and history of trauma.
2. Perform a clinical examination, including a periapical radiograph.
3. Pumice and dry the teeth.

4. Cut a sufficient amount of wire to splint from the maxillary right to maxillary left canine.
5. Contour the wire to conform to the arch.
6. Etch the teeth (primary teeth 30 to 45 seconds, permanent teeth 15 seconds), rinse and dry.
7. Place liquid bonding agent on the teeth and cure.
8. Place the wire in the proper position.
9. Lute the wire to the teeth with composite resin.
10. Place composite resin over the wire.
11. Remove the splint in 7 to 10 days.[10]

Orthodontic Ligature. As an alternative splinting procedure, orthodontic ligature wire can be twisted around the adjacent teeth and stabilized with auto-curing acrylic using a brush-on technique. Acrylic is used because it is easier to remove than composite resin.

Armamentarium:

- Standard dental setup (see the section on Class II Traumatic Injuries)
- Orthodontic ligature wire (0.008 in. to 0.011 in.) (Unitek/3M, Inc.)
- Auto-curing acrylic (L.D. Caulk/Dentsply)
- Brush
- Matthew needle holder
- Wire cutters
- Acrylic burs for trimming

Clinical Technique

1. Obtain a thorough medical history, neurological evaluation, and history of trauma.
2. Perform a clinical examination, including a periapical radiograph.
3. Pass the ligature wire around each tooth.
4. Using a Nealon technique, place acrylic over the wire to stabilize the teeth.
5. Adjust the occlusion to eliminate interferences.
6. Remove the splint in 7 to 10 days.[10]

Instruct the parent to limit the child to a diet of soft foods for a few days, and to prevent the child from incising food. Firm food should be cut into small bite-sized pieces.

Avulsed Teeth. If the primary anterior tooth is avulsed, no attempt should be made to replant it because it can damage the succedaneous tooth and result in ankylosis. If the primary tooth is lost in an accident, or must be subsequently extracted, it can be replaced with a prosthesis. (See the section on Anterior Fixed Space Maintainers later in this chapter.)

Class V Traumatic Injuries

Class V injuries consist of root fracture without loss of crown structure. This is an uncommon injury to the primary dentition because of the soft nature of the alveolar bone. If the radiograph reveals a root fracture of a primary incisor in the middle or coronal one-third of the root, the tooth should be extracted. If the fracture is in the apical one-third of the root, the tooth can be left in place and followed carefully for any clinical changes in the soft tissue, such as abscess formation, or for periapical radiolucencies or root resorption. Initially, the patient should be seen at 3 months, and subsequently at 6-month intervals. Biologic repair of the root can occur by a number of different modalities.[18]

1. Calcified tissue, similar to tooth structure, may form.
2. Healing with interposition of connective tissue, causing the root surface to be covered by cementum.
3. Healing with interposition of bone and connective tissue, and healing with interposition of granulation tissue.

If granulation tissue forms in the fracture site, the prognosis is poor.[19]

Class VI Traumatic Injuries

Class VI injuries consist of either vital or nonvital teeth that have been traumatized. This trauma causes an immediate inflammatory reaction and may result in discoloration. Vasodilation, edema, an ingress of inflammatory cells, and displacement of odontoblasts follows. If the fibroblasts and odontoblasts regenerate, the pulp will heal. Overwhelming inflammation leads to infarction and pulpal necrosis.[19] Vascular edema at the apical foramen occludes the apical vessels. If this occlusion continues, a slow generalized pulpitis leading to necrosis results.

Initial trauma will cause an escape of red blood cells from pulpal vessels into the dentin, with subsequent breakdown and bilirubin pigment formation. The tooth will become blue-gray in appearance (Fig. 20–14). This change may be reversible, but the injured tooth will retain some of the discoloration for an indefinite period.

A yellow opaque color appears with calcific degeneration. Secondary dentin is laid down obliterating the pulp chamber and canal. This is a degenerative process of a noninflammatory nature that takes place a few months after the injury.[20] Internal resorption is a result of odontoclastic activity. It can be seen radiographically within a few weeks or months of the injury. The tooth may appear translucent pink. Color is not an indication of the tooth's vitality.[7] Teeth can become nonvital at any time subsequent to traumatic injury, or they may repair themselves. Initially, the patient should be seen at 3 months, and subsequently at 6-month intervals. Changes in the soft tissue, periapical radiolucencies, and root resorption indicate devitalization.

If the parent is concerned about esthetics and the tooth remains vital, a thin veneer of composite resin can be applied. If the tooth is nonvital, it must be treated prior to restorative procedures (see the section on Nonvital Primary Teeth—Pulpectomy earlier in this chapter).

Armamentarium:

- Standard dental setup (see the section on Class II Traumatic Injuries)
- Acid etch gel
- Bonding agent of choice (see Chapter 3 Dentin Bonding Agents)

- Composite resin of choice (see Chapter 5 Composite Resin—Fundamentals and Direct Technique Restorations)

Clinical Technique:

1. Obtain a thorough medical history, neurological evaluation, and history of trauma.
2. Perform a clinical examination, including a periapical radiograph.
3. Remove a 0.5 mm layer of enamel from the labial portion of the teeth, etch, rinse, dry, and apply bonding agent.
4. Apply a layer of composite resin (microfilled) and build up to cover the discolored tooth.
5. A composite resin crown can also be placed for a more esthetic result. (See the section on Crowns for Primary Teeth later in this chapter.)

CARIES AND DEVELOPMENTAL DISTURBANCES

The morphology of the primary anterior dentition is unique and must be considered when restoring these teeth. The odontoblasts of primary teeth are active for less than half the time as the odontoblasts of the permanent teeth. Pulp chambers are larger and the enamel and dentin are half the thickness of the those of the permanent tooth.[21] This small crown size and large pulp chamber presents unique restorative problems.

The actual dimensions of the primary incisors offer little tooth structure for a permanent restoration.[22] The proportions shown in Table 20–2 may serve as a guide to the tooth structure present. In many instances, however, the tooth is smaller and less hard tissue is available for preparation.

The mandibular anterior teeth are extremely difficult to restore. The slightest amount of decay results in a preparation close to the pulp.

Repair of Interproximal Caries

Restoration of primary incisors with interproximal decay requires an exacting technique. Prudent evaluation of both the tooth to be restored and the procedure to be used is advised. The lesions should be small compared to the total tooth size. A lock must be placed in the labial or lingual portion of the preparation, rather than in

TABLE 20–2. AVERAGE SIZES OF PRIMARY TEETH

(From McBride, W.E. (ed): Juvenile Dentistry, 4th Ed. Philadelphia, Lea & Febiger, 1945.)

the proximal internal walls where there is a danger of pulp exposure.[23] The small size of the mandibular incisors makes it almost impossible to use this procedure without exposing the pulp.

Armamentarium:

- Standard dental setup (see the section on Class II Traumatic Injuries)
- High-speed bur, such as inverted cone No. 33½ or No. 34
- High-speed bur, such as pear-shaped bur No. 330 or No. 331
- Suitable liner material, such as calcium hydroxide (e.g., Dycal, L.D. Caulk/Dentsply) or glass ionomer cement (Keta-Cem, ESPE-Premier Sales Corp.)
- Polycarboxylate cement (Durelon, ESPE-Premier Sales Corp.)
- Acid etch gel
- Bonding agent of choice (see Chapter 3—Dentin Bonding Agents)
- Composite resin of choice (see Chapter 5—Composite Resin Restorations—Fundamentals and Direct Technique Restorations)
- Mylar strip and wooden wedge

Clinical Technique:

1. Administer local anesthesia.
2. Place a rubber dam.
3. Remove interproximal caries with a small inverted cone bur No. 33½ or No. 34 or pear shaped bur No. 330 or No. 331.
4. Add a labial or lingual lock for retention (Fig. 20–15 to 20–22). If there is both mesial and distal decay, these locks can be connected (Figs. 20–23 to 20–30). Remove the incisal angle if it is thin and undermined. If there is a small mechanical exposure, perform a vital formocresol pulpotomy. (See the section on Vital Primary Teeth–Pulpotomy earlier in this chapter.) Pulp capping primary teeth is contraindicated.[14]
5. Place a liner of calcium hydroxide or glass ionomer cement on the dentin. If a pulpotomy is performed, place a polycarboxylate or glass ionomer cement over the zinc oxide and eugenol which was placed during the pulpotomy procedure.
6. Acid etch the enamel for 30 to 45 seconds, rinse and dry.
7. Apply bonding agent. (See Chapter 3—Dentin Bonding Agents.)
8. Depending on the restorative situation:
   A. If the dental arch exhibits interdental space between the anterior teeth, place a bonded composite resin.
   B. If there is no interdental space, place a wedge and a mylar strip to aid in shaping the composite resin.
   C. If the incisal angle is missing, a plastic crown form (e.g., Ion Crown Form, 3M Inc.) may be used as an alternative to the mylar strip. Cut the form to fit the angle of the tooth and then fill it with a composite resin and bond it into place.

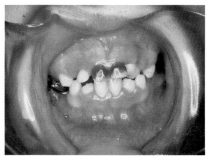

FIG. 20–14. Discoloration of primary teeth caused by blood pigments in the dentin.

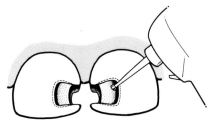

FIG. 20–15. Labial view of interproximal "through and through" decay requiring labial and lingual locks and peripheral undercuts for retention.

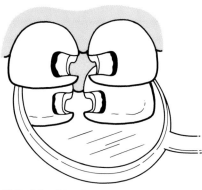

FIG. 20–16. Lingual view with a liner in place.

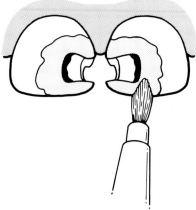

FIG. 20–17. Bonding agent is applied to etched enamel.

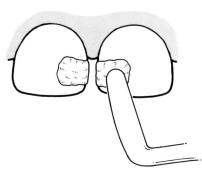

FIG. 20–18. Composite resin is placed.

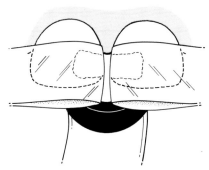

FIG. 20–19. Celluloid strips are used to stabilize the resin and the restoration is cured from the lingual direction.

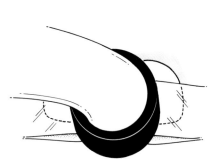

FIG. 20–20. The restoration is then light-cured from the labial direction.

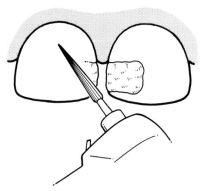

FIG. 20–21. The resin is trimmed with a 12-fluted bur and then polished.

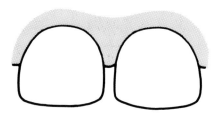

FIG. 20–22. The final restoration.

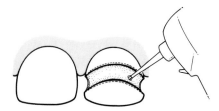

FIG. 20–23. Retentive locks can be interconnected when interproximal decay exists on both the mesial and distal surfaces.

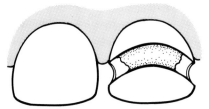

FIG. 20–24. Calcium hydroxide or glass ionomer liner is placed on dentin.

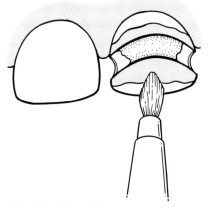

FIG. 20–25. Unfilled composite resin is applied to etched enamel.

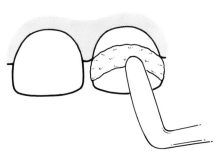

FIG. 20—26. Placement of composite resin.

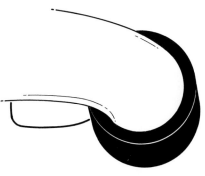

FIG. 20—27. The restoration is light-cured from the labial direction.

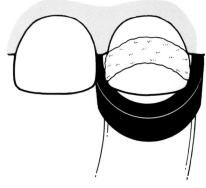

FIG. 20—28. The restoration is then light-cured from the lingual direction.

FIG. 20—29. The resin is trimmed and polished.

FIG. 20—30. The completed restoration.

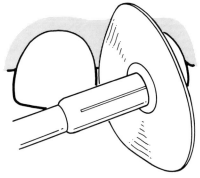

FIG. 20—29

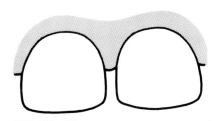

FIG. 20—30

Composite resins need adequate enamel for bonding and may not be strong enough to withstand constant occlusion pressures. If the anterior tooth is malformed, fractured, discolored, or has extensive caries, full coverage is indicated.

Repair of Buccal or Lingual Caries

The procedure for restoration of Class V caries on primary teeth is similar to that for permanent teeth. An undercut on the entire perimeter of the preparation ensures adequate retention of the composite resin.

Armamentarium:

- Standard dental setup (see the section on Class II Traumatic Injuries)
- High-speed bur, such as inverted cone No. 33½ or No. 34
- Suitable liner material, such as calcium hydroxide (e.g., Dycal, L.D. Caulk/Dentsply) or glass ionomer cement, (Keta-Cem, ESPE-Premier Sales Corp.)
- Acid etch gel
- Bonding agent of choice (see Chapter 3—Dentin Bonding Agents)
- Composite resin of choice (see Chapter 5—Composite Resin—Fundamentals and Direct Technique Restorations)

Clinical Technique:

1. Administer local anesthesia.
2. Place a rubber dam.
3. Remove buccal caries with a small inverted cone bur No. 33½ or No. 34.
4. Place an undercut within the entire perimeter of the preparation (Fig. 20—31). If there is a small mechanical exposure, perform a vital formocresol pulpotomy (see the section on Vital Primary Teeth—Pulpotomy earlier in this chapter). Pulp capping primary teeth is contraindicated.[14]
5. Place a liner of calcium hydroxide or glass ionomer cement on the dentin (Fig. 20—32). If a pulpotomy is performed, place a polycarboxylate or glass ionomer cement over the zinc oxide and eugenol which was placed during the pulpotomy procedure.
6. Acid etch the enamel for 30 to 45 seconds, rinse and dry.
7. Apply bonding agent (Fig. 20—33). (See Chapter 3—Dentin Bonding Agents.)
8. Place and light-cure the composite resin (Figs. 20—34).
9. Contour and finish the restoration (Figs. 20—35, 20—37).

CROWNS FOR PRIMARY TEETH

A number of different types of crowns exist for use on primary teeth. All are relatively inexpensive, available in different sizes, and can be placed in one visit.

Stainless Steel Crowns

Stainless steel crowns are manufactured for primary anterior maxillary teeth. They are strong, durable, and

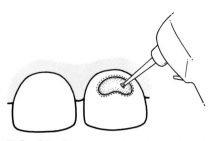

FIG. 20–31. An undercut is placed within the entire periphery of a Class V preparation.

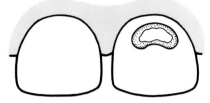

FIG. 20–32. A liner of calcium hydroxide or glass ionomer cement is placed on the dentin.

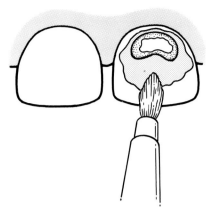

FIG. 20–33. Bonding agent is applied to etched enamel.

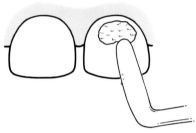

FIG. 20–34

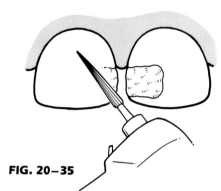

FIG. 20–35

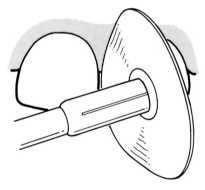

FIG. 20–36

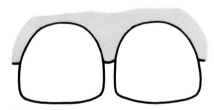

FIG. 20–37

FIG. 20–34. Composite resin is placed in the restoration.

FIGS. 20-35 AND 20–36. The restoration is contoured and polished.

FIG. 20–37. The final restoration.

easily adapted to a prepared tooth; however, they are not esthetically acceptable. Early attempts at cosmetic resin filled windows have been unsuccessful.

Celluloid Strip Crowns

Celluloid strip crowns are preformed plastic crown molds that are available in various sizes (e.g., Ion Crown Form, 3M, Inc.). They are used if the tooth is merely discolored and there are no occlusal interferences (e.g., an open bite). They are packaged in a kit of four sizes of right and left maxillary central and lateral primary incisors. The advantages of celluloid strip crowns are:

1. Esthetic appearance.

2. They require removal of only a small amount of tooth structure.
3. Supplemental retention can be gained by bonding to the remaining enamel.

   The disadvantages are:

1. The restoration often has an insufficient bulk of material to withstand occlusal stress.
2. They are only manufactured for the maxillary teeth and must be adapted to the mandibular anteriors.
3. They are difficult to use in tight contact cases.

Armamentarium:

- Standard dental setup (see the section on Class II Traumatic Injuries)

- High-speed bur, such as inverted cone No. 33½ or No. 34
- High-speed bur, such as pear-shaped bur No. 330 or No. 331
- High-speed bur, such as fine tapered diamond stone or No. 699 or No. 700 carbide bur
- Suitable liner material, such as calcium hydroxide (e.g., Dycal, L.D. Caulk/Dentsply) or glass ionomer cement (Ketac-Cem, ESPE-Premier Sales Corp.)
- Celluloid strip crowns (e.g., Ion Crown Form, 3M, Inc.)
- Acid etch gel
- Bonding agent of choice (see Chapter 3—Dentin Bonding Agents)
- Composite resin of choice (see Chapter 5—Composite Resin—Fundamentals and Direct Technique Restorations)

Clinical Technique:

1. Administer local anesthesia.
2. Place a rubber dam.
3. Remove interproximal caries with a small inverted cone bur No. 33½ or No. 34 or pear-shaped bur No. 330 or No. 331.
4. Perform pulp therapy, if necessary. (See the sections on Vital Primary Teeth—Pulpotomy and Nonvital Primary Teeth—Pulpectomy earlier in this chapter.)
5. If the tooth has been fractured, apply an adequate layer of calcium hydroxide.
6. Prepare the tooth using a fine tapered diamond stone or No. 699 or No. 700 bur, for the labial and proximal areas. A pear-shaped diamond can be used to reduce the lingual area.
7. Reduce the tooth as follows (Fig. 20–38):
   A. Mesial and distal, 1.0 mm
   B. Buccal, 0.5 mm
   C. Lingual, 0.5 mm
   D. Incisal, 0.5 mm
8. Create a feather-edged finishing line slightly subgingivally.
9. Fit and adjust the crown cervically.
10. Protect the dentin with calcium hydroxide
11. Acid etch the enamel for 30 to 45 seconds rinse, dry, and apply bonding agent.
12. Placed an air vent in the incisolingual area and fill the crown with composite resin.
13. Seat the crown.
14. Slit the celluloid cover with a scalpel along the lingual surface to avoid damaging the smooth surface on the labial portion and remove the celluloid material.
15. Adjusted the occlusion.
16. Finish and polish the composite resin.

Preformed Ceramo-Base Metal Crowns[25]

Preformed ceramo-base metal crowns (e.g., Childers' Crown, Keller Laboratories, Inc.) are the restoration of choice if the tooth has lost significant structure from decay or trauma or if occlusal stresses are high. Developed by Dr. Logan Childers, they are manufactured in five sizes that fit on either the left or right primary maxillary incisors (Fig. 20–39). Only light and universal shades of porcelain are available. They are contoured to the correct shape by the dentist. Advantages of preformed ceramo-base metal crowns are:[25]

1. Excellent esthetics.
2. Strength.
3. Durability.

Disadvantages are:[26]

1. Require extensive tooth reduction.
2. Time consuming.
3. High cost.
4. Difficult to fit because of hardness and lack of pliability.
5. Risk of porcelain fracture during placement.
6. Possible risk of allergy to nickel.
7. Questionable adverse effects of beryllium (1.8%).

As with the other crown techniques, the tooth must be fit to the manufactured crown. The preparation is similar to that for celluloid crowns, but more tooth structure must be removed. Porcelain-fused-to-metal crowns do not "spring" and conform to the tooth as do posterior stainless steel crowns, thus a tight fit is not always achieved. Attempts at cervical contouring may fracture the porcelain, therefore, marginal fit can only be obtained through proper tooth reduction.

Armamentarium:

- Standard dental setup (see the section on Class II Traumatic Injuries)
- High-speed bur, such as inverted cone No. 33½ or No. 34
- High-speed bur, such as pear-shaped bur No. 330 or No. 331
- High-speed bur, such as fine tapered diamond stone or No. 699 or No. 700 carbide bur
- Suitable liner material, such as calcium hydroxide

FIG. 20–38. A typical crown preparation.

FIG. 20–39. Ceramo-base metal crowns (Childers') are manufactured in five sizes in light and universal shades of porcelain.

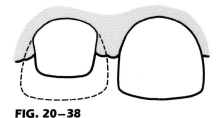

FIG. 20–38

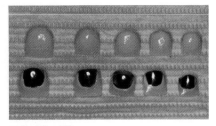

FIG. 20–39

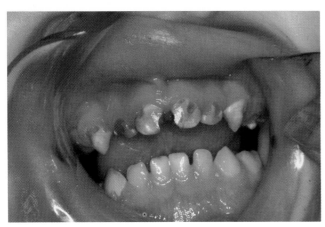

FIG. 20–40. Facial view of a patient with nursing bottle syndrome.

(e.g., Dycal, L.D. Caulk/Dentsply) or glass ionomer cement (Keta-Cem, ESPE-Premier Sales Corp.)

- Preformed ceramo-base metal crown kit (e.g., Childer's Crown, Keller Laboratories, Inc.)
- Suitable cementation medium, such as polycarboxylate cement (Durelon, ESPE-Premier Sales Corp.) or zinc phosphate cement, (Fleck's Cement, Mizzy, Inc.) or composite resin post and core material (Core Material, Henry Schein, Inc.)

Clinical Technique:

1. The initial preparation is identical to celluloid crowns (see step 1–6 under Celluloid Strip Crowns).
2. This preparation requires greater reduction than for a celluloid crown. Reduce the tooth as follows:
   A. Mesial and distal, 1.5 to 2.0 mm
   B. Buccal, 1.0 mm
   C. Lingual, 0.5 mm
   D. Incisal, 2.0 mm
   E. Occlusal, 2.0 mm
3. Create a feather-edged finishing line slightly subgingivally.
4. Select a suitable crown.
5. Fit the crown and adjust it cervically.
6. Contour and polish the crown with a porcelain finishing kit and diamond stones.
7. Cement the crown into place with a suitable luting agent.

POST AND CORES

The ravages of decay are most commonly seen with nursing bottle caries. The complete coronal portion of the crown can be destroyed by caries (Fig. 20–40). In many instances, these teeth can be salvaged if the root structure is sound (Fig. 20–41).

Armamentarium:

- Standard dental setup (see the section on Class II Traumatic Injuries)

- High-speed bur, such as No. 699, No. 330, or No. 331 Carbide bur
- Suitable post system (e.g., Flexi-Post, Essential Dental Systems, Inc)
- Preformed ceramo-base metal crown kit (Childer's Crown, Keller Laboratories, Inc.)
- Suitable cementation medium, such as polycarboxylate cement (Durelon, ESPE-Premier Sales Corp.) or glass ionomer cement (Keta-Cem, ESPE-Premier Sales Corp.)

Clinical Technique

1. Administer local anesthesia.
2. Place a rubber dam.
3. Remove all decay. Many times only the root structure remains (Fig. 20–42).
4. Perform a complete pulpectomy (see the section on Nonvital Primary Teeth—Pulpectomy earlier in this chapter) (Fig. 20–43).
5. Determine the length of the tooth radiographically.
6. Fit a stress-relieving post (e.g., Flexi-Post, Essential Dental Systems) to a depth of two-thirds the length of the canal. Clinical experience has shown that non-stress relieving brass screw posts are easily bent or broken and the chance of root fracture is high; thus these materials are not recommended.
7. The posts are held by friction and are not cemented.
8. Trim the post occlusally, leaving 3 to 4 mm of material above the gingiva (Fig. 20–44).
9. Fit and cement a preformed ceramo-base metal crown (Figs. 20–45 to 20–47). (See the section on Preformed Ceramo-Base Metal Crowns earlier in this chapter.)
10. Followup with a radiograph every 6 months to verify that no damage is occurring to the permanent tooth (e.g., as evidenced by a radiolucency).

These crowns can remain in place until just prior to the eruption of the maxillary permanent central incisors. This occurs when the mandibular permanent incisors have started to erupt or evidence of eruption of the maxillary permanent incisors is noted radiographically. The post has the potential of deflecting the succedaneous tooth as it erupts (Fig. 20–48). At this time, the crown is removed and the post is unscrewed (Fig. 20–49). or the entire tooth is extracted.

ANTERIOR FIXED SPACE MAINTAINERS

Anterior teeth can be decayed to a point where infection and resorption of the primary roots precludes endodontic therapy. Trauma and developmental disturbances can also cause early loss of the primary teeth. Anterior fixed space maintainers are the restoration of choice in this clinical situation. (Figs. 20–50, 20–51). Their advantages are:

1. Good esthetics.
2. Restored function.
3. Maintain space where necessary.

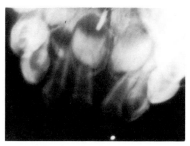

FIG. 20–41. Radiograph of a patient with nursing bottle syndrome. The teeth are vital and there is sufficient root structure to salvage them.

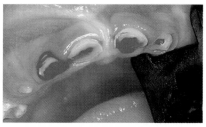

FIG. 20–42. Following the removal of all the decay, very little coronal tooth structure remains. Note that the deciduous molar was insufficiently erupted to allow for the placement of a rubber dam clamp.

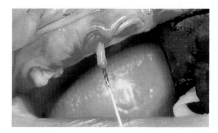

FIG. 20–43. Pulpectomies are performed on all of the anterior teeth. Note that the pulps of the teeth were vital.

FIG. 20–44. A second case showing the post trimmed occlusally, leaving 3 to 4 mm of material above the gingiva.

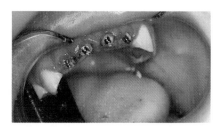

FIG. 20–44

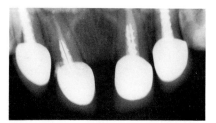

FIG. 20–45

FIG. 20–45. Radiograph of the patient shown in Figure 20-44 with nursing bottle syndrome whose teeth were restored with complete endodontics, preformed stress-relieving posts and porcelain-fused-to-metal crowns.

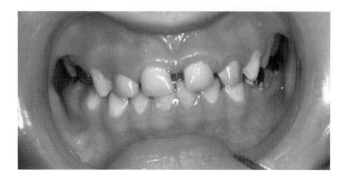

FIG. 20–46. Facial view of the patient shown in Figure 20-44, the completed restorations.

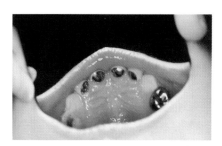

FIG. 20–47. Occlusal view of the completed restorations.

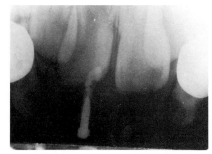

FIG. 20–48. Prior to the eruption of the maxillary permanent central incisors, the post should be removed or the tooth extracted to prevent deflection of the succedaneous tooth as it erupts. Note that the root paste is being resorbed.

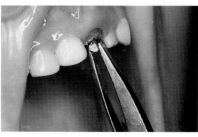

FIG. 20–49. The crown is removed and the post is unscrewed. Note the healthy appearance of the gingiva.

FIG. 20–50. The primary anterior teeth were removed because of nursing bottle syndrome.

FIG. 20–51. A fixed space maintainer was fabricated to replace the primary central and lateral incisors.

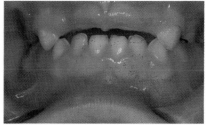

FIG. 20–50

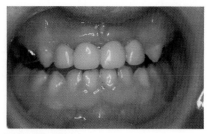

FIG. 20–51

4. Prevent supereruption of opposing dentition.

Their disadvantages are:

1. Possible inadvertent orthodontic movement if improperly fabricated.
2. Require cementation of bands or crowns, which may affect posterior teeth by causing decalcification or decay if the cement washes out.

Bands vs. Stainless Steel Crowns

Bands are fitted on healthy first or second primary molars. Bands do not require the removal of tooth structure and are therefore preferable to stainless steel crowns. However, stainless steel crowns are indicated in the following situations:

1. Where extensive decay is present.
2. When band retention proves to be insufficient.

CLINICAL TIP. Crowns must be used bilaterally. This avoids the difficulties of stainless steel crown removal should the band component dislodge unilaterally.

Armamentarium:

- Standard dental setup (see the section on Class II Traumatic Injuries)
- High-speed bur, such as No. 699, No. 330, or No. 331 carbide bur
- Dry angles (e.g., Dri-Aid, Lorvic Corp.)
- Stainless steel crowns or orthodontic bands
- Impression compound (Impression Compound, Kerr Manufacturing Co.)
- Irreversible hydrocolloid impression material (Jeltrate, L.D. Caulk/Dentsply)
- Stone
- 0.036 in. orthodontic wire (Unitek, 3M Inc.)

- Polycarboxylate cement (Durelon, ESPE-Premier Sales Corp.)

Clinical Technique

1. Fit the stainless steel crowns or bands on the maxillary primary first or second molars.
2. Capture the bands in a compound pick-up impression. Compound creates a firm seat to assure proper transfer.
3. Obtain a counter irreversible hydrocolloid impression and a wax wafer bite registration.
4. Using sticky wax, lute the bands or crowns into place in the compound impression.
5. Pour the models.
6. If the primary teeth were extracted recently, or at the same visit (i.e., when general anesthesia is used), remove a few millimeters of stone from the corresponding portion of the cast. This compensates for the tissue shrinkage that occurs after healing.
7. Adapt a wire to the dental arch.
8. Add acrylic to the wire to form the missing teeth (Figs. 20–52, 20–53).

CLINICAL TIP. To eliminate restoration breakage, solder an open-faced anterior stainless steel crown with the edges of the crown bent inward, or a solid direct bond pad with a mesh base and an eyelet tacked to the mesh for added retention. The retentive areas holding the teeth on the wire are usually stainless steel, not acrylic (Spacemaintainer Laboratories, Van Nuys, CA).

---

9. Try-in the case by seating the crowns or bands into place. Then adjust the wire holding the replacement teeth so the pontics rest passively on the gingiva. During use this will seat an additional 1 to 2 mm onto the ridge.
10. Isolate the teeth with a dry angle (e.g., Dri-Aids, Lorvic Corp.), dry the teeth with oil-free com-

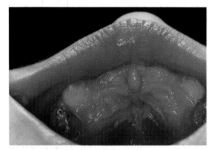

FIG. 20–52

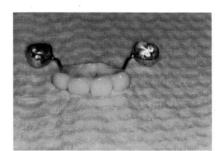

FIG. 20–53

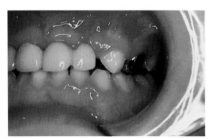

FIG. 20–54

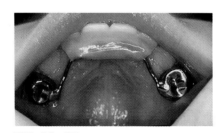

FIG. 20–55

FIG. 20–52. Occlusal view of an edentulous anterior maxilla requiring an anterior space maintainer.

FIG. 20–53. An anterior space maintainer is fabricated on the previously fitted stainless steel crowns.

FIG. 20–54. Three-quarter view of the fixed space maintainer in place.

FIG. 20–55. Occlusal view of the fixed space maintainer with acrylic teeth in place.

ESTHETIC DENTISTRY

pressed air, and cement the appliance into place with a polycarboxylate cement (Figs. 20–54, 20–55).

Follow these restorations closely to check for eruption of the anterior teeth. Take maxillary and mandibular radiographs at 6-month intervals. When the mandibular permanent incisors are about to erupt or when evidence of eruption of the maxillary permanent central incisors is noted radiographically, remove the appliance. If the restoration is placed with bands, remove the entire appliance. If crowns are used, cut the wire, leaving the crowns as final restorations.

REMOVABLE PROSTHETICS

Removable partial and complete dentures are necessary for children when fixed space maintainers are not adequate to replace teeth missing because of trauma and caries. Hereditary anomalies of tooth number also must be addressed. Anodontia, (complete lack of teeth) or oligodontia (partial lack of teeth) is seen in ectodermal dysplasia and Down's syndrome. Other diseases cause premature loss of teeth (e.g., histiocytosis X, Papillon-Lefevre syndrome, and hypophosphatasia). All of these conditions create the need for removable partial or complete dentures. The advantages of removable dentures are:

1. Good esthetics.
2. Restored function.

The disadvantages are:

1. Require a mature and compliant patient.
2. Easily lost.

The concept that the denture must be changed every year is a fallacy. There is essentially no interstitial growth in the anterior portion of the mouth from the age of 3 until the permanent anterior teeth erupt. There is only vertical growth.

The dentures remain stable, with little adjustment needed in the years prior to the eruption of the permanent dentition; however it is necessary to reline the dentures approximately every 12 or 18 months to accommodate vertical growth. With the eruption of the permanent teeth, there is a proliferation of alveolar bone. It is impossible to cut holes in the denture for these teeth to fit. New dentures must be fabricated at this time.

Armamentarium:

- Standard dental setup (see the section on Class II Traumatic Injuries)
- Irreversible hydrocolloid impression material
- Impression compound (e.g., Impression Compound, Kerr Manufacturing Corp.)
- Acrylic custom tray material (e.g., Formoatray, Kerr Manufacturing Corp.)
- Impression material (e.g. Reprosil, L.D. Caulk/Dentsply)

Clinical Technique

1. Make a preliminary irreversible hydrocolloid impression using stock trays.
2. Pour the impressions.
3. Fabricate custom trays.
4. Make muscle-trimmed impressions, as for adults.
5. Fabricate trays with wax occlusal rims on the master models.
6. If 1 or 2 teeth are present in the dental arch, it is not difficult to determine jaw relationships. (Figs. 20–56, 20–57) If no teeth are present, use the wax rim as a guide for proper orientation of the teeth. However, it is almost impossible to obtain a correct centric relationship from a child unless he is extremely cooperative.[27]
7. With the casts mounted on an articulator, arrange zero degree plastic denture teeth with a flat occlusal plane. Bambino Denture Teeth (OSE Dental Supplies and Equipment, Division Orthodontic Supply and Equipment Co., Inc. Gaithersburg, MD) can also be used.

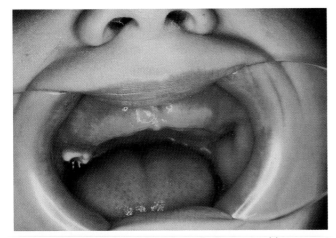

FIG. 20–56. A patient with a loss of primary dentition, except for maxillary second primary molars, because of caries.

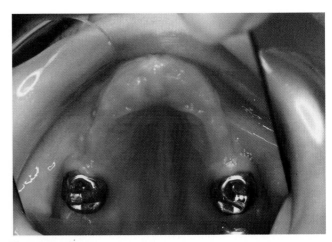

FIG. 20–57. Occlusal view of the patient shown in Figure 20–56.

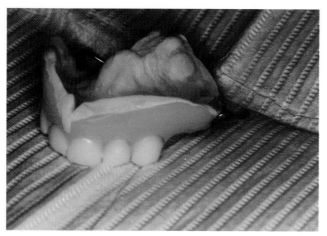

FIG. 20–58. A partial denture with full palatal coverage and labial flange to replace the missing anterior teeth.

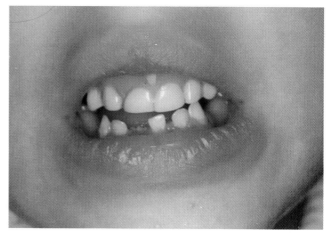

FIG. 20–59. A patient who had been wearing the same partial denture for 4 years. Note that the mandibular anterior permanent teeth are erupting. Although the denture does not fit completely, it is still functional.

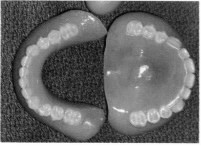

FIG. 20–60

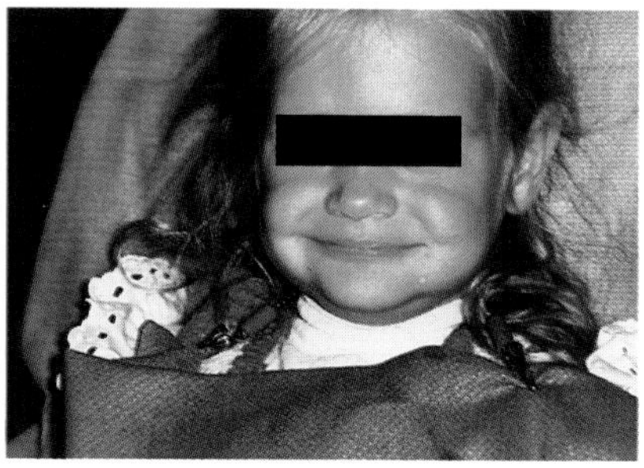

FIG. 20–61

FIG. 20–60. A complete maxillary and mandibular denture for a patient with Papillon-Lefevre syndrome.

FIG. 20–61. The patient with the denture in place.

8. If any primary teeth are present in the mouth, use them for retention by placing wrought wire clasps (Fig. 20–58).

9. Process and deliver the dentures to the patient.

10. Fit the dentures carefully. A child's vestibule is relatively shallow because there is no alveolar bone, only basal bone. In addition, follow the patient to determine when (and if) the denture must be replaced (Fig. 20–59).

Overlay complete or partial removable dentures can be fabricated over retained teeth or roots that are not specially prepared to accept copings.[28] These dentures can be used in patients with cleidocranial dysostosis, ectodermal dysplasia, and cleft palate, (Figs. 20–60, 20–61).

CONCLUSION

Esthetic restorations in the primary dentition are proper and necessary. With the many modalities available, children should have their mouths restored to proper form and function.

REFERENCES

1. Morrees, C.F., Fanning, E.A., and Gron, A.M.: The consideration of dental development in serial extraction. Angle Orthod 33:44, 1963.
2. Styczynski, L.E. and Langolis, J.H.: The effects of familiarity on behavioral stereotypes associates with physical attractiveness in young children. Child Dev 48:1137, 1977.
3. Dion, K.K. and Berscheid, E.: Physical attractiveness and peer perception among children. Sociometry. 1:1, 1974.
4. Landis, P. and Fleming, J.: The interrelationship of speech therapy and prostheses for the handicapped child. Dent Clin North Am 3:725, 1974.
5. Reikman, G.A. and Badrawy, H.G.: Effects of premature loss of primary maxillary incisors on speech. Pediatr Dent 2:119, 1985.
6. Baume, L.K.: Physiological tooth migration and its significance for the development of occlusion. J Dent Res 29:123, 1950.
7. Levine, N.: Injury to the primary dentition. Dent Clin North Am, 26:461, 1982.
8. Schreiber, C.K.: Effect of trauma on the anterior deciduous teeth. Br Dent J 106:340, 1959.
9. Ellis, R.G. and Davies, K.W.: The Classification and Treatment of Injuries to the Teeth of Children, 5th Ed. Chicago, Year Book Medical Publishers, Inc., 1970.
10. Hill, C.J.: Oral trauma to the preschool child. Dent Clin North Am, 28:177, 1984.
11. Croll, T.P., et al: Rapid neurological assessment and initial management for the patient with dental injuries. J Am Dent Assoc 100:530, 1980.
12. Citron, C.I.: The clinical and histological evaluation of cresatin with calcium hydroxide of the human dental pulp. J Dent Children, July-August:14, 1977.
13. Attalla, M.N., and Nowjaim, A.A.: Role of calcium hydroxide in the formation of reparative dentin. J Can Dent Assoc 35:268, 1969.
14. Camp, J.H.: Pulptherapy for primary and young permanent teeth. Dent Clin North Am 28:4, 1984.
15. Ranly, D.M. and Horn, D.: Assessment of systemic distribution

and toxicity of formocresol following pulpotomy treatment, part two. J Dent Children, 34:1, 1987.

16. Krakow, A.A. and Berk, H.: Efficient endodontic procedures with the use of the pressure syringe. Dent Clin North Am 387, July, 1965.

17. Andreasen, J.O. and Ravin, J.J.: Enamel changes in permanent teeth after trauma to their primary precessors. Scand J Dent Res 81:203, 1973.

18. Andreasen, J.O.: Traumatic Injuries of the Teeth. St. Louis, C.V. Mosby Co., 1972.

19. McDonald, R.E. and Avery, D.R.: Dentistry for the Child and Adolescent, 3rd Ed. St. Louis, C.V. Mosby Co., 1978.

20. Patterson, S.S., and Mitchell, D.F.: Calcific metamorphosis of the dental pulp. Oral Surg 20:94, 1965.

21. Schour, I.: Noyes' Oral Histology and Embryology. Philadelphia, Lea & Febiger, 1962.

22. Arnium, S.S., and Doyle, M.P.: Dentin dimensions of primary teeth. J Dent Children 26:191, 1958.

23. McAvoy, S.A.: Class III cavity preparation and composite resins. Dent Clin North Am 28:145, 1984.

24. Childers, L., Personal communication, 1989.

25. Christensen, G.: Esthetic pre-formed crowns. Clinical Research Associates Newsletter 11:1, 1987.

26. Jasmin, J.R. and Groper, J.N.: Fabrication of a more durable fixed anterior esthetic appliance. J Dent Children. 51:124, 1984.

27. Johnson, D.L., and Stratton, R.J.: Fundamentals of Removable Prosthetics. Chicago; Quintessence Publishing Co., Inc., 1980.

28. Schneidman, E., Wilson, S., and Spuller, R.L.: Complete overlay dentures for the pediatric patient: case reports. Pediatr Dent 10:222, 1988.

Edwin S. Rosenberg, D.M.D.
James Torosian, D.M.D.

ESTHETICS AND PERIODONTICS

21

Periodontal therapy plays an important role in esthetics, although the images invoked regarding conventional periodontal therapy (ugly spaces, gingival recession, tooth sensitivity) are anything but beautiful. The introduction of new surgical techniques and the adaptation of traditional periodontal procedures have led to a heightened esthetic awareness in periodontology. In addition, the recognition of the etiology and complicating factors underlying an esthetic periodontal problem is crucial. Often this identification alters or dictates the final treatment plan.

PERIODONTAL ALVEOLAR BONE DEFECTS

Differential Diagnosis

Traditional periodontal pocket elimination therapy causes unesthetic results, including large interdental spaces and long clinical crowns. However, without adequate access to deep lesions, a healthy periodontal environment cannot be achieved. There are several surgical solutions to this dilemma depending on whether the defect is anteriorly or posteriorly located.

Treatment Options

Retained Papilla. The retained papilla technique is an ideal treatment alternative for periodontal defects. The procedure provides adequate access to deep anterior defects, allowing for thorough surgical debridement of the area while maintaining the position of the free gingival margin. This is accomplished by including the entire interproximal tissue mass in the surgical flap. A straight line incision is made in the palate and the papilla reflected buccally with the flap. After thorough debridement of the defect and the root surfaces (and grafting, palatal ramping, and regenerative procedures, when necessary), the flaps are sutured. By including the papillary tissues (as opposed to removing them as with conventional pocket elimination) interproximal tissue height is maintained and there is little or no apical shrinkage. Thus, the physiologic needs of the periodontium are satisfied along with the esthetic demands of the patient.

Guided Tissue Regeneration. The goal of guided tissue regeneration is pocket elimination through reformation of the periodontal connective tissue attachment. It is applicable to both anterior and posterior sextants. Exclusion of the rapidly proliferating epithelial tissues from the defect allows regeneration of the connective tissue attachment by cells of the periodontal ligament. This epithelial exclusion is achieved by placing a semipermeable membrane (e.g., Gore-Tex, Gore and Assoc. Corp.) between the periodontal defect and the flap. This allows nutrients to reach the flap while preventing the formation of a long junctional epithelium. The membrane is removed via a simple gingival flap procedure after 4 to 5 weeks and reveals a dense connective tissue fill of the defect that may or may not be accompanied with bone regeneration. Alveolar bone is not always necessary to achieve pocket closure since the dense connective tissue attachment to the root surface can provide fill for the defect. It should be noted that not all defects are amenable to this type of procedure (Class II furcation defects and deep, narrow three-walled defects offer the best prognosis) and the results are not completely predictable.

Osseous Grafting. Osseous grafting is another alternative for the treatment of deep angular defects and is also applicable to both anterior and posterior sextants. The two primary types of materials used are decalcified freeze-dried cortical bone (DFDCB) and synthetic materials. With DFDCB, some regeneration is possible, whereas synthetic materials act as scaffolding to allow for osseous tissue ingrowth. The resultant pocket closure is via long junctional epithelial healing. Surgical access to the defects is gained via a flap designed to maintain the marginal tissues. Once the defects have been debrided, the graft material is placed into the defect. The flaps are replaced to cover the graft material (if primary closure is not achieved, exposed graft material may "fall out" of the defect). The end result is clinical pocket closure with maintenance of the free gingival margin. There must be adequate bony wall structure to contain and support the material because it will not remain in place as a free standing graft. As with guided tissue regeneration, the end results are not completely predictable. The criterion used to determine the appropriate procedure is the morphology of the alveolar defect. Guided tissue regeneration is best used in furcation involvements of mandibular molars, Class II buccal furcations of maxillary molars, and deep, narrow three-walled alveolar defects. Decreased predictability of results is seen with this procedure in two- and one-walled defects and in buccal and lingual dehissences. Allogenic bone grafts are best utilized in Class II furcations, three-walled defects, and craters. Also, in cases with interproximal craters and root proximity, a bone graft would be indicated because of the ease of placement. As with the guided tissue regeneration procedure, the success rate decreases with two- and one-walled alveolar defects and with lingual and buccal plate defects.

Another factor to consider is the ability to achieve primary closure of the flap margins. This is of utmost importance with bone grafts because the flap is needed for protection of the graft. Another factor is the need for a second surgical procedure with the Gore-Tex membrane; a minor flap procedure is needed to remove the membrane. All other factors being equal, a bone graft would be desirable in cases when a second stage would be a problem (e.g., difficult access, medical complications, patient cooperation).

The first procedure discussed above, the retained papillae technique, is used almost exclusively in the maxillary anterior sextant, and can be used in the presence or absence of alveolar bone defects. In addition, papillary retention in the flap does not preclude the use of guided tissue regeneration or bone grafts.

The decision to use the retained papillae technique is, obviously, made before the time of the procedure. However, the final decision to use guided tissue regeneration, bone grafting, or neither is made during the procedure.

Palatal or Lingual Ramping. Another esthetic option in the posterior sextant is palatal or lingual ramping of alveolar defects without involvement of the buccal bone. Ostectomy is done to remove the palatal or lingual wall of a crater-type defect. This results in increased crown length on the palatal or lingual aspect of the teeth, with the gingival tissues angled palatally or lingually. The buccal height of tissue remains relatively intact because the buccal bone is spared.

Open Debridement with Buccal Ostectomy. It should be noted that although the aforementioned procedures are designed to maintain buccal bone height, there are times when buccal ostectomy is necessary, such as in cases of a markedly uneven buccal bony profile. When this type of situation occurs, blending of the buccal alveolar crests is needed to ensure proper soft tissue healing and pocket closure. The patient must be made aware that despite best efforts to satisfy esthetic needs, physiologic demands may unfavorably affect the esthetics.

Clinical Case—Retained Papilla Technique

A 52-year-old male presented with deep periodontal pocketing of the anterior maxillary teeth (Figs. 21–1, 21–2). His medical history was noncontributory. Following initial periodontal therapy, a full thickness flap procedure was performed using the retained papilla technique (Figs. 21–3, 21–4). The interproximal tissues were kept in the buccal flap. The papillae were reattached with sutures through the tissue, not over the interproximal space (Fig. 21–5). Healing resulted in pocket reduction with maintenance of the gingival margin (Fig. 21–6).

Clinical Case—Retained Papilla Technique

A 19-year-old female presented with a maxillary midline diastema which had been closed by placing an orthodontic elastic around the two central incisors (Figs. 21–7, 21–8). Her medical history was noncontributory. Unfortunately, the ligature had not been removed and had migrated apically, resulting in a severe distal osseous defect (Figs. 21–9, 21–10). Because an ostectomy would have resulted in extremely long anterior teeth, a retained papilla full thickness flap procedure was performed (Fig. 21–11). Pocket reduction was achieved without sacrificing esthetics (Figs. 21–12, 21–13).

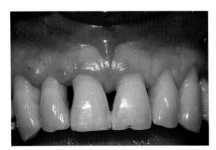

FIG. 21–1

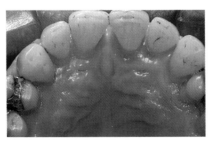

FIG. 21–2

FIG. 21–1. Facial view following initial therapy response in 52-year-old patient with deep periodontal pocketing.

FIG. 21–2. Palatal view of the patient shown in Figure 21–1.

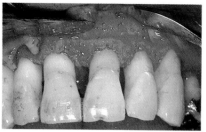

FIG. 21-3

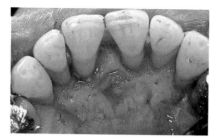

FIG. 21-4

FIG. 21-3. A full thickness flap was raised with complete retention of the papillae in the buccal flap.

FIG. 21-4. The osseous defects were exposed for thorough debridement.

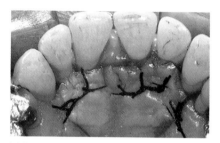

FIG. 21-5. The flaps were repositioned and sutured in place.

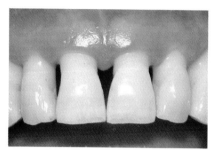

FIG. 21-6. At 6 months after surgery, pocket elimination has been achieved along with maintenance of the original tissue height.

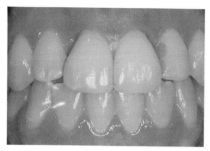

FIG. 21-7. The clinical appearance conceals severe angular defects that are present on the distal aspects of both central incisors. The defects were caused by apical migration of the orthodontic elastics, which were placed to close a previously existing diastema.

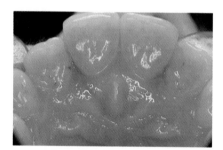

FIG. 21-8. Palatal view of the anterior teeth of the patient shown in Figure 21-7.

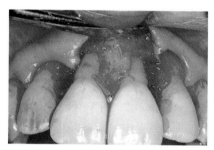

FIG. 21-9. Intraoperative view of the retained papillae technique used to gain access to the defects.

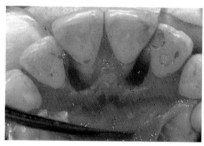

FIG. 21-10. Intraoperative palatal view of the patient shown in Figure 21-9.

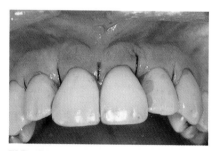

FIG. 21-11. The flap is sutured into place.

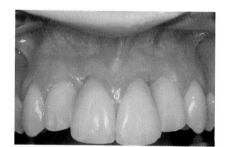

FIG. 21-12. Postoperatively, pocket depth was reduced while satisfying esthetic needs.

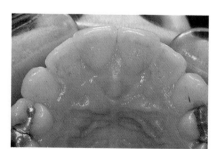

FIG. 21-13. Palatal view of the patient shown in Figure 21-12.

INADEQUATE TOOTH STRUCTURE FOR RESTORATION

Differential Etiology

1. Caries. Many patients are unaware of subgingival caries because the lesion is hidden under the gingiva and, therefore, they do not present for treatment until significant amounts of tooth structure have been destroyed.

2. Trauma. With traumatic injuries the patient is keenly aware of the problem. Teeth can be obliquely sheared, leaving margins below the alveolar crest. When the root fracture is horizontal or oblique, the longer the apical segment, the better the prognosis. Vertical fracture usually requires extraction.

Biologic Width

Proper margin placement of any type of restoration requires respect for the physiologic principle of biologic width: 1 mm of supracrestal connective tissue, 1 mm of junctional epithelium, and 1 to 2 mm of healthy sulcus. When a restoration is placed on a tooth in violation of this principle, a chronic inflammatory response occurs; the body is attempting to restore the dimensions required for periodontal health in the supracrestal attachment and sulcus. Histologically, crestal resorption is seen with apical migration of the connective tissue and junctional epithelium. Clinically, gingival redness, swelling, bleeding, and discomfort are present. Even the most natural looking restoration will fall short of the desired esthetic goals with such a gingival appearance. The inflammatory response will only cease when the biologic width has been re-established, a process that may take years. This inflammation is not bacterial in origin, and will not respond to gingival curettage or antibiotic therapy. Attempting to subgingivally "bury" a restoration margin in the hope of avoiding further treatment will only result in failure.

Treatment Options

Surgical Crown Lengthening. Surgical crown lengthening involves apical flap positioning with ostectomy around the involved tooth and the adjacent teeth. At least 3 to 4 mm of sound root structure must be exposed below the most apical extent of the proposed restoration. In addition, the alveolar crest of the adjacent teeth must be blended in with the involved tooth, otherwise an uneven, unesthetic gingival profile will result.

Forced Eruption with Fiberotomy. When ostectomy will result in extremely long clinical crowns and significantly weakened periodontal support (as with oblique fractures significantly apical to the alveolar crest), or when a surgical procedure is medically contraindicated, orthodontic forced eruption with a sulcular fiberotomy may be performed. Orthodontic force is applied to the involved tooth in an occlusal direction while the supracrestal connective tissue fibers are severed via fiberotomy every 4 days. The fiberotomy prevents the tooth and alveolar bone from erupting as a

unit, exposing sound tooth without changing the position of the alveolar crest or free gingival margin. The orthodontics will pull the root out of the bone, exposing the needed 3 to 4 mm of sound tooth structure, while the fiberotomy will prevent coronal reformation of the alveolar bone and maintain the free gingival margin at its original level. In addition to achieving the desired results, the crown to root ratio of the adjacent teeth remains intact and decreases for the involved tooth, thus improving the long-term periodontal prognosis.

Armamentarium

- Standard dental setup
  explorer
  mouth mirror
  periodontal probe
  high-speed handpiece
- Orthodontic brackets (optional), stainless steel, or clear plastic edgewise brackets (Unitek, 3M, Inc.)
- 0.036 orthodontic wire (Unitek, 3M, Inc.)
- 0.036 orthodontic eyelet (Unitek, 3M, Inc.)
- 0.20 rectangular arch wire
- Crown and bridge cement, zinc phosphate (Flecks' Cement, Mizzy, Inc.) or polycarboxylate cement (e.g., Durelon, ESPE-Premier Sales Corp.)
- Medium or heavy gauge orthodontic elastic or thread (Unitek Corp.)
- No. 15 surgical scalpel

Clinical Technique

1. Prepared a post preparation in the root.
2. Cement a 0.036" wire with an eyelet into the preparation with a zinc phosphate or polycarboxylate cement (Fig. 21–14).
3. When using orthodontic brackets, etch the teeth to be bracketed and apply orthodontic bonding resin to the bracket pad. Place the bracket on the tooth (Fig. 21–15).

   When using bonded arch wire, bond a heavy gauge wire (.030 to .040) across the portion of the labial surface edges of the anterior teeth or occlusal surfaces of the posterior teeth.

CLINICAL TIP. *A clear acrylic is the luting material of choice. Acrylic is strong enough to retain the wire under function and is easier to remove than composite resin.*

For posterior amalgam restorations, prepare the occlusal slots as for intracoronal splints (See A-Splint —Posterior) and bond the wire in the slots. The arch wire must be positioned directly over the root to be extruded.

4. Adapt a heavy (0.020) rectangular arch wire in the bracket slots and across the root to be erupted and position it directly over the root to be extruded (Fig. 21–16).
5. Thread a medium or heavy elastic through the eyelet and wrap it around the anchoring wire. Activate the elastic by pulling it taught and tieing it (Fig. 21–17).
6. Perform an initial fiberotomy with a No. 15 scalpel blade.

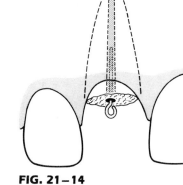

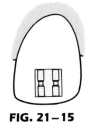

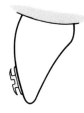

FIG. 21–14. Place a post preparation in the root and cement a 0.036 wire with an eyelet into the preparation with a zinc phosphate or polycarboxylate cement.

FIG. 21–15. Apply orthodontic bonding resin to the bracket pad and place the bracket on the tooth

FIG. 21–16. The arch wire is positioned directly over the root to be extruded.

FIG. 21–17. Activate the elastic by pulling it taught and tieing it

FIG. 21–14

FIG. 21–15

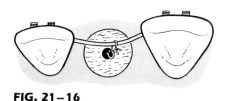

FIG. 21–16

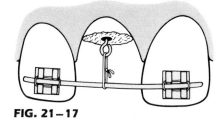

FIG. 21–17

A. Anesthetize the area.

B. Run the scalpel circumferentially in the sulcus around the root. This severs the supracrestal connective tissue fiber attachment.

7. Repeat the fibrotomy every 4 days to prevent the connective tissue fibers from reforming and also to prevent coronal reformation of the alveolar bone. Generally, eruption is accomplished at a rate of 0.5 mm to 1.0 mm per week. However, movements as slow as 1.0 mm per month is possible.

8. When the desired eruption is accomplished, stabilize the tooth for 2 to 3 months before fabricating the final restoration.

Clinical Case—Surgical Crown Lengthening

A 42-year-old female presented with a provisional restoration from the maxillary right canine to the maxillary left canine. Her medical history was noncontributory. Although the restoration was physiologically acceptable, the varied heights of the restored teeth were esthetically unacceptable (Fig. 21–18). Surgical crown lengthening was performed to correct this situation.

A submarginal incision was made at the desired height of the gingival margin (Fig. 21–19) and a full thickness flap reflected (Fig. 21–20). The disparity in the abutment crown length could be seen after reflection. Following the removal of some supporting bone, a more symmetric appearance was achieved (Fig. 21–21). The flaps were apically positioned and sutured into place (Fig. 21–22). This symmetry is reflected by the gingival margins of the final restoration (Figs. 21–23, 21–24).

Clinical Case—Forced Eruption With Fiberotomy

A 57-year-old male presented with a maxillary right lateral incisor root that had fractured at the gingival margin as a result of cervical caries. His medical history was noncontributory. The patient desired a tooth replacement but did not wish to have the root extracted. A post preparation was made in the root and an 0.036 wire with an eyelet was cemented into the preparation with zinc phosphate cement (Fig. 21–25). An 0.040 orthodontic wire was bonded to the incisal edges of the canine and central incisor over the root to be erupted (Fig. 21–26). This device was then engaged to the arch wire using a heavy elastic tie. A sulcular fiberotomy was performed at the time of activation and every 4 days throughout the time of tooth movement (Fig. 21-27). The desired eruption was achieved within 3 weeks (Figs. 21–28, 21–29), at which time a cast post and core was fabricated (Fig. 21–30) and a provisional restoration made. Using this technique, an excellent esthetic result was obtained (Fig. 21–31).

Clinical Case—Forced Eruption with Surgical Crown Lengthening

A 23-year-old male presented with subgingival caries on his mandibular right second premolar (Fig. 21–32). His medical history was noncontributory. After caries removal and endodontic therapy, an 0.036 orthodontic wire was formed into a loop and cemented into the post preparation (Fig. 21–33). A straight 0.040 orthodontic wire was bonded from the mandibular right first premolar to an occlusal slot prepared in the amalgam of the mandibular right first molar. An elastic thread was used to pull the tooth occlusally (Fig. 21–34). Because the patient could only come to the office twice a month, repeated fiberotomy was not possible. As a result, the gingival margin and the underlying attachment moved coronally with the root (Fig. 21–35). After adequate eruption, apical positioning of the tissues was performed (Figs. 21–36, 21–37), resulting in adequate tooth structure and an even gingival margin (Fig. 21–38). It should be noted that surgery without eruption would have resulted in an uneven gingival margin.

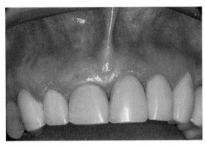

FIG. 21–18. An uneven free gingival margin is evident on the provisional restoration of this 36-year-old patient.

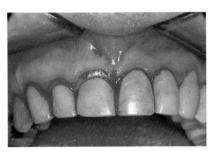

FIG. 21–19. A submarginal incision was made to even the gingival margins.

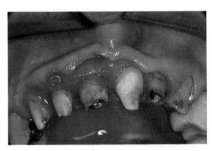

FIG. 21–20. Full thickness reflection revealed uneven alveolar crests on the abutment teeth.

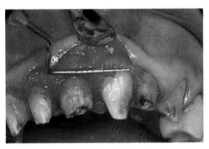

FIG. 21–21. An ostectomy was performed to even the alveolar crests.

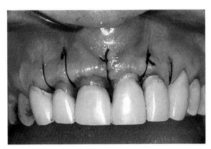

FIG. 21–22. The flaps were apically positioned and sutured into place.

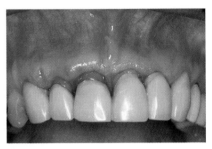

FIG. 21–23. The 3 week postoperative evaluation revealed an even free gingival margin.

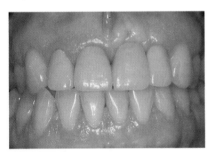

FIG. 21–24. An esthetic restoration after 2 months of healing.

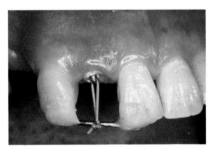

FIG. 21–25. The retained lateral incisor root posed a restorative problem. An eyelet post was cemented into the canal with activation to an incisal anchorage wire with elastic cord.

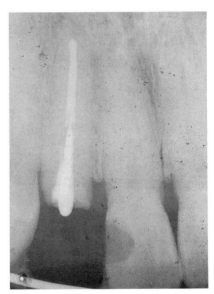

FIG. 21–26. Pre-eruption radiograph of the patient shown in Figure 21–25.

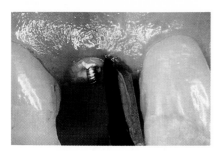

FIG. 21–27. A sulcular fiberotomy was performed every 4 days.

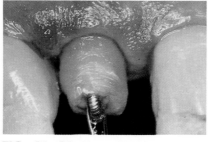

FIG. 21–28. Three weeks of rapid eruption exposed adequate root structure.

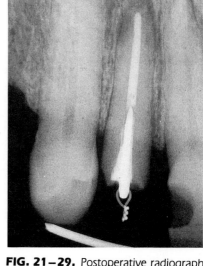

FIG. 21–29. Postoperative radiograph of the patient shown in Figure 21–28. Note the amount of eruption with maintenance of the coronal alveolar bone level.

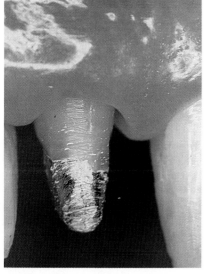

FIG. 21–30. A post and core was fabricated.

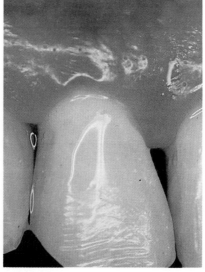

FIG. 21–31. An esthetic final restoration was inserted.

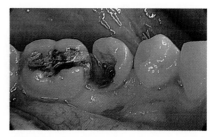

FIG. 21–32. Subgingival caries can be seen on the distal aspect of the second premolar.

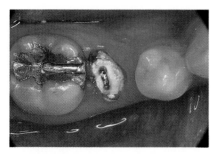

FIG. 21–33. After endodontic therapy was completed, an 0.036 eyelet was cemented into the canal.

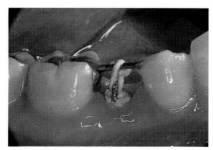

FIG. 21–34. An 0.040 straight wire was bonded directly over the root and activated with heavy elastic.

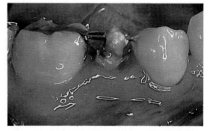

FIG. 21–35. Facial view 6 weeks after activation. Because a fiberotomy was not feasible, the tooth and attachment apparatus had erupted 3 to 4 mm.

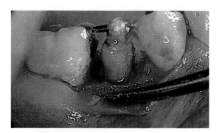

FIG. 21–36. Intraoperative view of the exposed flap.

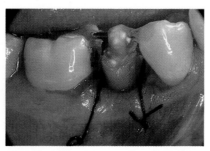

FIG. 21–37. The apically positioned gingiva is sutured into place.

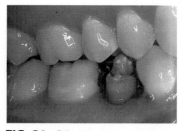

FIG. 21–38. Following healing, sound root structure is exposed while the free gingival margin is restored to a more esthetic level.

RECESSION

Differential Etiology

1. Abrasion. "Receding gums" will usually be diagnosed by a patient before presenting to the practitioner. The esthetic imbalance, particularly in the anterior sextants, is a common patient concern.

Overzealous brushing (even with a soft nylon toothbrush) is the predominant cause of mechanically abraded gingiva. Less frequently encountered causes include the use of an abrasive dentifrice, iatrogenic flossing, electric rotary tooth brushes improperly used at the highest setting, and intraoral foreign object habits.

2. Periodontitis. Periodontitis and acute periodontal abscesses will often destroy buccal attachment, resulting in recession.

3. Trauma. Intraoral trauma can result in severe defects, depending on the nature of the injury.

4. Inadequacy of attached gingiva. Inadequate gingiva may be caused by high frenal attachments, muscle pull, or scars.

Treatment Options

Free Gingival Grafts. Gingival grafting techniques have been used for the past 25 years to cover exposed root surfaces. Although grafts have been one of the most predictable and successful procedures for augmenting the zone of attached gingiva, success in covering exposed root surfaces is less predictable and dependent on several factors:

1. The dimension of the root surface to be covered.
2. The lateral probing depth.
3. The position of the tooth in the arch.

Grafts receive their primary nutrient supply from the underlying connective tissue of the recipient site, and donor tissue placed over the avascular root surface is fed solely by lateral circulation from the connective tissue bed. Because lateral circulation can maintain the viability of the donor tissue for only a limited distance, areas of narrow recession have better root coverage potential than deeper, wider areas of recession. Some areas that appear to be narrow actually have significant lateral probing depths and, therefore, have poorer root coverage potential than truly narrow areas.

CLINICAL TIP. Good results are obtained with widths of less than 2 mm and poor results with widths greater than 4 to 5 mm.

In addition, teeth that are prominent in the arch may have little or no buccal bone present with an underlying dehiscence presenting a major problem. Multiple procedures may be required for optimal results in these cases; however, performing multiple procedures does not guarantee total root coverage. In cases of very wide and deep recession, the purpose of multiple procedures is to achieve as much root coverage as possible. Tooth position and lateral bone support are two factors that could adversely affect the percentage of root coverage.

CLINICAL TIP. There is no formula that can accurately predict how much root coverage can be achieved, and this must be understood by the patient before beginning treatment.

A choice must be made between using a free gingival graft and a pedicle graft. Free gingival grafts are used in 90 to 95% of cases. When there are multiple roots to be covered, the free gingival graft (with or without subepithelial placement of connective tissue) is the procedure of choice. When there is a single tooth involved, the decision to use free gingival or pedicle grafting is primarily made based on the preference of the surgeon. A consideration concerning the free gingival graft is the need for palatal involvement; when a patient's gag reflex is severe, a pedicle graft would be the procedure of choice, if the necessary conditions exist.

Free gingival grafting, the most commonly performed procedure, involves three steps:

1. Preparing the recipient site.
2. Harvesting the donor tissue
3. Placing the graft.

A well vascularized connective tissue bed must be prepared around the graft site. If the goal is to augment the zone of attached gingiva, a submarginal incision can be made with apical dissection of the bed. This will maintain the existing free gingival margin, thus preventing possible postsurgical recession. However, if root coverage is desired, all marginal epithelium must be removed to create a connective tissue margin over which the graft is placed. Laterally the recipient site should extend a distance of at least one-half tooth in either direction to provide an adequate blood supply for the donor tissue.

Donor tissue is harvested from the palate. The anterior rugae must not be included in the graft because they will be visible at the recipient site. A 1 to 2 mm zone of marginal tissue should be maintained around the donor site to prevent recession. A surgical template should be made for the recipient site and transferred to the palate, thus minimizing and customizing the amount of tissue removed. Once the graft is harvested, a hemostatic dressing is placed in the donor site and a clear acrylic surgical stent is inserted. The stent applies constant pressure for hemostasis and covers the raw palatal tissue during healing to increase patient comfort. The donor tissue is sutured firmly to the recipient bed. Surgical dressing is applied to protect the recipient site. Postoperatively, a chlorhexidine rinse may be used for 3 to 4 weeks until proper oral hygiene can be performed without damaging the grafted site. A minimum of 6 weeks of healing is required before resuming or beginning any prosthetic work.

Lateral Pedicle Grafts. Several factors must be considered when a pedicle graft is contemplated:

1. The amount of keratinized tissue adjacent to the recipient site.
2. The existence of an adjacent edentulous ridge.

3. The existence of frena that could cause excessive pull.

4. The width of the recipient root surface.

When using lateral pedicle grafts, a well keratinized edentulous ridge or a wide zone of attached gingiva adjacent to the graft site is ideal. However, if the recipient area to be grafted is wide mesiodistally, excessive pull may occur on the donor tissue, causing strangulation and eventual failure. The lateral pedicle procedure involves bed preparation over the recipient root, partial thickness dissection of the donor tissue, and lateral positioning of the graft. The pedicle is sutured firmly and the donor area heals by granulation formation. With the double papilla procedure, a variation of the lateral pedicle procedure, both adjacent papilla are split thickness dissected and comprise the pedicle. Again, the donor site heals by granulation formation. As was the case with free gingival grafts, surgical dressing is placed over the surgical site, though no surgical stent is needed because no palatal tissue is involved. Postoperative care is similar for all three procedures. As with free gingival grafts, a minimum of 6 weeks of healing is needed before prosthetic work can begin.

Subepithelial Connective Tissue Graft. The above procedures all involve placing a graft or flap over an exposed root surface, with root coverage predicated on whether or not the donor tissues adhere to the denuded root surface. A variation of the pedicle graft and flap techniques, the subepithelial connective tissue graft, involves the placement of a strip of connective tissue from the palate under a partial thickness flap. The recipient site is prepared with a split thickness dissection, retaining all epithelium in the flap. An envelope procedure is performed on the palate to obtain the connective tissue. Two parallel horizontal incisions the length of the site to be grafted are made 3 mm apart near the palatal free gingival margin. Sharp dissection is performed vertically in the connective tissue to remove a strip of tissue similar in dimension to the graft site. The harvested donor tissue will be a "slab" of connective tissue with the 3 mm band of epithelium at one edge. This strip of connective tissue is then place over the exposed root surfaces, and the flap positioned over the donor tissue and sutured firmly. There are several advantages to this type of procedure, including no denuded palatal donor site, increased patient comfort during healing, and the double blood supply to the free connective tissue, which is fed by the underlying periosteum and the connective tissue of the flap. In addition, the connective tissue contains the genetic information that dictates the type of epithelium that will form, thus areas of the donor tissue that are not completely covered by the flap will form masticatory mucosa, aiding in healing and providing a much better blend of donor and recipient tissues.

Prosthetic Gingiva. When interdental spaces are a concern and no cosmetic prosthetic work is anticipated, artificial gingiva is an option. A border molded impression is made of the involved area and the laboratory fabricates a gingival veneer of pink denture acrylic, with the apical extent in the mucobuccal fold and the coronal extent restoring a normal free gingival margin appearance. There are some disadvantages to this procedure, such as inaccurate color matching and instability of the prosthesis. Before embarking on this course of treatment, the patient should see pictures of inserted prostheses and understand their limitations. Only then should fabrication of artificial gingiva begin.

Clinical Case—Free Gingival Graft

A 23-year-old male presented complaining of a frenal pull and stain on his buccal gingiva. His medical history was noncontributory. Eight years prior he suffered intraoral trauma caused by a hockey stick. Examination revealed scars extending from the buccal frenum onto the marginal gingiva of the right mandibular first and second premolar and a bluish tattoo in the alveolar mucosa around the right mandibular canine (Fig. 21–39). A free gingival graft was placed to apically position the frenum and remove the tattoo (Fig. 21–40). After uneventful healing (Fig. 21–41), both preoperative esthetic goals were met (Fig. 21–42).

Clinical Case —Free Gingival Graft

A 40-year-old woman presented with recession on the facial aspect of her anterior teeth, particularly over the canines (Fig. 21–43). Her medical history was noncontributory. After scaling and root preparation, a free gingival graft was placed over the right maxillary canine. A wide bed was prepared to provide adequate blood supply for the graft (Fig. 21–44). The area of recession to be covered was deep and wide and the facial root profile was flat. To help achieve maximal root coverage, the graft was made large enough to be placed over the cemento-enamel junction of the tooth, thus allowing for expected shrinkage (Fig. 21–45). The graft was sutured in place (Fig. 21–46). Even with the planned coverage of the graft, there still remained an area of recession over the root surface, although this was manageable with restorative dentistry. After 2 months, adequate healing had taken place and the patient was referred to the restorative dentist who placed a well contoured restoration to restore proper root form (Fig. 21–47).

Clinical Case—Free Gingival Graft, Double Papilla Graft, and Coronal Positioning of Keratinized Tissue

A 46-year-old woman complained of several areas of recession in both the mandibular and maxillary arches. Her medical history was noncontributory. The examination revealed multiple areas of recession and minimal zones of attached gingiva. In both arches, two-stage procedures were performed. In the mandible (Fig.

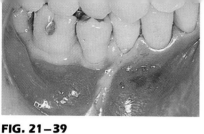

FIG. 21-39

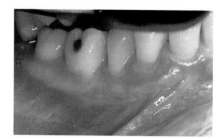

FIG. 21-40

FIG. 21-40. After bed preparation, a free gingival graft was placed to apically position the frenum and remove the tattoo.

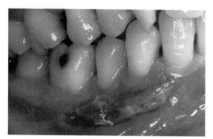

FIG. 21-41

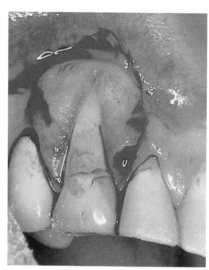

FIG. 21-42

FIG. 21-41. Facial view 10 days postoperatively.

FIG. 21-42. Facial view 2 years postoperatively. Note the restoration of normal frenal position and elimination of the tattoo.

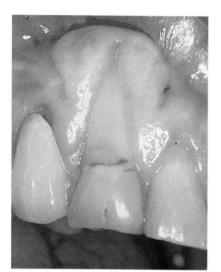

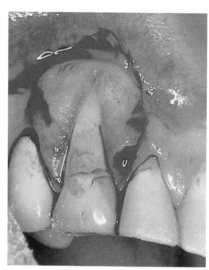

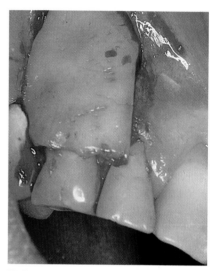

FIG. 21-43. A deep, wide zone of recession is seen on the facial aspect of the maxillary right canine.

FIG. 21-44. The incision was designed to remove a wide zone of tissue.

FIG. 21-45. The graft was placed over the cemento-enamel junction, allowing for expected shrinkage.

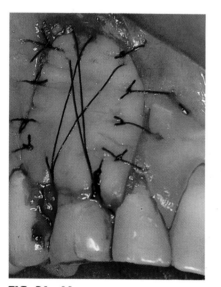

FIG. 21-46

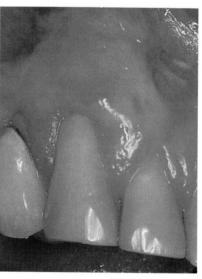

FIG. 21-47

FIG. 21-46. The graft is sutured firmly in place.

FIG. 21-47. Approximately 60% root coverage was achieved and a composite resin restoration was placed after 2 months healing. This satisfied the patient's esthetic demands.

21–48), the zone of attached gingiva was increased with a free gingival graft (Fig. 21–49). After waiting 2 month to allow for adequate healing (Fig. 21–50), the increased zone of keratinized tissue was coronally repositioned (Fig. 21–51), resulting in excellent esthetics (Fig. 21–52).

In the maxillary arch (Fig. 21–53), a double papilla graft was performed (Fig. 21–54). Again, after waiting 2 month to allow for adequate healing (Fig. 21–55), the increased zone of keratinized tissue was coronally repositioned (Fig. 21–56), resulting in excellent esthetics (Fig. 21–57).

FIG. 21–48. The preoperative evaluation revealed gingival recession and a narrow zone of keratinized tissue on the mandibular right premolars.

FIG. 21–49. Intraoperative view of the bed preparation for the first stage of the free gingival graft.

FIG. 21–50. Facial view 2 months postoperatively.

FIG. 21–51. The augmented zone of gingiva was coronally positioned in the second surgical phase. The flap was stabilized with cyanoacrylate tissue adhesive.

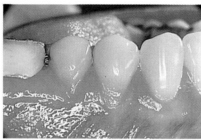

FIG. 21–48

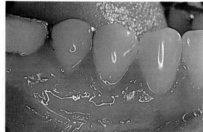

FIG. 21–49

FIG. 21–50

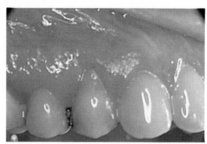

FIG. 21–51

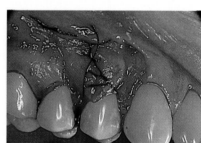

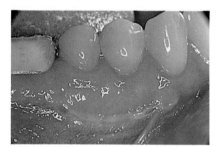

FIG. 21–52. One year postoperatively.

FIG. 21–53. The maxillary right first premolar had minimal attached gingiva, a wide zone of recession, and wide adjacent interdental papillae.

FIG. 21–54. The first surgical phase involved the double papilla technique to augment the zone of keratinized tissue.

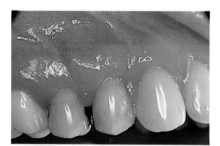

FIG. 21–55. Facial view 2 months postoperatively.

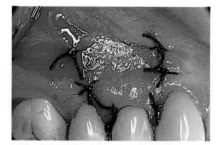

FIG. 21–56. After healing, the augmented tissue was coronally positioned to cover the remaining area of recession.

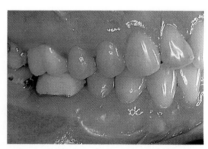

FIG. 21–57. The maxillary and mandibular areas 3 years postoperatively.

EDENTULOUS RIDGE DEFORMITIES

Differential Etiology

Trauma. Visible edentulous ridge defects and deformities are particularly challenging to treat both periodontally and prosthetically. The majority of these defects result from facial trauma sustained during motor vehicle accidents, contact sports, work related accidents, and other mishaps. Violent avulsion of one or more teeth and surrounding buccal or lingual bone segments often occurs. Healing of such injuries results in collapse of the overlying soft tissue into the depression created by the bony loss, leading to a buccolingual or crestal concavity of the edentulous ridge. If the overlying mucosa and connective tissue are also lost at the time of the injury, scarring of the vestibule and gingiva is a further complication.

Periodontitis and Juvenile Periodontitis. Other causes of edentulous ridge deformities include periodontitis and localized juvenile periodontitis (previously termed periodontosis). Periodontitis, a site specific disease, often presents with severe involvement of one or two anterior teeth. A jagged bony topography can be associated with this severe loss of attachment. When these hopeless teeth are extracted, soft tissue healing mimics the alveolar profile, with resultant defects. With localized juvenile periodontitis, severe bone loss often occurs around the central incisors. If extraction is required, similar defects result. Usually, buccal defects result from loss of the buccal plate, whereas, the apical extent of the defect is related to the amount of palatal bone loss.

Classification

Edentulous ridge deformities are classified according to their dimensions:

   1. Buccolingual. Buccolingual defects manifest as concavities on the buccal surface, brought about by loss of the buccal bone plate. Pontics placed in buccolingual defects appear unnaturally flat or thick.
   2. Occlusoapical. Occlusoapical defects are the easiest to see because there is an obvious discrepancy in the height of the gingival margin. In these cases, the pontics often are longer than the adjacent abutment teeth.
   3. Mesiodistal. The mesiodistal dimension indicates the width of the area to be reconstructed and aids in determining the number of procedures necessary to correct the problem (a wide span may involve multiple procedures). It is not a true classification of a defect type.
   4. Atrophied papilla. This defect involves loss of the papillae adjacent to an edentulous area. Usually caused by atrophy, this defect is not primarily traumatic or inflammatory in nature. These defects are highly visible and difficult to correct, and in many cases no change can be seen after multiple reconstructive attempts.

Treatment Options

Gingival Onlay Grafts. The primary technique used to correct buccolingual and occlusoapical defects is the gingival onlay graft or soft tissue augmentation procedure, which is an adaptation of the free gingival graft technique to this special case. Thick palatal donor tissue is used to fill the defect (the minimum thickness is the depth of the defect). The donor tissue is then tightly sutured into the prepared defect site. If a provisional restoration or transitional removable appliance is present, the pontics overlying the grafted site *must* be adjusted to allow 1 to 2 mm of clearance. This is necessary because the graft will swell during healing, and any excessive pressure can cause necrosis and failure. Once the graft has healed (approximately 6 to 8 weeks), a new provisional restoration can be made and an ovate pontic prepared to create the illusion of natural teeth emerging from their sockets.

Connective Tissue Augmentation. A subperiosteal tunnel can be created under the soft tissue of the defect and connective tissue placed to "plump out" the defect. The connective tissue graft is placed into the subperiosteal tunnel. The connective tissue can be obtained from an area of the palate distant to the defect (free connective tissue augmentation) or adjacent to the defect (connective tissue roll augmentation). This technique attempts to correct the defect by internal augmentation. This procedure can be used for occlusoapical, buccolingual and papillary defects. Pontics on provisional restorations must be adjusted to allow 1 to 2 mm of clearance over the surgical site during the 6 to 8 week healing period to compensate for postoperative tissue swelling.

Synthetic Bone Grafts. Synthetic bone graft material can also be placed under a ridge to "plump up" the defect. The graft material acts as scaffolding for connective tissue ingrowth and is not designed to regenerate the lost bone.

Ovate Pontics. Once the desired tissue reconstruction has been achieved, the area can be modified to allow for fabrication of ovate or bullet pontics. The advantage of this type of pontic design is that it creates the illusion of a natural tooth emerging from its socket and provides a more natural appearance to the adjacent "papillae." After adequate maturation of the grafted connective tissue (6 to 8 weeks), a round depression is placed into the augmented edentulous ridge crest with a round surgical diamond bur, the dimensions dependent on the tooth to be placed (i.e., a maxillary canine will require a larger preparation than a mandibular incisor). The provisional restoration is then relined so acrylic material fills the depression and the area heals by epithelialization around the pontic.

   The final prosthesis, thus, has apically tapered and rounded pontics that fit intimately into the tissue depression. This esthetic pontic design creates the appearance of a natural tooth emerging from a sulcus; the contours of the gingival aspects of the pontic are round without sharp or abrupt edges. Hygiene is easily performed by flossing under the pontic.

Clinical Considerations

There is some shrinkage involved with these procedures, sometimes necessitating a second procedure. In the case of occlusoapical and buccolingual defects, several procedures may be needed before the desired result is achieved. The long-term esthetic results are usually well worth the surgical time involved except for papillary reconstruction, which remains very unpredictable, and the patient should be made aware of the poor prognosis in these cases.

Clinical Technique—Ovate Pontic

Armamentarium

- High-speed handpiece
- Round, coarse surgical diamond bur (No. 4)
- Indelible ink marker (e.g., Dr. Thompson's Sanitary Color Transfer Applicators, Great Plains Dental Products Co., Inc.)
- Self-cure acrylic
- Periodontal pack (e.g., Coe-Pack, Coe Laboratories, Inc.)

Clinical Technique

1. Anesthetize the area with 2% lidocaine with 1/50,000 epinephrine (unless medically contraindicated) for hemostasis.
2. Outline the pontic form in indelible marker. The preparation should be approximately 5 mm in diameter.
3. Using light strokes of the high-speed handpiece and copious irrigation, prepare the tissue to the desired depth. Ideally, the pontic preparation should be 5 mm in diameter and 2 to 3 mm deep at the center. The preparation should not be cylindrical, but parabolic (ovate), in shape. Extreme care must be taken not to exceed the boundaries of the indelible ink and not to damage or involve the adjacent papillae.
4. Once the depth and lateral dimensions have been achieved, apply pressure with sterile gauze until hemostasis is achieved.
5. Reline the pontic area of the provisional restoration with a self-curing acrylic. Intimate adaptations should be achieved between the relined pontic and the prepared tissue.

CLINICAL TIP. A high polish must be placed on the relined surface to insure optimal healing and minimize patient discomfort.

---

6. Recement the provisional restoration with temporary cement and place periodontal packing around the surgical site.
7. Epithelization of the ovate preparation occurs in approximately 3 to 4 weeks. Completion of the final restoration can occur at that time. (See also Figs. 21–97 to 21–99 later in this chapter.)

CLINICAL TIP. The final restoration should lie passively on the tissue depression. Pressure may create an abscess with resultant necrosis.

Clinical Case—Connective Tissue Augmentation and Gingivoplasty

A 37-year-old woman presented with a cupped occlusoapical ridge defect resulting from the extraction of the maxillary left central incisor after an endodontic perforation (Fig. 21–58). Her medical history was noncontributory. The pontic was reduced in apical height before proceeding with connective tissue augmentation of the edentulous ridge (Figs. 21–59, 21–60). A partial thickness palatal flap was reflected (Fig. 21–61) to allow harvesting of the underlying connective tissue, which was left as a pedicle. This connective tissue roll was placed over the edentulous bony ridge and under the connective tissue of the defect (Fig. 21–62). The graft was sutured through to the buccal mucosa for stability (Fig. 21–63), the provisional restoration was recemented (Fig. 21–64), and the area was allowed to heal (Fig. 21–65). After 12 weeks of healing, most of the defect resolved (Fig. 21–66) and a new provisional bridge was fabricated (Fig. 21–67). At that time it was noted that the central incisors had a slightly uneven gingival margin (Fig. 21–68). A simple gingivoplasty was performed to even the facial margins of the central incisors (Fig. 21–69). The patient was referred for final restoration 4 weeks after this second surgery (Fig. 21–70) and the final restoration was fabricated (Figs. 21–71, 21–72).

Clinical Case—Multiple Free Gingival Grafts and a Synthetic Bone Graft

A 33-year-old female was involved in an automobile accident resulting in traumatic avulsion of the maxillary right central incisor (Fig. 21–73). Her medical history was noncontributory. The significant edentulous ridge defect required a multiple surgical approach (Fig. 21–74). First, the buccolingual aspect was corrected by placing a thick free graft. Only the outer epithelial layer was removed at the recipient site to maintain as much of the connective tissue as possible (Fig. 21–75). By removing only the epithelial layer, all existing connective tissue at the recipient site was maintained. Removing some of the connective tissue during bed preparation would result in increasing the dimension of the defect to be grafted (e.g., if there is 4 mm thickness of tissue at the recipient site and a 5 mm defect exists, removing the surface epithelium should maintain the defect dimensions, whereas removal of epithelium and 2 mm of connective tissue would increase the amount of defect to 7 mm). The graft (Fig. 21–76) was placed in the recipient site (Fig. 21–77) and the pontic trimmed (Figs. 21–78, 21–79) to avoid pressure necrosis. Healing was uneventful (Figs. 21–80, 21–81). After 2 months, a second procedure was performed to correct

(text continued on page 324.)

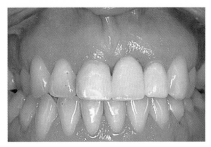

FIG. 21–58. A 3-unit provisional bridge was placed from the maxillary right central incisor to the left lateral incisor 3 months after removal of the left central incisor. Note the lack of an interproximal papilla adjacent to the pontic.

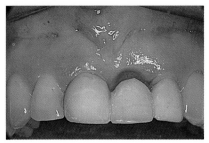

FIG. 21–59. The pontic is reduced in apical height before proceeding with connective tissue augmentation of the edentulous ridge.

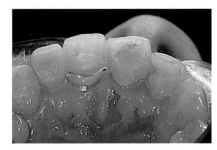

FIG. 21–60. Palatal view of the patient shown in Figure 21–59.

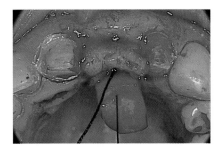

FIG. 21–61. A partial thickness flap is reflected toward the palate.

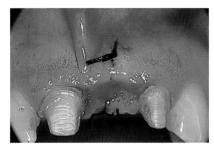

FIG. 21–62. The connective tissue pedicle is sutured through to the buccal aspect.

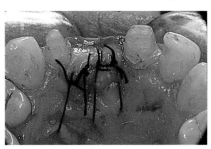

FIG. 21–63. The palatal flap is sutured over the area.

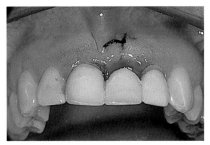

FIG. 21–64. The provisional restoration is recemented.

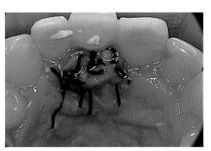

FIG. 21–65. Palatal view 10 days postoperatively.

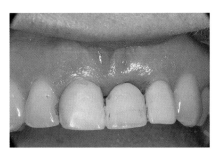

FIG. 21–66. Facial view after 3 months of healing.

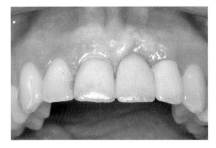

FIG. 21–67. A new provisional restoration was fabricated. Compare the interproximal papilla adjacent to the pontic with the preoperative view shown in Figure 21–58.

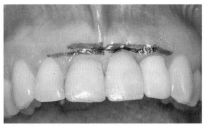

FIG. 21–68. A discrepancy in the free gingival margins of the central incisors was noted.

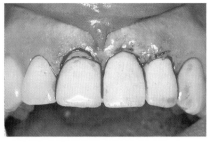

FIG. 21–69. A gingivoplasty was performed to even the margins.

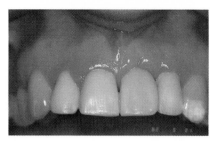

FIG. 21–70. Facial view after healing.

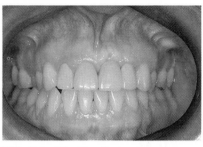

FIG. 21–71. The final restoration was inserted after adequate healing.

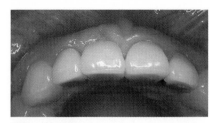

FIG. 21–72. Note the buccolingual papilla profile.

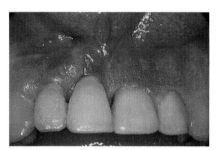

FIG. 21–73. Severe scarring and deformity of the maxillary anterior vestibule can be seen.

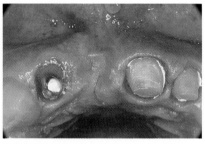

FIG. 21–74. The patient shown in Figure 21–73 without the provisional restoration.

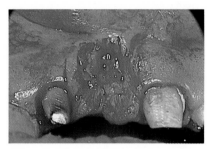

FIG. 21–75. The first surgical procedure addressed the buccolingual defect. The recipient bed preparation was done to conserve as much of the underlying connective tissue as possible.

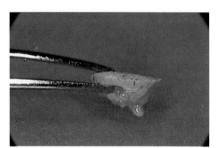

FIG. 21–76. A thick palatal graft was harvested.

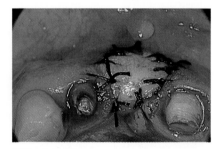

FIG. 21–77. The graft is sutured in the recipient bed.

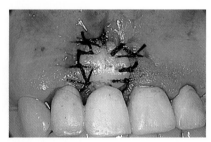

FIG. 21–78. The pontic is relieved and recemented.

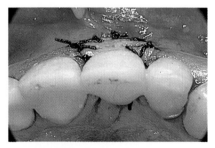

FIG. 21–79. Palatal view of the patient shown in Figure 21–78.

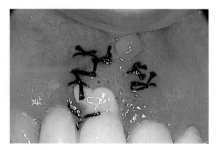

FIG. 21–80. The area 1 week postoperatively.

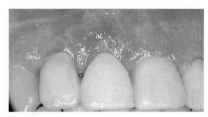

FIG. 21–81. The area 6 weeks postoperatively.

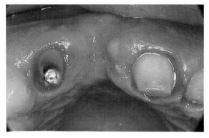

FIG. 21–82. The second surgical phase addressed the incisioapical defect. Palatal view of the site prior to bed preparation.

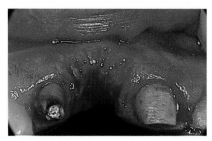

FIG. 21–83. The recipient bed is prepared.

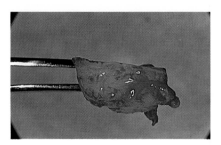

FIG. 21–84. A thick piece of donor palatal tissue is removed.

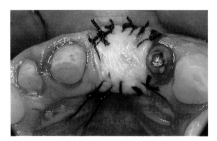

FIG. 21–85. The graft is sutured intimately into the defect.

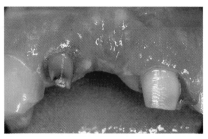

FIG. 21–86. Despite good healing, some residual defect remained.

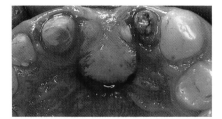

FIG. 21–87. A third procedure was performed. A full thickness palatal flap was created.

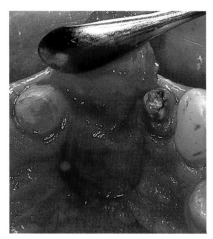

FIG. 21–88. The flap is reflected buccally.

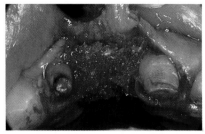

FIG. 21–89. A synthetic bone graft is placed beneath the graft to correct the residual defect.

the incisoapical defect (Fig. 21–82). The edentulous ridge was prepared (Fig. 21–83) and a thick palatal graft (Fig. 21–84) was sutured over the recipient site (Fig. 21–85). The graft was thick and included the fatty tissues. The graft was sutured in place and allowed to heal. After 8 weeks this area healed, but a slight depression remained (Fig. 21–86). To correct this incisoapical defect, a full thickness flap was reflected (Figs. 21–87, 21–88) and a synthetic bone graft was placed (Fig. 21–89). The provisional restoration was recontoured and recemented in place (Fig. 21–90). A pleasing esthetic result was thus achieved (Figs. 21–91, 21–92).

Clinical Case—Papillary Reconstruction via Connective Tissue Augmentation

A 22-year-old man presented with unesthetic replacement of both maxillary lateral incisors. His medical history was noncontributory. He was dissatisfied with the lack of papillae (Fig. 21–93). A connective tissue roll was used to "plump" the area (Fig. 21–94). The graft was taken from the palate directly behind the defect and sutured through the buccal mucosa for stability (Fig. 21–95). The pontic on the removable appliance was trimmed to prevent excessive pressure (Fig. 21–96). After healing, the ridge was reprepared to accept an ovate pontic (Figs. 21–97, 21–98). After 6 weeks the patient was referred for prosthetic restoration (Fig. 21–99). An acid etch retained fixed bridge was fabricated. Although the entire papilla could not be reconstructed, the patient was satisfied with the results (Fig. 21–100).

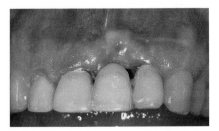

FIG. 21–90. The area is sutured and the provisional restoration is replaced.

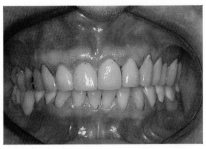

FIG. 21–91. After restoration of proper buccolingual and incisoapical dimensions apically and interproximally a final restoration was inserted.

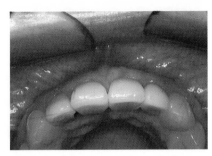

FIG. 21–92. Palatal view of the patient shown in Figure 21–91.

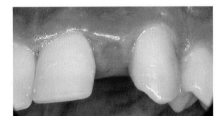

FIG. 21–93. This young male patient was dissatisfied with the lack of papillae around the missing lateral incisor.

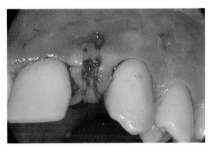

FIG. 21–94. A connective tissue roll was taken from the palate and sutured in place into a subperiosteal tunnel created under the edentulous ridge.

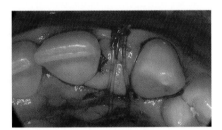

FIG. 21–95. Palatal view of the patient shown in Figure 21–94.

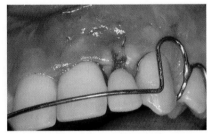

FIG. 21–96. The pontic on the removable appliance was trimmed to prevent excessive pressure.

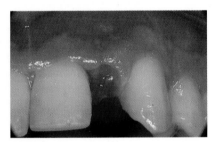

FIG. 21–97. After healing, an ovate pontic preparation was performed into the augmented edentulous ridge to allow for fabrication of an ovate pontic on the Maryland bridge.

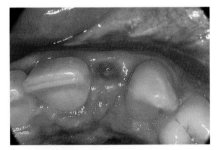

FIG. 21–98. Palatal view of the patient shown in Figure 21–97.

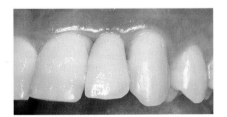

FIG. 21–99. One month following insertion of the Maryland bridge.

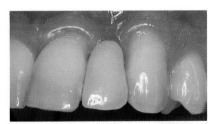

FIG. 21–100. Although tissue has regressed in the apical region, the interproximal papilla remains stable.

GINGIVAL OVERGROWTH

Patient dissatisfaction with the short appearance of the anterior teeth is commonplace. Identifying the underlying etiology is essential for proper treatment planning and prognosis.

Differential Etiology

1. Noninflammatory hyperplasia. Noninflammatory hyperplasia is a common cause for both local and generalized gingival overgrowth. The best known cause is Dilantin hyperplasia. Several other frequently prescribed drugs may cause a similar response (e.g., nifedipine, cyclosporine, and Inderal). Such an underlying cause should be discovered during the medical history. The hyperplasia observed may be localized to a sextant or an arch or generalized in both jaws. Another noninflammatory factor is irritation. This is seen with ill fitting removable partial dentures or overhanging margins of restorations. In these situations, the overgrowth is seen only at the site of the irritation. An uncommon cause is genetic predisposition to gingival overgrowth. This will present as generalized buccal and lingual hyperplasia. These noninflammatory conditions are usually accompanied by an inflammatory component, because of the difficulty in performing proper oral hygiene.

2. Inflammatory hyperplasia. In some situations gingival hyperplasia is purely inflammatory. This is usually observed in chronic gingivitis or periodontitis with severe gingival involvement. Localized inflammatory hyperplasia is also seen adjacent to caries.

3. Altered passive eruption. Altered passive eruption has neither an inflammatory nor an extrinsic noninflammatory etiology. During normal eruption of the permanent dentition, the tooth erupts coronally while the gingiva migrates apically (passive eruption). When insufficient apical migration occurs, the gingival margin appears as gingival overgrowth. Clinically, this appears as short crowns with the free gingival margin in the middle one-third of the enamel. Histologically, there are two distinct presentations of altered passive eruption. In both cases, the free gingival margin is coronally positioned, but the position of the alveolar crest is different. In the first case, the alveolar crest is at its normal level of more than 1 mm apical to the cemento-enamel junction. In the second case, the alveolar crest is at or above the cemento-enamel junction. Although both cases are clinically identical, the histologic differences dictate different surgical approaches. The differentiation between the two histologic types can be made radiographically only when the alveolar bone can be definitely seen below the cemento-enamel junction. Otherwise, it is often impossible to predict the position of the buccal or lingual bone radiographically, and the need for ostectomy can only be determined after flap elevation.

Treatment Options

Plaque Control. Plaque control is paramount in treating inflammatory hyperplasia. Oral hygiene instruction, scaling, and root planing or subgingival curettage should be performed prior to evaluating the need for surgical correction.

CLINICAL TIP. Often conservative, cause-related therapy will resolve inflammatory hyperplasia.

If the hyperplasia persists, surgical reduction is indicated. The choice of surgical procedure (i.e., gingivectomy vs. apically positioned flap) is determined by any underlying periodontal problems (e.g., pocketing, infrabony lesions.)

Gingivectomy or gingivoplasty.

In cases of noninflammatory gingival hyperplasia, gingivectomy is usually indicated. With irritation-induced overgrowth, local reduction or excision is performed in conjunction with removal of the irritant. These patients usually respond well, without recurrence. With drug or genetically induced hyperplasia, gingivectomy is still the procedure of choice, although the frequency of recurrence must be considered. Changing the patient's medication often results in eliminating recurrences, although it will not reverse any existing hyperplasia. If change in medication is contraindicated, retreatment of recurrent problems must be evaluated on an individual basis. Recurrence is also common with genetically predisposed hyperplasia. The patient's functional and esthetic needs must be considered in deciding how often to perform surgical reduction.

Apically Positioned Flap with or without Ostectomy.

Altered passive eruption is best treated with an apically positioned flap, which accomplishes two objectives: positions the gingival margin at a normal level and allows the evaluation of the alveolar crest. If the alveolar crest is correctly positioned, only apical positioning of the gingiva will be necessary. However, if the alveolar crest is at or above the cementoenamel junction, ostectomy is required to first achieve a normal physiologic relationship between tooth and bone before apically positioning the soft tissue. The purpose of bone removal is to establish a new biologic width (see the section on Inadequate Tooth Structure For Restorations earlier in this chapter) allowing the gingival margin to reform at an appropriate level. If a gingivectomy alone was performed in this situation, the gingiva would heal to its previous position, because the underlying bone dictates gingival margin position.

Clinical Case—Full Thickness Flap with Ostectomy

A 17-year-old female presented for correction of the esthetics of her maxillary anterior teeth. Her medical history was noncontributory. She desired bonding to make the teeth larger and to close the spaces between them. Clinically, she had short teeth occlusogingivally and she exhibited multiple diastemata (Fig. 21–101). The diagnosis was altered passive eruption and a tooth-arch size discrepancy. The case demanded an integration of periodontal and restorative therapy. Restorative diastema closure would have resulted in unnaturally wide teeth

ESTHETIC DENTISTRY

with an apparently overexaggerated incisal edge.

The anatomic crown was exposed with a full thickness flap (Figs. 21–102, 21–103). The alveolar crest was at the level of the cemento-enamel junction (Fig. 21–104), thus requiring ostectomy to allow for establishment of a proper biologic width (see the section on Inadequate Tooth Structure For Restorations earlier in this chapter). The tissue was apically repositioned and sutured into place (Figs. 21–105, 21–106). After 3 months of healing, the patient was referred for restorative treatment. A microfilled composite resin was used to close the diastema. The increased crown length permitted fabrication of an esthetic restoration (Fig. 21–107).

PATHOLOGIC MOBILITY

Differential Etiology

1. Periodontitis. Increased tooth mobility is a common problem of the adult periodontal patient. This results from the progressive loss of attachment.

2. Occlusal Trauma. Occlusal trauma with or without a coexisting periodontal condition often causes tooth mobility. Occlusal trauma causes increased osteoclastic activity, which results in decreased alveolar bone volume and widening of the periodontal ligament with a resultant increase in tooth mobility. This is particularly evident when trauma is superimposed on periodontal inflammation.

3. Post Orthodontics. Teeth sometimes have irreversibly increased mobility after orthodontic treatment. The mechanism for postorthodontic mobility is the same as that for occlusal trauma. It is impossible to predict this phenomenon, which occurs following "adult" orthodontics. If the patient is unaware of tooth mobility and mobility is not a symptom of untreated underlying disease and does not interfere with adequate function, no treatment is necessary.

Treatment Options

Cast Porcelain-Fused-to-Metal Splinting. The first choice of splints for treatment of pathologic mobility is cast porcelain-fused-to-metal, which would ideally sat-

FIG. 21–101. A 17-year-old female presented with altered passive eruption and a tooth/arch size discrepancy. She desired bonding to correct the unesthetic appearance of her teeth.

FIG. 21–102. The first phase of treatment required exposure of the anatomic crowns. A submarginal incision was made on the buccal mucosa and the marginal collar of tissue was removed.

FIG. 21–103. An additional incision was made on the palatal aspect of the six maxillary anterior teeth.

FIG. 21–104. Reflection of the flap revealed the alveolar crest at the level of the cemento-enamel junction.

FIG. 21–105. Minimal ostectomy was performed and the tissues sutured apically to reestablish the biologic width.

FIG. 21–106. Palatal view of the patient shown in Figure 21–105.

FIG. 21–107. The teeth were ultimately restored using a microfilled composite resin.

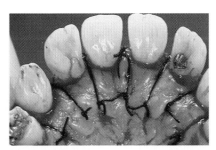
FIG. 21–101

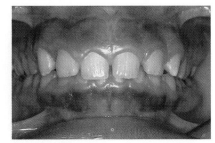
FIG. 21–102

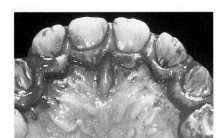
FIG. 21–103

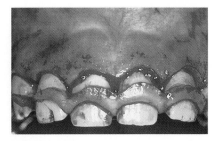
FIG. 21–104

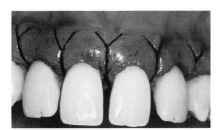

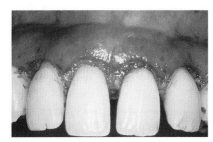

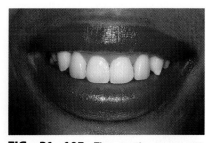

isfy both esthetic and functional demands. However, if financial limitations exist, intracoronal splinting is indicated.

Intracoronal Splinting. Intracoronal splinting involves preparing a channel in the occlusal surface of posterior teeth, or circumferentially in anterior teeth, to allow the placement of an anchoring wire. Composite resin is placed in the preparation to mask the wire and add strength. The advantage of these splints is the added reinforcement of the wire, coupled with the esthetics and repairability of the composite resins. The disadvantage is the irreversibility of the procedure (slot preparation), and the patient must be made fully aware of this before beginning. It is usually wise to have the patient examine photographs of these splints, because although the wire is hidden by composite resin, some shadowing may occur, making this esthetically unacceptable.

CLINICAL TIP. The use of clear nylon monofilament fishline (8 pound test) greatly reduces shadowing. Bury the knot carefully in composite resin because this ligature tends to untie.

A-splint—Anterior

Armamentarium

- Standard dental setup (see the section on Forced Eruption earlier in this chapter)
- No. ½ or No. 1 high-speed round bur
- No. 33½ high-speed inverted cone bur
- Monofilament fishline, 8 pound test or ligature wires
- Acid etch gel
- Enamel/dentin bonding agent (see Chapter 3, Dentin Bonding Agents)
- Anterior composite resin (e.g., Silux, 3M, Inc.)

Clinical Technique

1. Prepare a circumferential channel through the buccal

and lingual surfaces of the involved teeth with a No. ½ or No. 1 high-speed round bur, (Fig. 21-108).
2. Place a slight undercut lingually and facially with a No. 33½ high-speed inverted cone bur
3. Place a ligature wire through the channel around the involved teeth (Fig. 21–109).
4. Acid-etch the enamel margins.
5. Wash and dry the area.
6. Apply an appropriate bonding agent.
7. Restore with composite resin (Fig. 21–110).
8. Finish and polish (Fig. 21–111).

A-splint—Posterior

Armamentarium. The armamentarium is the same as that listed for A-Splint—Anterior, plus:

- No. 330 or No. 245 inverted pear high-speed bur
- No. 35 or No. 37 inverted cone high-speed bur
- No. 0.026" or 0.036" orthodontic wire (Unitek, 3M, Inc.)
- Posterior restorative material, such as posterior composite resin (e.g., P-50, 3M, Inc.), or powder/liquid composite resin (e.g., Super-C, AMCO) or acrylic (e.g., clear orthodontic resin, Caulk, Inc.)

Clinical Technique

1. Prepare a channel through the occlusal surface.
2. Place 0.036 orthodontic wire through the channel.
3. Acid-etch the enamel margins.
4. Wash and dry the area.
5. Apply an appropriate bonding agent.
6. Restore with acrylic or composite resin.
7. Finish and polish.

Extracoronal Splinting. Extracoronal splinting is only feasible in the anterior sextants. Composite resin is placed over and between the crowns of the anterior teeth. Because this splint does not involve tooth preparation into dentin, it is reversible. However, it does have

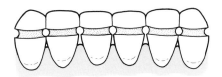

FIG. 21–108

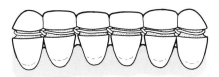

FIG. 21–109

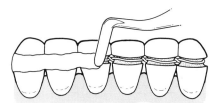

FIG. 21–110

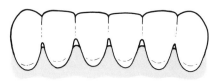

FIG. 21–111

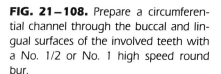

FIG. 21–108. Prepare a circumferential channel through the buccal and lingual surfaces of the involved teeth with a No. 1/2 or No. 1 high speed round bur.

FIG. 21–109. Place a ligature wire through the channel around the involved teeth.

FIG. 21–110. The channel is restored with composite resin.

FIG. 21–111. The finished restoration.

a greater tendency to fracture than intracoronal splinting. Should problems develop, conversion to a different kind of splint is possible.

Armamentarium

- Standard dental setup (see the section on Forced Eruption earlier in this chapter)
- Flame-shaped high-speed finishing bur
- Metal interproximal finishing strip (e.g., Lightening Strip, Moyco Industries, Inc.)
- Acid-etch gel
- Enamel/dentin bonding agent (see Chapter 3, Dentin Bonding Agents)
- Anterior composite resin (e.g., Silux, 3M, Inc.)

Clinical Technique

1. Acid-etch the enamel margins.
2. Wash and dry the area.
3. Apply an appropriate bonding agent.
4. Place composite resin over and between the crowns of anterior teeth (some stripping may be necessary with crowded teeth).
5. Finish and polish.

Clinical Consideration

Both intra and extracoronal procedures are intended as temporary stabilization. Frequently, they are used until a more permanent restoration can be made, or until stabilization occurs following surgery, orthodontics, or trauma.

CLINICAL TIP. When splints become long-term "permanent" restorations, it is imperative that the patient understands that frequent evaluation visits are required and that the splints will need repairs when they inevitably break.

Esthetic success can be achieved as long as the patient is aware of the maintenance involved and the limitations of these procedures.

CONCLUSION

Facial esthetics involves the interaction of many elements. The periodontium, which serves as a backdrop for the teeth, determines the environment in which any esthetic rehabilitation is seen. It is essential that periodontal procedures be considered an important part of any comprehensive esthetic treatment plan.

REFERENCES

1. Abrams, L.: Augmentation of the deformed residual edentulous ridge for fixed prosthesis. Comp Cont Ed 1:205, 1980.
2. Allen, E.P.: Use of mucogingival surgical procedures to enhance esthetics. Dent Clin N Am 32:307, 1988.
3. Allen, E.P. and Miller, P.D. Jr.: Coronal positioning of existing gingiva: short term results in the treatment of shallow marginal tissue recession. J Periodont 60:316, 1989.
4. Becker, B.E. and Becker, W.: Use of connective tissue autografts for treatment of mucogingival problems. Int J Periodont Rest Dent 6:88, 1986.
5. Becker, W., Becker, B.E., and Berg, L.: Repair of intrabony defects as a result of open debridement procedures. Report of 36 treated cases. Int J Periodont Rest Dent 6:8, 1986.
6. Bernimoulin, J.P., Luscher, B., and Muhlemann.: Coronally repositioned periodontal flap. J Clin Periodont 2:1, 1975.
7. Clark, J.W., Weatherford, T.W., and Mann, W.V. Jr.: The wire ligature-acrylic splint. J Periodont 40:371, 1969.
8. Cohen, D.W., and Ross, S.E.: The double papillae positioned flap in periodontal therapy. J Periodont 39:65, 1968.
9. deWaal, H., Kon, S., and Ruben, M.P.: The laterally positioned flap (review). Dent Clin N Am 32:267, 1988.
10. Dorfman, H.S., Kennedy, J.E., and Bird, W.C.: Longitudinal evaluation of free autogenous gingival grafts: a four year report. J Periodont 53:349, 1982.
11. Evans, C.A., and Schaff, H.A.: Acid etch technique adapted for splinting anterior teeth. Am J Orthodont 71:317, 1977.
12. Evian, C.I., Corn, H., and Rosenberg, E.S.: Retained interdental papilla procedure for maintaining anterior esthetics. Comp Cont Ed 6:58, 1985.
13. Gray, J.L., and Quattlebaum, J.B.: Correction of localized alveolar ridge defects utilizing hydroxyapatite and a "tunnelling" approach: a case report. Int J Periodont Rest Dent 8:72, 1988.
14. Grupe, H.E., and Warren, R.: Repair of gingival defects by a sliding flap operation. J. Periodont 27:92, 1956.
15. Ingber, J.: Forced eruption: part II. A method of treating non-restorable teeth—periodontal and restorative considerations. J Periodont, 47:203, 1976.
16. Kozlovsky, A., Tal, H., and Lieberman, M.: Forced eruption combined with gingival fiberotomy. A technique for clinical crown lengthening. J Clin Periodont, 15:534, 1988.
17. Langer, B., and Langer, L.: Subepithelial connective tissue graft technique for root coverage. J Periodontol, 56:715, 1985.
18. Langer, B., and Calagna, L.: The subepithelial connective tissue graft. J Prosthet Dent, 44:363, 1980.
19. Maynard, J.G. Jr., and Wilson, R.D.K.: Physiologic dimensions of the periodontium significant to the restorative dentist. J Periodontol 50:170, 1979.
20. Mellonig, J.T., et al: Clinical evaluation of freeze-dried bone allografts in periodontal osseous defects. J Periodontol, 47:125, 1976.
21. Mellonig, J.T.: Decalcified freeze dried bone allografts as an implant material in human periodontal defects. Int J Periodont Rest Dent 4:41, 1984.
22. Miller, C.J.: The smile line as a guide to anterior esthetics. Dent Clin North Am, 33:157, 1989.
23. Miller, P.D., Jr.: Regenerative and reconstructive periodontal plastic surgery. Mucogingival surgery (review). Dent Clin North Am, 32:287, 1988.
24. Miller, P.D. Jr., and Binkley, L.H. Jr.: Root coverage and ridge augmentation in Class IV recession using a coronally positioned free gingival graft. J Periodont 57:360, 1986.
25. Nelson, S.W.: The sub-pedicle connective tissue graft. A bilaminar reconstructive procedure for the coverage of denuded root surfaces. J Periodont 58:95, 1987.
26. Nevins, M.: Attached gingiva—mucogingival therapy and restorative dentistry. Int J Periodont Rest Dent 6:9, 1986.
27. Ochsenbein, C.: A primer for osseous surgery. Int J Periodont Rest Dent 6:1, 1986.
28. Ochsenbein, C., and Bohannan, H.M.: The palatal approach to osseous surgery: part II. Clinical application. J Periodont 35:54, 1964.
29. Pontoriero, R., et al: Guided tissue regeneration in the treatment of furcation defects in man. J Clin Periodont, 14:618, 1987.
30. Pontoriero, R., et al.: Guided tissue regeneration in degree II furcation-involved mandibular molars. A clinical study. J Clin Periodont, 15:247, 1988.
31. Pontoriero, R., et al.: Guided tissue regeneration in the treatment of furcation defects in mandibular molars. A clinical study of degree III involvements. J Clin Periodont 16:170, 1989.

32. Pontoriero, R., Celenza, F. Jr., Ricci, G., and Carnevale, G.: Rapid extrusion with fiber resection: a combined orthodontic-periodontic treatment modality. Int J Periodont Rest Dent 7:30, 1987.

33. Raetzke, P.B.: Covering localized areas of root exposure employing the "envelope" technique. J Periodont 56:397, 1985.

34. Ross, S.E., Crosetti, H.W., Gargiulo, A., and Cohen, D.W.: The double papillae repositioned flap—and alternative. I. Fourteen years in retrospect. Int J Periodont Rest Dent 6:46, 1986.

35. Saroff, S.A., et al.: Free soft tissue autografts: hemostasis and protection of the palatal donor site with a microfibrillar collagen preparation. J Periodont 53:681, 1980.

36. Seibert, J.S.: Reconstruction of deformed, partially edentulous ridges, using full thickness onlay grafts. Comp Cont Ed, 5:437, 1983.

37. Sepe, W.W., et al: Clinical evaluation of freeze-dried bone allografts in periodontal osseous defects. Part II. J Periodont 48:9, 1978.

38. Steinberg, A.D.: Office management of phenytoin-induced gingival overgrowth. Comp Cont Ed, 6:138, 1985.

39. Sullivan, H.C., and Atkins, J.H.: The role of free gingival grafts in periodontal therapy. Dent Clin North Am 13:133, 1969.

40. Takei, H., Yamada, H., and Hau, T.: Maxillary anterior esthetics. Preservation of the interdental papilla. Dent Clin North Am, 33:263, 1989.

41. Werbitt, M.: Decalcified freeze-dried bone allografts: a successful procedure in the reduction of intrabony defects. Int J Periodont Rest Dent 7:56, 1987.

Edward McNulty, D.M.D., M.D.S.

ESTHETICS AND ORTHODONTICS

22

The orthodontist, striving for excellent form and function, not only aligns the dentition and provides for good masticatory function, but concomitantly produces an esthetically pleasing result. Generalists and specialists in fields other than orthodontics, should be capable of diagnosing the need for orthodontic intervention and be competent in preforming simple orthodontic corrections. The orthodontist is called upon to correct complicated occlusal disharmonies, often using complex orthodontic mechanotherapy.

Prior to the introduction of more esthetic fixed appliances, patients, especially adults, often refused to accept full appliance mechanotherapy of even the shortest duration. The restorative dentist, thus limited by the patient's reticence to undergo prerestorative orthodontic correction, modified the treatment plan to accommodate the patient's wishes. This often compromised the success of the final restoration or placed its long-term stability in jeopardy.

RATIONALE FOR ORTHODONTIC INTERVENTION

An esthetic treatment plan must consider whether orthodontic movements will enhance the success or stability of the final restorations. Diagnostic determinations should be based on the following principles:

1. **Masticatory efficiency.** Proper occlusion and the development of proper interdigitation allows for enhanced masticatory efficiency.
2. **Periodontal protection.** Correct axial inclination of the teeth dissipates the forces of mastication and lessens trauma to the periodontium.
3. **Oral hygiene.** Corrective alignment of a crowded dentition eliminates food impaction, improves self-cleansing during normal masticatory movements, and permits easier oral hygiene by the patient.

4. **Temporomandibular joint protection.** Proper occlusion, which permits a good functional relationship between the maxilla and the mandible, mitigates strain of the masticatory muscles and the temporomandibular joint.
5. **Speech improvement.** Proper anatomic relationships between the teeth and the musculature of the orofacial complex enhances proper speech.
6. **Esthetics.** Orthodontic movement provides a dentition that is esthetically pleasing, and takes into consideration the soft tissue profile of the patient.

BASIC PREMISES FOR DIAGNOSTIC EVALUATION

Patients often have misconceptions regarding treatment results. Fundamentals should be discussed with the patient in order to base a diagnostic plan on a firm foundation of understanding.

1. **There must be a clear pathway for tooth movement** to take place when the patient is in maximum intercuspation. Interferences can be removed by selectively grinding the teeth, when function or esthetics permit, or by opening the vertical dimension of occlusion through fixed or removable appliance therapy. If the latter is attempted, a thorough evaluation of the effects of altering vertical dimension must be considered.
2. **Dentofacial harmony** can only be evaluated on a personal, subjective basis. The clinician, therefore, should be prepared to discuss with the patient, prior to commencing therapy, any profile or other facial changes expected to result from treatment. This is especially important when skeletal disharmonies will be altered by orthognathic surgery.
3. **There must be stability of the treated occlusion.** All orthodontic appliance therapy is planned

with this in mind. Overexpansion of the dental arch commonly results in relapse of crowding after retention is eliminated. Rotational discrepancies should be overcorrected because they also tend to relapse. This is also true of the correction of closed bites and Class III malocclusions.

4. **Orthodontic treatment has little effect on facial growth.** This applies primarily to full-banded mechanotherapy performed by an orthodontist. The facial pattern exhibited by the patient has to be accepted as the framework in which tooth movement must take place. In the mature adult, growth has obviously ceased. Although it is possible to effect some orthognathic changes in the maturing maxilla and local changes in the alveolar arches and lips, facial changes are the result of growth and not of treatment. Therefore, it is essential for the clinician to be well versed in predicting facial growth in the maturing patient or to send the patient for an orthodontic consultation. Predictions are based on the current conditions of the face and dental arch presented by the patient, correlated with statistical probabilities. Race, sex, and familial tendencies are also important factors.

5. **The mandibular dental arch provides the best starting point for diagnostic analysis** and treatment planning. This applies primarily to fixed appliance mechanotherapy performed by an orthodontist. The mandibular arch usually shows only slight growth changes after 9 or 10 years of age and is less amenable to mechanotherapeutic changes than the maxilla. Treatment, therefore, must be planned so the maxilla will conform to the therapeutic result that can be achieved in the mandible. An exception to this premise is Angle Class III malocclusions in which limitations in the treatment of the maxilla take on primary diagnostic and treatment priorities.

Some clinical problems may be corrected using one of several treatment modalities. It is essential to identify and compare therapeutic alternatives during the diagnostic evaluation so the most appropriate procedure can be selected.

DIAGNOSTIC EVALUATIONS

Malocclusions may result from skeletal, dental, or muscular disharmonies, or from a combination of these components. The origin of the problem often dictates the treatment modality. The mandible and maxilla should be evaluated separately, in addition to their relationship to each other, when making a differential diagnosis. A general outline is provided, however, the clinician must examine each case on its own merits and design a treatment plan accordingly.

When a therapeutic problem involving orthodontic principles appears beyond the scope of the clinician's knowledge, it should be referred to a specialist for a diagnostic opinion and, if needed, treatment. The orthodontist, in turn, must always consider whether restorative modalities may better serve a patient's needs than complicated orthodontic therapy.

Each case poses many questions and presents a set of different circumstances, which in themselves become self-limiting, making the differential diagnosis easier for the astute clinician.

Assessment of the Skeletal Component. Is the relationship of the bones of the face causing the malocclusion? Is a small mandible or a large maxilla causing the Class II or Class III protrusion, or is it caused by the dental or muscular component? Angle Class I bimaxillary protrusion is often seen in certain races (e.g., Australoid, Negroid, or Mongoloid) and must be evaluated on racial norms and patient preference, not on the clinician's preconceived notion of an orthognathically ideal profile. It should be determined if these skeletal disharmonies are mild enough to be masked by conventional orthodontic treatment, or if a surgical orthognathic approach should be undertaken? Many Class I bimaxillary protrusions can be treated orthodontically, but if there is a large overbite surgery may be indicated. Class II malocclusion has been successfully resolved orthodontically; however the clinician must take care when treating these cases that the midface or chin does not become too dominant in pursuit of a good dental correction. As a general rule, Class III relationships that allow the teeth to come into edge-to-edge contact when the mandible is placed in its most retruded position can be successfully treated with conventional orthodontics, but the resulting soft tissue profile must again be considered in evaluating the case. More severe Class III relationships often require a combined orthognathic surgical approach.

Assessment of the Dental Component. Spaces between the teeth or crowded teeth may be evidence of a poor tooth size to arch length ratio. The teeth may be too large or too small for the basal bone present. Other causes, such as early loss of primary teeth with resultant mesial migration of the posterior teeth, must be ruled out. Are some teeth missing? Are teeth missing because of impaction or congenital absence of the suspect tooth? Are there long-standing edentulous areas with resultant bite collapse? Has the periodontal integrity of the teeth been threatened by tipping or crowding?

Assessment of the Muscular Component. Are there cuspal interferences causing deviation of the mandible laterally, anteriorly, or posteriorly during closure? Are these caused by muscular imbalances, or are cuspal interferences causing the muscles to deflect the mandible on closure? Do any pernicious habits exert an undue influence on the dentition?

Evaluation of the Mandibular Arch. Do the present arch dimensions and any expected growth changes appear adequate to permit alignment of the teeth without expansion, or will space be required to properly align the teeth? Can any needed space be gained by interproximal reduction of enamel or are extractions necessary?

Evaluation of the Maxillary Arch and Its Relation to the Mandibular Arch. Are space requirements similar to those in the mandible? Acknowledging the mandibular molar position as a guide, do the maxillary molars need to be moved to provide a Class I interdigitation (Figs. 22–1 to 22–3). Accepting the mandibular incisors as a guide, what anteroposterior and vertical movements are required?

FUNDAMENTALS OF ORTHODONTICS

Types of Movement

1. **Bodily movement.** The tooth moves in a direction perpendicular to the occlusal plane.
2. **Tipping.** The crown of the tooth moves in an arc.
3. **Rotation.** The crown turns with a rotational movement around the vertical axis of the tooth.
4. **Torquing.** The tooth rotates around the cross-sectional axis of the arch wire.
5. **Uprighting.** The crown rotates around an axis located within the tooth. This axis is perpendicular to the cross-sectional axis of the arch wire and runs in a bucco-lingual direction.
6. **Extrusion.** The tooth moves in an incisal or occlusal direction along its long axis.
7. **Intrusion.** The tooth moves in an apical direction along its long axis.

Types of Appliances

1. **Anterior ceramic or plastic brackets.** Brackets are made of a clear material and can be bonded to the teeth.
2. **Metal brackets.** Brackets are made of metal and can be bonded to the teeth.
3. **Hawley appliance.** A removable appliance comprised of a labial wire with acrylic fitted against the palatal or lingual mucosa.
4. **Crozat appliance.** A removable appliance anchored to the first molars and made of orthodontic wire that fits in the labial vestibule and labial mucosa with extensions occlusally, which are activated to produce the desired movement.

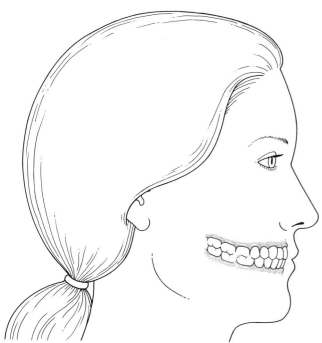

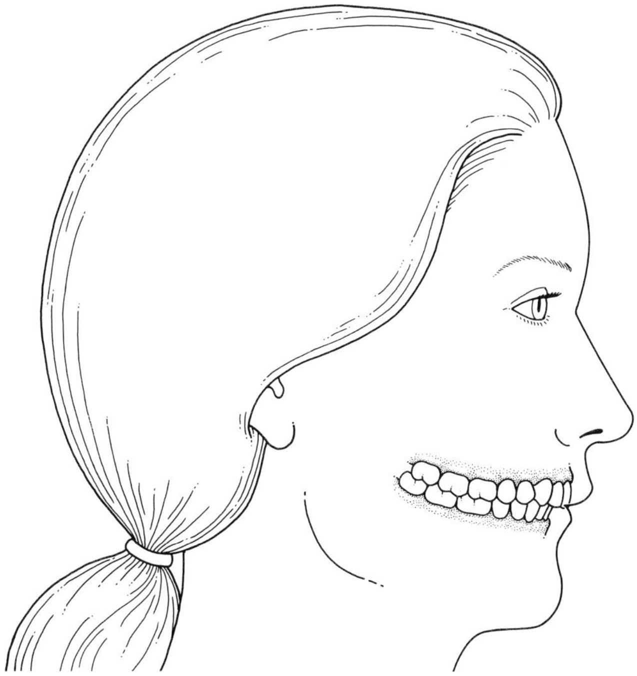

FIG. 22–1. Molar relationship in a normal Angle Class I occlusion.

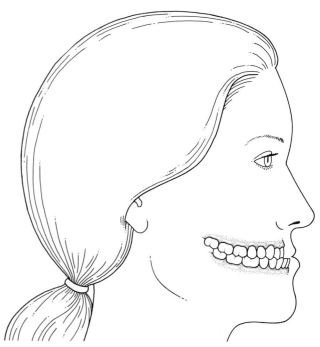

FIG. 22–2. Molar relationship in an Angle Class II malocclusion.

FIG. 22–3. Molar relationship in an Angle Class III malocclusion.

Types of Instruments

1. **Wire bending instruments.** No. 139 pliers are used to bend heavier wires. Light wire pliers are used to bend light wires.
2. **Ligature cutters.** These instruments are used to tie and cut the ligature wire (0.010″ soft round wire).

TREATMENT OF CLINICAL PROBLEMS—GENERAL CONSIDERATIONS

For the sake of simplicity, each type of malocclusion will be discussed as if it were a single entity. Often, however, the patient presents with a combination of disharmonies. The final treatment plan must account for all the factors causing a malocclusion, along with a selection of the most appropriate mechanotherapy to treat the particular case.

Placement of Edgewise Brackets

Armamentarium

- Standard dental setup
  explorer
  mouth mirror
  college pliers—non-locking
  low-speed dental handpiece
  periodontal scaler (optional)
- Pumice
- 30 to 50% phosphoric acid, liquid, or gel
- Edgewise brackets (Unitek/3M, Inc.) (brackets are available in metal, plastic, or ceramic and in assorted sizes to fit either 0.018 or 0.022 in. wire)
- Orthodontic composite luting agent (e.g., Concise, 3M, Inc.)
- Bracket positioning gauge (e.g., Boone bracket positioning gauge, Unitek/3M, Inc.)
- Bracket removing pliers (e.g., ETM 345RT Unitek/3M, Inc.) (if necessary).

Clinical Technique

1. Pumice the appropriate teeth.
2. Select the appropriate brackets and position them on the bracket table to allow for easy access during bracket placement.
3. Mix the orthodontic composite luting agent and apply it to the bracket according to the manufacturer's recommendations.
4. Center the bracket on the tooth so that the edges are "square" with the long axis of the tooth. The incisal edge of the bracket should be 3.5 mm from the incisal edge of the tooth. A bracket positioning gauge will assure uniform placement of the brackets.

CLINICAL TIP. Place the brackets digitally or with nonlocking pliers. Do not use locking pliers because they may cause unintended movement of the bracket when the lock is released.

CLINICAL TIP. If a band is improperly placed, detach it with bracket-removing pliers and remove any remaining resin with the chisel tip of the pliers or a periodontal scaler. Then repeat steps 1 to 4.

Placement of Orthodontic Bands

Armamentarium

- Standard dental setup
  explorer
  mouth mirror
  college pliers—non-locking
  low-speed dental handpiece
- Separating elastics (e.g., Ālastik S Modules, Unitek/3M, Inc.)
- Band pusher (e.g., band seater and pusher 811-003, Unitek/3M, Inc.)
- Nylon molar seater (Unitek/3M, Inc.)
- Assorted orthodontic bands (Unitek/3M, Inc.)
- Buccal tubes (if necessary) (Unitek/3M, Inc.)
- Spot welder (if necessary)
- Zinc phosphate cement (e.g., Fleck's Cement, Mizzy, Inc.)

Clinical Technique

1. Place separating elastics one day prior to insertion of orthodontic bands.
2. Remove the separating elastics.
3. Select the appropriate size band.
4. Place the band on the tooth seat with the band pusher.

CLINICAL TIP. Turn the head of the band pusher sideways and place it over the occlusal surface of the band. Apply thumb pressure to the band pusher until the band seats over the height of contour of the tooth.

---

5. Continue seating the band with the band seater.
6. Once properly seated, adapt (swedge) the band to cuspal and gingival anatomy with the band pusher.

CLINICAL TIP. Use the smallest band that fits the tooth. An ill-fitting band allows cement leakage, thus increasing the possibility of caries development.

---

7. Spot weld a buccal tube if required. Place the tube parallel to the occlusal surface and as close to the gingiva as possible. Align the mesial edge of the tube with the middle of the mesial cusp of the tooth.
8. Apply cement to the entire internal surface of the band and completely seat the band as described in steps 4 and 5 above.

CLINICAL TIP. Carefully place cement to prevent voids from forming, especially at the gingival edge. Cement voids increase the likelihood of leakage and subsequent caries development.

GENERALIZED SPACING

Diagnosis

Generalized spacing can be caused by:

1. Small teeth.
2. A large tongue.
3. Perverse sucking habits.
4. A component of a more severe syndrome, e.g., a Class II, Division 1 malocclusion.
5. A combination of one or more of the above.

Generalized spacing is confirmed by measuring the size of the teeth on study models. Little can be done orthodontically for these rare cases. They may be treated successfully with restorations by the general dentist.

If diastema are localized, the clinician should suspect sucking or tongue habits. A large tongue that is physiologically active usually has a scalloped edge because of constantly pushing against the teeth. Sucking habits can range from involvement of the thumb to several fingers turned in various positions when placed in the mouth. The fingers that are used in a sucking habit invariably are cleaner than their neighbors, and often exhibit a callus where the mandibular incisors contact them.

Treatment

Elimination of pernicious habits is never easy but can be accomplished if the clinician is patient, persistent, and most important, enlists the cooperation of the patient. The first step is to convince the patient that it is his responsibility to break the habit and that the doctor only offers assistance. In young patients, it is helpful to have patients give permission to the parents allowing the parents to remind the patient that the habit exists. However, parents should not force the patient to stop. Start with small successes and build on them. It is essential to avoid discouraging the patient if small episodes of "backsliding" occur.

The plethora of devices used to break sucking habits speaks for their lack of singular success. They may be used, but should be considered adjuncts to primary treatment stated above. Wearing cotton gloves is sometimes successful, as is the use of a bitter substance placed on the finger used during the habit. Success can often be obtained by asking the patient to wear an elastic bandage (ACE, Inc.) around the elbow during the times the patient is concentrating on breaking the habit (usually at bed time, reading time, and while watching television). It is important that the patient's parent place the bandage so that no pressure exists when the arm is extended, but it becomes tight when the elbow is bent. The resultant pressure on the elbow will remind the patient of the desire to stop the sucking habit. Fre-

quent office visits reinforce patient progress. Once the habit has been stopped, the spaces may self correct or orthodontic closure may sometimes be necessary.

Diastema Closure via Arch Contracture— Elastics

In order to treat multiple spacing via contraction of the maxillary arch, the mandibular antagonist must not interfere with the movement.

Armamentarium

- Basic bracket and band placement setup (see the previous section on Placement of Orthodontic Bands)
- 0.020 in. orthodontic elastic chord (Unitek/3M, Inc.)
- Orthodontic stress and tension gauge (Dontrix-Richmond)
- Orthodontic Stress and Tension Gauges (Unitek/3M, Inc.)

Clinical Technique

1. Place brackets on the labial surface of all teeth requiring diastema closure. (See the previous section on Placement of Orthodontic Bands.)
2. Place bilateral brackets (or bands) on the three teeth immediately distal to the teeth requiring movement (anchor teeth).

3. Ligate the three left anchor teeth together with elastic chord to create an anchor unit.
4. Repeat step 3 for the three right anchor teeth
5. If a single tooth must be move laterally, accomplish this before arch contraction begins. To activate the movement ligate, the single tooth with elastic chord to the anchor unit toward which the tooth must be move. The elastic should generate 1 ounce of force, as measured by an orthodontic stress and tension gauge. However, an arch wire must be placed to guide this movement (Fig. 22–5).
6. Ligate the left and right anchor unit to each other using elastic chord. The elastic should generate 1 ounce of force, as measured by an orthodontic stress and tension gauge (Fig. 22–6).
7. Additional therapy is discussed under the section on Localize Spacing of Maxillary Central Incisors, later in this chapter.

Multiple Diastema Closure—Removable Appliance

Armamentarium

- Irreversible hydrocolloid impression
- No. 139 pliers to activate Hawley appliance

FIG. 22-4. A fixed appliance used to close a diastema involving the central incisors.

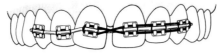

FIG. 22-5. A fixed appliance used to move a single tooth to close a diastema. Elastics are stretched from the tooth to be moved across multiple anterior teeth. Note the use of a stabilizing circumferential arch wire.

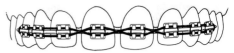

FIG. 22-6. A fixed appliance used to close multiple diastemata. Elastics are stretched from multiple teeth on either side of the midline. Note the use of a stabilizing arch wire.

NAME: _____ DATE: _____

ADDRESS: _____ PHONE: (___)_____

CITY: _____ STATE: _____ ZIP: _____

PATIENT NAME: _____

DATE NEEDED: _____ TIME NEEDED: _____

SPECIAL INSTRUCTION:

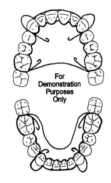

Please construct a maxillary Hawley appliance and a mandibular Hawley appliance with labial bows and circumferential clasps on the first molars. Slightly relieve the palatal and lingual acrylic to allow for the closing of multiple diastemata due to anterior flaring.

For Demonstration Purposes Only

Thank you.

SIGNATURE: _____ LICENSE: _____

FIG. 22-7. A sample prescription for the fabrication of maxillary and mandibular removable appliances for the correction of flared anterior teeth.

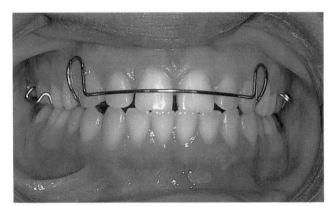

FIG. 22-8. Anterior view of a maxillary Hawley appliance inserted to reduce spacing between anterior teeth.

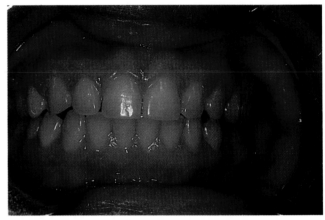

FIG. 22-9. Postoperative view showing the elimination of all the spaces between the maxillary anterior teeth.

Clinical Technique

1. Make an irreversible hydrocolloid impression.
2. Send the models to an orthodontic laboratory for fabrication of a Hawley appliance (Fig. 22-7).
3. Activate the springs on the Hawley appliance to increase pressure on the labial area of the teeth to be moved to decrease the labial circumference in working relationship with the mandibular anterior teeth.
4. Be sure that the opposing arch or the palatal aspect of the appliance will not interfere with the proposed movement.
5. Adjust the appliance every 2 weeks.
6. Space closure occurs at a rate of 1.0 to 1.5 mm per month (Figs. 22-8, 22-9).

LOCALIZED SPACING—CLINICALLY ABSENT TEETH

Diagnosis

Causes for the clinical absence of teeth include:

1. Congenitally missing teeth.
2. Unerupted teeth.
3. Premature loss of permanent teeth.
4. Perverse sucking habits.
5. Supernumerary teeth preventing normal eruption.
6. A combination of the above.

Overlong retention of primary teeth can cause ectopic impaction of the permanent successors. Congenitally

NAME: _____ DATE:_____

ADDRESS: _____ PHONE: (___)_____

CITY: _____ STATE: _____ ZIP: _____

PATIENT NAME: _____

DATE NEEDED: _____ TIME NEEDED: _____

SPECIAL INSTRUCTION:

Please construct a maxillary Hawley appliance with a labial bow and circumferential clasps on the first molars. Add coils springs coming from the palatal acrylic to move #6 distally and #8 mesially in order to gain space lost due to a congenitally missing #7.

Thank you.

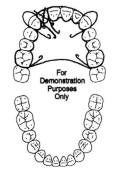

For Demonstration Purposes Only

SIGNATURE: _____ LICENSE:_____

FIG. 22–10. A sample prescription for the fabrication of a maxillary removable appliance for the correction of migrated teeth due to a congenitally missing lateral incisor.

missing lateral incisors are discussed with Localized Spacing of Maxillary Central Incisors later in this chapter. Diagnosis is ultimately confirmed by examination of the appropriate radiographs.

Sometimes prosthetic treatment is complicated by the mesiodistal drifting of teeth adjacent to the edentulous space. This drifting can occur through tipping or bodily movement. In the latter, the crown and the apex of the root move bodily through the bone with the long axis of the tooth remaining perpendicular to the occlusal plane. In the former, the crown tips mesially or distally ahead of the apex of the root. Radiographs confirm the type of movement that has occurred.

CLINICAL TIP. Tipped teeth always must be uprighted so that the crown is positioned over the apex. This provides stability to the result.

Attempts to correct a mesiodistally drifted tooth with an abnormally proportioned restoration often creates periodontal problems. Therefore, teeth should be orthodontically uprighted prior to prosthetic treatment.

Treatment

Ectopic impaction should be treated by extraction of the primary teeth. If less than one-half of the root has formed, the permanent tooth usually will be delayed in eruption. If more than one-half of the root is present and the tooth has failed to erupt despite the loss of the primary tooth, surgical exposure of the crown is required, often followed by mechanical therapy by an orthodontist to force eruption of the tooth.

Congenitally missing teeth are treated by prosthetic replacement, however orthodontic intervention often is necessary if adjacent teeth have shifted mesiodistally.

FIG. 22–11. Right labial view of a patient with spacing between the maxillary right lateral and central incisors.

FIG. 22–12. Palatal view of a maxillary Hawley appliance designed with a labial archwire and Adams clasps. Note also the auxiliary spring imbedded in the acrylic to move the maxillary right lateral incisor mesially.

FIG. 22–13. Occlusal view of a Hawley appliance placed passively over a model of the maxillary arch. Note that the palatal auxiliary spring in the passive position lies in the middle of the right maxillary lateral incisor.

FIG. 22–14. Occlusal view of a Hawley appliance placed actively over a model of the maxillary arch. Note that the palatal auxiliary spring is engaged on the distal surface of the right maxillary lateral incisor.

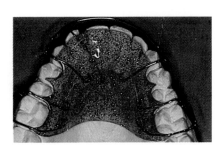

FIG. 22–11

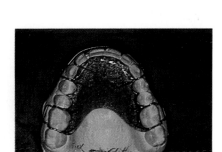

FIG. 22–12

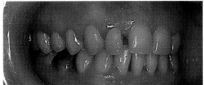

FIG. 22–13

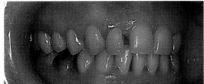

FIG. 22–14

Correction of Migrated Anterior Tooth—Removable Appliance

Armamentarium

- Irreversible hydrocolloid impression
- No. 139 orthodontic pliers

Clinical Technique

1. Make an irreversible hydrocolloid impression.
2. Send the models to an orthodontic laboratory for fabrication of a Hawley appliance, which will include uprighting springs imbedded in acrylic (Fig. 22–10).
3. Confirm that the labial arch wire lies passively against the teeth.
4. Activate the lingual springs against the interproximal surface of the tipped teeth.
5. Clinically evaluate the patient every 2 weeks.
6. Normal correction of a migrated tooth occurs 1.0 to 1.5 mm per month (Figs. 22-11 to 22-14).

Correction of Migrated Anterior Tooth—Fixed Appliance

Fixed appliances require that the generalist is absolutely familiar with all aspects of fixed orthodontic therapy. Failure to adhere to proper orthodontic technique could have adverse consequences.

Armamentarium

- Basic bracket and band placement setup (see the section on Placement of Orthodontic Bands earlier in this chapter)
- 0.016 in. round orthodontic wire (Unitek/3M, Inc.)
- 0.022 in. × 0.018 in. rectangular wire (Unitek/3M, Inc.)
- 0.010 in. diameter, 0.030 in. arbor diameter coil spring (Unitek/3M, Inc.)
- Orthodontic elastics (Unitek/3M, Inc.)
- Orthodontic stress and tension gauge (Dontrix-Richmond Orthodontic Stress and Tension Gauges, Unitek/3M, Inc.)

Clinical Technique

1. Acid-etch the anterior teeth and premolars.
2. Apply the orthodontic bonding resin.
3. Place the orthodontic brackets. (See the section on Placement of Orthodontic Bands earlier in this chapter.)

CLINICAL TIP. To ensure a satisfactory result, brackets must be placed perpendicular to the long axis of the tooth.

4. Construct an ideal arch wire to serve as a guide along which the teeth will be moved. Start with a thin (0.016 in.) round wire and finish with a 0.022 in. × 0.018 in. rectangular wire.

CLINICAL TIP. Coaxial wire provides a more gentle force and provides a relatively painless start to the therapy.

CLINICAL TIP. To achieve a satisfactory result, the arch wire must follow an ideal arch form.

5. Activate the appliance with a coil spring or orthodontic elastics. Position the coil spring between the teeth; attach elastics from the tipped teeth distally to the end of the archwire. The elastic should generate

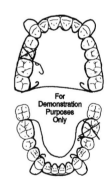

FIG. 22–15. An example of a fixed appliance used to correct a migrated anterior tooth. Note the elastics stretched over multiple anchors pull the lateral incisors distally while a coil spring between the central incisors is used to upright and move the inclined right central incisor distally.

NAME: _____ DATE:_____

ADDRESS: _____ PHONE: (___)_____

CITY: _____ STATE: _____ ZIP: _____

PATIENT NAME: _____

DATE NEEDED: _____ TIME NEEDED: _____

SPECIAL INSTRUCTION:

Please construct a maxillary Hawley appliance with a circumferential labial bow and a coil spring coming from the palatal acrylic to upright #3 distally which has migrated mesially due to the loss of #4. Also, construct a mandibular Hawley appliance with a labial bow and a coil spring coming from the lingual acrylic to tip #20 mesially which has migrated distally due to the loss of #19.

Thank you.

SIGNATURE: _____ LICENSE:_____

FIG. 22–16. A sample prescription for the fabrication of maxillary and mandibular removable appliances for uprighting of migrated teeth.

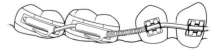

FIG. 22–17. A fixed appliance used to upright and align migrated premolars and molars. The coil springs help to upright molars and premolars while gaining space for future pontic placement and closing unwanted diastemata.

1 ounce of force, as measured by an orthodontic stress and tension gauge (Fig. 22-15).

6. Clinically evaluate the patient every 3 weeks.
7. Normal space closure occurs at the rate of 1.0 to 1.5 mm per month.

Correcting and Uprighting Migrated Premolars or Molars—Removable Appliance

Armamentarium

- Irreversible hydrocolloid impression
- No. 139 orthodontic pliers

Clinical Technique

1. Make an irreversible hydrocolloid impression.
2. Send the models to an orthodontic laboratory for fabrication of a Hawley appliance which will include uprighting springs embedded in the acrylic (Fig. 22–16).
3. Activate the springs on the Hawley appliance while keeping the labial archwire passive against the buccal surface of the mandibular teeth.
4. Clinically evaluate the patient every 2 to 3 weeks.
5. Normal uprighting occurs at a rate of 2° to 3° per month.
6. Conically shaped teeth are much harder to upright with removable appliances because the spring tends to slip off the tooth. In these type of cases, a fixed appliance should be used.

Correcting and Uprighting Migrated Premolars or Molars—Fixed Appliance

Fixed appliances require that the generalist is absolutely familiar with all aspects of fixed orthodontic therapy. Failure to adhere to proper orthodontic technique could have adverse consequences.

Armamentarium

- Basic bracket and band placement setup (see the section on Placement of Orthodontic Bands earlier in this chapter)
- Premolar orthodontic bands with edgewise brackets. (Brackets may also be bonded if the patient's esthetic concerns are paramount.)
- Molar orthodontic bands with tubes
- Orthodontic zinc phosphate cement (Fleck's Cement, Mizzy, Inc.)
- 0.016 in. round orthodontic wire (Unitek/3M, Inc.)
- 0.022 in. × 0.018 in. rectangular orthodontic wire (Unitek/3M, Inc.)
- 0.010 in. diameter, 0.030 in. arbor diameter open coil spring (Unitek/3M, Inc.)

Clinical Technique

1. Fit the orthodontic bands to the teeth. (See the section on Placement of Orthodontic Bands earlier in this chapter.)
2. Cement the bands into place. (See the section on

Placement of Orthodontic Bands earlier in this chapter.)

CLINICAL TIP. When uprighting premolar teeth it is important to incorporate the first molar teeth in the appliance for stability of the dental arch.

CLINICAL TIP. To achieve a satisfactory result, it is important that the bands are properly placed.

3. If the goal is simple correction of lost space, construct the wire into an ideal arch form to serve as a guide along which the teeth will move (Fig. 22–17). If uprighting is required include second order bends into the wire to create an uprighting action.

CLINICAL TIP. To ensure a satisfactory result, the arch wire must follow an ideal arch form.

4. If the goal is simple correction of lost space, place an open coil spring. If uprighting is required, activate the wire with second order bends.
5. Clinically evaluate the patient every 2 weeks.
6. Normal uprighting occurs at a rate of 3 to 5° per month.

Correction of Anterior Flaring of Teeth—Removable Appliance

Armamentarium

- Irreversible hydrocolloid
- No. 139 pliers (Unitek/3M, Inc.)

Clinical Technique

1. Make an irreversible hydrocolloid impression.
2. Send the models to an orthodontic laboratory for fabrication of a Hawley appliance.
3. Activate the labial arch wire to decrease the circumferences of the dental arch, thereby gently bringing the splayed teeth together.
4. Be sure that no occlusal interferences occur from the opposing arch as the teeth are brought together.
5. Clinically evaluate the patient every 2 weeks.
6. Normal correction of flaring occurs at a rate of 1.0 to 1.5 mm per month.

Correction of Anterior Flaring of Teeth—Fixed Appliance

Fixed appliances require that the generalist is absolutely familiar with all aspects of fixed orthodontic therapy. Failure to adhere to proper orthodontic technique could have adverse consequences.

Armamentarium

- Basic bracket and band placement setup (see the section on Placement of Orthodontic Bands earlier in this chapter)
- Bands for first molars
- Brackets for incisors, canines, and premolars (metal,

ceramic, or plastic depending on the esthetic needs of the patient)
- Orthodontic zinc phosphate cement (Fleck's Cement, Mizzy, Inc.)
- 0.016 in. round orthodontic wire (Unitek/3M, Inc.)
- 0.022 in. × 0.018 in. rectangular orthodontic wire (Unitek/3M, Inc.)
- 0.010 in. diameter, 0.030 in. arbor diameter open coil spring (Unitek/3M, Inc.)
- Orthodontic elastics
- Orthodontic stress and tension gauge (Dontrix-Richmond Orthodontic Stress and Tension Gauges, Unitek/3M, Inc.)

Clinical Technique

1. Fit and cement the molar orthodontic bands. (See the section on Placement of Orthodontic Bands earlier in this chapter.)
2. Acid-etch the anterior teeth and premolars.
3. Apply the orthodontic bonding resin.
4. Place the orthodontic bonded brackets. (See the section on Placement of Orthodontic Bands earlier in this section.)
5. Construct an ideal arch-wire to serve as a guide along which the teeth will be moved. Start with thin 0.016 in. round wire and finish with a 0.022 in. × 0.018 in. rectangular wire.
6. Activate the appliance with orthodontic elastic cord or orthodontic elastics worn from hooks bent in the arch wire mesial to the brackets on canines to the end of the molar tubes. The elastic should generate 1 ounce of force, as measured by an orthodontic stress and tension gauge.

CLINICAL TIP. Keep the hook on the arch wire far enough mesial to the canine brackets to allow for continued closure of spaces. Also, build in bite opening mechanics to open the bite if there are occlusal interferences.

7. Clinically evaluate the patient every 3 weeks.
8. Normal space closure occurs at a rate of 1.0 to 2.0 mm per month unless the bite must to be opened, in which case treatment time can increase by 3 to 6 months.

LOCALIZED SPACING OF MAXILLARY CENTRAL INCISORS

Because of the great esthetic impact of localized spacing of the maxillary central incisors, it will be described separately. The most common causes are:

1. Part of normal growth.
2. Imperfect fusion of the midline.
3. Enlarged labial frenum.
4. Congenitally missing lateral incisors.
5. Supernumerary teeth (mesiodens).
6. Anatomically small clinical crowns.

Differential Diagnosis

The space is localized between the central incisors.

CLINICAL TIP. Clinical examination of the frenum, along with lifting of the upper lip to note any blanching of the mucosa on the palate between the central incisors, will confirm an enlarged or malpositioned labial frenum.

Radiographic evidence will confirm a spade-shaped septum when there is a malpositioned labial frenum. This radiologic characteristic also is seen in imperfect fusion of the midline, but when the lip is stretched there will be no blanching of the frenum. Supernumerary teeth and congenitally missing lateral incisors will be confirmed with radiographs. Spacing as part of normal growth can also occur in patients with small bony bases and large teeth. The large crowns of the developing and unerupted lateral incisors and canines push the central incisor roots mesially toward each other, causing the central incisor crowns to erupt with a distal inclination and an accompanying diastema to be present. Anatomically small teeth may be confirmed by measurement.

Treatment

Normal Growth. If the spacing is determined to be part of normal growth, observe the patient until the lateral incisors and canines have erupted. In many instances, the diastema will close during the normal eruption process. However, this type of diastema may also be evidence of possible future crowding of the permanent dentition.

Imperfect Fusion of the Midline. In the primary and mixed dentition imperfect fusion of the midline becomes evident with the eruption of the permanent anterior teeth, including the canines, and should be treated in the permanent dentition stage.

Treatment of imperfect fusion of the midline in the permanent dentition consists of moving the teeth together and retaining the positions.

Diastema Closure—Removable Appliance

Simple closure of a maxillary midline diastema often creates spacing distally. Therefore, restorative dentistry may also be required to achieve proper esthetics (Figs. 22-18, 22-19).

Armamentarium

- Irreversible hydrocolloid impression
- No. 139 pliers (Unitek/3M, Inc.)

Clinical Technique

1. Make an irreversible hydrocolloid impression.
2. Send the models to an orthodontic laboratory for fabrication of a Hawley appliance (Fig. 22−20).
3. Activate the springs on the Hawley appliance to bring the central incisors together while increasing pressure on labial aspect to decrease the labial circumference in working relationship with the mandibular anterior teeth.
4. Be sure that no interference occurs in working rela-

FIG. 22–18. Anterior view of a patient with a diastema between the maxillary central incisors.

FIG. 22–19. Occlusal view of a maxillary Hawley appliance used to close the diastema for the patient shown in Figure 22–18.

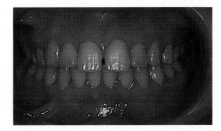

FIG. 22–18

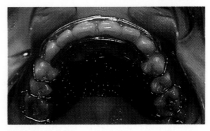

FIG. 22–19

tionship with the mandibular anterior teeth.
5. Adjust the appliance every 2 weeks.
6. Space closure occurs at a rate of 1.0 to 2.0 mm per month.

Diastema Closure—Fixed Appliance

Fixed appliances require that the generalist is absolutely familiar with all aspects of fixed orthodontic therapy. Failure to adhere to proper orthodontic technique could have adverse consequences. Simple closure of a maxillary midline diastema often creates spacing distally. Therefore, restorative dentistry may also be required to achieve proper esthetics.

Armamentarium

- Basic bracket and band placement setup (see the section on Placement of Orthodontic Bands earlier in this chapter)
- Anterior edgewise orthodontic brackets (metal, ceramic, or plastic depending on esthetic requirements)
- 0.016 in. round orthodontic wire (Unitek/3M, Inc.)
- 0.022 in. × 0.018 in. rectangular orthodontic wire (Unitek/3M, Inc.)
- Orthodontic elastics (Unitek/3M, Inc.)
- Orthodontic stress and tension gauge (Dontrix-Richmond Orthodontic Stress and Tension Gauges, Unitek/3M, Inc.)

Clinical Technique

1. Place the orthodontic brackets on the anterior teeth. (See the section on Placement of Orthodontic Bands earlier in this chapter) (Fig 22–21).

CLINICAL TIP. To achieve a satisfactory result, the brackets must be placed perpendicular to the long axis of the tooth.

---

2. Construct an ideal arch wire to serve as a guide along which the teeth will be moved.

CLINICAL TIP. To achieve a satisfactory result, the arch wire must follow an ideal arch form.

---

3. Activate the appliance with orthodontic elastics. The elastic should generate 1 ounce of force, as measured by an orthodontic stress and tension gauge.
4. Clinically evaluate the patient every 2 weeks.
5. Normal space closure occurs at a rate of 1.0 to 2.0 mm per month (Figs. 22-22 to 22-25).

NAME: _____ DATE:_____

ADDRESS: _____ PHONE: (___)_____

CITY: _____ STATE: _____ ZIP: _____

PATIENT NAME: _____

DATE NEEDED: _____ TIME NEEDED: _____

SPECIAL INSTRUCTION:

Please construct a maxillary Hawley appliance with a labial bow and circumferential clasps on the first molars. Please place coil springs coming from the palatal acrylic on the distal surface of both central incisors in order to close the diastema. Also, construct a mandibular Hawley appliance with a labial bow and circumferential clasps on the first molars to close anterior spaces. Slightly relieve the lingual acrylic to allow for the closing of the multiple diastemata.

Thank you.

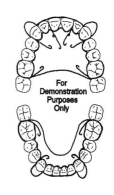

SIGNATURE: _____ LICENSE:_____

FIG. 22–20. A sample prescription for the fabrication of maxillary and mandibular removable appliances for the closure of multiple diastemata.

Diastema Closure—Retention
Armamentarium

- Irreversible hydrocolloid
- No. 128 pliers (Unitek/3M, Inc.)

Clinical Technique

1. Make an irreversible hydrocolloid impression.
2. Send the models to an orthodontic laboratory for fabrication of a Hawley appliance with a labial bow (Fig. 22–26).
3. Activate the labial bow to exert slight pressure on the labial surface of the teeth to retain the space clo-

sure. The patient must wear the appliance 24 hours a day for 3 months, then only at night for 3 to 6 months.

4. Clinically evaluate the patient in 3 weeks and then at intervals of 6 weeks.
5. If the space starts to reopen, the patient must wear the appliance more often. Check to see if the mandibular anterior teeth are pushing against the maxillary anterior teeth during working movements. If so, expand treatment to the mandibular arch.

Enlarged or Malpositioned Frenum

Treatment and retention is identical to that described in the section on treatment of normal growth, midline (earlier in this chapter) except that a frenectomy is necessary. A frenectomy is accomplished by:[1]

Armamentarium

- Standard dental setup
    explorer
    mouth mirror
    periodontal probe
    suitable anesthesia
- Curved hemostat
- Periodontal tissue scissors
- No. 15 Bard-Parker knife
- Needle holder
- 4-0 black silk sutures
- Periodontal dressing (e.g. COE-pak, Coe Laboratories, Inc.)

Clinical Technique

1. Obtain a proper medical history and presurgical evaluation.
2. Anesthetize the area.
3. Grasp the frenum with the curved hemostat.
4. Incise the upper margin of the frenum with a curved periodontal tissue scissor or a No. 15 Bard-Parker knife (Fig. 22–27).
5. Incise the lower margin of the frenum with a curved periodontal tissue scissor or a No. 15 Bard-Parker knife (Fig. 22–28).
6. Remove the incised wedge-shaped frenum.
7. If any mucosal tissue is under tension, place the curved periodontal tissue scissor beneath that tissue and release the fibers by blunt dissection (Fig. 22–29).
8. Suture the incision with 4-0 black silk sutures (Fig. 22–30).
9. After achieving hemostasis, place a periodontal packing on the area.
10. Leave the packing and sutures in place for 1 week.

Supernumerary Teeth

Supernumerary teeth (mesiodens) must be extracted.

Following removal of the supernumerary tooth in the primary and mixed dentition, normal tooth eruption may correct the situation. If spacing persists, use conventional orthodontic therapy.

In the permanent dentition, conventional orthodontic therapy is required.

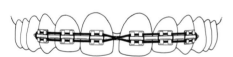

FIG. 22–21. A fixed appliance used to close a diastema through activation of elastic stretched over multiple teeth and a stabilizing arch wire.

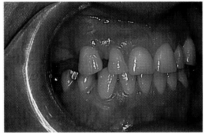

FIG. 22–22. Right labial view of a patient showing a diastema between the right lateral and canine teeth.

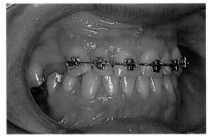

FIG. 22–23. Right labial view of the patient shown in Figure 22–22. The diastema between the right lateral and canine teeth was eliminated using bonded brackets and a segmented arch wire.

FIG. 22–24. Left labial view showing of a patient with a diastema between the left lateral and canine teeth.

FIG. 22–25. Left labial view of the patient shown in Figure 22–24. The diastema between the left lateral and canine teeth was eliminated using bonded brackets and a segmented arch wire.

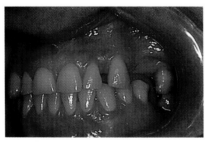

FIG. 22–24

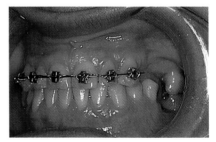

FIG. 22–25

NAME: _____ DATE: _____

ADDRESS: _____ PHONE: (___)_____

CITY: _____ STATE: _____ ZIP: _____

PATIENT NAME: _____

DATE NEEDED: _____ TIME NEEDED: _____

SPECIAL INSTRUCTION:

Please construct a maxillary Hawley appliance and a mandibular Hawley appliance with labial bows and circumferential clasps on the first molars to retain the teeth following space closure.

Thank you.

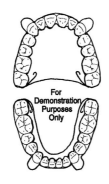

For Demonstration Purposes Only

SIGNATURE: _____ LICENSE: _____

FIG. 22–26. A sample prescription for the fabrication of maxillary and mandibular removable appliances to retain the position of the teeth after space closure.

Congenitally Missing Lateral Incisors

Congenitally missing permanent lateral incisors will not be clinically evident in the primary dentition. If suspected, (from familial history) radiographs may be taken.

In the mixed dentition, congenitally missing lateral incisors can be clinically distinguished from other causes of localized spacing of the maxillary central incisors by over-retention of the primary lateral incisors. Radiographs confirm the diagnosis.

In the permanent dentition, congenitally missing lateral incisors present the clinician with one of the greatest esthetic challenges. If the canines are slender, the spaces may be closed and the canines contoured to resemble the missing lateral incisors. This is often difficult because of the bulkiness of the canine. Several restorative approaches can be taken, dictated by the anatomic relationships present. Consultation and coordination of treatment objectives between the generalist and the orthodontic specialist is essential. The introduction of new esthetic materials has enhanced the resolution of these cases.

Anatomically Small Teeth

Anatomically small teeth are best treated with esthetic restorative materials.

It is essential to observe the occlusion whenever treating patients with space problems. Occlusal interferences from the mandibular dentition may cause spacing or prevent attempts at space closure. Both arches must be treated in order to resolve these cases properly.

FIG. 22–27. The upper margin of the frenum is incised with a curved periodontal tissue scissor or a No. 15 Bard-Parker knife.

FIG. 22–28. The lower margin of the frenum is incised with a curved periodontal tissue scissor or a No. 15 Bard-Parker knife.

FIG. 22–29. If any mucosal tissue is under tension the curved periodontal tissue scissor is placed beneath that tissue and the fibers are released by blunt dissection.

FIG. 22–30. The incision is sutured with 4-0 black silk sutures.

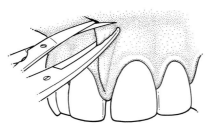

FIG. 22–27

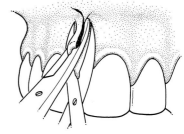

FIG. 22–28

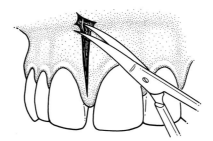

FIG. 22–29

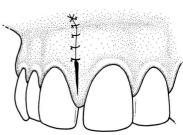

FIG. 22–30

LABIOVERSION OF THE MAXILLARY INCISORS

This type of malocclusion is usually caused by adverse oral habits, e.g., thumb or finger sucking. The generalist is likely to see these cases first, when palliative treatment of oral habits might prevent the condition from fully developing and reversal may occur. Therefore, early diagnosis and treatment or referral is essential. If serial extraction is selected, the clinician is committed to following the patient's treatment through the time of full eruption of the permanent dentition. The patient and the patient's parents should be advised of the extended nature of this type of correction and that treatment may include further fixed appliance therapy. However, such intervention usually tends to simplify and shorten the duration of active orthodontic appliance therapy, if it is required.

Diagnosis

Overjet of the maxillary anterior teeth often is combined with a Class I molar relationship. The amount of overbite varies, but a deep curve of Spee is common because the mandibular anterior teeth over-erupt when their antagonists' forward position cannot provide a normal occlusal stop relationship. It is important not to confuse this with the case of a Class II, Division 1 malocclusion in which the mandibular molars have moved mesially into a Class I position because of the early lost of the deciduous molars. Although the latter cases also exhibit both overbite and overjet, the mandibular anterior teeth also exhibit extreme crowding.

Treatment

In the primary dentition, palliative control of oral habits is indicated. (See the section on Generalized Spacing earlier in the chapter.)

In mixed dentition the elimination of oral habits also is indicated. Removable appliance therapy may be successful at this time. (See the section on Correction of Anterior Flaring of Teeth—Removable Appliance earlier in this chapter.) Selected serial extraction of the primary dentition may also influence the eruption pattern of the secondary teeth.

In the permanent dentition, full appliance mechanotherapy is used to open the bite and retract the anterior teeth. (See the section on Correction of Anterior Flaring of Teeth — Fixed Appliance earlier in this chapter.) Oral habits also must be corrected for treatment to be successful.

LABIOLINGUALLY MALPOSITIONED TEETH

Differential Diagnosis

Teeth may be labiolingually malpositioned for a number of reasons.

Normal Growth. Often no other malocclusion occurs except for a lingually or labially displaced tooth. This can be caused by over-retained primary teeth or by the individual growth pattern of the patient. If a simple labiolingual displacement is involved, a removable Hawley appliance is used. If the teeth are rotated or tipped, fixed orthodontic appliance therapy is indicated.

Crowded Teeth. Usually, crowded teeth result from teeth that are too large for the dental arch. Crowded teeth are discussed in the section on Lateral Disharmonies of the Teeth and Dental Arch later in this chapter.

Combined with Other Malocclusion. Labiolingual malpositioning of anterior teeth is seen in Class II and Class III malocclusions and is discussed in the sections on Class II Distoclusion and Class III Mesioclusion, respectively.

Treatment

CLINICAL TIP. Successful treatment of labiolingually malpositioned teeth requires adequate space within which to move the malpositioned tooth. If this space is not present, complete orthodontic therapy by a specialist is required.

Correction of Labially or Lingually Malpositioned Teeth—Removable Appliance

Armamentarium

- Irreversible hydrocolloid impression
- No. 139 pliers (Unitek/3M, Inc.)

Clinical Technique

1. Make an irreversible hydrocolloid impression of the dentition.
2. Send the models to an orthodontic laboratory for fabrication of a Hawley appliance (Fig. 22–31).
3. If lingual movement is required, activate the labial arch wire (Figs. 22-32, 22-33).
4. If labial movement is required, embed a finger spring in the palatal or lingual acrylic.
5. Normal movement occurs at a rate of 0.5 to 1.0 mm per month.

CLINICAL TIP. When labial movement is required it is important to position the labial arch wire so it does not inhibit movement of the tooth.

Correction of Labially or Lingually Malpositioned Teeth—Fixed Appliance

Fixed appliances require that the generalist is absolutely familiar with all aspects of fixed orthodontic therapy. Failure to adhere to proper orthodontic technique could have adverse consequences.

Armamentarium

- Basic bracket and band placement setup (see the section on Placement of Orthodontic Bands earlier in this chapter)
- Anterior edgewise orthodontic brackets (metal, ceramic, or plastic depending on the esthetics requirements)

ESTHETIC DENTISTRY

NAME: _____ DATE: _____

ADDRESS: _____ PHONE: (___)_____

CITY: _____ STATE: _____ ZIP: _____

PATIENT NAME: _____

DATE NEEDED: _____ TIME NEEDED: _____

SPECIAL INSTRUCTION:

Please construct a maxillary Hawley appliance with a labial bow and circumferential clasps on the first molars to move #8 palatally into proper alignment. Relieve the palatal acrylic around #8 to allow for this movement.

Also, please construct a mandibular Hawley appliance with a labial bow and circumferential clasps on the first molars. Add a spring coming from the lingual acrylic as shown to move #23 labially into proper alignment.

Thank you.

SIGNATURE: _____ LICENSE: _____

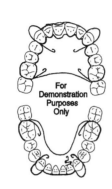

For Demonstration Purposes Only

FIG. 22-31. A sample prescription for the fabrication of maxillary and mandibular removable appliances to correct labially or lingually malpositioned teeth.

- 0.016 in. round orthodontic wire (Unitek/3M, Inc.)
- 0.022 in. × 0.018 in. rectangular orthodontic wire (Unitek/3M, Inc.)
- 0.010 in. diameter, 0.030 in. arbor diameter coil spring (Unitek/3M, Inc.)
- Orthodontic elastics (Unitek/3M, Inc.)
- Orthodontic stress and tension gauge (Dontrix-Richmond Orthodontic Stress and Tension Gauges, Unitek/3M, Inc.)

Clinical Technique

1. Place anterior orthodontic bonding brackets, including at least three teeth beyond the tooth to be brought into alignment. (See the section on Placement of Orthodontic Bands earlier in this chapter.)

CLINICAL TIP. To ensure a satisfactory result the brackets must be placed perpendicular to the long axis of the tooth.

2. Place a coil spring on the arch wire between the teeth adjacent to the malposed tooth or place elastics distally to the end of the arch if space is available to activate the appliance. The force on the tooth should be one ounce, as measured by an orthodontic stress and tension gauge (Fig. 22-34).
3. Clinically evaluate the patient every 2 weeks.
4. Normal movement occurs at a rate of 1.0 to 1.5 mm per month.

ROTATED TEETH

Diagnosis

When spaces are present, often the teeth will not only migrate mesiodistally, but may also rotate. In addition, over-retention of primary teeth may cause abnormal eruption patterns of the permanent tooth, causing abnormal rotational eruption.

Treatment

In the primary and mixed dentition, early diagnosis of over-retained primary teeth is imperative. Extraction of the offending tooth often leads to self-correction. Appliance therapy is not recommended at this time. In the permanent dentition, orthodontic correction is necessary.

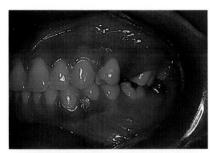

FIG. 22-32. Left buccal view of a patient with a crossbite of the maxillary first premolar.

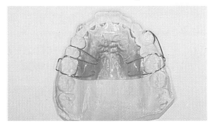

FIG. 22-33. Occlusal view of a maxillary Hawley appliance with an Adams clasp and auxiliary springs soldered at the left. The Adams clasp is coming mesially to engage the first premolar to push it palatally to eliminate the crossbite.

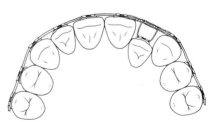

FIG. 22-34. A fixed appliance to correct a lingually malposed tooth. A coil spring is used to move the tooth. Space is gained by interproximal reduction of enamel. Note that the stabilizing arch wire extends three teeth or more past the affected tooth.

Rotated Teeth—Removable Appliance

Armamentarium

- Irreversible hydrocolloid impression
- No. 139 pliers (Unitek/3M, Inc.)

Clinical Technique

1. Make an irreversible hydrocolloid impression of the dentition.
2. Send the models to an orthodontic laboratory for fabrication of a Hawley appliance, which will include springs embedded in the lingual acrylic (Fig. 22–35).
3. Activate the lingual springs of the Hawley appliance while maintaining positive labial pressure with the labial wire.
4. Examine patients every 2 to 3 weeks.
5. Normal correction occurs at a rate of 2° to 3° per month.

Rotated Tooth—Fixed Appliance

Fixed appliances require that the generalist is absolutely familiar with all aspects of fixed orthodontic therapy. Failure to adhere to proper orthodontic technique could have adverse consequences.

Armamentarium

- Basic bracket and band placement setup (see the section on Placement of Orthodontic Bands earlier in this chapter)
- Anterior edgewise orthodontic brackets (metal, ceramic, or plastic, depending on the esthetics requirements)
- 0.016 in. round orthodontic wire (Unitek/3M, Inc.)
- 0.022 in. × 0.018 in. rectangular orthodontic wire (Unitek/3M, Inc.)
- 0.010 in. diameter, 0.030 in. arbor diameter coil spring (Unitek/3M, Inc.)
- Orthodontic elastics
- Orthodontic stress and tension gauge (Dontrix-Richmond Orthodontic Stress and Tension Gauges, Unitek/3M, Inc.)
- No. 128 pliers (Unitek/3M, Inc.)

Clinical Technique

1. Place the orthodontic brackets or bands on at least 3 teeth (or up to the first molar) on each side of the rotated tooth. (See the section on Placement of Orthodontic Bands earlier in this chapter.)
2. Place a lingual button on the tooth to be rotated. (See the section on Placement of Orthodontic Bands earlier in this chapter.) (Fig. 22–36).

CLINICAL TIP. To ensure a satisfactory result, the brackets must be placed perpendicular to the long axis of the tooth.

3. Construct an ideal arch wire to serve as a guide for the rotation of the malposed tooth.
4. Activate the appliance with orthodontic elastics.

CLINICAL TIP. The arch wire must follow ideal arch form, otherwise migration of other teeth could occur.

5. Clinically evaluate the patient every 2 weeks.
6. Normal rotation occurs at a rate of 3 to 5° per month (Figs. 22-37 to 22-39).

CLINICAL TIP. Relapse is common after rotational correction of malpositioned teeth. Over-correction is recommended to compensate for this relapse. Permanent retention can be achieved by bonding the lingual surface of the tooth to the adjacent teeth with a thin orthodontic wire embedded in composite resin.

EXTRUDED TEETH

Diagnosis

An extrusion occurs when a tooth has over-erupted past the normal plane of occlusion. It is most commonly seen in middle aged or older patients who have lost opposing teeth. Most cases also have periodontal involvement.

Treatment

Correction of Extruded Teeth—Removable Appliance

Armamentarium

- Irreversible hydrocolloid impression
- Orthodontic elastic (Unitek/3M, Inc.)
- No. 128 pliers (Unitek/3M, Inc.)

Clinical Technique

1. Make an irreversible hydrocolloid impression of the dentition.
2. Send the models to an orthodontic laboratory for fabrication of a Hawley appliance (Fig. 22–40).
3. The Hawley appliance should be modified with both a labial and palatal hook.
4. Following placement of the appliance stretch the elastic over the labial and palatal hooks. This serves as a sling to intrude the tooth. Use the smallest elastic that will fit on the hooks.
5. Examine the patient every 2 weeks.
6. The normal rate of correction of extrusion is 0.1 to 0.25 mm per month.

Correction of Extruded Teeth—Fixed Appliance

Fixed appliances require that the generalist is absolutely familiar with all aspects of fixed orthodontic therapy. Failure to adhere to proper orthodontic technique could have adverse consequences.

Armamentarium

- Basic bracket and band placement setup (see the section on Placement of Orthodontic Bands earlier in this chapter)
- Anterior edgewise orthodontic brackets (metal, ce-

NAME: _____ DATE: _____

ADDRESS: _____ PHONE: (___)_____

CITY: _____ STATE: _____ ZIP: _____

PATIENT NAME: _____

DATE NEEDED: _____ TIME NEEDED: _____

SPECIAL INSTRUCTION:

Please construct a maxillary Hawley appliance with a labial bow and circumferential clasps on the first molars. Add springs coming from the lingual acrylic as shown to rotate #7 mesiolabially and #9 distolabially.

Also, please construct a mandibular Hawley appliance with a labial bow and circumferential clasps on the first molars. Add a spring coming from the lingual as shown to rotate #26 distolabially.

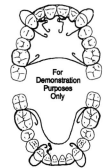

For Demonstration Purposes Only

Thank you.

SIGNATURE: _____ LICENSE: _____

FIG. 22–35. A sample prescription for the fabrication of maxillary and mandibular removable appliances to correct rotated teeth.

ramic, or plastic, depending on the esthetics requirements)
- 0.016 in. round orthodontic wire (Unitek/3M, Inc.)
- 0.022 in. × 0.018 in. rectangular orthodontic wire (Unitek/3M, Inc.)
- Orthodontic elastics (Unitek/3M, Inc.)
- Orthodontic stress and tension gauge (Dontrix-Richmond Orthodontic Stress and Tension Gauges, Unitek/3M, Inc.)

Clinical Technique

1. Place orthodontic bonded brackets on malposed tooth and on at least 3 teeth on each side of the tooth to be moved. (See the section on Placement of Orthodontic Bands earlier in this chapter.)

CLINICAL TIP. It is important that the brackets are placed perpendicular to the long axis of the tooth and at the central part of the crown. Because the tooth requiring intrusion is at a different level than the adjacent teeth, the bracket must also be at the corresponding level. Following the completion of therapy all brackets will line up.

2. Construct an ideal arch wire.

CLINICAL TIP. To ensure a satisfactory result the arch wire must follow ideal arch form.

3. Crimp and tie the labial arch wire to allow for ligation of the teeth.
4. The crimped arch wire will intrude the teeth as it returns to ideal form.
5. Clinically evaluate the patient every 2 weeks.
6. The normal rate of correction of extrusion is 0.25 to 0.5 mm per month.

FIG. 22–36. A fixed appliance that is used to correct a rotated tooth. Note the use of elastic ligature attached to a lingual button to help rotate the tooth.

FIG. 22–37. Occlusal view of a mandibular archwire with elastic "lig-o-ring" ligature placed on an archwire prior to the placement of the archwires into the molar tubes.

FIG. 22–38. Occlusal view of a patient's left buccal area. The ligature is being stretched and attached to a button on the lingual side of a mesiolingually rotated second premolar.

FIG. 22–39. Occlusal view of the left buccal area of the patient shown in Figure 22–38. The ligature is in place on the lingual side of the second premolar and rotation is taking place.

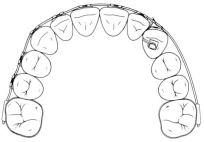

FIG. 22–36

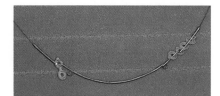

FIG. 22–37

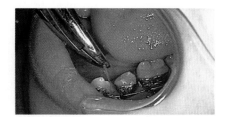

FIG. 22–38

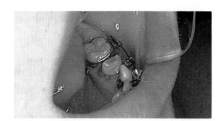

FIG. 22–39

INTRUDED TEETH

Intrusion of teeth is caused by either ankylosis or trauma. Ankyloses are impossible to orthodontically move and often require prosthetic treatment to correct esthetic problems. Traumatically intruded teeth or teeth that require extrusion because of traumatic loss of the clinical crown can be extruded orthodontically. The principles discussed in the section on Extruded Teeth apply, except that the forces are reversed as discussed under the section on Crown Lengthening Procedures in Chapter 21—Esthetics and Periodontics. (Figs. 22–41 to 22–43).

SIMPLE ANTERIOR CROSSBITE

Diagnosis

First molars are often in a Class I relationship with one or more of the maxillary anterior teeth inclined lingually. The simpler cases involving only one or two teeth can be treated by the generalist, however, the more complicated cases involving multiple teeth and an extreme lack of space should be referred to a specialist. These cases can normally be diagnosed on clinical examination, but space requirements are easier to determine when study models are utilized.

Tongue Depressor Therapy

When the patient is cooperative and only a single tooth is involved, the simplest solution is to use a tongue depressor to leverage the tooth into correct alignment.

Armamentarium

- Tongue depressor

Clinical Technique

1. Instruct the patient to hold the tongue blade at a 45° angle against the lingual surface of the maxillary incisor.
2. Caution the patient not to impinge on the soft tissue of the palate with the tip of the blade while biting down.
3. Instruct the patient to execute this biting maneuver 50 times, twice a day, for 2 weeks. This is usually sufficient for the tooth to move labially into its correct position.

CLINICAL TIP. This technique works rapidly, provided enough space is available. The patient experiences some pain, however. Therefore, this technique is usually unsuccessful with sensitive patients or those with a low level of pain tolerance.

Appliance Therapy

An alternative to tongue depressor therapy is the use of a removable appliance. This is indicated when space is sufficient, but the patient either cannot use or cannot tolerate tongue blade therapy or when several teeth are involved. A Hawley appliance with either an acrylic inclined plane or a finger spring to push the tooth into

NAME: _____ DATE:_____

ADDRESS: _____ PHONE: (___)_____

CITY: _____ STATE: _____ ZIP: _____

PATIENT NAME: _____

DATE NEEDED: _____ TIME NEEDED: _____

SPECIAL INSTRUCTION:

Please construct a maxillary Hawley appliance with a labial bow and circumferential clasps on the first molars. Solder a hook onto the labial bow by tooth #9. Imbed a hook in the acrylic palatal to #9 so that an elastic can be placed to intrude the tooth.

Also, construct a mandibular Hawley appliance in a similar manner to allow for the intrusion of #26.

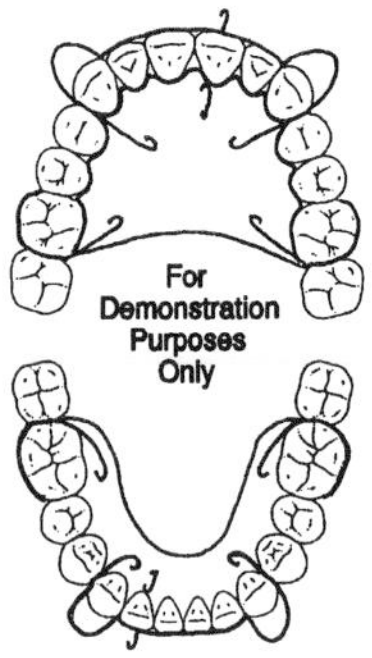

Thank you.

SIGNATURE: _____ LICENSE:_____

FIG. 22–40. A sample prescription for the fabrication of maxillary and mandibular removable appliances to intrude teeth.

position is used. The finger spring appliance incorporates an occlusal plane to prevent the mandibular incisors from occluding. This type of appliance is used when a true cross bite relationship exists. The inclined plane appliance is utilized when the patient can incise in an edge-to-edge relationship when closing into the most retruded mandibular position but the mandible slips anterior into a bite of convenience during mastication. Sometimes, especially when space is insufficient, it is necessary to use full appliance therapy with Class III mechanics to correct the cross bite.

Correction of Anterior Crossbite— Removable Appliance

Armamentarium

- Irreversible hydrocolloid impression
- No. 139 orthodontic pliers (Unitek/3M, Inc.)

Clinical Technique

1. Make an irreversible hydrocolloid impression.
2. Send the models to an orthodontic laboratory for fabrication of a Hawley appliance (Fig. 22–44).
3. Insert the Hawley appliance.
4. For the inclined plane appliance, adjust the acrylic so the mandibular incisors are forced to occlude lingually and cannot position labially into a bite of convenience.

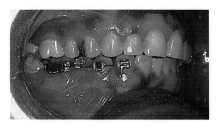

FIG. 22–41. Right buccal view of a patient with a fixed segmented arch wire on the mandibular right canine through the first molar to elevate the crown of the mandibular right second premolar.

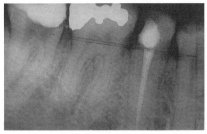

FIG. 22–42. Dental radiograph of the patient shown in Figure 22–41 at the beginning of treatment.

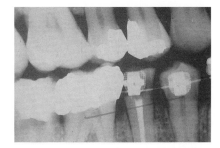

FIG. 22–43. Radiograph of patient shown in Figure 22–41 demonstrating elevation of the mandibular second premolar.

NAME: _____ DATE:_____

ADDRESS: _____ PHONE: (___)_____

CITY: _____ STATE: _____ ZIP: _____

PATIENT NAME: _____

DATE NEEDED: _____ TIME NEEDED: _____

SPECIAL INSTRUCTION:

Please construct a maxillary Hawley appliance with a labial bow and circumferential clasps on the first molars. Place springs palatal to #9 and #10. Build an occlusal table palatal to #6 through #11 to open the bite to allow for the correction of the crossbite of #9 and #10.

Also, construct a mandibular Hawley appliance with a labial bow and circumferential clasps on the first molars. Build up occlusal acrylic with a lingual inclination over the incisal edges of #22 through #27 to correct the crossbite.

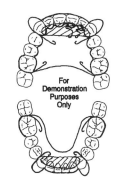

For Demonstration Purposes Only

Thank you.

SIGNATURE: _____ LICENSE:_____

FIG. 22–44. A sample prescription for the fabrication of maxillary and mandibular removable appliances to correct an anterior crossbite.

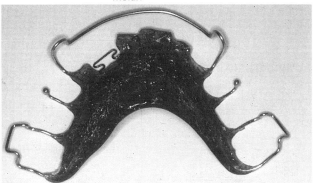

FIG. 22–46. Occlusal view of a Hawley appliance with an Adams clasp on the first molars and a palatal spring imbedded in the acrylic to move the lateral incisor out of crossbite.

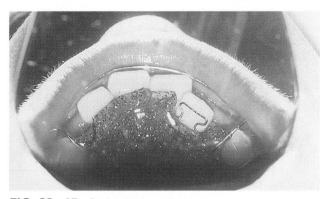

FIG. 22–47. Occlusal view of the patient shown in Figure 22–45 with the Hawley appliance engaged.

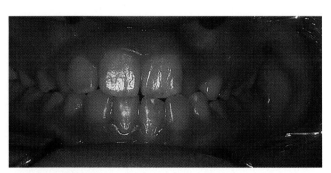

FIG. 22–45. Anterior view of a patient with a crossbite on the maxillary lateral incisor.

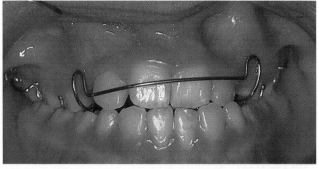

FIG. 22–48. Anterior view of the patient shown in Figure 22–45 with correction of the crossbite of the maxillary left incisor.

5. For the lingual finger spring appliance, adjust the spring so the lingually tipped maxillary anterior teeth are pushed labially. The occlusal plane prevents the mandibular anterior teeth from occluding with the maxillary anterior teeth, which would inhibit therapeutic correction.
6. Clinically evaluate the patient every 2 week.
7. Therapy is usually completed in 2 to 3 months (Figs. 22-45 to 22-48).

Correction of Anterior Crossbite—Fixed Appliance

Fixed appliances require that the generalist is absolutely familiar with all aspects of fixed orthodontic therapy. Failure to adhere to proper orthodontic technique could have adverse consequences.

Armamentarium

- Basic bracket and band placement setup (see the section on Placement of Orthodontic Bands earlier in this chapter)
- Anterior edgewise orthodontic brackets (metal, ceramic, or plastic depending on the esthetics requirements)
- 0.016 in. round orthodontic wire (Unitek/3M, Inc.)
- 0.022 in. × 0.018 in. rectangular orthodontic wire (Unitek/3M, Inc.)
- 0.010 in. diameter, 0.030 in. arbor diameter coil spring (Unitek/3M, Inc.) (optional)
- Orthodontic elastics (Unitek/3M, Inc.)
- Orthodontic stress and tension gauge (Dontrix-Richmond Orthodontic Stress and Tension Gauges, Unitek/3M, Inc.)

Clinical Technique

1. Place anterior orthodontic brackets on all anterior teeth; place bands on the first molars. (See the section on Placement of Orthodontic Bands earlier in this chapter.)

CLINICAL TIP. To ensure a satisfactory result, the brackets must be placed perpendicular to the long axis of the tooth.

---

2. Place bilateral Class III elastics from the mandibular canines to the maxillary first molars, in order to move the mandibular anterior teeth lingually. In addition, bilateral coil springs may be placed between the maxillary canine and the first molar brackets if the maxillary anterior teeth must be moved labially. The elastic should generate 1 ounce of force as measured by an orthodontic stress and tension gauge.
3. Clinically evaluate the patient every 2 weeks.
4. Normal movement occurs at a rate of 1.0 to 1.5 mm per month (Figs. 22-49 to 22-54).

ANTERIOR OPEN BITE

An open bite occurs when teeth of the opposing arches do not meet in a centric occlusion position (Fig. 22–55). This can occur with any type of molar rela-

tionship. Treatment is often complicated and diagnosis usually requires clinical evaluation along with examination of study models, cephalometric and panoramic radiographs. The generalist may wish to consult a specialist about these cases. Ankylosed teeth may require alternative treatments.

Diagnosis

Deleterious habits, such as finger or tongue sucking, are the cause of anterior open bites in children. Constant biting on pencils or on the stem of a pipe can be the cause in adults. Sometimes the problem persists when the tongue fills the void. Gross osseous dysplasia, such as seen in maxillary micrognathia, mandibular hypertrophy, or rickets, can give rise to an open bite, but this is usually a minor manifestation of the gross discrepancy.

Treatment

Treatment requires habit elimination. (See the section on Generalized Spacing earlier in this chapter.) Conventional orthodontic fixed appliance therapy with vertical elastics may be necessary to close the bite. In extreme cases, a surgical orthognathic approach may be indicated. It is important to provide adequate stabilization of the teeth following orthodontic therapy.

POSTERIOR OPEN BITE

Diagnosis

Tongue thrusting is often the suspected cause of a posterior open bite, but it is rarely the primary cause; it merely allows the problem to persist. Abnormal skeletal development is the primary cause of a bilateral posterior open bite. Ankyloses of primary or permanent teeth may also be the cause of a localized posterior open bite.

Treatment

The etiology of the open bite must be considered when treatment planning.

Muscular. Although the tongue is rarely the primary cause of a posterior open bite, an appropriate appliance often must be constructed to keep the tongue from interfering with bite closure.

Dental. If the posterior open bite is caused by ankylosis of a primary tooth, radiographs must be taken to verify that a permanent tooth is present. If it is present, the primary tooth should be extracted and the permanent successor must be brought into position by an orthodontic specialists. If it is not present, alternative therapy includes attempting to rebuild the primary tooth to proper occlusion or extracting the tooth and constructing a fixed bridge. If a permanent tooth is ankylosed, it cannot be moved orthodontically. The ankylosed tooth must be restored to proper occlusion prosthetically. If the ankylosed tooth cannot be restored, it should be extracted and prosthetically replaced.

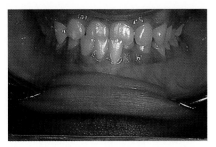

FIG. 22–49. Frontal view of a patient with an anterior crossbite involving the maxillary central and lateral incisors and the mandibular right lateral, right central, and left central incisors.

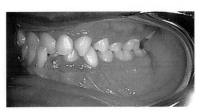

FIG. 22–50. Left labial view of the patient shown in Figure 22–49.

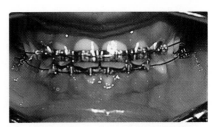

FIG. 22–51. Frontal view of the patient shown in Figure 22–49 with the fixed appliance in place. The first molars and all anterior teeth are banded. Ceramic, plastic, or even metal brackets could be substituted for bands if esthetics is a concern.

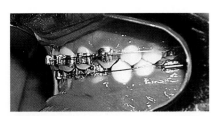

FIG. 22–52. Left labial view of the patient shown in Figure 22–51.

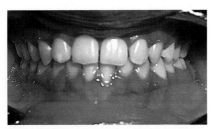

FIG. 22–53. Frontal view following the completion of orthodontic treatment.

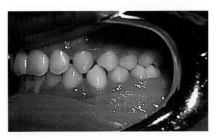

FIG. 22–54. Left labial view following the completion of orthodontic treatment.

Skeletal. A bilateral posterior open bite of skeletal origin must be treated with orthodontic mechanotherapy alone or combined with a surgical orthognathic approach.

EXCESSIVE OVERBITE

Excessive overbite can occur with all types of molar relationships. Dental factors are often the cause in Class I malocclusions, whereas skeletal factors are often combined with dental factors in Class II or III malocclusions. The generalist most commonly will work with a specialist to diagnose these cases, with the orthodontist treating the more complicated types.

Diagnosis

Cephalometric analysis is necessary to confirm whether the problem is skeletal or dental in nature.

Treatment

In the primary dentition, eliminate occlusal interferences; otherwise, treatment is postponed until further growth has occurred.

In the mixed and permanent dentition, if there is a Class I molar relationship, use a bite plate to allow the first molars to erupt and the curve of Spee to decrease. If there is a Class II molar relationship, extensive appliance therapy is indicated.

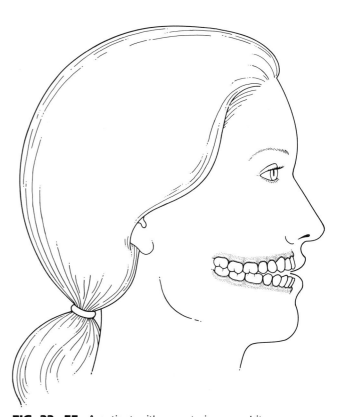

FIG. 22–55. A patient with an anterior open bite.

CLOSED BITE

Usually seen in adults with any molar relationship, a closed bite is best diagnosed and treated through a team approach. Diagnosis can often be made clinically, but it is confirmed with study models and radiographic evidence.

Diagnosis

Commonly, in cases involving areas that have been edentulous for a long duration, teeth have tipped into a neighboring extraction site or super-erupted from the opposing dental arch. A loss of arch length and posterior bite collapse, resulting in a closing or deepening of the bite, results in an exaggerated curve of Spee.

Treatment

The bite is opened by orthodontic movement of tipped and intruded teeth in preparation for prosthetic rehabilitation. The removal of the orthodontic appliances should occur on the same day as preparation for fixed prosthetic replacements because the provisional restoration acts as a retainer.

LATERAL DISHARMONIES OF THE TEETH AND DENTAL ARCHES

Lateral disharmonies of the teeth and dental arches appear in patients of all ages, without regard to anteroposterior molar relationships. Lateral disharmonies result in excess wearing of the cusps that normally maintain a functional occlusal relationship. Since cuspal wear is generally a function of time, the earlier the treatment is instituted, the more successful and stable the final result.

Differential Diagnosis

Lateral disharmonies involving single or multiple teeth and can be unilateral or bilateral. The generalist should have little difficulty diagnosing those of dental origin, whereas those of muscular and skeletal origin are usually diagnosed by a specialist. Study models will show cuspal wear but a clinical examination is required to determine whether the disharmony is unilateral or bilateral, and whether it is caused by a skeletal or muscular deviation from normal development.

Skeletal. There is a gross disharmony between the bony bases. Unilateral crossbites exhibit a deviation of the midline of the two jaws when the teeth are in occlusion. Bilateral crossbites may have a normal midline relationship or may mimic a unilateral crossbite with a shifted midline. The difference is that this shift is one of convenience and occurs at the last moment of mandibular closure. If the mandible is placed in its most retruded position and slowly closed, the midline will be centered until just before occlusal contact is made.

Muscular. Occlusal interferences develops because of an aberrant muscular closing pattern.

Dental. Often caused by lack of space in the dental arch, it usually involves tipped teeth and is sometimes accompanied by a muscular shift.

Treatment

Treatment of these conditions can be handled by the experienced generalist, especially when dealing with the dental type. Those caused by skeletal or muscular deviations probably should be referred to a specialist for treatment.

Skeletal. If the crossbite is slight, a maxillary lingual arch may be used to expand the maxilla, or a Hawley appliance with an inclined plane may be used if only one or two teeth are involved. (See the section on Correction of Anterior Crossbites earlier in this chapter; modify the appliance to move involved buccal teeth.) In more severe cases, the treatment of choice would be a rapid palatal expansion appliance.

Muscular. In the primary or mixed dentition occlusal grinding often allows the proper closing pattern to resume.

In the permanent dentition occlusal grinding may allow for a proper closing pattern, however appliance therapy may be necessary.

NAME: _____ DATE: _____

ADDRESS: _____ PHONE: (___) _____

CITY: _____ STATE: _____ ZIP: _____

PATIENT NAME: _____

DATE NEEDED: _____ TIME NEEDED: _____

SPECIAL INSTRUCTION:

Please construct a maxillary rapid palatal expansion appliance. Add labial wires to the bands on #3 and #5 and #12 and #14. Note that the bands placed on #3, #5, #12 and #14 were removed with the impression.

Thank you.

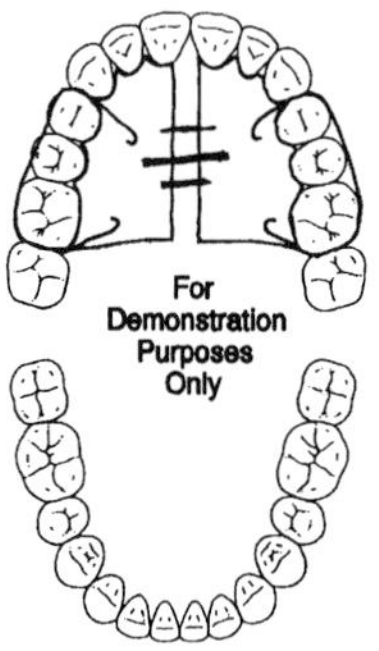

For Demonstration Purposes Only

SIGNATURE: _____ LICENSE: _____

FIG. 22—56. A sample prescription for the fabrication of a maxillary rapid palatal expansion appliance to correct a buccal crossbite involving all teeth distal to the canine.

Dental. Treatment involves regaining space for the tooth or teeth to fit into the arch, by expanding the arch or interproximal stripping.

The crossbite is eliminated by banding or bonding brackets onto the teeth in the opposing arches and having the patient wear through-the-bite elastics attached from buttons or hooks placed on the side of the tooth opposite the direction of desired tooth movement. If an anterior tooth is involved, a Hawley appliance with a finger spring to push the tooth labially and an occlusal plane to prevent the opposing arch from making contact during the time of movement may be used. (See the section on Correction of Anterior Crossbites earlier in this chapter.)

Correction of Posterior Crossbite—Palatal Expansion—Removable Appliance

A fixed appliance is the preferred method of palatal expansion because removable appliances tend to dislodge during therapy.

Armamentarium

- Irreversible hydrocolloid impression
- Adjustment instrument for palatal expansion device (supplied by laboratory)

Clinical Technique

1. Make an irreversible hydrocolloid impression.
2. Send the models to an orthodontic laboratory for fabrication of a Hawley appliance modified with an expansion screw to expand the palate laterally. (Fig. 22–56).
3. Insert the Hawley appliance.
4. Instruct the patient to adjust the palatal expansion device one-quarter turn twice daily.
5. Clinically evaluate the patient every 2 week.
6. Expansion occurs at a rate of 2.0 to 3.0 mm per month.
7. Once palatal expansion is complete, securely lock the expansion mechanism by applying auto-cured acrylic. Leave the appliance in place an additional 6 to 8 weeks to allow for adequate healing and retention.

Correction of Posterior Crossbite—Palatal Expansion—Fixed Appliance

Fixed appliances require that the generalist be absolutely familiar with all aspects of fixed orthodontic therapy. Failure to adhere to proper orthodontic technique could have adverse consequences.

Armamentarium

- Basic bracket and band placement setup (see the section on Placement of Orthodontic Bands, earlier in this chapter)
- Orthodontic bands (Unitek/3M, Inc.)
- Irreversible hydrocolloid impression
- Adjustment instrument for palatal expansion device (supplied by laboratory)

Clinical Technique

1. Fit the bands onto the maxillary first premolars (or first deciduous molars) and molars. (See the section on Placement of Orthodontic Bands earlier in this chapter.) *Do not* cement the bands.
2. Make an irreversible hydrocolloid impression with the bands in place. If the bands do not come out with the impression they should be removed from the teeth and set into the impression prior to the impression being poured up with dental stone.
3. Send the models to an orthodontic laboratory for fabrication of the fixed rapid palatal expansion appliance.
4. Cement the appliance in place with zinc phosphate cement.
5. Instruct the patient to adjust the palatal expansion device one-quarter turn twice daily.
6. Clinically evaluate the patient every 2 week.
7. Expansion occurs at a rate of 2.0 to 3.0 mm per month. Active expansion is usually completed in 4 to 6 weeks.
8. Once palatal expansion is complete, securely lock the expansion mechanism by applying auto-cured acrylic. Leave the appliance in place an additional 6 to 8 weeks to allow for adequate healing and retention (Figs. 22-57 to 22-67).

CLASS II DISTOCLUSION

A normal relationship, i.e., neutroclusion (Angle Class I), exists when the mesial buccal cusp of the maxillary molar occludes between the mesial and distal buccal cusps of the mandibular first molar (see Fig. 22–1). A Class II distoclusion occurs when the mandibular first molar occludes posterior to its normal relationship with the maxillary first molar (see Fig. 22–2). This is easily ascertained on clinical examination and is well documented on study models or cephalometric radiographs. Some simpler cases, especially in young patients, can be treated by a clinician who is well versed in orthodontic treatment procedures, however, referral to an orthodontist is usually indicated.

Differential Diagnosis

Skeletal. These distoclusions are caused by inherent growth patterns within the facial skeleton. Sometimes it is possible to mask these skeletal disharmonies with conventional orthodontic therapy. Occasionally orthognathic surgery is the treatment of choice. Clinically, these patients present with a large overjet of the maxillary anterior teeth.

Muscular. These distoclusions are caused by learned neuromuscular reflexes that can be altered in the primary and mixed dentition. The overjet is usually slight and functional appliances are sometimes successful in correcting the malocclusion.

Dental. These distoclusions involve mesial drifting of the teeth in the maxilla. Often, teeth exhibit edge-to-edge occlusion with severe crowding in the maxillary arch and distoclusion of the mandibular first molars.

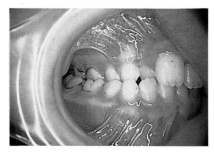

FIG. 22–57. Right lateral view of a patient with a buccal crossbite involving all the maxillary teeth distal to the right central incisor. There is also palatal crowding of the right lateral incisor.

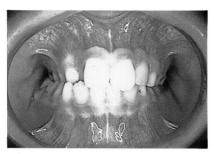

FIG. 22–58. Frontal view of the patient in Figure 22–57. There is a midline shift of the mandibular anterior teeth, which indicates that the maxilla is narrowed bilaterally and that the patient shifts to the right side into a "bite of convenience."

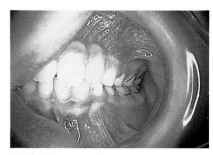

FIG. 22–59. Left lateral view of the patient shown in Figure 22–57.

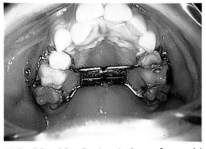

FIG. 22–60. Occlusal view of a rapid palatal expansion appliance at the beginning of treatment.

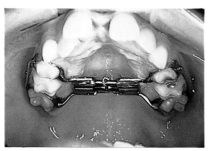

FIG. 22–61. Occlusal view of the rapid palatal expansion appliance during treatment. Note the amount of spacing between the central incisors is less than the space between the halves of the open appliance due to the action of the transeptal fibers pulling the central incisors together.

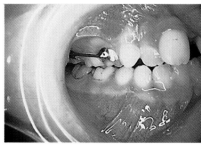

FIG. 23–62. Right lateral view of the patient shown in Figure 22–61 at the end of palatal expansion.

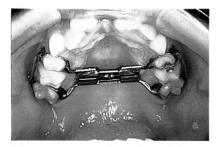

FIG. 24–63. Occlusal view of the patient shown in Figure 22–61 at the end of palatal expansion. The appliance is left passively in the mouth for six to eight weeks while calcification of the increased arch width takes place.

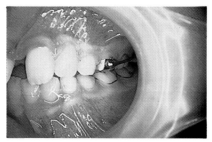

FIG. 24–64. Right lateral view of the patient shown in Figure 22–61 at the end of palatal expansion.

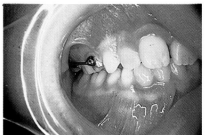

FIG. 22–65. Right lateral view of the patient shown in Figure 22–61 following the completion of orthodontic treatment. Both the midline and the palatally crowded right lateral incisor have been corrected. The diastema between the central incisors closed without intervention due to the action of the transeptal fibers.

FIG. 22–66. Frontal view following the completion of orthodontic treatment.

FIG. 22–67. Left lateral view following the completion of orthodontic treatment.

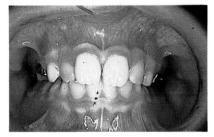

FIG. 22–66

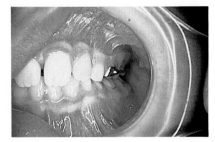

FIG. 22–67

Treatment

Skeletal. In the primary dentition palliative treatment involves control of deleterious sucking habits and elimination of any tooth interferences that might inhibit mandibular growth. Judicious occlusal equilibration at an early age allows free anterior growth of the mandible if it has been forced distally because of occlusal interferences. Many appliances and techniques have been advocated for controlling sucking habits, but the most important factor is patient cooperation. No appliance can overcome a patient who is determined to continue a pernicious habit. (See the section on Generalized Spacing earlier in this chapter.)

Palliative treatment of distoclusion in a mixed dentition usually is beyond the scope of the generalist. However, the following procedures are normally undertaken by the orthodontist. If there is a good tooth size to arch length ratio, headgear will allow growth of the mandible, while retaining the maxilla in place. A functional appliance may also be used. Many of these patients require full appliance mechanotherapy. If there is an unfavorable tooth size to arch length ratio, the patient most likely will require the extraction of teeth and full appliance therapy.

In the permanent dentition comprehensive orthodontic therapy is usually necessary.

Muscular. In the primary dentition treatment involves elimination of cuspal interferences. This often can be accomplished by the generalist, and allows the jaw to assume its normal occlusal position. If a patient requires treatment by an orthodontist, an Andresen or Frankel functional appliance could be used successfully at this stage of development.

The same therapeutic measures are used for treatment of distoclusion in the mixed dentition as in the primary dentition. Because the harmful habits are now longer standing, they are harder to correct.

In the permanent dentition the distoclusion has commonly progressed to a locked-in bite so that full orthodontic appliance therapy is usually needed.

Dental. Distoclusion is rarely seen in the primary dentition because there has not been time for mesial drifting of the teeth to take place.

In the mixed dentition of persistent thumb or finger suckers all the teeth are tipped forward, with the distal cusp of the molar positioned more occlusally than the mesial cusp. Treatment, usually undertaken by the orthodontist, entails uprighting the molars, which in turn, opens the bite and allows the anterior teeth to move distally. Head gear is usually used in the treatment of these cases.

Distoclusion in the permanent dentition is more difficult to treat because all growth potential has been lost. Often full orthodontic appliance therapy is necessary.

Special Considerations for Class II Malocclusions

Certain situations can affect the prognosis of a Class II case and may require treatment by a specialist.

Tooth Size to Alveolar Arch Length Ratio. Large teeth may require therapeutic extractions, making the case more difficult to treat.

Nasorespiratory Function. Poor nasal breathing habits cause a narrow underdeveloped palate, often rendering treatment and retention more difficult.

Parental and Patient Interest in Treatment. Enthusiastic cooperation is essential for good results

ANGLE CLASS III MESIOCLUSION

The mandibular first molars are mesial of their normal occlusal relationship in an Angle Class III malocclusion (see Fig. 22–3). Although true Class III cases represent only about 3% of the malocclusions seen in the United States, they are among the most difficult to treat. Referral to a specialist for diagnosis and therapy is indicated. When the cause is skeletal, it can be due to either a micromaxilla or mandibular hypertrophy. If the cause is functional in nature, tooth interferences cause the mandible to be moved forward of its normal position. This also is called an apparent or pseudo Class III occlusion. If the cause is dental in nature, linguoversion of the maxillary anterior teeth exists with a Class I molar relationship. (See the section on Correction of Anterior Crossbites earlier in this chapter.)

Differential Diagnosis

A differential diagnosis requires cephalometric radiographs, study models and clinical examination of the patient both at rest and during function.

Skeletal (True Class III). The characteristics of the skeletal or true Class III malocclusion follow.

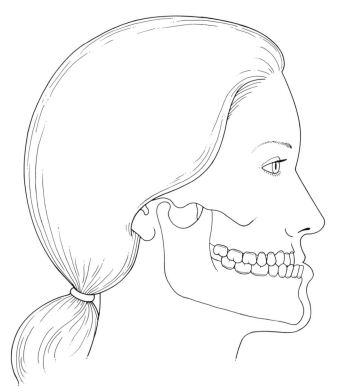

FIG. 22–68. Patient with a true Angle Class III skeletal relationship.

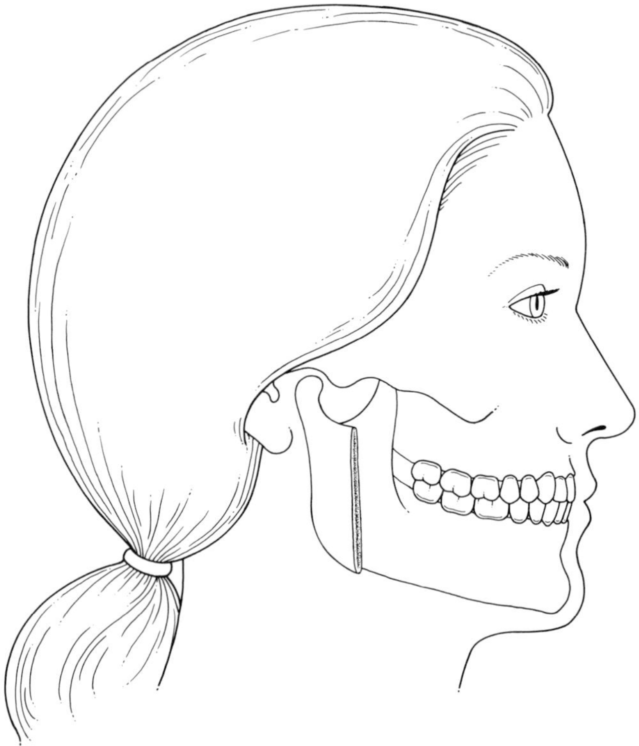

FIG. 22–69. Surgical correction of a true Angle Class III skeletal relationship.

Profile. The mandible is dominant and cannot be retruded (Fig. 22–68). This can be caused either by a large mandible or by a small maxilla. The patient will have a "dished in" appearance of the midface, especially in cases caused by a small maxilla.

Mandibular angle. A mandibular angle of 130 to 140° is present.

Mandibular incisal Angle. The mandibular incisors are often crowded and in linguoversion.

Mandibular Closing Pattern. An even closing pattern occurs (not a "hit and slide" pattern because of cuspal prematurities).

Molar Relationship. The molars will always be in a Class III relationship; when the teeth are in centric relation, when they are together in maximum intercuspation, and when the mandible is in postural rest position.

Dental (Pseudo Class III). The characteristics of the dental or pseudo Class III malocclusion follow.

Profile. The mandible is in a Class I relationship posturally at rest, but exhibits the full Class III face when the teeth are in occlusal contact.

Mandibular Angle. A mandibular angle close to 120° is present.

Mandibular Incisal Angle. The mandibular incisors are vertical or slightly in labioversion.

Mandibular Closing Pattern. When closing into maximal intercusapation, the mandible slides anteriorly because of cuspal interference.

Molar Relationship. The pseudo Class III relationship sometimes demonstrates molars in either a Class I or Class III alignment, with the mandible in maximum intercuspation and postural rest positions; therefore, one cannot rely solely on the molar position for the diagnosis. In some cases there will be a shift from a Class I to a Class III relationship on closing of the mandible.

Treatment

The etiology of the malocclusion must be considered when treatment planning.

Skeletal (True Class III). Referral to a specialist is indicated in true Class III malocclusions. Active intervention with full appliance mechanotherapy is often delayed until the permanent teeth are present. It may be necessary to include a surgical orthognathic approach (Fig. 22–69).

Dental (Pseudo Class III). In the primary or mixed dentition it is sometimes possible to correct the bite by removing any tooth interferences. This could be accomplished in the primary or mixed dentition phase with a mandibular Hawley appliance, having an anterior inclined plane. (See the section on Correction of Anterior Crossbites earlier in this chapter but modify the appliance to move the inclined plane in the opposite direction because the appliance is now on the mandible). Fixed orthodontic appliances may be used in some instances, with the use of Class III elastics to encourage a new closing pattern.

In the permanent dentition this is always treated with full appliances, and often requires orthognathic surgery.

BIMAXILLARY PROGNATHISM

In bimaxillary prognathism, the molars are in an Angle Class I relationship. Careful evaluation of the cephalometric radiograph and study models to determine the true nature of the problem is essential. The generalist should refer these difficult cases to a specialist.

Differential Diagnosis

The three types of bimaxillary prognathism follow.

Skeletal Bimaxillary Prognathism. In these cases both the mandible and the maxilla are anterior to the cranial base. Usually, it is a hereditary growth pattern. It is a racial characteristic of the Australoid, Mongoloid, and Negroid races.

Dental Bimaxillary Prognathism. In these cases, the maxillary and mandibular teeth are positioned anteriorly in their bony bases. It is often seen in patients with large teeth.

Combined Bimaxillary Prognathism. In these cases, the mandible, maxilla, and teeth are anteriorly positioned.

Treatment

The etiology of the malocclusion must be considered when treatment planning.

Skeletal Bimaxillary Prognathism. Treatment planning is complicated in these cases because it is difficult to predict growth. Maxillary growth ceases at approximately 12 years of age, but mandibular growth continues into young adulthood. These patients are difficult to treat, despite extractions, using conventional orthodontic appliances. An orthognathic surgical approach is often indicated.

Dental Bimaxillary Prognathism. These patients are difficult to treat during growth. Treatment is not possible during the primary or early mixed dentition stages because all the first premolars have not yet erupted. These patients can be treated in the late mixed dentition stage once the first premolars have erupted since these teeth must be extracted. The teeth are usually mesially inclined on their bony bases, therefore, treatment is successful in young adults with the extraction of four teeth and the use of conventional fixed appliance mechanotherapy.

Combined Bimaxillary Prognathism. Treatment of these patients consists of correcting both the skeletal and dental components of the prognathism (see above).

CLINICAL TIP. The clinician's personal esthetic preferences must not be imposed in cases of bimaxillary prognathism. Genetic and racial factors must be respected and the desires of the patient must be solicited and taken into consideration.

GROSS FACIAL DEFORMITIES

Although a wide variety of facial dysplasias may be encountered in association with congenital deformities, only two are seen frequently enough to be discussed in this chapter. All gross facial deformities should be referred to specialists for treatment.

Mandibular Prognathism. In this condition the mandible is proportionately too large for the rest of the face. It may be caused by mandibular hypertrophy, midface deficiency, or a combination of the two. Clinical examination is sufficient to diagnose the condition, but radiographs and study models will be necessary to ascertain the cause and the preferred treatment modality. (See the section on Angle Class III Mesiocclusion earlier in this chapter.)

Cleft Lip and Palate. Diagnosis of cleft lip and palate is made at birth when the lip is involved. Cases involving only the hard or soft palate are discovered later and may be brought to the dentist for diagnosis. There are several popular approaches to therapy of this condition and much research is being carried out at several cleft palate centers. Referral is indicated.

CONCLUSION

The goal of the dentist is to provide a stable and maintainable occlusion. An occlusion that cannot be maintained and is unstable will fail.[2] If restorations can be avoided by moving the teeth into a correct relationship, orthodontics is the method of choice.[3] Collaboration between the general dentist, the orthodontist, the periodontist, or any appropriate specialist is essential.[4]

Orthodontic treatment has traditionally been limited to correcting malocclusions in children or adolescents. Advances in esthetic appliance design have made adult esthetic orthodontic care feasible and commonplace.[5]

Removable appliances may be used in some cases, however, fixed appliances offer more predictable and faster results.[6] With an enlightened introduction to modern orthodontic treatment, adults will happily accept it as part of their restorative plan.

Color figures courtesy of Joy Hudecz, D.D.S., Clinical Instructor, and Malcolm E. Meistrell, Jr. D.D.S., Associate Clinical Professor of Dentistry, Orthodontic Department, Columbia School of Dental and Oral Surgery, New York, NY.

REFERENCES

1. Ward H.L., Simring, M.: Manual of Clinical Periodontology, 2nd Ed. St. Louis, C.V. Mosby, 1978.
2. LaSota, E.P.: Orthodontic considerations in prosthetic and restorative dentistry. Dent Clin North Am 32:447, 1988.
3. Dawson, P.E.: Evaluation, Diagnosis, and Treatment of Occlusal Problems. St. Louis, C.V. Mosby, 1974.
4. Baker, I.A., Stewart, A.V.: Adult orthodontics services. J Am Coll Dent 57:16, 1990.
5. McNulty, E.C.: Appliance Selection. Dent Clin North Am 32:571, 1988.
6. DeAngelis, V.: Integration of orthodontics with prosthodontics and reconstructive dentistry. J Mass Dent Soc 30:130, 1981.

David Beller, D.M.D.
Marc R. Leffler, D.D.S.

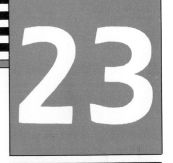

ESTHETICS AND ORAL SURGERY

Recognition by the general practitioner of an existing abnormal state is the cornerstone of patient satisfaction, for without it, appropriate treatment can never be implemented. Some oral and maxillofacial surgery procedures create better esthetics in and of themselves. Other procedures make it possible for the general practitioner to complete the esthetic restoration. An understanding of these surgical procedures will broaden the scope of possible treatments a general practitioner can present to a patient for consideration.

FACIAL DISHARMONY

The assessment of facial harmony has a significant subjective component, and is, to an extent, determined by the likes and dislikes of each individual. However, in addition to soft tissue profile and frontal esthetic considerations, the skeletal configuration of the maxilla and mandible must allow for a dental relationship amenable to chewing and the teeth within each arch must align with respect to each other to achieve true harmony (Figs. 23–1, 23–2).

Facial disharmony refers to dentofacial abnormalities involving facial contours, skeletal relationships, and occlusion. To facilitate the recognition and diagnosis of a facial skeleton that is unharmonious, the following definitions and examples are presented.

1. **Prognathism** refers to excessive jaw growth in the horizontal plane. It most often occurs in the mandible, such as in Class III malocclusion (Figs. 23–3, 23-4) but maxillary prognathism is also possible, as is prognathism of both jaws (bimaxillary prognathism).
2. **Retrognathism** refers to insufficient horizontal growth of the mandible or maxilla (Figs. 23–5, 23–6).
3. **Apertognathisim** refers to an anterior open bite (Figs. 23–7, 23–8).
4. **Vertical maxillary excess** refers to excessive growth of the maxilla in the vertical plane. It frequently manifests as a "gummy smile" (Figs. 23–9, 23–10).
5. **Lip incompetence** refers to the inability of the lips to passively appose one another at rest with an unstrained perioral musculature. It is a soft tissue result of an underlying skeletal problem. Lip incompetence is commonly seen in vertical maxillary excess (Fig. 23–11).
6. **Orthognathism** refers to the appropriate relationship between the facial bones, the teeth, and the associated soft tissue structures to achieve proper masticatory function and esthetics (see Figs. 23–1, 23–2).

Sometimes these conditions are accompanied by asymmetries, (differences between the facial midlines and the dental midlines, or a lack of coordination of the midlines of one or both jaws), malocclusions, or temporomandibular joint pain and dysfunction.

The potential orthognathic surgery patient presents to the general practitioner for several reasons. Many complain of difficulty in eating, chewing, or speaking. Others are unable to fully occlude their teeth. Temporomandibular joint pain or dysfunction is a frequent complaint accompanying skeletal malocclusions. Some patients are unhappy with the appearance of their facial contours. The general practitioner is often the first professional in a position to recognize abnormalities. Problem recognition and appropriate referral increases the patient's confidence in the general practitioner's knowledge of all aspects of dentistry.

ORTHOGNATHIC SURGERY

Orthognathic surgery is a specific area of oral and maxillofacial surgery that deals with the correction of dentofacial abnormalities involving facial contours, skeletal relationships, and occlusion. The goal of these surgical procedures is to create orthognathism.

(text continues on page 361)

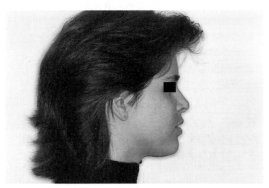

FIG. 23–1. Orthognathism or normal profile.

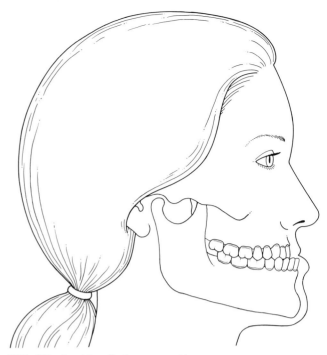

FIG. 23–4 . Mandibular prognathism.

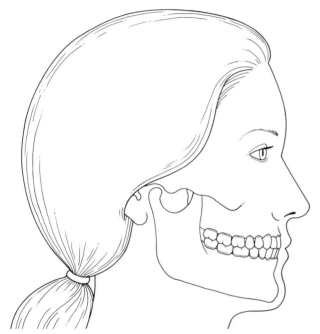

FIG. 23–2. Normal skeletal configuration of the maxilla and mandible with the teeth within each arch in proper alignment.

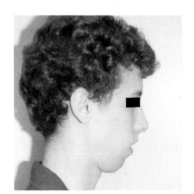

FIG. 23–5 . Mandibular retrognathism.

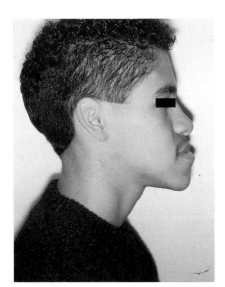

FIG. 23–3. Mandibular prognathism.

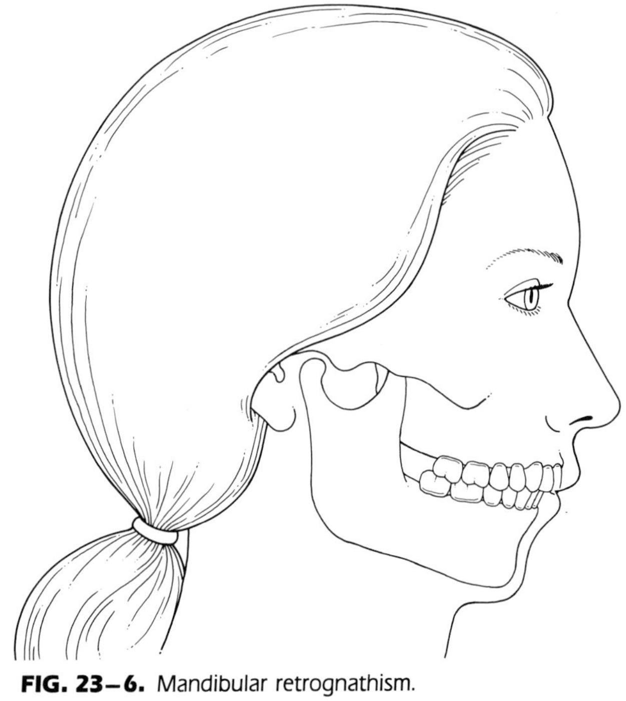

FIG. 23–6. Mandibular retrognathism.

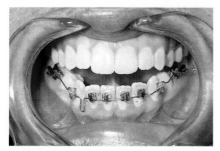

FIG. 23−7. Apertognathism (anterior open bite).

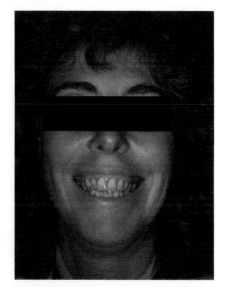

FIG. 23−9. Vertical maxillary excess.

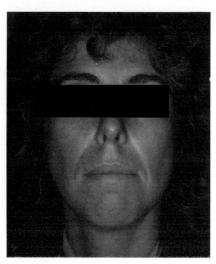

FIG. 23−11. Lip incompetence.

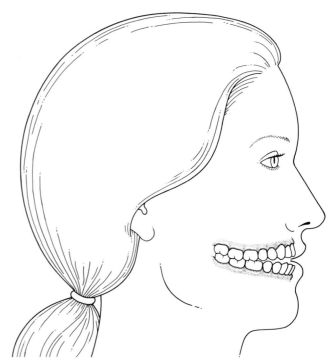

FIG. 23−8. Apertognathism (anterior open bite).

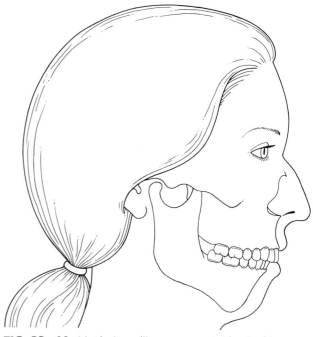

FIG. 23−10. Vertical maxillary excess combined with a mandibular retrognathia.

After the general practitioner diagnoses an abnormal situation and refers the patient to an oral and maxillofacial surgeon, additional workup is performed to confirm the diagnosis and formulate a tentative treatment plan. A lateral cephalometric radiograph (Fig. 23−12) and other radiographs are used to analyze the patient's hard and soft tissue profile measurements against a standard. The standard is a combination of several methods of numerical assessment that compare the various distances and angles within the patient's facial skeleton to the averages for the patient's race and sex. When a diagnosis is made, a prediction cephalogram is drawn so that both patient and surgeon may visualize the planned new contours. The proposed surgery is performed on articulator-mounted study models to assure that desired skeletal movements are compatible with the occlusal changes that occur simultaneously.

From this "model surgery," an acrylic occlusal registration wafer is fabricated to serve as the surgical stent. At the time of surgery, when the bones are mobilized, the teeth are placed and ligated onto the stent to assure that the occlusion predicted on the articulator is established in the patient. When this is accomplished, the

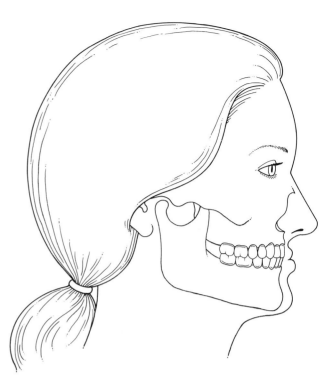

FIG. 23–13. Vertical maxillary deficiency.

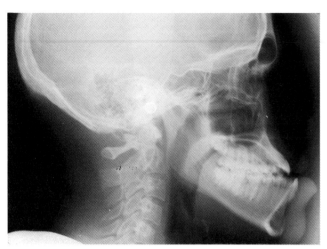

FIG. 23–12. Cephalometric radiograph.

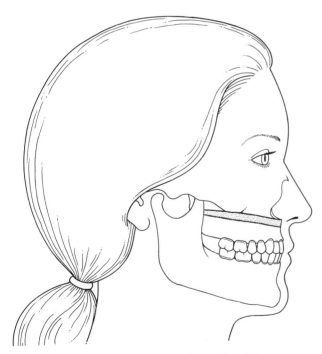

FIG. 23–14. The maxilla shown in Figure 23–13 is separated (downfractured) from the skull at a level immediately below the floor of the nose and repositioned into correct alignment.

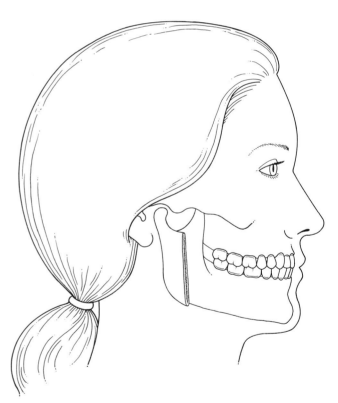

FIG. 23–15. A vertical oblique osteotomy of the ramus allows the mandible to be pushed posteriorly while maintaining the condyles in the correct position within the articular fossae.

bones are secured to the stable portion of the skeleton by whichever means of fixation is chosen by the surgeon.

This diagnosis and treatment planning phase is one of the most important aspects of treatment. Without meticulous care in treatment planning, the best of skilled surgeons may achieve only mediocre results.

SURGICAL PROCEDURES

Maxillary Surgery

The most frequently performed maxillary procedure is the LeFort I osteotomy, either involving the entire maxilla or one or more maxillary segments. The maxilla is separated from the skull at a level immediately below the floor of the nose via a method known as the "downfracture technique" (Figs. 23–13, 23–14). When the maxilla is in the downfractured position, it can be placed superiorly, inferiorly, anteriorly, posteriorly, or mediolaterally, or rotated to correct asymmetries, or positioned with any combination of these movements. The osteotomized segments are held in their new positions by intermaxillary fixation (the immobilization of the mandible via ligation to the maxilla), stents, bone wires or screws, bone plates, or a combination of these.

Mandibular Surgery

The two most common mandibular procedures involve surgery of the ramus of the mandible. The vertical oblique osteotomy of the ramus involves vertically sectioning the ramus from a point in the sigmoid notch to a point near the angle of the mandible (Fig. 23–15). When performed bilaterally, the mandible may be pushed posteriorly, to correct a prognathism, while maintaining the current condylar position within the articular fossae (Figs. 23–16, 23–17).

The sagittal split ramus osteotomy (Fig. 23–18) allows the surgeon the latitude of moving the mandible forward to correct a retrognathism or posteriorly to correct a prognathism while maintaining the current condylar position. (The choice of which procedure to use to correct a prognathism is the surgeon's.) Stabilization methods are the same as for maxillary surgery.

Combination Surgery

Simultaneous or sequential surgery of both the maxilla and the mandible may be indicated when a severe anterior-posterior discrepancy exists between the jaws, when a severe open bite exists, and when surgery of one jaw alone cannot provide the desired result (Fig. 23–19).

Segmental Surgery

Orthognathic surgery can correct segments of the jaw rather than the whole jaw. Patients who present with unilateral or bilateral crossbites, extruded posterior

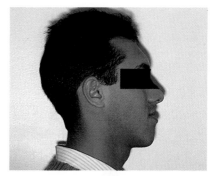

FIG. 23–16. Preoperative view of a prognathic patient.

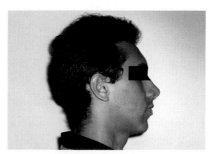

FIG. 23–17. Postoperative view of the patient shown in Figure 23–16.

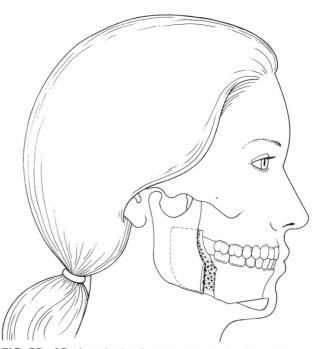

FIG. 23–18. A sagittal split ramus osteotomy allows the surgeon the latitude of moving the mandible anteriorly to correct a retrognathism or posteriorly to correct a prognathism, while again maintaining condylar position. Often a genioplasty is performed in conjunction with this procedure.

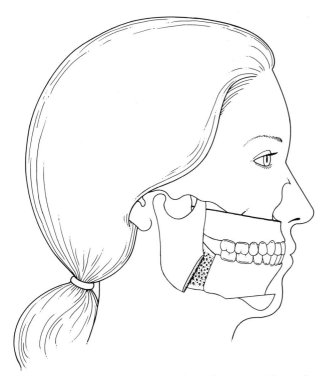

FIG. 23–19. Combination surgery is used to correct the problem shown in Figure 23–10.

maxillary segments, or large diastemata may be candidates for surgical osteotomies.

Inferior border sliding osteotomies, or genioplasties, are generally performed for cosmetic purposes and may be combined with other procedures. The bony chin is sectioned through an incision in the anterior vestibule and moved in the direction dictated by esthetics. It is then stabilized. The sliding osteotomy replaces the chin implant, which may become infected, wander from its intended position, or extrude completely through the skin or mucosa.

POSTOPERATIVE HEALING

Hospital postoperative care generally lasts 1 to 3 days. The patient, in most cases, has minimal pain or swelling and is discharged when food and liquid intake is sufficient to meet caloric and nutritional demands.

Stabilization continues until approximately 6 weeks after surgery. During this period, excessive physical activity is limited and a liquid and puree diet is prescribed. Weight loss of 10 to 15 pounds is common.

Following the 6-to 8-week healing period, the patient approaches the return to a normal diet slowly, as the associated musculature regains its preoperative strength and function.

TEAM APPROACH

The need to determine whether or not orthodontic therapy is necessary prior to surgery illustrates the importance of a team approach to diagnosis and treatment planning. When jaw segments are moved on the articu-

lator-mounted study casts and it is determined that the proposed new occlusion will be unstable, orthodontic treatment is indicated prior to surgery. Final orthodontic adjustments can be accomplished after surgery. Once the surgery and orthodontics are completed, the patient returns to the general practitioner for restorative treatment.

TREATMENT PLANNING CRITERIA FOR THE GENERAL PRACTITIONER

In cases involving a diastema, the general practitioner must determine if the space can be closed by orthodontic or restorative dentistry. If neither procedure is indicated, such as in the case of an extremely wide diastema, orthognathic surgery may be indicated (Figs. 23–20, 23–21).

The case of a large diastema serves as an example that the general practitioner, as the primary care provider, must be able to recognize situations that are potentially amenable to surgical management. Although it may be readily apparent that significant prognathism and retrognathism are surgically treatable, it may not be as obvious that less global occlusal discrepancies are frequently correctable.

Overextended dentulous posterior maxillary segments, that oppose mandibular edentulous areas and provide little or no interocclusal distance can be corrected by superiorly repositioning the extruded segments. Regional crossbites, which might otherwise require full-banded orthodontics, are often corrected by surgically moving segments in a medial or lateral direction. Multiple level occlusal planes may be leveled by surgery.

Though only several situations have been noted for exemplifications, it is most important that the general practitioner assess each patient who is to undergo prosthodontic treatment to consider what effect, if any, malocclusion will play in the restoration of the dentition. Initially, the usual methods of clinical and radiographic analyses are used. An ideal treatment plan should be formulated using both the existing occlusal relationship and a more favorable skeletal-occlusal relationship. If the latter provides the dentist and patient with a superior functional and esthetic result, the practitioner should consider referral for orthodontic or surgical correction.

It is incumbent upon the general practitioner to advise the patient that the more ideal treatment modalities often require a greater commitment in terms of time and finances to obtain a more stable, lasting and attractive result. This should be discussed in detail prior to embarking on any course of treatment, especially those involving a multidisciplinary approach.

SOLVING A PROSTHETIC DILEMMA

A 42-year-old female presented for cosmetic improvement of her dentition. Her medical history was noncontributory. The patient appeared much older than 42 years of age. She had a severe Class III relationship (Fig. 23–22) with an 18 mm negative overjet measured between the maxillary and mandibular incisal edges. She also had significant mandibular prognathism and a deficient maxillary "nose-to-lip-to-mandible" relationship. The mandibular dentition consisted of the six anterior teeth in various states of disrepair. Multiple silicate restorations and the clasps of a bilateral free end saddle removable partial denture were visible. The maxilla consisted of a removable partial denture and six periodontally involved anterior teeth with 2 to 3 + mobilities. Restoration of this case would have been simple if not for the marked skeletal abnormality. The cosmetic replacement of the teeth alone would not have been acceptable functionally or esthetically. The general practitioner referred the patient for periodontal and surgical evaluation.

It was determined that the anterior maxillary teeth were hopelessly periodontally involved and extractions were recommended. The mandibular anterior teeth required restoration after periodontal treatment.

Both maxillary and mandibular surgery were indicated because of the severe Class III discrepancy. Forward maxilla repositioning would also correct the collapsed appearance around the maxilla. The patient, however, expressed a fear of maxillary surgery and opted only for a mandibular procedure. It was expected that a satisfactory result could still be obtained in this way. The fabrication of a maxillary denture would "plump" the upper lip enough to provide an esthetic result.

Surgery consisted of bilateral vertical oblique osteotomies, which were performed extraorally. After a healing period of approximately 8 weeks, the patient was referred back to the general practitioner (Fig. 23–23) Final treatment consisted of crown placement on the mandibular anterior teeth and a new removable partial denture. The maxilla was treated with a full denture (Figs. 23–24, 23–25).

IMPLANTS

For centuries, dentistry has been searching for innovations in the treatment of edentulous regions of the mouth. Although fixed and removable prostheses have been the traditional modalities for the replacement of missing teeth, the quest for root and supportive structure replacement has continued. Treatment of the patient who is physically or psychologically incapable of accepting a removable prosthesis has also been problematic.

Types of Implants

Four types of implants are currently in use. The general practitioner must determine whether the patient needs an implant and which implant system is most applicable.

The four types of implant systems in use today are the endosseous blade implant, osseointegrated cylinder implant, subperiosteal implant, and synthetic bone im-

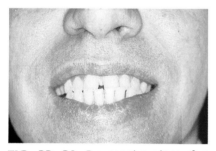

FIG. 23–20. Preoperative view of a large diastema.

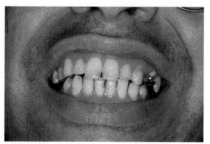

FIG. 23–21. Postoperative view of surgical closure of the diastema with orthodontic brackets in place.

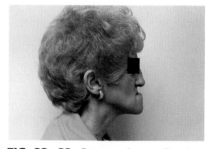

FIG. 23–22. Preoperative profile view of a prognathic patient.

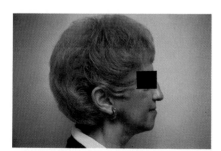

FIG. 23–23. Postoperative profile view of the patient shown in Figure 23–22.

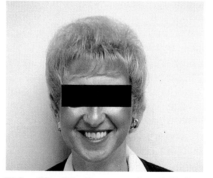

FIG. 23–24. Postoperative full face view of the patient shown in Figure 23–22.

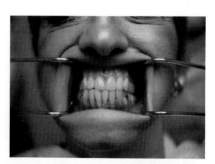

FIG. 23–25. Postoperative view of occlusion following dental treatment.

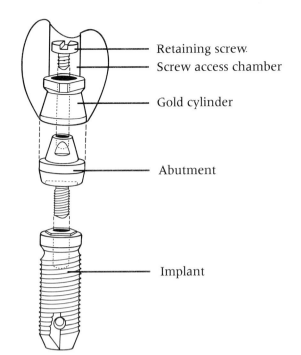

Retaining screw
Screw access chamber

Gold cylinder

Abutment

Implant

FIG. 23—26. Typical screw-type implant.

plant.[1] Synthetic bone is addressed separately.

The blade or cylinder implant is indicated when alveolar bone is sufficiently wide and deep. However, if one or both dimensions are lacking, a subperiosteal framework or synthetic bone buildup, is often preferred.[1]

Endosseous Blade Implants. In the 1960s, Dr. Leonard Linkow developed the endosseous blade implant. This system is used primarily as an intermediate abutment in a long span bridge or in free end saddle situations. The recipient bony site should be at least 8 mm wide and 8 to 12 mm deep. These implants are contraindicated in the presence of a bruxism.

Subperiosteal Implants. Subperiosteal implants are used when bone is inadequate to meet the width and depth requirements for "within the bone" (endosseous) types of implants. Three new developments have given the subperiosteal implant a more popular place in treatment planning.

First, better framework design ensures that the extensions of the framework are firmly placed over basal bone. Many earlier implants rested on alveolar bone, which was subject to resorption under masticatory pressure.

The second improvement, coating of the subperiosteal metal with hydroxyapatite, helps create a stronger bonding of soft tissue to the implant, decreases healing time, and stimulates the formation of denser bone at the implant junction.[2]

A third development, the advent of the prefabricated framework, eliminates one surgical procedure. Until recently, an initial surgical procedure was required to enable making an impression of the bone. After frame-

work fabrication, a second procedure was necessary for placement of the implant. Today CT scans and CAD/CAM multiplanar diagnostic imaging permits framework fabrication without surgery.[3] Subperiosteal implants offer an additional advantage of virtually no waiting period between implant placement and restoration fabrication.

Osseointegrated Cylinder Implants. Osseointegrated cylinder implants (Fig. 23-26) were developed by a Swedish team under the direction of P-I. Branëmark.[4] Several manufacturers have since made additional modifications to the system, such as the introduction of hydroxyapatite coating of the titanium surface. This coating is thought to allow an actual biologic bond between bone and metal.[1] The hydroxyapatite may increase the success rate when these implants are placed into fresh extraction sockets.

Other uses include situations requiring overdentures, unilateral free end prostheses, and multiple abutments for stabilization of full arch reconstruction. It is recommended that the bony recipient site measure 10 to 12 mm in depth and 7 to 8 mm in width.[5] Implant placement is a two-step procedure. The implant fixtures are entirely submerged under the oral mucosa for 4 to 6 months to allow time for osseointegration. After this healing period, the implants are surgically exposed and the abutment hardware attached. Two weeks later prosthesis construction may begin. (See also Chapter 19, Esthetics and Implant Prosthetics.)

Stent Use and Fabrication

One of the main advantages of the cylinder endosseous implant is the ability to place multiple units in an edentulous arch as abutments for full mouth fixed reconstruction. When the need for multiple units in an arch arises, it is advisable for the general practitioner to communicate to the surgeon exactly where the fixtures should be placed. This is accomplished through the use of stents. (See Chapter 19, Esthetics and Implant Prosthetics, for a complete discussion of different types of stents.) An impression of the arch is made and a model fabricated (Fig. 23—27). It is not necessary to make a full arch stent if a small section is being restored (e.g., distal free end saddle case). It is only necessary to capture the edentulous ridge and a few teeth in order to seat the stent correctly. Marks are made on the study cast to indicate the location of the implants (Fig. 23—28). A clear plastic stent (Fig. 23—29) is fabricated from any in-office system (such as an Omnivac, Buffalo Dental Mfg. Co., Inc.) or may be fabricated by a commercial laboratory. Holes are then placed in the stent to correspond with these markings (Fig. 23—30). The surgeon places the stent in the mouth and marks the tissue with an appropriate marking unit (such as methylene blue) in order to ensure correct placement of the implants. In small cases requiring one or two implants, stent use may be unnecessary because fixture placement may be clinically determined at the time of surgery. However, if more units are anticipated, stent use is recommended. This ensures that the general practitioner's

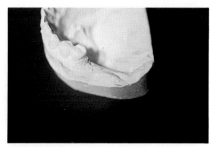

FIG. 23–27

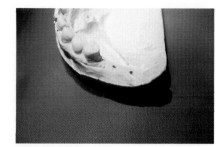

FIG. 23–28

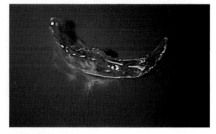

FIG. 23–29

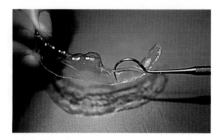

FIG. 23–30

FIG. 23–27. Model for construction of a stent.

FIG. 23–28. Model with marks placed.

FIG. 23–29. Clear plastic stent.

FIG. 23–30. Stent with holes placed.

prosthetic requirements are fulfilled. (See also Chapter 19, Esthetics and Implant Prosthetics.)

BONE GRAFTS

Bone grafts provide an additional esthetic treatment mode, i.e., ridge augmentation. This is helpful in the following situations:

1. Narrow ridges.
2. Bony undercuts.
3. Deficient vertical height.
4. Buccal plate collapse secondary to tooth removal or trauma.

Types of Bone Grafts

There are a number of different materials available for bone grafting.

Autologous Iliac Crest Cortical and Cancellous Bone. This is harvested from the patient's own hip at the time of augmentation surgery.

Autologous Rib. This may be used as an onlay graft, but it is subject to severe resorption. Again, the donor and recipient are the same patient.

Banked Freeze-Dried Bone. This is reconstituted with saline immediately prior to use. It can be placed in block or particulate form.

Synthetic Bone. A nonresorbable form is well suited for these procedures.

Hydroxyapatite. Hydroxyapatite comprises over 60% of the cortical bone of the skeleton and more than 95% of dental enamel. When used to augment a maxilla or mandible, it is shown to be both osteophilic, (chemical-

ly and mechanically "bone-liking") and osteoconductive, (fostering host bone growth by allowing normal physiologic mechanisms of bone formation to occur, i.e., no barriers are placed in the way of new bone formation), but not osteogenic (inducing host bone growth by actively assisting in the normal physiologic growth mechanisms).[6] For this reason, when building the height of a jaw by more than 6 to 8 mm, it is recommended that the hydroxyapatite is mixed with cancellous bone and marrow so that the host bone may aid in induction of new bone growth. Not only is the hydroxyapatite component not osteogenic, but when the vertical build-up above exceeds 6 to 8 mm, the ratio of the horizontal surface area (at the implant interface) to height increase becomes undesirable. This adversely affects prosthesis-bearing strength when subjected to functional and parafunctional conditions. On the other hand, if only autogenous bone is used for augmentation, the final result may be unsatisfactory. Post surgically there is approximately a 20% loss of graft height when autogenous bone is mixed with hydroxyapatite, a 10% loss of height when using hydroxyapatite alone, and a 50% loss of height with autogenous bone grafts alone.

Others. A number of other synthetic graft materials are available. A plasticized particulate formulation marketed as HTR (hard tissue replacement) has been used similarly to hydroxyapatite. Block synthetic materials including Proplast, Silastic and Teflon have been used to augment facial bones and to replace large regional defects.

Surgical Technique for Bone Graft

Surgical ridge aumentation can be achieved via a vertical incision anteriorly or via two incisions in the canine region. A tunnel is initially made superficial to the periosteum as a space-gaining mechanism. Then the incision is carried through the periosteum and a subperiosteal tunnel is formed, pushing the periosteum outward into the previously gained space. Then using a syringe, augmentation material is placed into this tunnel beneath the periosteum, so that it is in direct contact with the underlying bone. Following the surgery, a prefabricated clear acrylic stent is placed over the surgical site to assist in control of particle movement and to promote good sulcus depth. When anything more than an isolated, non-force-bearing area is augmented, the stent is ligated into position using circumosseous wires or sutures. If the augmentation is minimal, a removable stent may be used. Dentures are rarely appropriate because it is difficult to modify them sufficiently to accommodate the surgical changes.

The decision regarding the type of stent to be used, or whether to use a stent, is made by the surgeon based on preoperative assessment of the patient, personal preference, experience, and, when appropriate, patient concerns and desires.

A good surgical stent possesses many characteristics. Ideally, it is transparent, so that deleterious internal tissue compression can be noted at the time of placement, however, this is not mandatory. It should passively fit the surgical site, providing adequate support without excessive pressure on the postoperative morphology. It should be firm enough to allow for external wire placement and should be easily adjusted the operating room so that material may be readily added or removed. Clear acrylic meets all of these criteria.

Fabrication of the stent is usually the responsibility of the surgeon, and it is made upon a stone model after "model augmentation surgery" demonstrates a prosthetically satisfactory and surgically feasible result. However, in large augmentations, the general practitioner can assist in stent fabrication by providing the surgeon with a border-molded, muscle-trimmed cast on which the stent can be fabricated. This step greatly aids postoperative patient comfort by assuring ideal extension into tissue borders. Because the stent should remain in place for approximately 2 to 3 weeks it may be made with teeth in the anterior region for esthetic purposes. The stent is then relined or a temporary denture fabricated. After 4 to 6 weeks, a permanent denture may be fabricated. If it is found that the augmentation has caused too much of the vestibular sulcus to be obliterated, a corrective vestibuloplasty should be performed 8 weeks after the initial surgery. Vestibuloplasty consists of a mucosal flap extending from the alveolar crest to the depth of the vestibule. In maxillary vestibuloplasties, skin grafting is not always necessary. In the mandible, the same incision and flap can be performed but a skin graft is indicated because otherwise regression will occur due to strong perimandibular muscle pull. Dentures can then be constructed 1 month after vestibular surgery.

Case Presentations

A 25-year-old patient presented with a small defect in the maxillary ridge (Fig. 23–31). Excessive bone loss occurred after extraction of the maxillary canine and first premolar following a traumatic injury. The desired ridge shape and height was simulated using acrylic on a study model. Then, via a small incision and tunnelling, hydroxyapatite was packed in an attempt to duplicate the model. A stent was not necessary and the material was placed by "freehand" (Fig. 23–32). Approximately 1 month later prosthetics were constructed.

A 26-year-old female presented with a severe Class II malocclusion. Her medical history was noncontributory. A sagittal split osteotomy was performed (Fig. 23–33). Postoperatively, the occlusion was in excellent relationship but the patient still desired more fullness to her lower lip (Fig. 23–34). An hydroxyapatite augmentation of the mandibular vestibule below the incisor teeth protruded the lower lip and resulted in improved esthetics (Fig. 23–35).

SUBMENTAL LIPOSUCTION

Submental liposuction is frequently performed as an adjunct to rhytidoplasty (face-lift)[8–10] and to head and neck flap procedures.[11] It should be considered as possible treatment for a "double chin" deformity as a single procedure or in combination with orthognathic surgery of the mandible. Liposuction has been performed in Europe for nearly 20 years with results that are predictable and favorable.[12]

Evaluation and preparation for liposuction is similar to that for orthognathic surgery and involves visual analysis and palpation of the neck, cephalograms, frontal and lateral photographs, and study casts. These allow the surgeon to differentiate purely bony deformities from those combined with a soft tissue component and to be able to predict the proposed soft tissue alignment. Palpation of the region enables evaluation of the amount of excess fat to be removed. Removal of an inadequate amount of fat will result in continued sagging, whereas excessive fat removal may cause a concave or invaginated defect. Intra- and postoperative complications are rare.[12] The procedure is commonly performed using general anesthesia or intravenous sedation in an operating room and healthy patients are often discharged the day of surgery.

Surgical Technique for Submental Liposuction

A blunt-ended suction cannula attached to a vacuum pump is placed into the area of excessive fat accumulation. Overabundant fat is removed via the negative pressure gradient created by the pump. The placement of the incision is important because it determines access to the prepared site.

Submental liposuction is frequently performed via a small extraoral skin incision made inconspicuously in normal skin folds. However, an entirely intraoral approach, which totally eliminates even the smallest of scars on the face, has been developed. After making an incision deep in the mandibular anterior muccobuccal fold, tunneling proceeds below and behind the bony chin until the pocket of fat is carefully located. The suc-

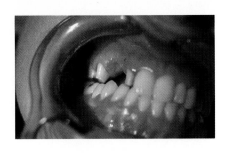

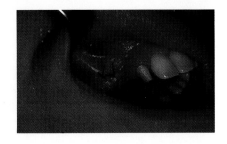

FIG. 23–31. Preoperative view of a small maxillary alveolar ridge defect.

FIG. 23–32. Postoperative view following hydroxyapatite placement.

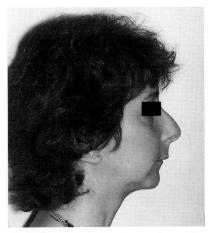

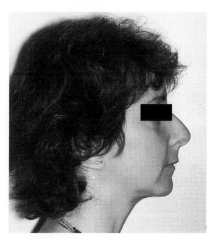

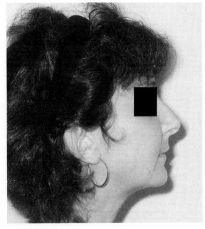

FIG. 23–33. Preoperative view of a patient with a severe Class II malocclusion.

FIG. 23–34. Postoperative view following a sagittal split osteotomy.

FIG. 23–35. Postoperative view of the patient shown in Figure 23–33 following hydroxyapatite placement to "plump" lower lip.

tion catheters are placed and operated in the usual manner.

CONCLUSION

Complex esthetic problems often require a multidisciplinary approach. The inclusion of oral and maxillofacial procedures often allows a dentist to achieve esthetic results that otherwise would not be possible.

REFERENCES

1. Golec, T.S.: Implants, what and when. J Can Dent Assoc 15:49, 1987.
2. Golec, T.S.: The use of hydroxyapatite to coat subperiosteal implants. Oral Implantol 1:21, 1985.
3. Golec, T.S.: CAD-CAM multiplanar diagnostic imaging for subperiosteal implants. Dent Clin North Am 30:85, 1986.
4. Balkin, B.: Implant dentistry: historical overview with current perspective. J Dent Educ 52:683, 1988.
5. Shulman, L.: Surgical considerations in implant dentistry. J Dent Educ 52:712, 1988.
6. Kent, J., et al.: Hydroxyapatite alveolar ridge reconstruction. J Oral Maxillofac Surg 44:37, 1986.
7. Kent, J.: Reconstruction of the alveolar ridge with hydroxyapatite. Dent Clin North Am 30:231, 1986.
8. McCurdy, J.: A rational approach to the neck in cervicofacial rhytidectomy—a guide to planning skin undermining, platysma surgery, and lipectomy. Laryngoscope 94:1383, 1984.
9. Teimourian, B.: Face and neck suction-assisted lipectomy associated with rhytidectomy. Plast Reconstr Surg 72:627, 1983.
10. Dolsky, B.: Innovations in platysma rhytidectomy. Arch Otolaryngol Head Neck Surg 109:337, 1983.
11. Hallock, G.: Defatting of flaps by means of suction-assisted lipectomy. Plas Reconstr 76:9, 1985.
12. Kennedy, B.: Suction assisted lipectomy of the face and neck. J Oral Maxillofac Surg 46:546, 1988.

Saul Hoffman M.D.

ESTHETICS AND PLASTIC SURGERY

24

There can be no standard definition of beauty because it varies among individuals, cultures, and races, and over time. When there is a significant deviation from what is considered normal, a deformity exists. However, a deformity may exist only in the person's mind. An individual may view himself as different and seek cosmetic surgery when psychiatric help is needed to correct his distorted body image. It is important for the professional who treats facial esthetics to be able to evaluate not only the anatomic defect, but also the patient's concept of the deformity and the expectations for correction.

Anthropologists have established criteria and standardized landmarks that enable measurement of facial dimensions. A range of normal can be established for any group. Although beauty cannot be measured numerically, gross deviations from normal can. These measurements are also helpful in planning surgical corrections of deformities.

Leonardo da Vinci sketched and analyzed the relationships of facial structures and determined geometrically "the divine proportions." His measurements are still used to teach art students to draw. He noted that "from the edge of the orbit to the ear, there is the same distance as the length of the ear, in other words, one-third of the head." He wrote "the distance from the chin to the nose and from the hairline to the eyebrows are equal, each of them to the height of the ear and one-third of the face."

Other significant proportions are that the distance between the eyes is equal to one eye and that, in the ideal Caucasian nose, the width of the nostril shall be confined within the lines drawn vertically from the medial canthus. Also, the mouth extends laterally to a line dropped from the medial margin of the limbus. A beautiful face, however, does not always conform to these proportions.

The American Society of Plastic and Reconstructive Surgery has defined cosmetic surgery as "that surgery which is done to revise or change the texture, configuration or relationship with contiguous structures of any feature of the human body which would be considered by the average prudent observer to be within the range of 'normal' and acceptable variation for the age and ethnic origin and, in addition which is performed for a condition which is judged by competent medical opinion to be without potential jeopardy to physical or mental health." (The American Medical Association has accepted this definition.)

RHINOPLASTY

The earliest plastic surgical operations in recorded history were for reconstruction of the nose. These operations were generally performed following amputation, which was a common form of punishment in ancient India.

Rhinoplasty can do more to enhance the appearance of the face than almost any other procedure in plastic surgery. The nose is the center of the face, and when unusually large or distorted, can significantly detract from an otherwise attractive face (Figs. 24–1, 24–2). The surgeon performing the rhinoplasty must keep in mind that the nose should be in harmony with the other facial features (Figs. 24–3, 24–4). For example, in most cases rhinoplasty is a reduction in the size of the nose, but in some patients it may be necessary to augment the nose with additional bone or cartilage (Figs. 24–5, 24–6).

Rhinoplasty is performed through intranasal incisions in which the skin is undermined and separated from the underlying cartilaginous and bony structures. These structures can then be altered with fine rasps and osteotomies. The skin then adjusts to the new underlying

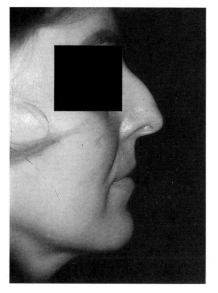

FIG. 24–1.

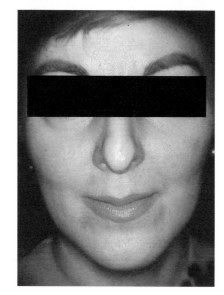

FIG. 24–2.

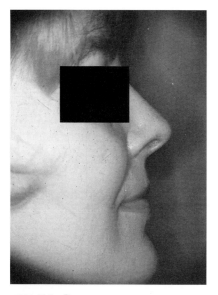

FIG. 24–3.

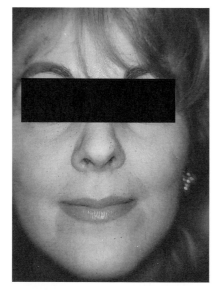

FIG. 24–4.

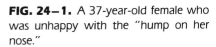

FIG. 24–1. A 37-year-old female who was unhappy with the "hump on her nose."

FIG. 24–2. Frontal view of the patient shown in Figure 24–1.

FIG. 24–3. Postoperative lateral view of the patient shown in Figure 24–1.

FIG. 24–4. Postoperative frontal view of the patient shown in Figure 24–1.

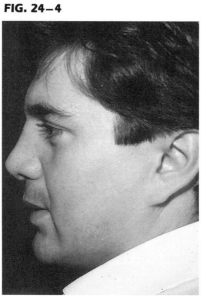

FIG. 24–5.

FIG. 24–6.

FIG. 24–5. A 30-year-old male who had previously undergone a rhinoplasty for a traumatic nasal deformity. He complained that "too much was removed" making his nose appear flat.

FIG. 24–6. Appearance after augmentation of the dorsum with septal cartilage graft.

framework. The bony dorsum is rasped to remove a hump, and the cartilage is trimmed to improve the profile line and reduce the prominence of the nasal tip. It is usually necessary to perform osteotomies and fracture the nose in order to narrow it. Bone and cartilage grafts may be necessary when the nose is too flat or damaged by trauma. When the tip lacks projection, grafts of cartilage from the septum or ear are necessary.

CHIN AUGMENTATION

Because proportions are important in facial harmony, when one feature is out of proportion, it affects all other features. For example, an underdeveloped chin can make a normal nose appear too large. Patients may ask for a rhinoplasty when what is really needed is correction of a hypoplastic chin.

Preoperative evaluation is extremely important for this group. There is a tendency for chin implants to be overutilized because the procedure is simple compared to the more complex operations of the mandible. When a hypoplastic chin is associated with labial incompetence, a chin implant is usually contraindicated. The overactive mentalis muscle forces the implant into the bone, causing erosion with distortion of the implant and possibly damage to the dentition. These patients require orthognathic surgery to correct the problem. When indicated, however, chin augmentation with silicone implants can be an important adjunct to rhinoplasty, as well as face-lifting (Figs. 24–7, 24–8).

BLEPHAROPLASTY

In our youth-oriented society, many people become concerned about appearing younger and seek procedures to improve their appearance. One of the most common procedures in plastic surgery is blepharoplasty. In this operation, varying amounts of excess skin and fat are removed from the eyelids (Figs. 24–9, 24–10). Excess periorbital fat can be hereditary and can affect young people. As one ages and the soft tissue around the eyes begins to relax, the fatty tissue (or "bags" as it is commonly referred to) becomes more obvious. Patients with this problem complain of looking sad and tired. Correction involves removing the excess fat, skin, and sometimes muscle in the periorbital region.

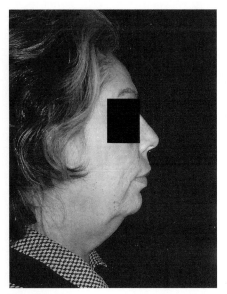

FIG. 24–7

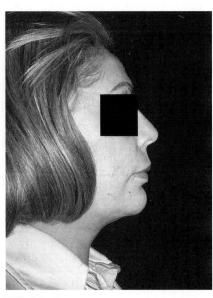

FIG. 24–8

FIG. 24–7. A 60-year-old female with severe submental skin and fat excess accentuated by hypoplasia of chin.

FIG. 24–8. Postoperative view of the patient in Fig. 24–7 after facelift and chin augmentation.

FIG. 24–9. Preoperative view of a patient with fatty deposits under the eyes.

FIG. 24–10. Postoperative view of the patient in Fig. 24–9 following blepharoplasty.

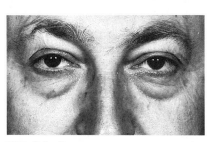

FIG. 24–9

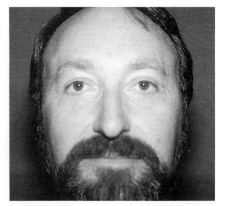

FIG. 24–10

BROWLIFT

The eyebrows are important features of facial expression. With age they tend to become ptotic and droop and this, combined with wrinkling of the forehead and glabella, makes the patient appear angry. Laxity of the upper eyelid skin will be accentuated by this condition. Care must be taken to evaluate the position of the eyebrows before resecting the upper eyelid skin because removal of too much skin can pull the eyebrows down and accentuate the problem. In these cases, a browlift must be considered. The brows are repositioned by removing forehead or scalp skin. A coronal incision is generally preferred because the resultant scar can be covered by the hair. In balding men and in women with a high forehead, it may be necessary to make an incision at the frontal hairline or directly in the forehead skin, a procedure that results in a more visible scar than a coronal lift. The incision is made behind the hairline to the galea and the flap undermined to the supraorbital ridge. The flap is then pulled back, the brows repositioned, and the excess skin removed. Care must be taken not to over correct because an unnatural, surprised look will result.

FACELIFT (RHYTIDECTOMY, MELOPLASTY)

The cheeks, perioral tissue, and submental tissue are affected by aging and gravity. As the skin loosens, the oral commissures descend and the nasolabial groove deepens, becoming more prominent. These effects can be temporarily reversed by lifting and tightening up the soft tissues, a procedure commonly known as a face-lift (see Figs. 24–7, 24–8). The changes associated with aging are aggravated by sun-induced pigmentation and fine wrinkling of the skin. The lips are a common site of fine vertical wrinkles, which are caused by loss of collagen, and often can be improved by dermabrasion or a chemical peel.

A chemical peel is generally effective in improving perioral wrinkles. An 88% solution of phenol, to which has been added croton oil, water, and Septisol, is applied to the wrinkled skin, covered with adhesive tape for 48 hours and allowed to heal (similar to a second degree burn). When the crust comes off in 3 to 5 days, a reddish discoloration is seen. This gradually fades but sometimes leaves a permanent discoloration. Patients with dark complexion are more prone to develop this discoloration, thus patient selection is extremely important. In addition, patients must be warned about permanent color changes.

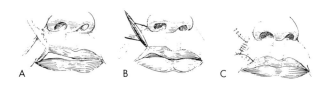

FIG. 24–11. A Z-plasty consists of the repositioning of triangular flaps of normal tissue adjacent to the scar.

CHEILOPLASTY

Reduction of prominent lips is achieved by making a transverse elliptical incision in the mucosa down to the muscle. The scar is placed behind the free border of the lip so it remains inconspicuous. Care must be taken to remove a uniform width of mucosa to avoid creating irregularities of the free border of the lip.

COLLAGEN INJECTIONS

For years physicians have been trying to correct wrinkles and contoural depressions by injecting various materials. Autologous fat injections were unsuccessful because the fat was absorbed. Collagen injections were similarly disappointing due to eventual absorption. Some clinicians claim that there can be permanent improvement with these techniques, which they continue to utilize. Silicone injections offer a more permanent solution, but because it is a synthetic material that remains in the tissue, it also presents a potential problem (i.e., foreign body reactions, cellulitis, or nodularity).

SCAR REVISION

When incisions are made electively, the scars can be minimized by placing them within the wrinkle lines. Scars resulting from trauma usually do not follow these natural lines and will therefore be more conspicuous. It is impossible to completely remove scars, and patients must be made to understand this in order to avoid disappointment. However, cosmetic improvements are feasible. Simple excision of the scar, undermining the adjacent tissue, and resuturing may result in improvement of a spread or irregular scar. In some cases, it may be necessary to change the direction of a scar or to elongate it to release a contracture. This is done by a technique called Z-plasty in which triangular flaps of normal tissue adjacent to the scar are interpolated to form a Z (Fig. 24–11). This allows the scar to elongate, and at the same time changes its direction (Figs. 24–12, 24–13). As much of the revised scar as possible is placed within the natural wrinkle lines.

COMPUTER IMAGING

Computers have added an exciting dimension to facial plastic surgery. By manipulating facial features with the computer, one can achieve some idea of what looks esthetic to the physician and, more important, to the patient. The danger lies in the fact that it is not always possible to duplicate computer predictions surgically because of the many variables that the computer does not reveal. In addition, showing the patient a computerized result may imply a guarantee, which is medicolegally dangerous. Nevertheless, when properly utilized computers can be useful tools for educating patients.

CONCLUSION

Esthetic surgery of the face may involve the soft tissues alone, as in a blepharoplasty or face-lift, or may include the bony skeleton. As previously mentioned, patients may request rhinoplasty when what is really needed is

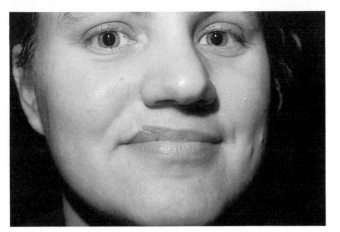

FIG. 24–12. Scar contracture of the upper lip.

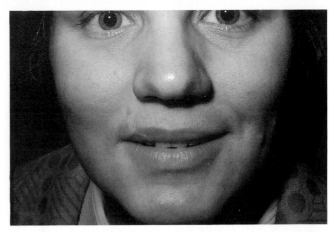

FIG. 24–13. Postoperative view of patient in Fig. 24–12 following Z-plasty surgery.

a genioplasty. Maxillary deficiency may be corrected by osteotomies with advancement of the maxilla or by on-lay grafts of bone or synthetic material. Because these deformities are often accompanied by malocclusion, it is important for the plastic surgeon to consult with dental colleagues in order to properly evaluate the optimum method of treatment.

Complex maxillofacial and craniofacial deformities are usually treated through a team approach. Members of the team include plastic surgeons and dental specialists. Planning and performing the operation as a team offers the patient the best chance of obtaining a satisfactory result.

Michael J. Pertschuk, M.D.
Albert M. Kligman, M.D., Ph.D.

ESTHETICS AND DERMATOLOGY

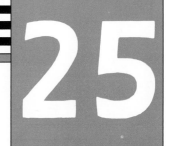

The skin is a multipurpose organ that isolates the internal organs from the external environment. It is a marvelous barrier that assures homeostasis. The skin responds to heat, cold, pressure, and pain. It plays an important role in temperature regulation. The skin is also the most visible organ of the body. It has a rich repertoire of emotional expressions and serves important esthetic and social functions.

In all animals, the skin provides useful information regarding general state of health and reproductive potential. For some mammals, specific skin pigment and secretory changes are associated with estrous and sexual availability. For humans, the social function of skin as an explicit sexual signal has been superseded by its role as a major factor in determining appearance. There is massive psychosocial literature demonstrating the importance of appearance in virtually all social interactions. Social scientists have clearly demonstrated the importance of appearance in self-esteem and self-concept.

SKIN

To understand how skin changes in response to various physical and chemical stimuli, it is essential to appreciate its structure (Fig. 25–1). The skin is composed of three layers: epidermis, dermis, and subcutis. The epidermis is the outermost layer and is composed of three basic cell types: keratinocytes, melanocytes, and Langerhans' cells. The epidermis is itself composed of four layers. Beginning with the innermost they are: basal layer, malpighian or prickle layer, granular layer, and horny layer or stratum corneum. The undulating basal layer is composed of keratinocytes, which have the capacity to divide. The daughter keratinocytes change in size and shape during the course of their upward journey to the stratum corneum. By the time the

cells enter the horny layer they have lost their nuclei and organelles and have developed a thick cell wall. The dead keratinocyte is called a corneocyte. The cell is densely packed with keratin filaments. The corneocytes are organized into a fabric of cells that serves as a barrier to water and chemicals. Keratin is also the structural protein of hair and nails.

The melanocytes are the pigment-producing cells of the epidermis and are located in the basal layer. The ratio of melanocytes to keratinocytes in the basal layer is approximately 1 to 10 and is the same regardless of race. It is the number and size of the melanosomes, melanin-containing granules that are synthesized by melanocytes, that determines differences in skin color. Chronic sun exposure causes melanocytes to manufacture larger melanosomes, darkening or tanning the skin. The melanosomes are transferred to neighboring keratinocytes, which serve as reservoirs for pigment granules. Langerhans' cells are scattered throughout the midepidermis and are now recognized as antigen imprinting cells. Their key role is in immune surveillance, recognizing foreign allergens and antigens.

Eccrine sweat glands, apocrine glands, and hair follicles with their associated sebaceous glands, are all derived from the epidermis. Apocrine glands are largely vestigial in humans, though they serve as a source of odor in the axilla. It is theorized that they produce chemical messengers called pheromones. Man has been called a naked ape owing to involution of hair follicles over most of the body surface. What remains, primarily scalp hair, has considerable psychosocial significance.

The dermis is composed primarily of collagen synthesized by fibroblasts. Collagen bundles give the skin its tensile strength and prevent overstretching. Fibroblasts also produce elastic fibers. These enable the skin to snap back after it has been stretched, providing resilience. A third component of the dermal tissue matrix is the

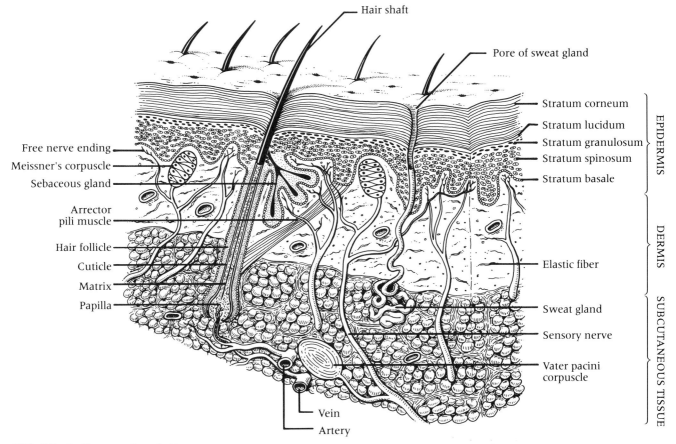

FIG. 25–1. Cross-section of skin.

Labels on figure:
Hair shaft
Pore of sweat gland
Stratum corneum
Stratum lucidum
Stratum granulosum
Stratum spinosum
Stratum basale
EPIDERMIS
Free nerve ending
Meissner's corpuscle
Sebaceous gland
Arrector pili muscle
Hair follicle
Cuticle
Matrix
Papilla
DERMIS
Elastic fiber
Sweat gland
Sensory nerve
Vater pacini corpuscle
SUBCUTANEOUS TISSUE
Vein
Artery

structureless ground substance. This is composed of proteoglycans and glycosaminoglycans. Abundant in fetal skin, ground substance decreases rapidly in infancy and is a minor but functionally important component of the dermis in adult skin.

The deepest layer of skin, the subcutis, consists of lobules of fat cells separated by fibrous septa of collagen. It serves as a shock absorber against trauma and as thermal insulation. It is also a storage depot for nutrients.

The thickness of the epidermis, dermis, and subcutis varies throughout the body, as does the thickness of each of these individual layers. The dermis in males is demonstrably thicker than in females.[1]

SKIN PATHOLOGY

"Old" skin comes in two varieties: thin, pale, and finely wrinkled; and thick, leathery, dry, discolored, and deeply furrowed. In reality only the former is truly old skin, the latter is a result of photodamage. They are both perceived as "old" because culturally we identify both with age. The former is genetically based and unavoidable. The latter is entirely preventable and to some extent reversible. Accordingly, we now differentiate between innate or biologic aging, a chronologic process evident in sun-protected skin, and photoaging, a result of cumulative damage by solar radiation.

Biologic Aging

Much of our understanding of the innate aging process of skin is limited, based on information gleaned from extremely small patient samples and, therefore, of questionable validity.[2] Nonetheless, it is possible to characterize some of the changes.

Aging involves a deterioration in cellular organization. The orderly progression of cellular morphologic change within the epidermis is lost.[3,4] Epidermal cell replacement is slowed, although not until after age 50. Turnover times in the stratum corneum average 14 days in young and middle aged adults. In the elderly, turnover may be 24 days or more.[5] The relative lack of change in the width of the stratum corneum with age, however, may account for the stability of the barrier function of skin over time.[5,6]

The basal layer is composed of relatively uniform basal keratinocytes in youth. In the elderly the basal cells vary considerably in size, shape, and staining qualities. The undulations of the basal layer are lost with age. The epidermis then rests on a flat epidermal-dermal junction and is, therefore, more easily dislodged by shearing forces.

Aging causes qualitative functional changes in the melanocytes and a diminution in their number,[7] and may play a role in the overall decreased pigmentation of aging skin.[2] The dermis thins considerably and the

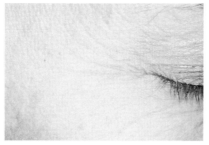 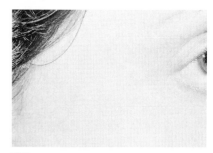

FIG. 25–2. Periocular wrinkling.

FIG. 25–3. Postoperative appearance following treatment with topical all-trans-retinoic acid (Tretinoin).

FIG. 25-2 **FIG. 25-3**

number of dermal cells diminishes by perhaps by as much as 50% by age 80.[8]

The absolute amount of collagen in the skin decreases with age. The neat meshwork of bundles in young skin are replaced with clumps of thickened collagen fibers.[9] Changes in elastin are detectable between the ages of 30 and 50 and are characterized by small spaces or vacuoles within the fibers.[6] Over the next two decades elastin becomes riddled with more and larger vacuoles. By age 70 most of the elastic fibers are abnormal.[10] The subepidermal elastic fibers are lost.[4] There is an increase of elastin in the underlying reticular dermis. The fibers are thicker and structurally abnormal.[2] The ground substance, which controls the percentage of water in the skin, probably decreases.[11]

The subcutaneous tissue decreases, but not uniformly throughout the body.[2] The microvasculature degenerates. Many capillaries and vessels disappear entirely[4] and venules may be reduced by at least 30%.[12]

The shrinking of the dermis and subcutis causes thinner skin. The loss of melanocytes and microvasculature leads to pallor. The epidermis, tenuously connected to the dermis, is more fragile. The decrease in amount and quality of elastin leaves the skin lax and contributes to fine wrinkling. This is the picture of old, but sun-protected, skin. The picture of chronically sun-exposed skin is different.

Photodamage

Sun exposure produces great size and shape variability in the basal cells of the epidermis,[13] along with cellular atypia.[14] There is loss of the normal orderly keratinocyte progressive maturation. More impressive are the changes in the dermis. The amount of mature collagen decreases.[15] There is a massive proliferation of tangled, degraded elastic fibers, which eventually degenerate into an amorphous mass.[16] There is an increase in ground substance.[17] Fibroblasts are numerous and appear in a hypermetabolic state. Mast cells and other inflammatory cells are also seen in abundance. There is reactive hyperplasia and hypertrophy of melanocytes.[18] The microvasculature degenerates. Vessels become dilated and tortuous and appear on the skin surface as telangiectasias.[13]

With increased elastic mass in the dermis, sun damaged skin is thicker than both old and young skin. The degradation of elastin contributes to the deep furrowing

and wrinkling. The mottled coloration is secondary to the abnormalities of the melanocytes.

Unlike intrinsic aging which is unavoidable, photodamage is caused by exposure to ultraviolet light, specifically in the 290 to 315 nm range (UVB) and the 315 to 400 nm range (UVA). UVB is directly responsible for the discomforts of sunburn, causes dermal thickening and abnormal elastin synthesis.[19,20] UVA is much lower in energy then UVB and requires a 500 to 1000 times greater dose to produce an erythema.[21] Unfortunately, UVA radiation is more prevalent than UVB, occurring during daylight in all seasons. In animal models, UVA exposure has been associated with abnormal elastin synthesis and an increase in ground substance, but little collagen damage.[20]

Photodamage can be prevented by avoiding direct exposure to sunlight. This is not always practical or socially desirable. A less effective option is to use sunscreen. Paraaminobenzoic acid (PABA) and benzophenone derivatives, such as oxybenzone, have been shown to effectively absorb UV radiation.[22,23] In studies with hairless mice, sunscreens with a sun protection factor (SPF) of 15 were found to significantly diminish UVA and UVB induced photodamage and to prevent progression of photodamage in previously photodamaged skin. Sunscreens allow for some early repair and the generation of new subepidermal collagen.[24]

No sunblock is complete, and current sunscreens only modestly protect against UVA. With consistent use, however, they offer significant protection against photodamage and also allow the skin an opportunity for self repair.

Another approach to correcting established photodamage, at least partially, is to topically apply vitamin A acid. Topical all trans-retinoic acid (tretinoin) had been used for 20 years as a treatment for acne (see below). Serendipitously, some patients reported that the medication also seemed to make their skin look younger. Investigation of tretinoin has borne out these initial impressions.[25,26] Tretinoin unequivocally promotes the repair of photodamage.[27] It causes a diminution of fine wrinkling and, to some extent, of coarse wrinkling. The skin becomes pinker and areas of discoloration fade (Figs. 25–2, 25–3). On a histologic level, changes occur primarily in the epidermis. Epidermal thickness almost quadruples, mean granular layer thickness more than doubles, and mitotic activity of the keratinocytes increases. The stratum corneum becomes compact and

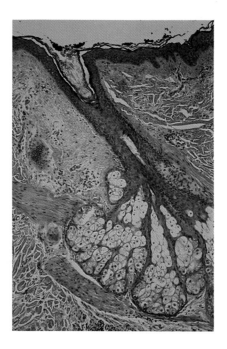

FIG. 25–4. Photomicrograph of a sebaceous gland.

FIG. 25–5. Cross-section of a sebaceous gland.

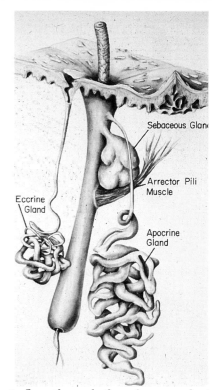

uniform and melanocytic hypertrophy and hyperplasia diminish. The formation of both new collagen and new blood vessels (angiogenesis) occurs.[26]

The face is the most exposed part of the body and, therefore, subject to the severest photodamage. It is also the most socially significant region and the one most closely identified with a sense of self. The current state of knowledge offers nothing biologic to combat the ravages of intrinsic aging; however, many of these intrinsic changes do not become significant until the seventh or eighth decade of life. By contrast, photodamage may be clinically manifest by the second decade. Avoidance of excessive sunlight is the lifelong prescription for good-looking skin. The use of physical shade and chemical shade (sunblocks) can prevent photoaging. Tretinoin can offer at least partial remedy to the current generations that did not know enough to come in out of the sun.

Acne

Acne derives from the interaction of sebaceous glands, sebum, bacteria, and the immune system. It effects up to 90% of adolescents to some extent and can continue well into adult life, especially in women. Acne can be significantly disfiguring, thereby diminishing quality of life and negatively influencing psychologic well being.

The skin of the face, especially around the nose, cheeks, and forehead, contains the largest and most numerous sebaceous glands on the body (Figs. 25–4, 25–5). They consist of clusters of lipid-filled cells. Cells on the periphery of the gland resemble epithelial basal cells. These cells divide and migrate into the interior of the glands. As they do so, they begin to synthesize lipid. With further differentiation, cell membranes, nucleic acids, and proteins are broken down. The cell ruptures

and the lipid contents flow through the sebaceous duct into the follicle and then to the surface of the skin. The function of this lipid substance, sebum is uncertain, but may be a vestige of our furrier ancestors.[28]

Sebaceous glands begin secreting sebum at puberty in response to increased levels of circulating androgens. Acne is associated with particularly high levels of sebum production.[29] This may be a necessary, but not sufficient, condition for acne.

An anaerobic diphtheroid, *Propionibacterium acnes*, is found to reside within sebaceous follicles in adults.[30] Colonization of the skin begins in adolescence. Teenagers with acne appear to have both higher levels of sebum and *P. acnes*, which nourishes on the fatty acids in the sebum.[31] It is theorized that a critical level of sebum is required before *P. acnes* can successfully colonize sebaceous glands.[32]

Hyperplasia of the follicular epithelium results in lipid engorgement and cohesion of horny cells, which distends the follicle and creates the initial lesion of acne: a microcomedo.[33] As the follicle continues to distend with sebum, follicular horny cells, and bacteria it forms a comedo. Young comedones are called white heads or closed comedones. Older comedones are bigger and are termed blackheads or open comedones. *P. acnes* produces chemotactic factors that attract neutrophils,[34] and microscopically breaks down the follicle wall.[35] Inflammation results in the formation of pustules, papules, and cysts. If the lesions are sufficiently deep within the dermis, they heal with scar formation.

There are many different treatment strategies for acne. Sebum can be reduced by estrogens. *P. acnes* can be controlled through antibiotics or benzoyl peroxide. Abnormal follicular keratinocyte production can be altered through retinoids. Inflammatory reactions can be limited with steroids. Despite the variety of options, no single treatment has proven entirely satisfactory or to be without side effects.

Sebum production is stimulated by androgens and inhibited by estrogens. Estrogens probably exert their effects on sebaceous glands indirectly by suppressing androgen synthesis.[36] Oral contraceptives have been shown to both decrease sebum production and reduce acne lesions.[37]

Systemic tetracycline and erythromycin and topical clindamycin and erythromycin antibiotics have been used to reduce the number of *P. acnes* present in the sebaceous glands. Antibiotics work by preventing new lesions and have little effect on lesions present at the initiation of treatment. Side effects with topical antibiotics are fewer, but these medications may be less effective than the systemic formulations.

Topical retinoic acid has been one of the more successful treatments for acne. It acts by reducing the formation of microcomedones. Retinoic acid increases the turnover of the follicular epithelial cells and reduces the cohesiveness of the horny cells. Follicles are less prone to blockage, and lesions are thus prevented.[38] Retinoic acid is locally irritating, requires at least 6 weeks to achieve visible benefits, and may initially aggravate the condition.

An oral retinoid, isotretinoin, has been available for treatment of acne since 1982. It inhibits the sebum production,[39] reduces the *P. acnes* population (probably as a result of decreased sebum),[40] and has some anti-inflammatory properties.[41]

These drugs have numerous side effects including cheilitis, scaly skin, erythema, pruritus, dry mucous membranes, angular stomatitis, gingivitis, epistaxis, nausea, vomiting, bone, muscle and joint pain, and triglyceride elevation. The most serious problem with isotretinoin is its considerable teratogenic potential. Women of childbearing age who are taking tretinoin, must use contraception. The risk-benefit ratio of this medication has limited its use to the most severe cases of cystic acne.

Systemic steroids have been used with limited success in the short-term control of severe acne flare-ups. Improvements have been seen within days of initiating treatment. Steroids have been injected directly into individual nodular or cystic lesions. The response is often dramatic, with rapid resolution of the local inflammation. This approach is limited by the necessity of direct physician involvement in treatment and by the risk of steroid atrophy of the subdermal tissue.

With the array of treatments available and the often fluctuating chronic course of the condition, management requires considerable expertise and understanding on the part of the physician. Added to the medical care is the frequent need for at least informal supportive counseling. In a study of psychologic sequelae of skin disease, acne patients were found to score significantly lower on a measure of psychologic adjustment than malignant melanoma patients.[42] Another psychobehavioral factor to be considered is the tendency of many patients to pick at their lesions in order to reduce the immediate visibility of pustules. Unfortunately, this further damages surrounding tissue and intensifies inflammation with potential scarring. Counseling and some simple self-monitoring techniques can significantly alter this pattern.

COSMETIC PROCEDURES

Tretinoin Therapy

Numerous strategies have evolved to repair damage caused by sun, acne, and aging. One of the simplest treatments is the use of topical tretinoin. Tretinoin acts primarily in the epidermis and papillary dermis. It can help with discolorations and fine wrinkles, but will do little for deeper wrinkles.

Chemical Peels

An alternative approach to removing or ameliorating somewhat deeper wrinkles, as well as discoloration, is chemical skin peeling. Chemical peeling is not a new technique. It dates to the early days of this century, and has been commonly used for more than 30 years.[43] There are multiple variations involving different chemicals, applied according to different schedules, with or without occlusion of treated skin. Peels are classified according to depth, i.e., how deeply the applied substance penetrates and damages skin. The goal is to cause sloughing of old damaged tissue with replacement by healthier new tissue. At the level of the epidermis, replacement tissue exhibits good cellular differentiation with a well developed stratum corneum. Pigment and keratin irregularities are removed. At the level of the dermis, new collagen is laid down, which results in wrinkle reduction. In general, deeper peels are associated with greater cosmetic change, more significant morbidity, and higher complication rates.

Superficial peels are usually accomplished with trichloroacetic acid (TCA) in concentrations between 15 and 35%, or with Jessner's solution (resorcinol, salicylic acid, lactic acid, and ethanol). Applications are often repeated with gradually increasing concentrations over a period of weeks. Indications include fine wrinkling, acne, and pigmentary changes. Exfoliation involves primarily epidermis. There may be associated inflammation of the papillary dermis. The procedures are at most mildly uncomfortable and do not involve anesthesia or sedation. Although skin-peeling achieves more rapid results than topical retinoids, it is not clear that the cosmetic outcome of superficial peels is any better than the outcome of daily application of tretinoin.

Medium depth chemical peels utilize TCA in concentrations between 35 and 50%, often in combination with Jessner's solution or dry ice, to first remove the stratum corneum and improve absorption. Indications are essentially the same as for superficial peels. A better cosmetic outcome is anticipated as the TCA penetrates into the papillary dermis, resulting in the destruction of this layer with subsequent synthesis of new collagen. The procedure is performed with sedation or local nerve blocks. There is erythema and edema immediately following the peel. The erythema typically intensifies after

3 or 4 days and then gradually fades. Healing is usually complete within 10 days. Complications include prolonged erythema, hyperpigmentation, herpes simplex virus I infection, bacterial infection, and scarring. Scarring occurs if the solution penetrates through the entire dermis.

Deep peels are used to remove fine to medium wrinkles and pigmentary changes. Phenol or Baker-Gordon phenol (88% phenol, water, soap, and croton oil) are the chemical agents used. Tape is often applied immediately following treatment to promote absorption. Penetration is to the upper reticular dermis. Sedation, analgesia, and local or sometimes general anesthesia are required. Edema is severe. An exudate develops within 24 hours and forms a crust if allowed to dry. The skin is very erythematous. Re-epitheliazation is usually complete within 10 days. Edema can persist for several weeks and erythema for up to 3 months. Complications include those listed for medium depth peels. With deeper peels there is increased risk of scarring since the potential for dermal full-thickness damage is greater. Hypopigmentation occurs with some frequency. In addition, phenol is absorbed through the skin and can cause cardiac arrhythmias. Other infrequent but reported complications include laryngeal edema and toxic shock syndrome.[44]

Long-term histologic followup of deep phenol peels has shown the presence of new, well organized collagen, 2 to 3 mm wide, with a network of fine elastic fibers.[45] This was in marked contrast to the histology of adjacent nonpeeled dermis. The latter showed typical actinic changes, including reduced collagen and thickened amorphous masses of elastin. Although the patient sample in this study was small, 10-year followup suggests that positive changes with deep peels endure.

Dermabrasion

Dermabrasion is the mechanical equivalent of medium to deep chemical peels resulting in the removal of the epidermis and the upper to middle dermis layers. As a mechanical procedure, it has the advantage of being highly controllable. Specific areas of skin with deeper lesions, can have more tissue removed; areas with minimal defects can be treated more superficially.

Although applicable to the reduction of wrinkles, dermabrasion is used primarily in the treatment of acne scars. Scars that appear to improve when the skin is stretched tend to be the those that improve with dermabrasion.[46] These usually are the broader, more shallow scars. Narrow, deeper scars may require excision and grafting.

General anesthesia is not required. Most patients can be treated with oral or parenteral analgesics and local nerve blocks. A refrigerant is applied to local areas of skin immediately before abrasion. Superficial freezing enhances anesthesia, reduces bleeding, and makes the tissues more rigid. The abrasion itself is accomplished by means of rapidly rotating wire brushes or sandpaper pads. More pressure is applied to areas requiring deeper removal of tissue. As with peels, there is the risk of removal of too much dermis, resulting in scar formation rather than regeneration of normal dermis and epidermis.

Recuperation takes about a week to 10 days. Edema is invariably present for the first 48 hours. An antibiotic ointment is applied to reduce the risk of infection and to keep the skin supple. After about 5 days, warm water soaks are used to gradually remove the serous gel that forms over the treated areas. Erythema is always present and can last from weeks to months. Milia (small keratin producing cysts) formation may occur and 10% of patients experience eczematous changes, which may require topical steroids.[46] Hypopigmentation is common and persists for 4 to 6 weeks, and occasionally much longer. Ten percent of patients develop hyperpigmentation, which may last several weeks or months. Hypertrophic healing occurs in approximately 1% of treated acne patients.[46]

Dermabrasion can be repeated in localized areas after 6 to 8 weeks to reduce deeper scars. Changes accomplished through dermabrasion are lasting, and repeat procedures are rarely required unless subsequent flare-ups of acne result in additional scarring.

Collagen Implants

The strategy of peels and dermabrasion is to destroy the outer layers of the skin so that new and healthier cells might regenerate from the underlying dermis and epidermal appendages. An alternative approach has been to build-up the dermis directly underneath identifiable "faults," such as wrinkles and scars. This is not an entirely new technique. In the 1960s silicone injections were used as "fillers" for facial defects until well publicized medical misadventures, most likely the result of using impure silicone, effectively put an end to the procedure.[47] In the 1970s, injectable collagen first became available and has since found a niche as a safe and relatively easy "touch up" technique for wrinkles and scars. Collagen implants are derived from bovine dermal collagen.

Prior to treatment, a skin test is performed for possible allergic reaction. If the patient is determined to be hypersensitive to the materials, treatment is not pursued. Approximately 1 to 3% of patients exhibit hypersensitivity.[48,49]

Collagen implants have been used to treat glabellar creases, nasolabial folds, and perioral and periorbital wrinkles (Fig. 25−6). The last of these may be somewhat problematic because the periorbital dermis is particularly thin; there is little to hold the collagen implant and prevent its spreading. Shallow acne scars can be successfully filled with collagen. Deeper, pitted scars are not helped cosmetically by collagen.

Duration of cosmetic change is a function of the patient's skin and the practitioner's skill. For reasons that are not well understood, cosmetic changes tend to outlast the histologically demonstrable presence of the implant. Depending on the rate of resorption of the implant and the patient's awareness of deterioration of cosmetic results, repeat collagen injections for correc-

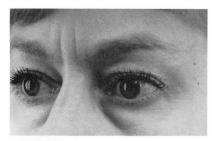

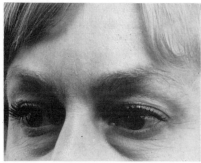

FIG. 25—6. Top, before collagen injections. Bottom, after collagen injections.

tion of wrinkles or scars may be necessary every 4 to 24 months. At this time, there is no established limit on the number of repeat procedures on the same tissues.

Complications due to bovine collagen have been limited to local allergic response. These are manifested by erythema and induration. In patients experiencing an allergic reaction, circulating antibodies to bovine collagen have been identified. There is no evidence of systemic complications or increased collagen vascular disease with collagen implants.[51]

Less traumatic than either a deep peel or dermabrasion, collagen implants offer temporary esthetic improvement for relatively discrete facial imperfections. The transiency of the benefits requires an ongoing relationship between the practitioner and the patient. As with other "beauty treatments," the serious collagen patient must followup with the practitioner for periodic, perhaps annual or semiannual, touchups. It is likely that only a small subset of the general population would have the concern and motivation to pursue these procedures on a regular basis. To date, there have been no psychologic studies to better characterize this group.

FUTURE TRENDS

The term "cosmeceuticals" has been used to describe prescription medications with cosmetic applications. Tretinoin (Retin-A, Ortho Pharmaceutical Corp.) and topical minoxidil (Rogaine, Upjohn Co.), which is used to treat male pattern baldness, fall into this category.

Another trend affecting all medical and dental specialities involved with appearance is a move toward better coordination of treatment. There are a growing number of possible interventions for a range of appearance defects. Although it is possible to deal with each esthetic problem individually, care can be provided in a far more rational manner when it is organized among

specialists according to a considered plan. Such coordination may be relatively simple. A face-lift patient with obvious actinic changes is referred to a dermatologist for counseling regarding sun exposure and use of tretinoin to reduce photodamage.

CLINICAL TIP. Planning can be far more complex for the aging face with mandibular and maxillary alveolar bone resorption secondary to the loss of dentition. Treatment may need to be coordinated between the oral surgeon, plastic surgeon, dermatologist, and restorative dentist.

If interventions are extensive and the potential cosmetic changes considerable, a psychiatric consultant may be needed as well to assess the patient's ability to cooperate with treatment and the potential psychologic costs and benefits.

This interdisciplinary cooperation can be partially achieved through routine referrals among specialists or through a team approach in a university or hospital setting. Under optimal conditions, dermatologists, plastic surgeons, oral surgeons, oculoplastic surgeons, psychiatrists, dermohygienists, orthodontists, maxillofacial prosthodontists, and restorative dentists work together in the management of appearance-related problems.

REFERENCES

1. Tan, C.Y., Statham, B., Marks, R., and Payne, P.A.: Skin thickness measurement by pulse ultrasound: its reproducibility and validation. Br J Dermatol 106:657, 1982.
2. Kligman, A.M. and Balin, A.K.: Aging of human skin. *In* Balin, A.K. and Kligman, A.M. (eds): Aging and the Skin. New York, Raven Press, 1989.
3. Montagna, W. (ed.): Advances in the Biology of the Skin. New York, Pergamon Press, 1965.
4. Montagna, W. and Carlisle, K.: Structural changes in aging human skin. J Invest Dermatol 73:47, 1979.
5. Grove, G.L., and Kligman, A.M.: Age-associated changes in human epidural cell renewal. J Gerontol 38:137, 1983.
6. Lavker, R.: Structural alterations in exposed and unexposed skin. J Invest Dermatol 73:59, 1979.
7. Gilchrest, B.A., Blog, F.B., and Szabo, G.: The effect of aging and chronic ultraviolet light on melanocytes in human skin. J Invest Dermatol 73:141, 1979.
8. Andrew, W., Behnke, R., and Sato, T.: Changes with advancing age in the cell populations of human dermis. Gerontol 10:1, 1964.
9. Kohn, R.R. and Schnider, S.L.: Collagen changes in aging skin *In* Balin, A.K., and Kligman, A.M. (eds.): Aging and the Skin. New York, Raven Press, 1989.
10. Braverman, I.M. and Fonferko, E.: Studies in cutaneous aging: I. The elastic fiber network. J Invest Dermatol 78:434, 1982.
11. Fleischmajer, R., Perlish, J.J., and Bashey, R.I.: Aging of human dermis. *In* Pobert, C.L. (ed.): Frontiers of Matrix Biology, Vol I. Basel, S. Karger, 1973.
12. Gilchrest, B.A., Stoff, J.S., and Soter, N.A.: Chronologic aging alters the response to UV-induced inflammation in human skin. J Invest Dermatol 79:11, 1982.
13. Kligman, A.M.: Perspectives and problems in cutaneous gerontology. J Invest Dermatol 73:39, 1979.
14. Kligman, L.H.: Photoaging manifestations, prevention and treatment. Dermatol Clin 4:517, 1986.
15. Smith, J.G. Jr., Davidson, E.A., Sams, W.M. Jr., and Clark, R.D.: Alterations in human connective tissue with age and chronic sun damage. J Invest Dermatol 39:347, 1962.

16. Kligman, A.M.: Early destructive effects of sunlight on human skin. J Am Med Assoc 210:2377, 1969.
17. Sams, W.M. and Smith, J.G.: The histochemistry of chronically sundamaged skin. J Invest Dermatol 37:447, 1961.
18. Gilchrest, B.A.: Relationship between actinic damage and chronologic aging in keratinocyte cultures of human tissues. J Invest Dermatol 75:219, 1979.
19. Kligman, L.H., Akin, F.J., and Kligman, A.M.: Prevention of ultraviolet damage to the dermis of hairless mice by sunscreens. J Invest Dermatol 78:181, 1982.
20. Kligman, L.H., Akin, F.J., and Kligman, A.M.: The contributions of UVA and UVB to connective tissue damage in hairless mice. J Invest Dermatol 84:272, 1985.
21. Gilchrest, B.A., Stoff, N.A., Hawk, J.L.M., et al.: Histologic changes associated with ultraviolet A induced erythema in normal human skin. J Am Acad Dermatol 9:213, 1983.
22. Pathak, M.A., Fitzpatrick, T.B., and Frenk, E.: Evaluation of topical agents that prevent sunburn: superiority of para-aminobenzoic acid and its ester in ethyl alcohol. N Engl J Med 280:1459, 1969.
23. Sayre, R.M., Marlowe, E., Poh Agin, P., et al.: Performance of six sunscreen formulations on human skin. Arch Dermatol 115:46, 1979.
24. Kligman, L.H., Akin, F.J., and Kligman, A.M.: Sunscreens promote repair of ultraviolet radiation-induced dermal damage. J Invest Dermatol 81:98, 1983.
25. Kligman, L.H., Chen, H.D., Kligman, A.M.: Topical retinoic acid enhances the repair of ultraviolet damaged dermal connective tissue. Connect Tissue Res 12:139, 1984.
26. Kligman, A.M., Grove, G.L., Hirose, R., and Leyden, J.J.: Topical tretinoin for photoaged skin. J Am Acad Dermatol 15:836, 1986.
27. Weiss, J.S., Ellis, C.N., Headington, J.T., et al.: Topical tretinoin improves photoaged skin A double blind vehicle-controlled study. JAMA.
28. Kligman, A.M.: The uses of sebum? In Montagna, W., Ellis, R.A., and Silver, A.F. (eds.): Advances in the Biology of Skin Volume 4. Oxford, Pergamon Press, 1963.
29. Harris, H.H., Downing, D.T., Stewart, M.E., et al.: Sustainable rates of sebum production in acne patients and matched normal controls. J Am Acad Dermatol 8:200, 1983.
30. Montes, L.F. and Wilborn, W.H.: Anatomical location of normal skin flora. Arch Dermatol 101:145, 1970.
31. Leyden, J.J., McGinley, K.J., Mills, O.H., et al.: *Propionibacterium* levels in patients with and without acne vulgaris. J Invest Dermatol 65:382, 1975.
32. Leyden, J.J.: Follicular microflora in acne vulgaris. Dermatol Clin 1:345, 1983.
33. Knutson, D.D.: Ultrastructural observations in acne vulgaris: the normal sebaceous follicle and acne lesions. J Invest Dermatol 62:288, 1974.
34. Puhvel, S.M. and Sakomoto, M.: The chemoatractant properties of comedonal contents. J Invest Dermatol 71:324, 1978.
35. Webster, G.F., Leyden, J.J., and Tsai, C.C., et al.: Polymorphonuclear leukocyte lysosomal release in response to *Propionibacterium acnes* in vitro and its enhancement by sera from patients with inflammatory acne. J Invest Dermatol 74:398, 1980.
36. Pochi, P.E. and Strauss, J.S.: Endocrinologic control of the development and activity of the human sebaceous gland. J Invest Dermatol 62:191, 1974.
37. Pochi, P.E. and Strauss, J.S.: Sebaceous gland suppression with ethinyl estradiol and diethylstilbestrol. Arch Dermat 108:210, 1973.
38. Kligman, A.M., Fulton, J.E. Jr. and Plewig, G.: Topical vitamin A acid in acne vulgaris. Arch Dermatol 107:551, 1973.
39. Strauss, J.S., Stranieri, A.M., Farrell, L.N., et al.: The effect of marked inhibition of sebum production with 13-cis-retinoic acid on skin surface lipid composition. J Invest Dermatol 74:66, 1980.
40. Weissman, A., Wagner, A., and Plewig, G.: Reduction of bacterial skin flora during treatment with 13-cis-retinoic acid. Arch Dermatol Res 270:179, 1981.
41. Plewig, G., Nikolowski, J., and Wolff, H.H.: Action of isotretinoin in acne rosacea and gram-negative folliculitis. J Am Acad Dermatol 6:766, 1982.
42. Cassileth, B.R., Lusk, E.J., and Tenaglia, A.N.: A psychological comparison of patients with malignant melanoma and other dermatologic disorders. J Am Acad Dermatol 7:742, 1982.
43. Brody, H.J.: The art of chemical peeling. J Dermatol Surg Oncol 15:918, 1989.
44. Brody, H.J.: Complications of chemical peeling. J Dermatol Surg Oncol 15:1010, 1989.
45. Kligman, A.M., Baker, T.J., and Gordon, H.C.: Long term histologic follow-up of phenol face peels. Plast Reconstr Surg 75:652, 1985.
46. Orentreich, N. and Durr, N.P.: Rehabilitation of acne scarring. Dermatol Clin 1:405, 1983.
47. Shumrick, K.A. and Kridel, R.W.H.: Comparison of injectable silicone versus collagen for soft tissue augmentation. J Dermatol Surg Oncol 14:66, 1988.
48. Kligman, A.M.: Histologic responses to collagen implants in human volunteers: comparison of Zyderm collagen with Zyplast implant. J Dermatol Surg Oncol 14:35, 1988.
49. Balin, P.L. and Balin, M.D.: Collagen implantation: clinical applications and lesion selection. J Dermatol Surg Oncol 14:21, 1988.
50. Stegman, S.J., Chu, S., and Armstrong, R.C.: Adverse reactions to bovine collagen implant: clinical and histologic features. J Dermatol Surg Oncol 14:39, 1988.
51. Klein, A.W.: Indications and implantation techniques for the various formulations of injectable collagen. J Dermatol Surg Oncol 14:27, 1988.

ESTHETICS AND COSMETOLOGY

Mark Lees, Ph.D.

26

The profession of esthetics involves the art and science of skin care, make-up, and facial cosmetology. Practitioners of esthetics, called estheticians or dermohygienists, are licensed in most states by the state board of cosmetology. Estheticians are to dermatologists and plastic surgeons what dental hygienists are to dentists.

Estheticians treat such problems as minor acne, blemish-prone skin, oily skin, dry skin, the appearance effects of aging, superfluous hair, blackheads, and clogged pores. Estheticians also help maintain skin in healthy condition. They teach patients how to care for their skin, and how to prevent acne, sun damage, and skin cancer. Most estheticians have training in basic cosmetic chemistry. They can help acne patients avoid comedogenic ingredients, and can offer helpful advice regarding skin that is hypersensitive to certain cosmetic ingredients.

Most estheticians are also make-up artists and specialists. They teach patients make-up application techniques, ranging from simple fashion make-up to corrective and paramedical camouflage make-up for conditions such as vitiligo, hyperpigmentation, perioral wrinkling, aging, and surgical reconstruction.

Estheticians practice in free standing salons or in clinics. However, there is a trend toward paramedical esthetics, in which the esthetician shares an office with the dermatologist or plastic surgeon.

CLEANSING

The proper use of cleansers and soaps is fundamental to any skin care regime. Healthy skin is clean skin. Patients are taught elementary cleansing procedures, which can be adapted to individual problems such as oiliness, sensitivity, make-up use, aging, use of topical and systemic drugs (e.g., retinoic acid, Accutane), dis-

tended capillaries, and erythemic conditions. Proper pH levels are maintained by the use of toners and astringents. Plain soap and water is not for everyone when skin appearance is considered. Highly alkaline soaps can dehydrate the skin and cause xerosis (dryness) and flaking, and can accentuate the superficial appearance of lines and wrinkles.[1]

PROTECTION

Sealant Creams

Sealant creams protect against superficial moisture loss and irritation due to cold or dry air and climatic conditions. Protective products also aid make-up adherence and evenness.

Moisturizers

Moisturizers may or may not contain sealant ingredients. Moisturizers contain hydrating agents that help water adhere to the skin, helping to "plump" the epidermis and create a younger, smoother, less wrinkled appearance. Hydration is the secret to the controversial "anti-aging" products. Whether or not these products have any long-term effect on aging is yet to be documented. Nevertheless, they do help skin look better.

Sunscreens

Sunscreens are now produced for lips, face, and body. Many protectants and make-up products also contain sunscreen. It has been accepted that the appearance of aging is directly proportional to the amount of sun exposure.[2]

Specialty Cosmetic Treatments

Moisturizers of various densities and hydrating levels, treatment preparations for hyperpigmentation, excess

Portions of this chapter were adapted from *Milady's Standard Textbook of Cosmetology,* Milady Publishing Company, Tarrytown, NY, 1991.

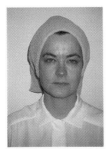

FIG. 26–1. Preoperative view prior to camouflage make-up placement. Note the red blemish on the forehead.

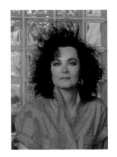

FIG. 26–2. Postoperative view following camouflage make-up placement.

oil control products, acne products containing benzoyl peroxide, salicylic acid, or resorcinol, and special products for hypersensitive and hyperallergic skin are included in this group.

MAKE-UP

Two types of make-up services of interest to the cosmetic dentist are corrective make-up and paramedical camouflage. Corrective make-up, most often used as a basic cosmetic fashion technique, is the art of sculpting the face with make-up to produce illusions based on light reflection.

Paramedical camouflage make-up is used for persons suffering from more esthetically devastating afflictions, such as those caused by skin or oral cancer, accidents, burns, congenital esthetic defects, or facial reconstruction (Figs. 26–1, 26–2). In severe cases, facial esthetic prostheses may also be included in this type of make-up artistry.

CORRECTIVE MAKE-UP PRINCIPLES

CLINICAL TIP. The actual application of corrective make-up is obviously outside the parameters of cosmetic dentistry. However, the cosmetic dentist should have an understanding of the basic principles and goals of corrective make-up application. After successful esthetic correction of the dentition, patients are often desirous, to varying degrees, of extending cosmetic improvement to other facial areas. The dentist may be in a position to offer preliminary guidance to the patient. Of course, this must be approached with considerable sensitivity to avoid embarrassing a patient who may consider discussions in this area to be overly intrusive. In these cases broaching the subject is inappropriate.

The principles behind corrective make-up are similar to those used in cosmetic dentistry (see Chapter 2—Fundamentals of Esthetics). Make-up that is lighter than the original foundation highlights a feature. Creating shadows on the face diminishes the impact of an area. These principles allow the corrective artist to create an illusion by "evening out" facial features. By using light and dark shades of foundations, powders, contours, eye shadows, and other make-up products, the face is "corrected" by detracting from overly prominent features, scars, blemishes, and imperfections. The pleasing features of the face are accented or highlighted. For example, a prominent nose may appear less noticeable by applying a *slightly* darker cosmetic. If the make-up is

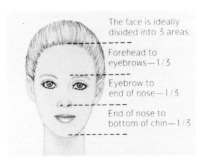

FIG. 26–3. The face is divided into three horizontal sections. (From Milady's Standard Textbook of Cosmetology, Milady Publishing Co., Tarrytown, NY. Copyright 1991.)

carefully blended, noticeable lines of demarcation are eliminated.

Terminology

A number of terms, products, and instrumentations are commonly used by make-up artists and estheticians.

1. **Contouring** refers to the overall procedure of creating an illusion with make-up.
2. **Shading** is the procedure of applying darker shades to make a facial area appear less prominent.
3. **Highlighting** accentuates and calls attention to a particular area or feature and involves the application of lighter shade.
4. **Foundation** is a flesh-colored cosmetic make-up. It is usually a cream or liquid which is used to cover and blend uneven facial colors, such as freckles or solar pigmented areas. Loose powder, applied with a brush, helps to "set" the foundation and provides a surface that allows easy blending of other powders.
5. **Concealer** is a heavier, flesh-colored cream foundation that is used to cover extremely dark or light areas of the face which cannot be covered by a foundation. It is used to cover blemishes, hyperpigmented areas, vitiligo, or scars. Concealer may vary in color and opacity so that it may also be used to shade and highlight areas.
6. **Contouring creams and powders** are used to highlight areas of the face for corrective make-up. They are available in a wide variety of skin colors.
7. **Color toners or veils** are similar to foundations,

    ESTHETIC DENTISTRY

but are actually colors, rather than flesh tone shades. They are used to neutralize the dominance of a color in the skin (e.g., a green toner is used to cover redness) and to help blend foundations to a more precise shade. (See Chapter 2—Fundamentals of Esthetics, Complementary Colors).

8. **Color corrective products** are also made for specific areas, such as lips and eyes, to help neutralize color abnormalities.

9. **Color or glamour products** include lipstick, mascara, liner pencils, blush, eye shadows, lip gloss, and other decorative products.

10. **Tools of the make-up artist** include sponges of various texture and absorbency levels and brushes of various size, texture, bristle length, and shape, which are used to contour and adapt to different facial features and angles.

Corrective Make-up for Different Facial Shapes

Prior to the application of corrective make-up, it is important to determine overall facial shape. The face is divided into three horizontal sections (Fig. 26—3). The top section is measured from the hairline to a point between the beginning of the eyebrows. The middle section is measured from the bottom of the first section to the end of the nose. The bottom section is measured from the end of the nose to the bottom of the chin. The seven basic facial configurations follow.[3]

1. **Oval-shaped face.** The oval face is considered the esthetically ideal shape. The ideal oval face is approximately three-fourths as wide as it is long. The forehead is slightly wider than the chin and the distance between the eyes is the width of one eye. The three horizontal sections are equal in height (Figs. 26—4, 26—5).

2. **Round-shaped face.** The round face is similar to the oval face, except that it is much wider in propor-

tion to its length. In addition, the hairline and chin are rounded. The goal of corrective make-up is to lengthen and slenderize the round face (Figs. 26—6, 26—7).

3. **Square-shaped face.** The square face is composed of comparatively straight lines with a wide forehead and square jawline. The goal of corrective make-up in this case is to soften the lines around the face and offset the squareness (Figs. 26—8 to 26—11).

4. **Pear-shaped face.** The pear-shaped face is characterized by a forehead that is narrower than the jaw. In this situation, the goal of corrective make-up is to slenderize the jaw line, widen the forehead, and lengthen the face (Figs. 26—12, 26—13).

5. **Heart-shaped face.** The heart-shaped face is characterized by a wide forehead. The goal of corrective make-up in this case is to reduce the width across the forehead and widen the jawline (Figs. 26—14 to 26—17).

6. **Diamond-shaped face.** The diamond-shaped face has the narrow features of both the pear-shaped and heart-shaped face; i.e., a narrow chin and forehead. The greatest width is across the cheekbones. Here, the goal of corrective make-up is to slenderize the cheekbone line and widen the chin and forehead (Figs. 26—18, 26—19).

7. **Oblong-shaped face.** The oblong face is characterized by greater length in proportion to its width than the square or round face. It is long and narrow. The goal of corrective make-up in cases of oblong-shaped faces is to create the illusion of width across the cheekbone line and to make the entire face appear shorter (Figs. 26—20 to 26—23).

As with the frontal view, an oval is considered an ideal shape when viewed from a profile. The goal when designing hairstyles should be to create the illusion of an oval shape (Figs. 26—24 to 26—29).

(text continued on page 391.)

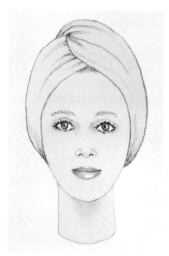

FIG. 26—4. An oval-shaped face. (From Milady's Standard Textbook of Cosmetology, Milady Publishing Co., Tarrytown, NY. Copyright 1991.)

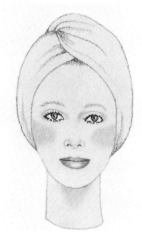

FIG. 26—5. An oval-shaped face with corrective make-up applied. (From Milady's Standard Textbook of Cosmetology, Milady Publishing Co., Tarrytown, NY. Copyright 1991.)

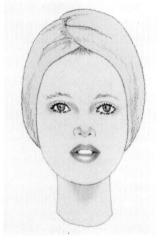

FIG. 26—6. A round-shaped face. (From Milady's Standard Textbook of Cosmetology, Milady Publishing Co., Tarrytown, NY. Copyright 1991.)

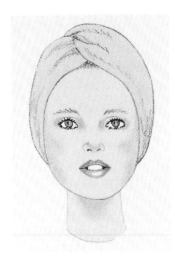

FIG. 26–7. A round-shaped face with corrective make-up applied. (From Milady's Standard Textbook of Cosmetology, Milady Publishing Co., Tarrytown, NY. Copyright 1991.)

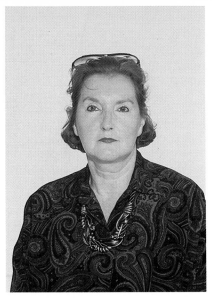

FIG. 26–8. This patient exhibited facial flaws that included a square face, small eyes, a thin upper lip, and a broad nose. (Hairstylists, Josey Leech and Miki Callahan; photographer, Carter Hawkins; make-up designer, Charlotte Hopkins.)

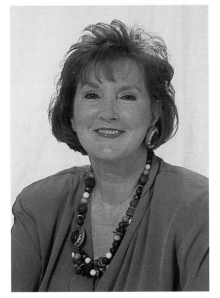

FIG. 26–9. After make-up and hairstyling the face appears considerably more oval. The eyes are accentuated in order to focus attention away from the lower face. (Hairstylists, Josey Leech and Miki Callahan; photographer, Carter Hawkins; make-up designer, Charlotte Hopkins.)

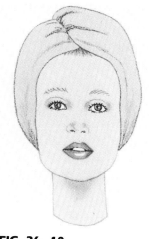

FIG. 26–10

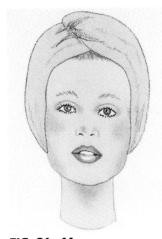

FIG. 26–11

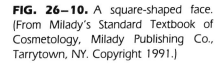

FIG. 26–10. A square-shaped face. (From Milady's Standard Textbook of Cosmetology, Milady Publishing Co., Tarrytown, NY. Copyright 1991.)

FIG. 26–11. A square-shaped face with corrective make-up applied. (From Milady's Standard Textbook of Cosmetology, Milady Publishing Co., Tarrytown, NY. Copyright 1991.)

FIG. 26–12. A pear-shaped face. (From Milady's Standard Textbook of Cosmetology, Milady Publishing Co., Tarrytown, NY. Copyright 1991.)

FIG. 26–13. A pear-shaped face with corrective make-up applied. (From Milady's Standard Textbook of Cosmetology, Milady Publishing Co., Tarrytown, NY. Copyright 1991.)

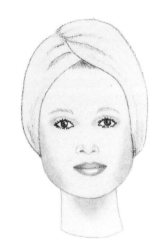

FIG. 26–12

FIG. 26–13

FIG. 26—14. This patient exhibited circles around the eyes, a narrow chin, and a thin face. (Hairstylists Josey Leech and Miki Callahan; photographer, Carter Hawkins; make-up designer, Charlotte Hopkins.)

FIG. 26—15. Corrective make-up "reversed her color" by replacing dark areas with light shades and light areas with darker contour. The upswept hair creates a more balanced appearance. (Hairstylist Josey Leech and Miki Callahan; photographer, Carter Hawkins; make-up designer, Charlotte Hopkins.)

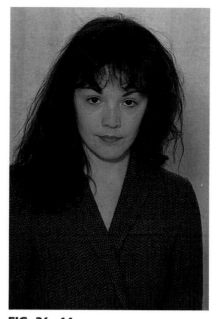

FIG. 26—14

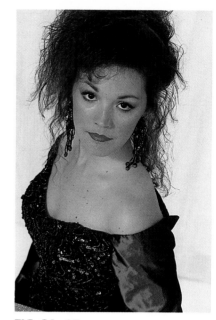

FIG. 26—15

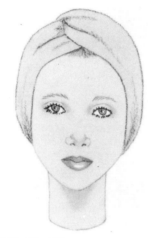

FIG. 26—16

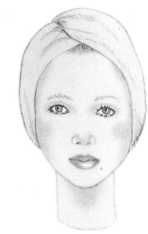

FIG. 26—17

FIG. 26—16. A heart-shaped face. (From Milady's Standard Textbook of Cosmetology, Milady Publishing Co., Tarrytown, NY. Copyright 1991.)

FIG. 26—17. A heart-shaped face with corrective make-up applied. (From Milady's Standard Textbook of Cosmetology, Milady Publishing Co., Tarrytown, NY. Copyright 1991.)

FIG. 26—18. A diamond-shaped face. (From Milady's Standard Textbook of Cosmetology, Milady Publishing Co., Tarrytown, NY. Copyright 1991.)

FIG. 26—19. A diamond-shaped face with corrective make-up applied. (From Milady's Standard Textbook of Cosmetology, Milady Publishing Co., Tarrytown, NY. Copyright 1991.)

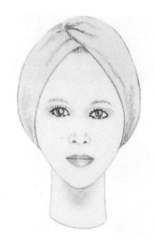

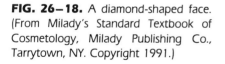

FIG. 26—18

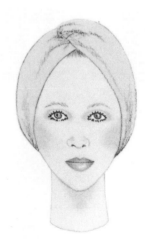

FIG. 26—19

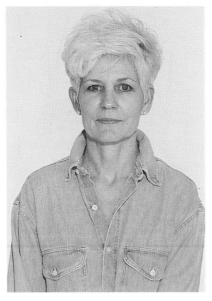

FIG. 26—20

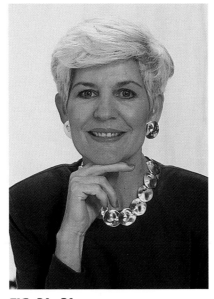

FIG. 26—21

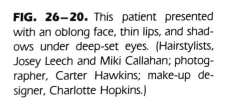

FIG. 26—20. This patient presented with an oblong face, thin lips, and shadows under deep-set eyes. (Hairstylists, Josey Leech and Miki Callahan; photographer, Carter Hawkins; make-up designer, Charlotte Hopkins.)

FIG. 26—21. By adding corrective make-up to create contours and by altering the patient's hairstyling, the oblong face appears more oval. Bright lipstick adds size and fullness to the lips and highlighting eliminates shadows from around the eyes. Proper eyeshadow placement corrects the deep-set look of the eyes. (Hairstylists, Josey Leech and Miki Callahan; photographer, Carter Hawkins; make-up designer, Charlotte Hopkins.)

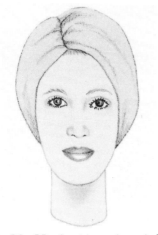

FIG. 26—22. A oblong-shaped face. (From Milady's Standard Textbook of Cosmetology, Milady Publishing Co., Tarrytown, NY. Copyright 1991.)

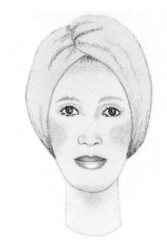

FIG. 26—23. A oblong-shaped face with corrective make-up applied. (From Milady's Standard Textbook of Cosmetology, Milady Publishing Co., Tarrytown, NY. Copyright 1991.)

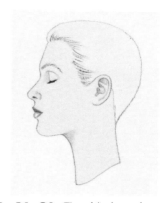

FIG. 26—24. The ideal oval profile. (From Milady's Standard Textbook of Cosmetology, Milady Publishing Co., Tarrytown, NY. Copyright 1991.)

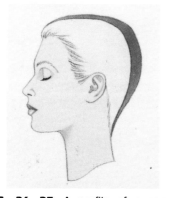

FIG. 26—25. A profile of a narrow head with a flat back. (From Milady's Standard Textbook of Cosmetology, Milady Publishing Co., Tarrytown, NY. Copyright 1991.)

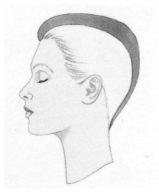

FIG. 26—26. A profile of a flat crown. (From Milady's Standard Textbook of Cosmetology, Milady Publishing Co., Tarrytown, NY. Copyright 1991.)

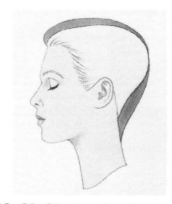

FIG. 26—27. A profile of a pointed head and a hollow nape. (From Milady's Standard Textbook of Cosmetology, Milady Publishing Co., Tarrytown, NY. Copyright 1991.)

FIG. 26—28. A profile of a "flat top". (From Milady's Standard Textbook of Cosmetology. Milady Publishing Co., Tarrytown, NY. Copyright 1991.)

FIG. 26—29. A profile of a small head. (From Milady's Standard Textbook of Cosmetology, Milady Publishing Co., Tarrytown, NY. Copyright 1991.)

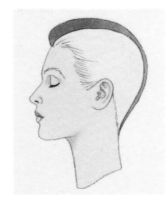 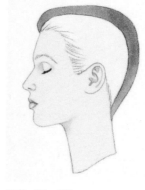

FIG. 26—28   **FIG. 26—29**

FIG. 26—30. This patient exhibited a thin lower lip, circles under the eyes and an uneven complexion. (Hairstylist, Robert Palumbo; assistant hairstylist, Holly Fay; photographers, James Dombrowski and Gene Rizzutto; make-up designers, Larry Fallon and Lisa Duryea.)

FIG. 26—31. The thin lower lip is extended with liner pencil and filled in with harmonizing color. The circles under the eyes and the uneven complexion are concealed with foundation. (Hairstylist, Robert Palumbo; assistant hairstylist, Holly Fay; photographers, James Dombrowski and Gene Rizzutto; make-up designers, Larry Fallon and Lisa Duryea.)

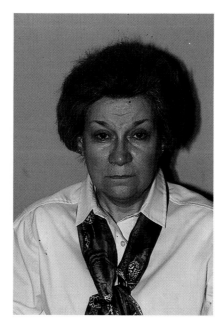 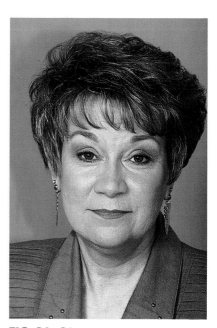

FIG. 26—30   **FIG. 26—31**

Corrective Make-Up for Eyes

CLINICAL TIP. Improvements of identical facial flaws can be accomplished in numerous ways. The effectiveness of different techniques which are designed to accomplish the same goal will vary from patient to patient.

The appearance of the eyes is crucial to correct facial balance. Eye colors and shadows can create the illusion of changes in eye shape and enhance the overall attractiveness of the face.

1. **Dark circles under eyes.** Make-up foundation is applied to the face as usual. Light colored concealer is applied to the circle area to reduce light absorption. Dark liner is avoided around the eyes because of the possibility of drift, the tendency of a color product or cosmetic to move because of gravity into areas of the face other than where initially applied. Foundation is blended in order to avoid a line of demarcation around the eye caused by lighter concealer. An attempt is made to create the illusion of a wider eye by applying a liner to the outer corners to make the eye look less round. Light, flat eye shadow colors are used because eyes with dark circles are often deep-set and need lighter muted shades to detract from shadow created by a protruding brow bone or a sagging upper lid. Color products are emphasized on the cheeks and lower face to focus attention away from the eye area in general (Figs. 26—30 to 26—32). (See also Figs. 26—20, 26—21.)

2. **Bags under eyes and sagging lower eyelids.** Skin care treatment in a clinic may help reduce puffiness. Compress lotions may be recommended for use at home. Make-up technique is much the same as for dark circles except that light concealer is applied and blended only into the lower ridge, just under the bag and not directly on the protruding area. Stress avoidance is advised and referral to a dermatologist or plastic surgeon is advised if fluid retention persists.

3. **Round eyes.** Round eyes can be lengthened by extending the shadows beyond the outer corner of the eyes (Figs. 26—33, 26—34).

4. **Close set eyes.** Close set eyes can be improved by applying shadow lightly with progressive darkening towards the temples (Figs. 26–35 to 26–38).

5. **Bulging eyes.** Bulging eyes can be minimized by blending a dark shadow carefully over the prominent part of the upper lid and carrying it lightly to the line of the brow (Figs. 26–39, 26–40).

6. **Heavy lidded eyes.** Heavy lidded eyes should be shadowed evenly and lightly across the lid from the edge of the eyelash line to the small crease in the eye socket. Frosted shades should be avoided (Figs. 26–41, 26–42).

7. **Small eyes.** To make small eyes appear large, shadow is extended slightly above, beyond and below the eye. Medium colors are preferable (see Figures 26–8, 26–9).

8. **Wide set eyes.** Wide set eyes can be improved by applying darker shadow on the upper inner side of the eyelid.

9. **Deep set eyes.** Deep set eyes require very little shadow on the lids. The part next to the nose and inner corner of the eyes should either be left untouched or flesh colored shadow may be used, darkening slightly as the temple is approached (Fig. 26–43). (See also Figures 26–20, 26–21.)

Strip Eyelashes. Strip eyelashes are available in a variety of types, sizes, and textures. They can be made from human hair, animal hair, such as mink, or synthetic fibers. Synthetic fiber eyelashes are made with a permanent curl and do not react to changes in weather conditions. Artificial eyelashes are available in colors ranging from light to dark brown and black or light to dark auburn to coordinate with hair and brow color. Black and dark brown are the most popular choices. Care should be taken so that false eyelashes are not too large for the eyes and face.

CLINICAL TIP. Strip eyelashes should be used with caution to avoid a "hard" or "over-done" appearance. This is especially true for women over the age of thirty-five.

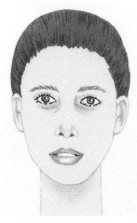

FIG. 26–32. Dark circles under the eyes. (From Milady's Standard Textbook of Cosmetology, Milady Publishing Co., Tarrytown, NY. Copyright 1991.)

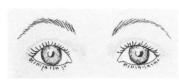

FIG. 26–33. Round eyes. (From Milady's Standard Textbook of Cosmetology, Milady Publishing Co., Tarrytown, NY. Copyright 1991.)

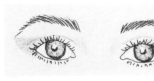

FIG. 26–34. Round eyes with corrective make-up. (From Milady's Standard Textbook of Cosmetology, Milady Publishing Co., Tarrytown, NY. Copyright 1991.)

FIG. 26–35. This patient exhibited facial flaws that included close-set eyes and a high forehead. (Hairstylist, Robert Palumbo; assistant hair designer, Holly Fay; photographers, James Dombrowski and Gene Rizzutto; make-up designers, Larry Fallon and Lisa Duryea.)

FIG. 26–36. Close-set eyes are treated by applying shadow lightly and carrying it up from the outer edge of the eyes. A suitable hairstyle draws attention away from the high forehead. (Hairstylist Robert Palumbo; assistant hair designer, Holly Fay; photographers, James Dombrowski and Gene Rizzutto; make-up designers, Larry Fallon and Lisa Duryea.)

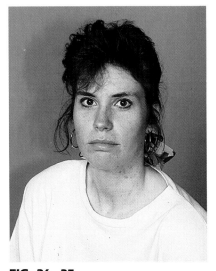

FIG. 26–35

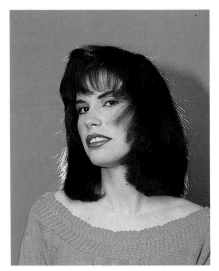

FIG. 26–36

ESTHETIC DENTISTRY

FIG. 26—37. Close-set eyes. (From Milady's Standard Textbook of Cosmetology, Milady Publishing Co., Tarrytown, NY. Copyright 1991.)

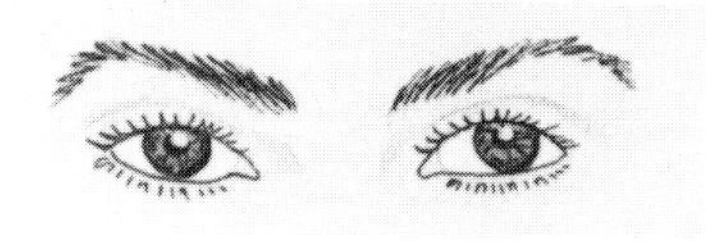

FIG. 26—38. Close-set eyes with corrective make-up. (From Milady's Standard Textbook of Cosmetology, Milady Publishing Co., Tarrytown, NY. Copyright 1991.)

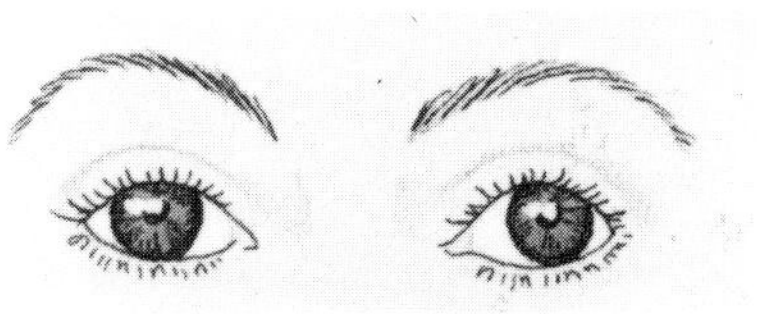

FIG. 26—39. Bulging eyes. (From Milady's Standard Textbook of Cosmetology, Milady Publishing Co., Tarrytown, NY. Copyright 1991.)

  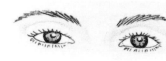 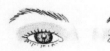

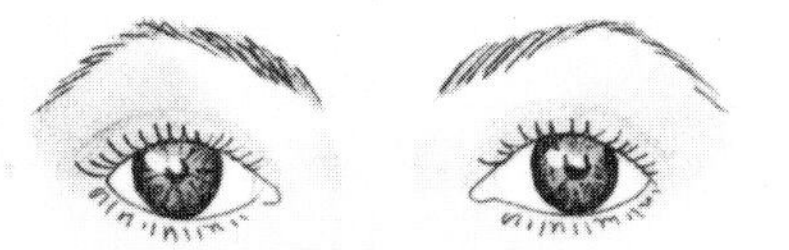

FIG. 26—40. Bulging eyes with corrective make-up. (From Milady's Standard Textbook of Cosmetology, Milady Publishing Co., Tarrytown, NY. Copyright 1991.)

FIG. 26—41. Heavy-lidded eyes. (From Milady's Standard Textbook of Cosmetology, Milady Publishing Co., Tarrytown, NY. Copyright 1991.)

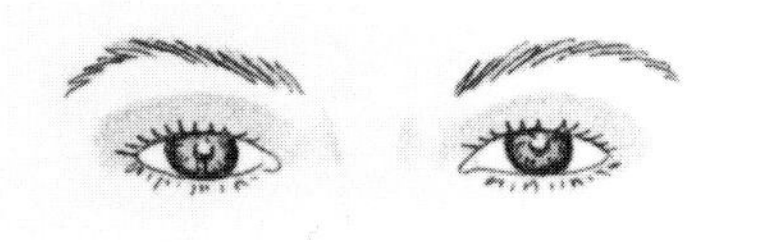

FIG. 26—42. Heavy-lidded eyes with corrective make-up. (From Milady's Standard Textbook of Cosmetology, Milady Publishing Co., Tarrytown, NY. Copyright 1991.)

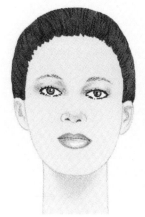 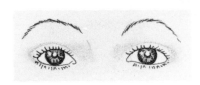 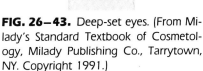 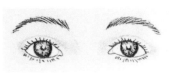 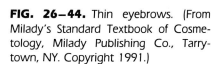

FIG. 26—43. Deep-set eyes. (From Milady's Standard Textbook of Cosmetology, Milady Publishing Co., Tarrytown, NY. Copyright 1991.)

FIG. 26—44. Thin eyebrows. (From Milady's Standard Textbook of Cosmetology, Milady Publishing Co., Tarrytown, NY. Copyright 1991.)

FIG. 26—45. Corrective technique for thin eyebrows. (From Milady's Standard Textbook of Cosmetology, Milady Publishing Co., Tarrytown, NY. Copyright 1991.)

Corrective Make-Up for Eyebrows

CLINICAL TIP. Patients should be advised to have eyebrows shaped by professionals. Badly arched brows are worse than untouched brows.

1. **Brow devoid of hair.** When there are spaces in the brow devoid of hair, they can be filled in with hairlike strokes of an eyebrow pencil. An eyebrow brush is used to soften the pencil marks (Figs. 26—44, 26—45).
2. **High arch.** When the arch is too high, the superfluous hair from the top of the brow is removed and the lower part is filled in with pencil.
3. **Low arch.** When the arch is too low, the superfluous hair from the lower part of the brow is removed and the shape of the brow is built up using the eyebrow pencil.
4. **High forehead.** In the case of a high forehead, the eyebrow arch may be slightly elevated to detract from a high forehead. A too thin, too round line, however, creates a "surprised" look.
5. **Low forehead.** A low arch gives more height to a very low forehead.
6. **Wide set eyes.** The eyes can be made to appear closer together by extending the eyebrow lines to the inside corners of the eyes. However, care must be taken to avoid creating a frowning look.
7. **Close set eyes.** To make the eyes appear farther apart, the distance between the eyebrows is widened; the brows are slightly extended outward. Dark shadows on inner corners should be avoided (Figs. 26—46, 26—47). (See also Figs. 26—35, 26—36).
8. **Round face.** High arching of the brows makes the face appear narrower. A line is started directly above the inside corner of the eye and extended to the end of the cheekbone.

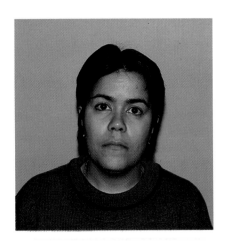

FIG. 26-46

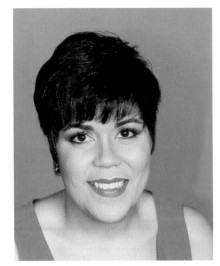

FIG. 26-47

FIG. 26-46. This patient presented with an uneven blemished complexion, a broad nose, close-set eyes, and a thin upper lip. (Hairstylist, Robert Palumbo; assistant hairstylist, Holly Fay; photographers, James Dombrowski and Gene Rizzutto; make-up designers, Larry Fallon and Lisa Duryea.)

FIG. 26-47. The uneven, blemished complexion is covered with base. The broad nose is slenderized with darker base placed on both sides of the nose. The close-set eyes are treated by tweezing the brows above the inner corners of the eyes and the lower lip is extended with liner pencil and filled in with harmonizing color. (Hairstylist, Robert Palumbo; assistant hairstylist, Holly Fay; photographers, James Dombrowski and Gene Rizzutto; make-up designers, Larry Fallon and Lisa Duryea.)

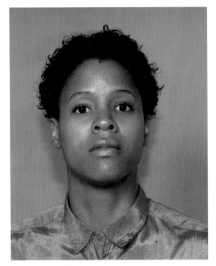

FIG. 26-48

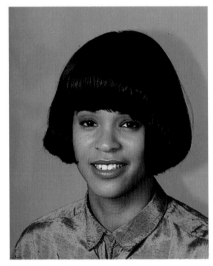

FIG. 26-49

FIG. 26-48. This patient presented with an oblong face and a high forehead. (Hairstylist, Robert Palumbo; assistant hairstylist, Holly Fay; photographers, James Dombrowski and Gene Rizzutto; make-up designers, Larry Fallon and Lisa Duryea.)

FIG. 26-49. Alteration of the hairstyle creates a more appealing look. (Hairstylist, Robert Palumbo; assistant hairstylist, Holly Fay; photographers, James Dombrowski and Gene Rizzutto; make-up designers, Larry Fallon and Lisa Duryea.)

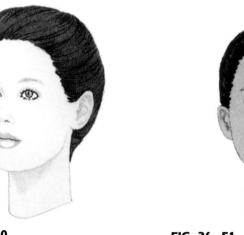

FIG. 26-50

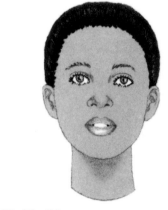

FIG. 26-51

FIG. 26-50. Protruding forehead. (From Milady's Standard Textbook of Cosmetology, Milady Publishing Co., Tarrytown, NY. Copyright 1991.)

FIG. 26-51. Short flat nose. (From Milady's Standard Textbook of Cosmetology, Milady Publishing Co., Tarrytown, NY. Copyright 1991.)

ESTHETIC DENTISTRY

Corrective Make-Up for Forehead

For a low forehead, applying a lighter foundation cream creates a broader appearance between the brows and hairline. For a bulging forehead, a darker foundation applied over the prominent area gives the illusion of fullness to the rest of the face and minimizes the bulging forehead. With a suitable hairstyle, attention can be drawn away from the forehead (Figs. 26–48 to 26–50). (See also Figs. 26–35, 26–36.)

Corrective Make-Up for Nose and Chin

1. **Large nose.** For a large protruding nose, darker foundation is applied on the nose and a lighter foundation on the cheeks at the sides of the nose. This creates fullness in the cheeks and makes the nose appear smaller. Placing cheek color close to the nose should be avoided.
2. **Short flat nose.** For a short flat nose, a lighter foundation is applied down the center of the nose, ending at the tip. This makes the nose appear longer and larger. If the nostrils are wider, a darker foundation is applied to both sides of the nostrils (Fig. 26–51).
3. **Broad nose.** For a broad nose, a darker foundation on the sides of the nose and nostrils is used. This dark tone should not be carried into the laugh lines because it will accentuate them. The foundation must be carefully blended to avoid visible lines (Figs. 26–52, 26–53). (For a preoperative view of the patient in Figure 26–52 see Figure 26–8.) (See also Figs. 26–46, 26–47.)
4. **Protruding chin and receding nose.** For a protruding chin and receding nose, the chin is shadowed with a darker foundation and the nose is highlighted with a lighter foundation.
5. **A receding (small) chin.** For a receding (small) chin, the chin is highlighted by using a lighter foundation than the one used on the face (Fig. 26–54).
6. **A sagging double chin.** For a sagging double chin, a darker foundation is used on the sagging portions and a natural skin tone foundation is used on the face (Fig. 26–55).

FIG. 26–52. This is the same patient shown in Figure 26–8. The use of an upswept evening hairstyle and darker eye make-up creates a different appearance from that seen in Figure 26–9. The bridge of the nose appears narrower through the use of proper make-up. (Hairstylist, Josey Leech and Miki Callahan; photographer, Carter Hawkins; make-up designer, Charlotte Hopkins.)

FIG. 26–53. Broad nose. (From Milady's Standard Textbook of Cosmetology, Milady Publishing Co., Tarrytown, NY. Copyright 1991.)

FIG. 26–54. Receding chin. (From Milady's Standard Textbook of Cosmetology, Milady Publishing Co., Tarrytown, NY. Copyright 1991.)

FIG. 26–55. Double chin. (From Milady's Standard Textbook of Cosmetology, Milady Publishing Co., Tarrytown, NY. Copyright 1991.)

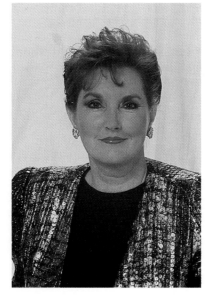

FIG. 26–52

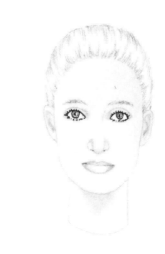

FIG. 26–53

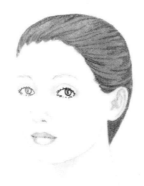

FIG. 26–54

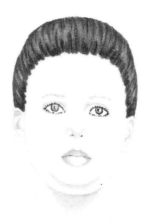

FIG. 26–55

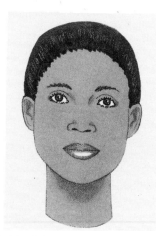

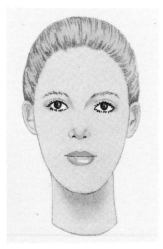

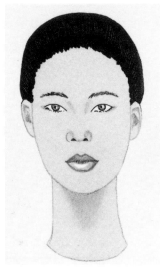

FIG. 26–56. Broad jawline. (From Milady's Standard Textbook of Cosmetology, Milady Publishing Co., Tarrytown, NY. Copyright 1991.)

FIG. 26–57. Narrow jawline. (From Milady's Standard Textbook of Cosmetology, Milady Publishing Co., Tarrytown, NY. Copyright 1991.)

FIG. 26–58. Long, thin neck. (From Milady's Standard Textbook of Cosmetology, Milady Publishing Co., Tarrytown, NY. Copyright 1991.)

Corrective Make-Up for the Jawline and Neck

The neck and jaws are as important as the eyes, cheeks, and lips. When applying make-up, the foundation cream is carried down below the neckline of the patients clothing to prevent the appearance of a line of demarcation.

1. **Broad jaws.** For broad jaws, a darker shade of foundation is applied over the heavy areas of the jaws beginning at the temples. This minimizes the lower part of the face and creates the illusion of width in the upper part (Figs. 26–56).
2. **A narrow jawline.** A narrow jawline may be highlighted by using a lighter shade of foundation than the one used on the rest of the face (Fig. 26–57).
3. **A round, square, or triangular face.** For a round, square, or triangular face, a darker shade of foundation is applied over the prominent area of the jawline. By creating a shadow over this area, the prominent part of the jaw will appear softer and more oval.
4. **A small face and a short, thick neck.** For a small face and a short, thick neck, a darker foundation is used on the neck than the one used on the face. This will make the neck appear thinner.
5. **A long thin neck.** For a long thin neck, a lighter shade and foundation is applied to the neck than the one used on the face. This will create fullness and counter the long thin appearance of the neck (Fig. 26–58).

Corrective Make-Up for Perioral Flaws

Frequently, conditions of the perioral area require cosmetic correction.

Upper Lip Recession. An illusion may be produced by applying a slightly lighter foundation color to the center of the upper lip. Because a recessed upper lip also has a flat and widened appearance due to lack of support from the teeth, care must be taken to apply a slightly darker foundation to the outside edges of the upper lip to reduce the effect of this "widening." Recession of the mandible and lower lip can be treated in the same manner. Focusing attention toward the eyes, cheekbones, and more attractive areas of the face by accentuating these areas with color cosmetics will also help to detract from the mouth (Fig. 26–59).

Perioral Wrinkling. Perioral wrinkling should initially be treated with appropriate moisturizers and corrective skin care products that make the skin smoother and more hydrated. Wrinkles around the mouth are mitigated by the application of light color concealer applied with a fine brush directly to the wrinkle. Flesh-colored foundation can then be blended in over this area (Fig. 26–60).

Sagging Nasolabial Areas. The same technique used for the correction of lines around the mouth can be used on the nasolabial folds. Again, detraction from the oral area to other areas of the face helps to soften the appearance of these lines. Shifting the visual focus to the cheekbones also results in detraction from the nasolabial areas (Fig. 26–61).

Thin Lips. To correct thin lips, a bright lipstick which adds size and fullness to the lips is used. (See Figs. 26–8, 26–9, 26–30, 26–31, 26–46, 26–47.)

Lipstick "Bleeding". Lipstick sometimes drifts or "bleeds" into small wrinkles in the perioral area. A number of commercial products are designed to provide a protective sealant to the lips and wrinkle areas to prevent this problem. In addition, frequent maintenance of

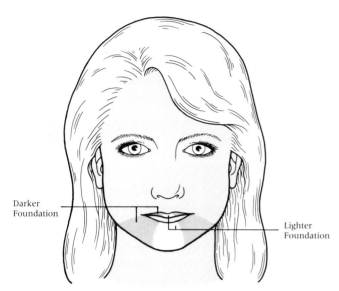

FIG. 26–59. *Visual correction of upper lip recession. The philtrum of the lip and the chin are highlighted with lighter foundation to focus attention upward and outward. This detracts from the recession of the mandible. The lower lip is also highlighted with a slightly lighter lipstick, creating a more youthful appearance.*

the lipstick and avoidance of deep lipstick colors lessens the chance of "bleeding."

Lip Dryness. The lips should be treated frequently with emollient products, particularly when the patient lives in a sunny, cold, or windy climate. If the skin exhibits excessive chronic peeling the patient should be seen by a physician. Sunscreens help decrease dryness by reducing sun damage, as well as reducing the risk of skin cancer.

Creases in the Lower Corners of the Mouth. Creases in the lower corners of the mouth can be corrected by the judicious use of dark and light shaded cover-up make-up. (See the section on Corrective Make-Up Principles earlier in this chapter.)

Make-Up Induced Tooth Discoloration. To avoid make-up induced tooth discoloration, very dark lipstick combined with very light foundation should be avoided (Fig. 26–62). Women with yellow teeth should avoid amber or gold-toned shades of lipstick and foundations with warm gold or sallow undertones (Fig. 26–63). Application of a lilac or lavender color toner underneath the foundation helps cut yellow or sallow tones (Fig. 26–64). Hair color with gold or yellow tones should also be avoided.

FIG. 26–60. *Perioral wrinkling without nasolabial sagging. Perioral wrinkling in younger patients usually occurs without nasolabial sagging. These lines can be caused by sun damage or facial expression, such as those that occur while smoking. Use of a good moisturizing treatment will help mitigate the appearance of these lines. Corrective make-up procedures are the same as for perioral wrinkling with nasolabial sagging (see Figure 26–61).*

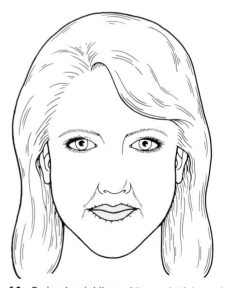

FIG. 26–61. *Perioral wrinkling with nasolabial sagging. Perioral wrinkling is caused by solar (environmental) exposure and intrinsic aging. The nasolabial sagging can be visually corrected by applying light concealer directly to the wrinkles and blending it with flesh-colored foundation. Use of a good hydrating moisturizer will also help improve the appearance of these lines. Protective sealants are commercially available to help keep lipstick from "bleeding" or seeping into these fine perioral lines.*

ESTHETICS AND COSMETOLOGY

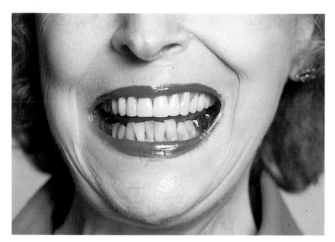

FIG. 26–62. Lipstick that is too dark frames the mouth and accentuates dental discoloration. The teeth appear darker because of the dark lipstick and relatively light foundation.

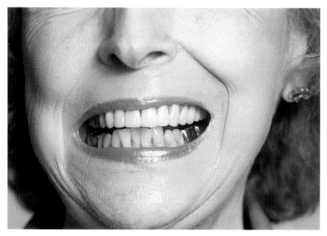

FIG. 26–63. Gold lipstick causes the teeth to appear yellower.

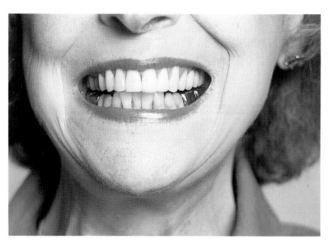

FIG. 26–64. Correct color foundation and proper lipstick color facilitate the esthetic improvement gained from the placement of porcelain laminate veneer restorations.

HAIR STYLING

CLINICAL TIP. The actual application of hairstyling techniques is obviously outside the parameters of cosmetic dentistry. As with the use of make-up, the cosmetic dentist should have an understanding of the basic principles and goals of corrective hairstyling. However, some patients may consider discussions in this area to be overly intrusive. (See also the Clinical Tip in the section on Make-Up.)

As with corrective make-up, hairstyling involves an assessment of overall facial type (Table 26–1). The goal of corrective hairstyling is to create the illusion of the ideal facial shape. Facial profile, including the shape of the nose, eyes, and head, racial consideration, and even the use of glasses, can influence the esthetic effect of a particular hairstyle.

Profiles

The profile can be a good indicator of the correct shape for a hairstyle (Table 26–2).

Nose Shapes

Nose shapes are closely related to profile. When selecting a hairstyle, the nose should be considered both in profile and from the full face view (Table 26–3).

Eyes

Because the eyes are the focal point of the face, hairstyles must complement the patient's eyes. The effects of wide set eyes, which are usually found on a round or square face, can be minimized by lifting and fluffing the top of the hair and the bang area (Figs. 26–65, 26–66). A side bang helps draw attention away from the space between the eyes. Close-set eyes are usually found on long narrow faces. In these cases the hair should be styled fairly high with a side movement to create the illusion of more spaces between the eyes. The hair ends should turn outward and upward (Figs. 26–67, 26–68).

Styling for People Who Wear Glasses

People who wear glasses have special considerations regarding hairstyle and make-up. Following are some basic rules that should be followed by those who wear glasses.

1. Glass frames should be up-to-date with large lenses for good vision.
2. Gaudy, over-jewelled, frames should not be worn.
3. Strip false eyelashes should not be worn; they are too long and will contact the lens.
4. Heavy makeup should not be used; heavy makeup is not necessary to bring out the color and best features of the eyes.
5. Hairstyles should fall naturally around the face and not interfere with putting on and removing glasses.
6. Overstyled hair with many tight curls is impractical for people with glasses.

TABLE 26–1. HAIRSTYLING FOR DIFFERENT FACIAL TYPES

FACE TYPE	GOAL	METHOD	SHAPE
Oval-shaped	Considered the ideal facial shape	A person with an oval-shaped face can wear any hairstyle unless there are other considerations, such as eye-glasses, length and shape of nose, or profile.	
Round-shaped	To add length to the face	Create a hairstyle with height by arranging the hair on top of the head. Some hair can be placed over the ears and cheeks or hair can be kept on one side exposing the ears. Bangs should be styled to one side.	
Square-shaped	To add length and offset the square features	Treat the square face similar to the round face. Asymmetrical hairstyles that lift the hair off the forehead and forward of the temples and jaw, create the illusion of narrowness and softness in the face.	
Pear-shaped	To add width to the forehead	Build a semi-curl or soft wave effect hairstyle that is fairly full and high. Partially cover the forehead with a fringe of soft hair. The hair should be cropped over the ears.	
Heart-shaped	To decrease the width of the forehead and increase the width of the lower part of the face	To reduce the apparent width of the forehead, the hair should be parted in the center with bangs flipped up. Alternatively, a hairstyle slanted to one side can be used.	
Diamond-shaped	To decrease the width across the cheekbone lines	To create an oval appearance, increase the fullness across the jawline and forehead and keep the hair close to the head at the cheekbone line. Avoid hairstyles that lift away from the cheeks or move back from the hairline.	
Oblong-shaped	To decrease the length and increase the width of the face	The hair should be styled fairly close to the top of the head with a fringe of curls and bangs combined with fullness to the sides. Drawing the hair out from the cheeks creates the illusion of width.	

(Adapted from Milady's Standard Textbook of Cosmetology, Milady Publishing Co., Tarrytown, NY, 1991.)

TABLE 26-2. HAIRSTYLING FOR DIFFERENT FACIAL PROFILES

PROFILE	METHOD	SHAPE
Straight	This profile, which is neither concave nor convex, is considered ideal; thus, all hairstyles usually work well.	
Concave (prominent chin)	The hair at the nape should be styled softly with a movement upward. Hair should not be built out onto the forehead.	
Convex (receding forehead, prominent nose, and receding chin)	Place curls or bangs over the forehead. Keep the style close to the head at the nape.	
Low forehead, protruding chin	Build a fluffy bang with height to create the illusion of fullness to the forehead. An upswept temple movement will add length to the face. Soften the chin line with soft curls in the nape area. Do not end the style line at the nape—this draws attention to the chin line. Rather, create a line that is either higher or lower than the chin line.	

(Adapted from Milady's Standard Textbook of Cosmetology, Milady Publishing Co., Tarrytown, NY, 1991.)

FIG. 26-65. Wide-set eyes—improper hairstyling. (From Milady's Standard Textbook of Cosmetology, Milady Publishing Co., Tarrytown, NY. Copyright 1991.)

FIG. 26-66. Wide-set eyes—correct hairstyling. (From Milady's Standard Textbook of Cosmetology, Milady Publishing Co., Tarrytown, NY. Copyright 1991.)

FIG. 26-67. Close-set eyes—improper hairstyling. (From Milady's Standard Textbook of Cosmetology, Milady Publishing Co., Tarrytown, NY. Copyright 1991.)

FIG. 26-68. Close-set eyes—correct hairstyling. (From Milady's Standard Textbook of Cosmetology, Milady Publishing Co., Tarrytown, NY. Copyright 1991.)

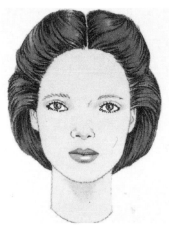

FIG. 26-65

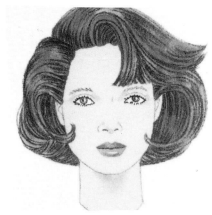

FIG. 26-66

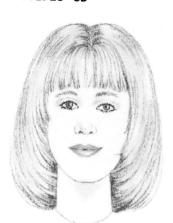

FIG. 26-67

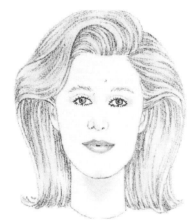

FIG. 26-68

TABLE 26—3. HAIRSTYLING FOR DIFFERENT NOSE

TYPE OF NOSE	GOAL	WRONG WAY	RIGHT WAY
Turned-up nose	This type of nose is usually small and accompanied by a straight profile. The small nose is considered to be a childlike quality; therefore, it is best to design a hairstyle that is not associated with children. The hair should be swept off the face, creating a line from the nose to the ears. This adds length to the short nose. The top hair should move off the forehead to give the illusion of length to the nose.		
Prominent (hooked, large, or pointed) nose	In order to draw attention away from the nose, bring the hair forward at the forehead with softness around the face.		
Crooked nose	To minimize the conspicuous crooked nose, style the hair in an off-center manner, which attracts the eye away from the nose. Asymmetrical styles work best. Any well-balanced hairstyle accentuates that the face is uneven.		
Wide flat nose	A wide flat nose tends to broaden the face. In order to minimize this effect, the hair should be drawn away from the face. In addition, a center part tends to narrow the nose, as well as draw attention away from the nose.		

(Adapted from Milady's Standard Textbook of Cosmetology, Milady Publishing Co., Tarrytown, NY, 1991.)

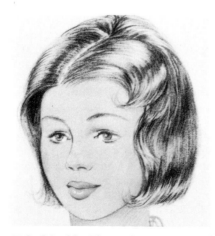

FIG. 26—69. Diagonal parts are used to give height to a round or square face. (From Milady's Standard Textbook of Cosmetology, Milady Publishing Co., Tarrytown, NY. Copyright 1991.)

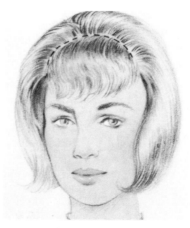

FIG. 26—70. Curved rectangular parts are used for a receding hairline or a high forehead. (From Milady's Standard Textbook of Cosmetology, Milady Publishing Co., Tarrytown, NY. Copyright 1991.)

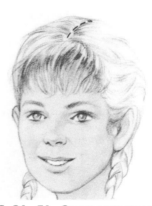

FIG. 26—71. Center parts are used for popular children's hairstyles with bangs. (From Milady's Standard Textbook of Cosmetology, Milady Publishing Co., Tarrytown, NY. Copyright 1991.)

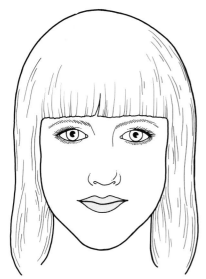

FIG. 26-72. *Youthful hairstyles are* not *appropriate for patients with perioral esthetic problems. This style "frames" the face, focusing too much attention on the center of the face* and *the mouth area.*

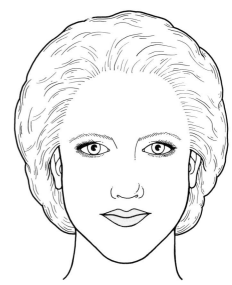

FIG. 26-73. *Upswept, off the face hairstyles are more appropriate for the dental patient with perioral appearance problems. The visual center of the face is raised, focusing attention away from the mouth.*

A combination of proper hairstyle, proper make-up, and the correct glasses helps to accentuate the wearers best features (Table 26-4).

Hair Parting

Hair parting can be the focal point of a hairstyle. Because the eye is drawn to a part it must be neat, without hairs straggling from one side or another, and it must be straight and directed positively. If possible, a natural part should be used. However, it may be necessary to create a part according to the specific head shape, facial features, or desired hairstyle. Unfortunately, it is often difficult to create a lasting hairstyle when working against the natural crowning parting.

Following are suggestions for suitable hair partings for various facial types.

Parting for bangs

1. Rectangular to triangular partings are most commonly used for children's bangs. The triangular part distributes more hair to the temple area, which is often sparse in children.
2. Diagonal parts are used to give height to a round or square face (Fig. 26-69).
3. Curved rectangular parts are used for a receding hairline or high forehead (Fig. 26-70).
4. Center parts are popular for children's hairstyles with bangs (Fig. 26-71).

Hairstyles and Oral Considerations

Hairstyles for persons with oral esthetic problems should not "frame" the face. Avoidance of bangs, bob cuts, and other styles that focus and accentuate the cen-

ter of the face will help to lessen the appearance of perioral features. Upswept, off the face hairstyles will be more attractive for these individuals (Figs. 26-72, 26-73).

SPECIAL CONSIDERATIONS

Few, if any, individuals have a perfect set of features. The goal is to analyze specific features and accentuate the favorable ones (Table 26-5).).

Aging

Following are some rules for the aging patient regarding make-up techniques.

1. **Choose flat colors rather than frosted.** Frosted or "pearlized" powders settle in facial lines. They are generally intended for younger people because they have a higher amount of light reflection and accentuate aging skin rather than make it appear more youthful.
2. **Bright colors should not be worn on mature skin.** Bright colors are not as easily blended as less vivid shades and may accentuate an aging appearance.
3. **Use a foundation color that perfectly matches skin color.** Many patients choose foundation colors that are darker than their skin, mistakenly believing that they cover blemishes better. The viscosity, pigment, and talc levels of the product are the factors that determine coverage. Patients with sun damaged skin have a tendency to incorrectly choose dark foundation colors that match the hyperpigmented solar freckles and splotchiness, rather than the actual color of the skin.
4. **Blend make-up properly.** Improperly blended make-up creates lines that often run parallel to skin

FACE	GLASSES	MAKE-UP	HAIRSTYLE	BANGS	WRONG WAY	RIGHT WAY
ound, oval or square face	Choose slender frames with large visual lenses. Match the frame color with the hair color.	Blend dark eye shadow over the prominent part of the upper lid in patients with large eyes.	Use a simple, uncluttered, casual bouffant hairstyle in natural balance.	Slashed bangs that freely touch the eyebrows.		
eart-shaped or diamond-shaped face	Frames should be slender, of medium thickness, and should follow the eyebrows and rest against the face.	Wear light make-up shades and delicate eye make-up.	A full page boy style or other hairstyle with increased width in the lower part of the face.	Open bangs harmonize and balance with the lower part of the face.		
nall, narrow or oval face	Select large up-to-date frames that are not too gaudy.	Use natural tones of make-up. Since eyes are magnified through the glasses proper eye make-up is essential.	The hairstyle should be short, with deep wave shapings on the sides leaving freedom for control of glasses.	Side wave bangs touching one eyebrow can complement the eyes.		
ar-shaped face	Wear large, oval-shaped frames to let the glasses reveal eyes.	Place the appropriate eye shade depending on patient eye type (see preceding section on Corrective Make-Up for Eyes)	The hair should be worn up and out of the face to emphasis length. Soft bouffant styling around the face, with softness brushed forward on the cheeks will reduce width.	Side wave bangs over one eye add expression and interest.		

pted from Milady's Standard Textbook of Cosmetology, Milady Publishing Co., Tarrytown, NY, 1991.)

lines. This accentuates wrinkles. Good quality brushes and proper technique are important when blending out edges of colors, especially of eye-liner and eyeshadow.

5. **Less is better.** This is a good rule of thumb when applying make-up to an aging patient. This rule particularly applies to color products.

6. **Hair color should be lighter than the patient's original color.** This is especially true if the hair is artificially colored. Dark hair creates shadows and edges that make the perimeter of the face look older.

PARAMEDICAL CAMOUFLAGE

Paramedical camouflage make-up involves many of the same principals of corrective make-up. Paramedical camouflage make-up, however, is used for persons suffering from more esthetically devastating afflictions such as scars, skin or oral cancer, accidents, burns, congenital esthetic birth defects, or facial reconstruction. In severe cases, facial esthetic prostheses may also be included in this type of make-up artistry.

Scars

Scars vary greatly in texture, color, size, depth, shape, location, and age. Therefore, many different disguise techniques may be implemented. Small scars are obviously easier to cover than large ones, however, a small scar on otherwise beautiful skin can be more esthetically detrimental than a large scar on an imperfect complexion.

The appearance of a scar may change with time. Redness associated with a recent injury or surgical procedure often fades over time. In order to avoid applying make-up or any chemical to a healing area (i.e., scabs or areas of recently removed sutures), estheticians frequently obtain clearance from the physician or dentist.

The texture of a scar, as opposed to its color, usually cannot be covered completely. Raised or indented scars are much harder to hide than flat scars. Basic corrective principals are appropriate for textured scars; light colors are applied to indentions and darker contours to raised scars. Foundation is then blended to detract from scar perimeters. "Ice pick" scars are extremely difficult to

TABLE 26–5. HAIRSTYLING FOR SPECIAL CONSIDERATIONS

FEATURE	GOAL	HAIRSTYLE	STYLE
Plump with short neck	To create the illusion of length	Sweep the hair up to give length to the neck. Build height on top. Avoid hairstyles that give fullness to the back of the neck and hairstyles with horizontal lines.	
Long thin neck	To minimize the appearance of the long neck	Cover the neck with soft waves. Avoid short or sculptured necklines. Keep the hair long and full at the nape.	
Thin features	To give width to the face and neck	Lift sides up and away from the hairline, but keep the style soft and loose. The nape hair should be long and full to fill in at the neck.	
Uneven features	To minimize imperfect features	Any style that draws attention away from the imperfect features. If a face is smaller on one side than the other, an asymmetrical style may balance it.	

(Adapted from Milady's Standard Textbook of Cosmetology, Milady Publishing Co., Tarrytown, NY, 1991.)

conceal and are best treated by skin conditioning treatments and the use of astringent foundations. Patients with scarred skin often are referred to a plastic surgeon for evaluation of surgical possibilities.

Bruising

Redness on the perimeter of a surgical site or injured area can be neutralized with the application of a green colored toner or foundation, followed by the application of a flesh colored foundation. Multiple colors appear as the bruise ages. The typical progression of bruise colors is black to purple to blue to green and finally to yellow. Yellow or white toners are used for black, purple, and blue bruises; mauve is used for green bruises; and lilac is used for yellow bruises and sallow skin tones. Patients are most concerned with the darkest bruises, however, the use of make-up immediately postoperatively on a bruise is often contraindicated. The usual exception to this rule is a dental procedure in which the outside of the skin is bruised as a result of surgery on the inside of the oral cavity. The doctor usually allows make-up application as soon as the patient is no longer sensitive to touch. Bruises associated with sutures usually require more time to heal.

As large facial bruises dissipate, they may appear to "drift," often moving to the neck, collar, and chest. The areas can be covered with either make-up or scarves and high neckline garments.

It is often advisable for patients to undergo a series of skin cleansing and skin conditioning treatments prior to elective surgery. Cleansing treatments help to rid the skin and follicles of debris, fatty deposits, comedones (skin lesions which may contribute to acne), blackheads, and whiteheads. Conditioning treatments improve the softness and surface texture of the face. These treatments improve skin circulation and general appearance. On average, patients who undergo these procedures show less postoperative bruising and redness and the scar textures are more even in appearance. It is theorized that healthy skin heals better than skin that is not well cared for, although there are no controlled scientific studies in this area.

DISORDERS AND TREATMENTS
Perioral Dermatitis

Perioral dermatitis, found predominantly in women, is characterized by papular erythemic eruptions in the

ESTHETIC DENTISTRY

perioral area.[4] Because it is a dermatitis, rather than a cosmetic disorder, it should be treated by a dermatologist.

Heavy make-up and foundations may be irritating or may produce comedones.[5] The esthetician may be consulted to teach the patient to conceal the condition using noncomedogenic foundations that may be less irritating and still provide adequate cosmetic coverage of the area.

Chin Acne

"Chin acne," also predominant in women, is characterized by large inflamed nodules in the cheeks, chin, and jawline. Often associated with menstrual cycles, researchers theorize that an elevation of androgenic hormones may aggravate the condition.[5] The biochemical mechanics of this theory are not fully understood, however, clinical evidence supports this theory. The appearance of large, sore papules in the chin and lower facial areas during the third week of the menstrual cycle, a similar occurrence in females using androgen-dominant oral contraceptives, and evidence of acne flare-ups associated with stress-induced adrenal testosterone production, all implicate androgens as an aggravating factor.[5]

Patients with chin acne are normally treated by a dermatologist, however the esthetician plays an important role in topical cleansing and cosmetic treatment of this affliction. Cleansing treatments help to rid the skin of acne-causing clogged follicles. Counseling in external factors, such as proper home cleansing and the use of noncomedogenic cosmetics, can be beneficial. Noncomedogenic cosmetics are preparations that have been formulated to eliminate large amounts of irritating fatty acids and other known follicle-clogging ingredients.[6-8] Proper cleansing procedures, the use of noncomedogenic preparations, and professional cleansing treatments and care help to control *external* factors that can aggravate acne flare-ups. Although medical care and drug therapy is necessary for some patients, controlling external factors often is sufficient in persons with minor blemish problems.

Perioral Wrinkling and Aging

There is a genetic component of susceptibility to wrinkling and aging of the face, but this can be prematurely activated by many external and environmental factors. The professional esthetician can help reduce the appearance of premature aging characteristics and help to eliminate, through patient preventive education, external factors that cause aging.

The most preventable cause of premature aging is sun overexposure. Sun exposure causes damage to the collagen and elastin fibrils in the dermis, which in turn causes wrinkles and loss of elasticity.[2] The esthetician is in a position to educate the patient about the proper use of sunscreens and sunblocks to help prevent this damage. Proper use of hydrating treatments and moisturizers can help to soften and reduce the appearance of lines, wrinkles, and loss of elasticity. Today's sophisticated cosmetic preparations can help to significantly reduce these visual flaws.

The Use of Retinoids

The use of topical retinoids, particularly tretinoin (Retin-A, Ortho Pharmaceutical Corp.), shows promise in reducing the affects of photoaging. While the actual mechanisms of tretinoin therapy are not fully understood, routine use significantly decreases tactile roughness, fine lines, and photoinduced hyperpigmentation. Histologic improvements include enhanced blood vessel formation, increased "turnover" rate of epidermal cells, and increased layering of the epidermal strata.[9] (See Chapter 25-Esthetics and Dermatology.)

The esthetician's role in working with tretinoin treated patients is multifaceted. Cosmetic regimes may need to be significantly altered due to the side effects of tretinoin use. Elimination of strong astringents, alcoholic topical products, keratolytic creams and lotions, and harsh abrasives is recommended.[10]

Increased use of intensive nonirritating hydrating or moisturizing products, and in-clinic hydrating and soothing treatments may be necessary to aid the tretinoin patient in controlling the irritation and dehydration caused as a side effect of tretinoin treatments. These topical therapies will help to comfort the skin, aid in the appearance of a smooth texture, and improve the skin surface so that make-up can be applied in a normal manner.[11]

The use of sunscreens is essential for patients using tretinoin. Due to its irritating effects on the skin, patients using the drug are more susceptible to sun damage, sunburn, and sun irritations.[11]

Additionally, cleansing treatments may be necessary to help rid the skin of comedones brought to the surface by the tretinoin therapy or by the use of comedogenic moisturizers.

Estheticians should be well trained in the procedures involved with tretinoin therapy. It is important that the esthetician contact the prescribing dermatologist or plastic surgeon concerning care for retinoic patients. Even though tretinoin is a prescription drug, estheticians should be aware of correct procedures for application and usage, and how tretinoin, as a topical agent, fits within a normal cleansing, skin hygiene, and cosmetic regime. In this way, estheticians may give proper counsel to their cosmetic patients.

Hirsutism

Hirsutism is the superfluous growth of excess hair. It is most often caused by an imbalance of hormones and occurs predominantly in females. Excessive hair growth may affect any area of the body but is most often a concern to the female patient when it involves the face.[1] Hirsutism of the face most often involves the lip and chin area. The hair growth is often self-treated by tweezing, shaving, or clipping. Improper tweezing and shaving often result in irritations, in-grown hairs, and subsequent localized infection.

Professional salon waxing techniques are a more efficient, albeit still temporary, treatment for hirsutism. Waxing involves the application of a warm wax to the skin, which adheres to the exposed hair. The wax and hair are then removed by pulling the wax off the skin, usually with a cloth or cellophane strip. This method, if performed correctly by a licensed professional, produces a much smoother result than tweezing or shaving. Correct and aseptic procedures control irritation and reduce the risk of infection or ingrown hairs. Because waxing treatment removes the hair from the bottom of the follicle rather than the skin surface, the results are longer-lasting than shaving.

The only scientifically accepted method of permanent hair removal, electrolysis, involves the insertion of a small filament (needle) into the ostium of the hair follicle.[12] A small amount of current is passed through the filament, which cauterizes the papilla (growth cells) of the hair, inhibiting further growth.

There are two types of electrolysis current which, when combined, create both heat and chemical reactions. Galvanic current produces a chemical reaction that causes an ionization of the moisture and body salts in the tissue creating sodium hydroxide (lye) which destroys the papillae of the hair. Short-wave current kills the cells with heat.

Electrolysis requires time and a financial commitment on the part of the patient. It is impossible to exactly determine how much of the papilla is damaged or destroyed, therefore, the hair may grow back. It is usually smaller in diameter, and lighter in texture and treatment is repeated until the final results are achieved.

Temporary irritation, swelling, scabbing, and occasional ingrown hairs may occur. Scarring is very unlikely when electrolysis is performed by a competent electrologist.

Hair on the upper lip, a frequent complaint, is treated in a scattered pattern on a weekly basis until the area is "clean."

Occasionally, hair will grow in an unnatural area due to reconstructive surgery. For example, skin grafted from the leg to the lip may include hair follicles. This type of growth may be treated with electrolysis at a time deemed suitable by the surgeon. Certain drugs, such as steroids, hormones, oral contraceptives, and antihypertensives, may also result in superfluous hair growth.

CONCLUSION

The licensed esthetician can play an important role in the comfort, appearance, health, and psychological well being of the cosmetic dental patient. For more information regarding esthetic referrals contact dermatologists or the National Cosmetology Association, Division of Esthetics, 3510 Olive Street, St. Louis, MO, 63103.

REFERENCES

1. Gerson, J.: Standard Textbook for Professional Estheticians. Tarrytown, NY, Milady, 1980.
2. Smith, J., et al.: Alterations in human dermal connective tissue with age and chronic sun damage. J Invest Dermatol 39:347, 1962.
3. Milady's Standard Textbook of Cosmetology. Tarrytown, NY, Milady, 1991.
4. Fitzpatrick, T.B.: Dermatology and General Medicine. New York, McGraw-Hill, 1987.
5. Fulton, J.: Step-by-Step Program for Clearing Acne. New York, Harper & Row, 1983.
6. Kligman, A. and Mills, O.: Acne Cosmetica. Arch Dermatol 112:482, 1972.
7. Fulton, J.: Comedogenicity of current therapeutic products, cosmetics, and ingredients in the rabbit ear. J Am Acad Dermatol 10(1):96, 1984.
8. Lanzet, M.: Comedogenic effects on cosmetic raw materials. Cosmetics Toiletries 101:63, 1986.
9. Voorhees, J., et al.: Topical tretinoin improves photoaged skin. JAMA 259:527, 1988.
10. Rohlfing, C.: Retin-A: the real scoop. Self, May, 1988.
11. Kligman, A.: The use of retinoic acid as a topical anti-aging ingredient. Les Nouvelle Estheiques, Feb, 1989.
12. Hinkle, A. and Lind, R.: Electrolysis, Thermolysis, and the Blend. Los Angeles, Arroway, 1968.

Phillip Bonner, D.D.S.

ESTHETICS AND DENTAL MARKETING

27

The concept of marketing elicits a variety of responses from dental professionals ranging from total opposition to enthusiastic acceptance and use of marketing techniques within the dental practice setting. All acknowledge, however, that the recent emphasis on marketing results from such factors as increased dental manpower, changing disease patterns, cost containment policies by business and government, and the rise of consumerism. These powerful factors, although sometimes cyclical in nature, will continue to impact upon the profession for some time. As a result, competition among dentists for patients, or for the discretionary income of consumers, has reached historically high levels. In a free market society, marketing is a logical by-product of increasing competition.

HISTORY

Prior to 1977, when the U.S. Supreme Court Bates decision legalized advertising by attorneys, professional marketing was essentially limited to word-of-mouth patient referrals and fundamental in-office patient relations techniques.[1] Active marketing by dentists was discouraged by organized dentistry, both nationally and at the local level. Soon after the Bates decision, however, dentistry and other health professions were required by law to allow advertising. The Federal Trade Commission (FTC) applied pressure to state dental boards and other dental organizations to alter professional ethics standards and other rules that restricted or prohibited advertising. The FTC's position was that advertising that was not false or misleading would stimulate competition and lower the cost of dental care for consumers. This ushered in a controversial era of conflict between those dental professionals and organizations who felt that advertising was unprofessional, and those in dentistry and government who felt that it was beneficial and acceptable.

Today, the furor over advertising in particular, and marketing in general, has abated, although strong differences of opinion still remain. The marketing of dental services has become an accepted and integral part of the practice of dentistry for thousands of dentists. With the rapid advances in dental materials and techniques, particularly in the area of cosmetic dentistry, the role of marketing is likely to expand.

WHAT IS MARKETING?

Marketing encompasses a variety of disciplines and techniques that are intended to motivate a targeted individual or group to take an action that is desired by the marketer. This action may be, for example, to purchase a product or service, attend a specific event, vote for a particular candidate, or visit a dental office.

The two major disciplines within marketing are advertising and public relations. Advertising involves a marketing message that is made possible by direct payment from the advertiser to the specific advertising medium. Examples of advertising media are television, radio, magazines, and newspapers.

There are many variations within advertising. Direct mail involves designing a marketing message that is delivered to targeted recipients via the U.S. Postal Service or other delivery service. Another form of advertising, specialty advertising, involves the distribution of various specialty items, such as pens or calendars, with a marketing message imprinted on them.

Public relations involves the dissemination of information through a variety of channels without payment for the media space. For example, a dentist-marketer may write an article on some aspect of cosmetic dentistry, and due to the informational value of the article, it is published in a magazine. Although the article may contain information that is beneficial to the dentist's practice, the educational value of that information is sufficient to result in publication without payment for advertising space. As with advertising, there are many public relations techniques, including a variety of patient relations activities in the dental office setting. For the purposes of this chapter, the basic difference between the two disciplines is that direct payment for media space is required for advertising messages, but is not required for public relations messages.

The Bates decision focused on only one marketing technique: advertising. As a result of the controversy generated by this decision, many dentists equate marketing with advertising. However, there are many marketing methods in addition to advertising that can be used to reach a specific audience. Of particular relevance to dentists are two basic marketing approaches: external marketing and internal marketing. An understanding of these two approaches will aid in designing a marketing program that is in harmony with the individual dentist's philosophy.

EXTERNAL AND INTERNAL MARKETING

Two basic goals of dental marketing are to attract new patients to the practice and keep existing patients active within the practice. Marketing techniques designed to attract new patients to the practice can be categorized as external techniques, and those designed to keep existing patients active and motivate them to refer others to the practice are internal techniques.

External Marketing

External marketing techniques encompass any marketing activities designed to attract consumers into the dental office so that they can become active patients. A few examples of external marketing techniques dentists can use are:

1. Advertising, such as magazines, newspapers, radio, television, Yellow Pages, and direct mail
2. Community programs, such as health fairs and lectures to schools and civic groups
3. Dental article writing for newspapers or magazines
4. Communication with referral sources, such as health professionals, cosmetologists, and realtors

Internal Marketing

Internal marketing techniques encompass any marketing or communication activities that take place within the practice setting or are directed at active or inactive patients with the objective of retaining these patients in the practice and stimulating referrals. A few examples of internal marketing techniques dentists can use are:

1. Case presentation techniques
2. Office decor and design
3. Staff-doctor-patient interaction (patient relations)
4. Office newsletter, brochure, and educational aids
5. "Patient friendly" management and clinical systems

OBJECTIVES OF PROFESSIONAL MARKETING

One concern about the use of marketing is that it will tarnish the professional image of dentistry. To avoid this potential problem, it is imperative that dental personnel understand the true objectives of professional marketing. These are: consumer and patient education and motivation of consumers and patients to seek and accept needed dental services and take responsibility for their oral health. If these objectives are the focus of all marketing efforts by dentists, marketing will serve a beneficial function for both the public and the dental profession.

Trends Affecting Marketing

A number of major trends that affect our society have been identified.[2] Three have particular significance to dentists who wish to educate and motivate patients with marketing techniques.

Self-help movement. People have become more concerned with helping themselves rather than relying on institutions. Self-help groups in a variety of specialized areas have materialized across the country and self-help books routinely top the bestseller lists. The strong interest in physical fitness is one example of consumers assuming a more active role in their own healthcare. Dentists must understand this trend and refrain from dictating to the patient; dentists must work *with* patients to help them improve their oral health.

High touch and high tech. People seek personal interactions to counter the current impersonal, highly technological environment. If this need for "high touch" is not met by the dentist and staff, clinical expertise alone may not retain patients in an office they perceive as "unfriendly."

The age of information. The world's database is growing exponentially. People increasingly demand information about oral health. Much of this information is provided by sources outside the dental profession. Dentists and staff must also become a source of accurate information that the patient can personally use to improve oral health.

Marketing that is focused on education and motivation and that is based on these and related trends can be a powerful force. Marketing that educates the public about oral health satisfies society's need for information. Marketing that motivates people to participate with dental professionals in establishing and maintaining optimum oral health meets people's need for self-determination or self-help. When accomplished in an atmosphere of professional caring and concern for the needs of the individual, marketing becomes "high touch." Marketing as an educational and motivational process can thus become an ethical practice building tool that enhances rather than tarnishes the image of dentistry.

PRODUCT VS. SERVICE MARKETING

In order to properly focus marketing programs on education and motivation and to meet the needs and wants of individuals, it is important to distinguish between product marketing and service marketing.

Product marketing focuses on the actual products being sold. For example, in a television or magazine advertisement for an automobile, the focus of the visual, auditory, and written message is the particular car being marketed, including its most prominent features. In dentistry, product-focused marketing would emphasize the actual "product" being delivered to the patient, such as a crown, veneer, or composite resin restoration. Many dentists and staff, in their marketing materials and case presentations, focus on the actual restoration.

Service marketing focuses on the actual service being provided. The product being sold is secondary to the service and attendant benefits that the product provides. In the dental setting, the "services" and benefits of cosmetic dentistry might include: a more attractive smile, a better chance for career advancement, a better social life, and more self-confidence. The actual "product," the veneer or crown, is merely the vehicle for providing that service and achieving a benefit.

CLINICAL TIP. Dental marketing should primarily be service-focused marketing, because a service approach more clearly focuses on the individual needs and wants of the patient and how treatment can meet those needs and wants.

In the world of marketing, perception is reality in the mind of the patient. If a patient perceives that he has a need, then he definitely does have that need, even if the dentist does not have the same perception. The public is generally not as interested in the product, or type of restoration, that is to be provided as they are in the benefits of treatment. These benefits must be tailored to individual needs and wants.

The correct focus can mean the difference between gaining patient acceptance of treatment and losing the patient's interest (and thus losing the patient). For example, a product-focused brochure, which simply lists the "products" available, forces the patient to take that information and somehow determine if these products meet his needs. In contrast, a service-focused approach does not demand extrapolation by the reader. It explains the benefits of cosmetic services in lay terms. It shows how cosmetic dentistry is the means to an end. It motivates the patient to accept treatment because such treatment is the answer to personal wants and needs.

Following are brief examples of product-focused and service-focused marketing statements.

Example A (excerpted from a product-focused brochure)

Our office is proud to provide the most advanced cosmetic dental technology. Ask Dr. Jones or our staff about the latest direct bonding procedures, tooth-colored crowns, porcelain veneers and bleaching.

Example B (excerpted from a service-focused brochure)

Our office can give you a beautiful smile using the latest cosmetic dental technology. Ask Dr. Jones or our staff how we can work together to create an attractive smile that can help your career and your social life.

These are simple examples, but they illustrate the difference in approach between product and service marketing. Example A focuses on specific procedures and restorations, whereas example B focuses on the patient's needs. Specific individual needs can be determined during patient interviews and in-office discussions, and can then be addressed during the case presentation. Each staff member, as well as the dentist, should pay close attention to what patients say from the moment they come into the office. A great deal of information about individual needs and desires can be gained from patients' comments about their teeth and what they expect from the dental visits. (See the sections on Patient Motivation Profile and Case Presentation Using the Patient Motivation Profile later in this chapter.)

DESIGNING A MARKETING PROGRAM

The business community often uses a well structured business plan. Such a plan sets short- and long-term goals and provides a well defined program for reaching those goals. Dental offices also should have an overall business plan that incorporates a marketing plan. In order to design a cosmetic dentistry marketing plan appropriate for an individual dental office, basic market research must first be undertaken. Market research will delineate:

1. the goals and objectives of the practice and its personnel
2. the profile of existing active patients
3. the profile of the surrounding community

Goals and Objectives of the Dental Practice

The foundation of any marketing program is a clear understanding of goals and objectives. People perform at their best in an environment compatible with their needs and talents, and when they are performing tasks they enjoy and believe in. If the dentist and staff do not have a clear conception of what they want the practice to be, it is impossible to design a marketing program that will help them achieve that image.

Therefore, the first task in designing a marketing program is for the dentist and each staff member to write down their own personal goals and the goals they seek for the practice. Do they want to provide only cosmetic dental services, or do they want to provide a range of general dental services, including cosmetic procedures? Do they want to focus only on the upper economic group of patients in the community, or on a broader economic range? Do they want to focus on any particular age group of patients? Is the practice in an expansion or growth mode in terms of anticipating more personnel, or is the goal to maintain current patient load and practice size?

There are many such questions that should be addressed prior to designing a marketing plan. After written answers are provided by all personnel, a staff meeting should be held to discuss everyone's views and arrive at a definitive mission statement that will govern the philosophy and direction of the practice.

Patient Assessment

After determining practice direction, the types of patients already in the practice must be identified. The dentist and staff are usually surprised at how erroneous their perceptions are in this area. An assessment of existing patients may show that the practice philosophy and direction are not compatible with the majority of patients.

Dental practices take on "personalities" of their own and, ideally, this personality should coincide with the general characteristics of the patient base. If the office is not in tune with the majority of patients, this will inevitably be reflected in the overall success of the practice. Similarly, if the existing patient base is out of tune with the true goals and objectives of the office personnel, the practice is misdirected and stress and unhappiness can result.

No dental practice can be all things to all people. The most successful practices are those that first determine the type of patients they wish to treat and the guiding philosophy of the practice and then create an overall office environment that appeals to this type of patient. A patient assessment can help put the practice in perspective and guide the design of a marketing program.

Conducting the Patient Assessment. Compare the following data from a random sampling of 100 active patient records (certain data may require direct questioning of the patients if it is not included in the record).

1. Sex
2. Age
3. Marital status
4. Number of children
5. Education
6. Family income
7. Occupation
8. Frequency of dental visits
9. Driving time from work to dental office
10. Preferred times for dental visits
11. Types of dental procedures completed

Other questions may be added to answer individual practice questions. The objective of the assessment is to gain insight into the general characteristics of the active patient base. If this patient base is consistent with the practice's goals and objectives, then a marketing program can be designed that will appeal to this type of patient both within and outside the practice. If the patient base is inconsistent with practice ideals, serious thought must be given to slowly shifting the patient base in the desired direction.

The Community Profile

Conducting a community profile can help both new and established dental practices focus properly for future growth. In today's mobile society, the makeup of a community can change dramatically in a few short years. A patient base acquired and courted over time will often cease to represent the predominant type of patient currently living in the community. Future practice growth may be generated by appealing to the typical community resident. This may require physical changes within the office.

Conducting the Community Profile. A number of companies offer demographic studies for a fee. The report furnishes a breakdown of the population by criteria such as age, sex, family income, travel time to work, ethnic groups, marital status, and other demographic characteristics. A community profile helps establish criteria for developing a marketing program that meets the needs and expectations of the local population. Demographic data about the community can be compared to data obtained from the patient profiles to determine compatibility.

CLINICAL TIP. Some demographic studies rely on older census information. Local organizations, such as the Chamber of Commerce and government agencies, can provide supporting data that will help fine tune the community profile.

Elements of the Marketing Plan

After preliminary market data has been collected and the practice's goals and objectives are clear, a definitive marketing plan should be designed. The following elements should be included in a marketing plan.

1. Goals and objectives
2. Target audience
3. Budget
4. Specific marketing techniques to be used
5. Time frame for implementation
6. Monitoring of results

The contents of the marketing plan should be decided in staff meetings specifically devoted to this purpose. After the plan has been designed, one or more staff members should be assigned the task of organizing and recording the plan in writing.

Goals and Objectives. The goals and objectives of the marketing plan are related to the goals and objectives of the practice as a whole, but consist of the specific goals and objectives of the office's marketing program (i.e., exactly what is to be accomplished with the use of marketing techniques). Are you trying to attract a specific number of new patients each month? Are you trying to target a specific age category of patient, such as the elderly? Are you trying to increase the number of veneers placed per month by a specific amount? It is crucial to identify specific rather than general marketing goals and objectives.

Target Audience. The target audience most likely to satisfy the marketing goals must be identified. For example, if one goal is to add 20 new elderly patients to the practice each month, then individuals over the age of 55 would constitute the target audience. If the goal is to increase the number of veneers placed per month, the primary target audience might be women age 18 to 55. A secondary target audience might be men age 21 to 55. This does not mean that people older than 55 do not want veneers, or that men aren't interested in veneers; it simply means that it is more likely that women age 18 to 55 will make the decision to invest in veneers for cosmetic reasons. If the surrounding community is comprised predominantly of one demographic group, for example a retirement community, the target audience must necessarily reflect that fact (or marketing to other communities may be necessary). Often, a target market not normally considered "primary" requires a different marketing focus to motivate them to take action. The purpose of determining a target audience is to provide a tangible, well defined "target" for the marketing efforts, a target with the highest likelihood of response.

Budget. Marketing plans are "budget-driven." The techniques to be used and the size of the target market depend on available funds. Two to five percent of gross practice revenues is a typical budget for marketing. Aggressive dental marketers budget 6 to 8% of revenues or more. A budget sufficient to accomplish the goals and objectives of the marketing plan must be allocated in the written plan, and must be dispensed according to a time schedule as determined by the plan.

Specific Marketing Techniques to be Used. Within the confines of the plan's budget, specific marketing techniques should be selected that will best accomplish the marketing goals. Both internal and external marketing techniques can be used, depending on the marketing plan and the philosophy of the practice.

Time Frame for Implementation. A written marketing plan must contain a specific time frame for implementation. For example, if a direct mail campaign is budgeted and targeted for a specific number of patients within certain demographic parameters, a target date for implementation of the campaign should be included in the marketing plan. This date, and any dates required for various steps involved in the campaign, should be adhered to, with reports given by the responsible person at periodic staff meetings.

Monitoring of Results. Many dentists institute impressive marketing programs but fail to monitor the results of individual elements within the program. Monitoring systems that record results are imperative if the program is to be evaluated and improved. For example, if a Yellow Pages advertisement is used, the person answering the telephone for new patient appointments should ask the caller how he or she selected the office. All Yellow Pages respondents should be recorded, and the fees generated by these respondents logged as treatment proceeds. In this manner, the cost of the adver-

tisement program can be weighed against the income generated.

CLINICAL TIP. If, after a predetermined period of evaluation (perhaps 6 to 12 months) the advertisement does not generate sufficient fees, it should be either altered or replaced by another marketing technique.

Ongoing monitoring of the marketing program is essential if the program is to optimize cost-effectiveness.

SAMPLE MARKETING PLAN

Individual marketing plans for dental practices can be lengthy, or they can be concise to the point of being an outline. If the elements listed previously are addressed in enough detail to ensure implementation, the format and length of the plan are inconsequential. The following outline of a sample marketing plan includes both internal and external marketing techniques. This outline is intended as a guide for the development of an individually tailored plan for marketing cosmetic dental services, and as such its content is intentionally concise. Many of the indicated steps can be more detailed and can be intended to accomplish a broader goal. Actual dollar figures used are examples and are not intended as accurate estimates.

1. **Goals and objectives.** (Based on a patient profile and community profile that showed a significant portion of the patient and community population to be families with children and both spouses working): to attract 20 new patients who need cosmetic bonding and veneering services per month. Average income goal per patient is $500, for a total increase in income of $10,000 per month derived from cosmetic services.
2. **Target Audience.**
   A. Primary audience—women age 18 to 55.
   B. Secondary audience—men age 21 to 55.
3. **Budget.** (Based on present practice gross revenues of $250,000 annually): $12,500 or 5% of annual gross revenues.
4. **Marketing Techniques to be Used:**
   A. Participation in two community health fairs to be held in the fall and spring at the local shopping mall. Exhibit table with color photograph album of cosmetic dental cases and display board with color photographs of cosmetic results and explanatory text. Table to be manned by Kathy and Sharon. Budget allocation for album development, table, display board: $750.
   B. Civic lectures by Dr. Jones. Sharon will book one lecture every two months at the Rotary Club, Lion's Club, Men's Club, Garden Club, Chamber of Commerce meeting, Businessmen's Club. Lecture plus slide presentation. Time of presentation 20 to 30 minutes. Budget allocation for slide development: $50.
   C. Yellow Pages ad. One-quarter page black and white advertisement. Kathy to contact graphic artist for design and camera-ready art. Budget al-

location for advertisement design and space in Yellow Pages directory: $2000.

D. Office brochure on cosmetic services and benefits available from our office. Brochure to be given to all active patients at their next visit; sent to new patients who appoint by phone; placed in local beauty shops, and health clubs. Kathy to contact graphic artist and work with her on design. Sharon to work with printer to produce brochures. Budget allocation for design and production of initial print run of 5000 brochures: $2750.

E. Direct mail package to local residents, to include the office brochure and a cover letter explaining our cosmetic services and how they can benefit the reader. Sharon to write the letter, to be signed by Dr. Jones. Budget allocation for 1000 mailings: $400.

F. Four in-office color photograph albums of cosmetic cases for patient education. Kathy in charge of reproducing the photograph album used in the health fair exhibit. Budget allocation for four albums: $160.

G. Practice newsletter. Joanne in charge of writing quarterly newsletter, 4 pages, 2 colors. Content: dental education articles, with emphasis on cosmetic services available at our office. Joanne will send newsletter to all active patients, plus copies to all local beauty shops. Annual budget allocation for printing and mailing 2000 copies quarterly: $3800.

H. Development of office logo, business cards, stationery. Logo to reflect modern cosmetic-oriented dental practice. Kathy to work with graphic artist to develop logo. Each staff member to have business cards. Budget allocation for logo development and printing: $1750.

Total Budget Allocation: $11,660.
Contingency funds: $840.

CLINICAL TIP. Contingency funds should be 5 to 10% of the total budget allocation

---

5. Time Frame for Implementation.
A. Health fair exhibit materials ready by September 1.
B. Slide presentation for civic lectures ready by September 1. Lectures booked every two months, starting in October. Sharon will log each lecture appointment on office calendar and post on bulletin board.
C. Kathy will meet with artist on August 1 to design Yellow Pages ad. First concept art due from artist on August 15. Final concept decision by September 1. Camera-ready art and copy due September 20. Kathy to meet with Yellow Pages representative on October 1.
D. Kathy to meet with graphic artist on August 1 (same time as Yellow Pages meeting) to discuss concepts for office brochure. First concept art due from artist on August 20. Sharon will coordinate the written copy with her freelance writer friend.

Final art and copy due September 28. Final art and copy to printer on October 5. Kathy to deliver to beauty shops and discuss with owners on October 15.
E. Sharon will write direct mail letter by December 1 and get Dr. Jones' approval. Direct mail package mailed on January 10.
F. Kathy will reproduce photograph albums and have assembled and ready for office use by October 15.
G. Target date for first issue of newsletter is January 1. Subsequent issues to be ready on April 1, July 1, October 1. Joanne will write newsletter, with the rest of the staff contributing, and have copy to the printer no later than two weeks prior to target dates. Joanne will set an editorial calendar and discuss at staff meeting on August 10, and at subsequent staff meetings prior to quarterly publication.
H. Kathy will meet with graphic artist on November 15 to begin design of logo, business cards, and stationery. Initial concept review on December 5. Final art by December 20. Printing of cards and stationery completed by January 20.

6. Monitoring Results. Sharon will coordinate all monitoring activities. All new patients calling the office will be questioned about how they heard about the office. Answers will be recorded and categorized according to response. Direct mail response cards and newsletter response cards will be recorded. Response statistics will be evaluated quarterly and discussed at appropriate staff meetings.

CASE PRESENTATIONS

Many marketing techniques can be used to build the cosmetic dental practice. Because there are advantages and disadvantages to each technique, the final choice depends on many factors. Each practice must decide which techniques are consistent with its philosophy and are appropriate for the goals and objectives of the practice.

One technique that is common to all practices, however, is the individual patient case presentation. Many dentists do not equate the case presentation with marketing. Some use a formal case presentation, which takes place in an area of the office specially designed for maximum patient comfort and communication. The case presentation follows a specific format and every aspect of the presentation is planned to gain patient acceptance of treatment. Some dentists approach case presentation informally and with little preplanning or prescribed format. However, case presentations, in whatever form they take, represent one of the most powerful types of internal marketing available to every dentist.

It is during the case presentation that the dentist and staff must educate the patient about his or her individual oral health needs, and most importantly, motivate the patient to accept and pay for needed treatment. If the patient leaves the case presentation without a firm commitment to treatment, that patient may be lost.

Patient Motivation Profile

Use of the patient motivation profile can greatly increase the patient's motivation and treatment plan acceptance. Addressing these concerns may motivate a patient to undergo necessary treatment.

From the time a patient first enters or telephones the office, each staff member, as well as the dentist, should carefully monitor the importance to the patient of each of these four areas of concern:[3]

1. Money
2. Romance
3. Self-preservation
4. Appearance

CLINICAL TIP. By classifying patients as closely as possible into one or more of these primary areas, it becomes possible to "target" the case presentation to the individual, thus greatly improving the chances for patient acceptance of treatment.

Case Presentation Using the Patient Motivation Profile

For example, an elderly gentleman presents with some missing teeth and one fractured tooth. The dentist has not taken the time to analyze the patient's motivating emotions, so he stresses the economic advantages of his treatment plan, emphasizing that it will save the patient money in the long run by preventing further deterioration of his oral health. The dentist takes this approach because currently his own personal concerns center on money and achieving financial independence. He assumes the patient is thinking in the same terms, particularly because of his age and the need for financial security in his retirement years. The dentist is surprised when the man shifts uncomfortably in the chair and says he will "think about it" and call him later.

If the dentist, receptionst, or other staff members had noticed that during the initial office contact the man did not mention money or financial concerns, but did mention a magazine article he had read about "dental cripples" who had lost all their teeth, a clearer picture of the patient's emotional "trigger" would have been possible. When the man pointed out that his own mother had "pyorrhea" and had lost all her teeth, and he did not want to lose his teeth too, this should have alerted the dentist to the fact that this person's emotional profile was "self-preservation," not money. Knowing this, the dentist would logically take another approach during the case presentation. He would explain that treatment would prevent further tilting of the teeth adjacent to the missing spaces and would prevent the fractured tooth from breaking more extensively. His chewing would be more efficient, thus aiding in overall systemic health, and his entire mouth would be healthier. With proper home care, as instructed by the hygienist, the patient would significantly increase the likelihood of retaining his teeth for the rest of his life.

When the case presentation is keyed to the patient's motivation profile, it is far more likely that the patient will respond positively to the treatment plan. For the cosmetic dentist, the emotions associated with money, appearance, and romance can be targeted in a powerful way during case presentation. A more attractive smile can enhance one's career, thus providing the opportunity for more money, and it can improve one's social life, thus meeting a patient's need to appear attractive or for romance.

MARKETING TECHNIQUES

Many marketing techniques can be used by dentists in a professional manner. The number of techniques available is limited only by the imagination of the marketer.

Referrals

Referrals are historically, and still remain, the most effective marketing tool available. Special effort and a definitive plan should be devoted to stimulating referrals from patients as well as outside sources. Good outside referral sources include related health professionals, cosmetologists, realtors, and local businesspersons who meet the public and are often asked for recommendations concerning dentists and community services. Strong referral sources should be thanked in a noticeable way. A first- or second-time referral source may simply be sent a personalized thank you note. Those who continue to refer patients can be sent a special gift, such as flowers, concert tickets, or other tasteful gifts. In the case of flowers, it is especially effective if they are sent directly to the place of business of the referring person. Everyone in the referring person's office will see the flowers and notice who sent them, which expands the marketing effort.

Civic Lectures by Dentists and Staff

An external public relations technique, the civic lecture is highly educational in nature and benefits the entire profession as well as the individual office. It is a strong marketing tool if the dentist or staff member is enthusiastic and a good speaker. Effective public speaking can be learned through practice.

Practice Newsletter

An internal and external public relations technique, a newsletter's effectiveness can be reduced if a large number of dental offices in the area are using them. The content should be focused on services and benefits offered by the practice.

CLINICAL TIP. Avoid sections such as "Did You Know?," which are mainly filler material with little practical use for patients.

A good idea before launching a newsletter is to survey a random sampling of perhaps 500 active patients via postcard, asking them if they would be interested in receiving a newsletter that educates them about cosmetic dental services and oral health. Base the decision to launch the newsletter on the strength of the response. Always adhere to a publication schedule, and do not publish erratically. With any type of publication, consistency is important because it imparts a sense of continuity and dependability to the reader. If patients come to expect a dental practice newsletter at a certain time, such as every quarter, it becomes part of their routine. This consistency will reinforce the doctor's name in the minds of the patients and hopefully translate into consistency of office visits. From an in-office standpoint, if a fixed publication schedule is not established, the newsletter will quickly become a task that "we will get to when we can." This usually means that it will cease publication after a few erratically timed issues. A quarterly publishing schedule is usually sufficient and is not too burdensome for the office.

Direct Mail

An external advertising technique, direct mail can be expensive if not properly targeted.

CLINICAL TIP. Direct mail experts usually agree that a 1% response is strong, although this can vary according to how well the mailing is targeted.

Best results are obtained if target groups are clearly defined and the contents of the direct mail package are focused on the needs of that group. A response mechanism, such as a reply card or a request to call the office for more information, should be included.

Yellow Pages Advertisement

An external advertising technique, the results from Yellow Pages advertisements vary across the country. Dentists interested in this technique should try a test advertisement and monitor the results closely. The decision to renew should be based on results. As a general rule, larger advertisements work better, but it is important to determine the size of other advertisements that will be run on the same page. In a page full of large advertisements more graphic creativity is required if the advertisement is to stand out. Consult with the Yellow Pages representative or a graphic artist for various graphic techniques to improve the response.

In-Office Educational Materials (brochures, photograph albums of cosmetic cases, and video or slide presentations)

An internal marketing technique, in-office educational materials are highly effective if combined with direct dentist-staff-patient interaction. Whenever possible, use the dentist's own treatment results in photograph albums. These aids represent an excellent patient education opportunity.

Radio and Television Advertisements

Although some large dental clinics have successfully used the external advertising technique of radio and television commercials, their effectiveness and feasibility for the average dental practice is questionable. Creation of an advertisement that maintains professionalism and generates new patients requires special talent, such as a professional advertising agency. This can be expensive.

Staff as Marketers

A motivated, enthusiastic staff is one of the most powerful internal and external marketing tools a practice can utilize. Dentists should make a special effort to train the staff in proper telephone technique and patient interaction techniques. Each staff member should have a business card to distribute at outside functions. Regular staff meetings should be devoted to improving staff-patient relations.

CONCLUSION

In the purest sense, marketing is education and motivation. As cosmetic dental technology continues to advance at a truly staggering rate, techniques for educating the public about the benefits of cosmetic dental services must keep pace with dentists' ability to deliver these services. The most successful dental practices are those that effectively educate patients about available dental services and motivate them to accept needed treatment.

REFERENCES

1. *Bates v. State Bar of Arizona,* 433US350 (1977).
2. Naisbitt, J.: Megatrends. New York, Warner Books, 1982.
3. Garn, R.: The Magic Power of Emotional Appeal. Englewood Cliffs, NJ, Prentice-Hall, 1960.

Burton R. Pollack, D.D.S., M.P.H., J.D.

ESTHETICS AND DENTAL JURISPRUDENCE

28

A BRIEF HISTORY OF RISK MANAGEMENT

Until the mid 1970s the term "risk management" was not included in the dental lexicon. Today it is part of everyday conversation in dental circles. Interest in risk management began for the health professions as an outgrowth of the medical malpractice crisis in the early 1970s. Hospitals could no longer afford the rapid rise in professional liability premiums. Many resorted to bearing their own litigation and liability loss costs through self-insurance. To decrease their exposure, hospitals adapted a system which had long been used by industry—risk management. This involved instituting in-house programs to reduce liability, providing quality assurance in the provision of health care, identifying risk areas, changing hiring policies, reviewing patient complaints, studying incident reports, and purchasing insurance.

Reducing legal exposure in the hospital setting protected resources from loss due to legal actions. Eventually, laws were enacted to require health facilities to institute formal programs in risk management. Some laws required periodic review of the credentials of physicians and dentists.

The concept of risk management spread from hospitals to physicians' and dentists' offices. Programs for dentists began in the late 1970s and early 1980s, when legal actions against them increased dramatically, settlements and jury awards escalated beyond any expectation, and premiums rose to a level few could have anticipated. In addition, access to liability insurance in general, and malpractice insurance in particular, became a problem for many practitioners.

LOSS WITHOUT FAULT

In a study conducted by the author, 60% of several hundred malpractice claims were settled by the insurance company without evidence of negligence on the part of the dentist. These cases could not be successfully defended because the defendant dentist's records were poor, there was no documentation that consent was obtained, or other office practices were sufficiently deficient to make it difficult to defend the claim. Thus, the concept of loss without fault emerged.

DENTAL RISK MANAGEMENT

Risk management adapted to dental practice appeared to be a reasonable means of controlling the increased incidence of litigation. The literature was flooded with risk management articles. Risk management presentations were included at most dental meetings. Insurance companies began risk management educational sessions, either as a benefit for the insured dentist or to qualify clients for premium discounts. Continuing dental education and risk management became inexorably linked. From the ashes of a profession threatened by litigation arose a program of office management that has raised the quality of dental care, provided the practitioner with a sense of security against legal claims, and created a profession that is more careful and caring than before.

Professional Responsibility

To ensure a legally worry-free professional life, the practitioner has some new responsibilities including:

1. Knowing and obeying the laws that regulate dental practice, and remaining current about changes.
2. Continuing education and remaining knowledgeable of technical advances in the profession through membership in professional organizations, continuing dental education programs, professional journals, and joining hospital staffs and the faculty of dental schools.
3. Being aware of areas of legal vulnerability in dental practice by reading appropriate literature, exchanging information with colleagues, and attending continuing dental education courses.
4. Purchasing professional liability insurance.

CLINICAL TIP. Purchase as much professional liability insurance as can be afforded.

---

5. Carefully hiring, training, and supervising competent personnel.
6. Keeping proper records on each patient. (See the section on Records later in this chapter.)
7. Limiting care to areas of competence.
8. Referring appropriate patients.
9. Maintaining good interpersonal relationships with patients: showing care and ensuring that the staff does the same by monitoring what they say and how they relate to patients.
10. Being careful during treatment.
11. Obtaining proper consent prior to initiating treatment. (See the section on Consent and Informed Consent later in this chapter.)
12. Fastidiously documenting everything. (See the section on Records later in this section.)
13. Keeping patients informed about their oral health status and of problems that arise during treatment.
14. Carefully considering what the patient's response would be if he or she were sued by the dentist in order to collect a fee. (This is one of the major causes of malpractice suits.)
15. Taking careful health histories, and updating them at appropriate intervals as determined by the "prudent" dentist.
16. Keeping patient records forever or for as long as possible.
17. Never parting with the original record or radiograph.
18. Never altering a patient's record after becoming aware that a malpractice suit is contemplated or initiated by a patient or by the patient's attorney.
19. Notifying the insurance carrier at the earliest time after becoming aware that a patient intends or threatens to sue, or after becoming aware that treatment may result in a malpractice suit. This is a provision in all professional liability policies.

High Risk Treatment Areas

A study by the author of allegations brought against dentists reveals some interesting trends during the past decade of dental malpractice litigation.

Traditional Causes of Malpractice Suits

1. Extraction of wrong teeth.
2. Dentures that do not fit.
3. Bridges that must be redone because another dentist says so.
4. Broken root tips left in the bone.
5. Infections following extractions.
6. Adverse outcomes from the administration of general anesthesia or intravenous sedatives.

Recent Causes of Malpractice Suits

Plaintiff attorneys have become sophisticated about dentistry since the proliferation of dental malpractice claims. New areas of dental vulnerability are constantly being "discovered." They include:

1. Failure to obtain informed consent.
2. Failure to diagnose, refer, or treat a disease or condition (notably periodontal disease).
3. Faulty history taking resulting in allergic responses, drug incompatibilities, paralysis, and, in rare cases, death.
4. Problems associated with the temporomandibular joint.
5. Implant failures.
6. Treating a patient in areas beyond the competence of the practitioner.
7. Administering wrong or inappropriate medication.
8. Failure to inform the patient of an untoward event occurring during treatment, such as root tip fracture or an irretrievable broken instrument tip lodged within a root canal.
9. Failure to inform the patient of the consequences of refusal to follow professional advice.
10. Abandonment by prematurely discontinuing care or not attending to the needs of a patient under treatment.

Breaking a file within a root canal or the fracture of a root tip may not constitute negligence, however, failure to inform the patient of the event is negligence. It may also be considered fraudulent concealment, thus falling within the statute of limitations for fraud, which is considerably longer than the statute of limitations for malpractice. This provides the patient more time to enter suit against the dentist. In addition, fraudulent concealment may not be covered by malpractice insurance.

Oral and maxillofacial surgeons continue to be at highest insurance risk in terms of the dollar amount of settlements and awards. Problems associated with the temporomandibular joint, implants, and medical problems following dental care, such as drug incompatibilities and subacute bacterial endocarditis (SBE), also bring large settlements and awards. However, the greatest number of suits are brought against general practitioners. Orthodontists have recently become targets of lawsuits because of bad results, periodontal and caries neglect, and root resorption. The practice of adult orthodontics has substantially increased the risks.

THE LAW AND DENTAL PRACTICE

The Doctor-Patient Relationship: A Brief Review of Contract Law

The relationship between a treating health professional and a patient has its foundation in contract law, which governs when the relationship begins, when it ends, how to end it, breaches actionable at law, express terms, implied terms and warranties or, as used in the health care field, duties.

When the Contract Begins. The doctor-patient relationship begins whenever the doctor, in his or her professional capacity, expresses a professional opinion, or recommends to a specific individual a course of health action upon which the individual may rely. The locale in which the opinion is expressed or the recommendation made (be it curb-side, at a social event, or elsewhere) is of no consequence. Whether a fee was charged does not affect the relationship. Once the doctor-patient relationship begins, contract law applies.

Oral vs. Written Contracts. The contract of care between a dentist and patient does not have to be written to be enforceable. However, when disputes arise, the written contract will serve as evidence that the parties reached an agreement, and its terms. Except in the practice of orthodontics, written contracts are rare.

When the Contract Ends. The doctor-patient relationship ends when:

1. The patient is cured.
2. The patient dies.
3. The doctor dies.
4. The patient voluntarily seeks the services of another provider.
5. The doctor unilaterally terminates the care.

Abandonment. One of the implied duties in the doctor-patient relationship is for the doctor to continue treatment until one of the above five conditions occurs. When accepting a patient for care, the doctor automatically warrants not to abandon the patient. In order to unilaterally discontinue treatment and avoid liability for abandonment, the following generally accepted rules apply.

1. Do not discontinue treatment at a time when the patient's health may be compromised. This is a professional judgment, not a legal one.
2. Recommend that the patient seek care elsewhere. It is best not to recommend another dentist, or even to supply the patient with a list from which to choose. To do so may link the two dentists in future liability should the new dentist be accused of malpractice.
3. Inform the patient that you will be available to provide emergency care for a reasonable time during the period in which the patient is seeking care elsewhere. What is reasonable depends upon the availability of dentists in the community.
4. Inform the patient that you will cooperate with the new dentist by making copies of your records, radiographs, reports, and other information about the patient available. Never send the original records or radiographs.
5. Inform the patient that seeking care elsewhere is in the *patient's* best interest, not the dentist's.

It is recommended that the patient is first informed orally regarding the above, then by a signed receipt certified letter that includes the same information. One may refuse to accept a patient and may discontinue the care of a patient for any reason, without fear of abandonment, except for reasons of race, color, religion, or national origin. As a result of the enactment of the Americans With Disability Act of 1990, declaring a health practitioner's private office as a "place of public accommodation," a dentist who refuses to treat a patient solely because the patient has AIDS, is HIV-positive, or is disabled in any other way, may be found guilty of discrimination and subjected to severe penalties, i.e., a large fine and possible restriction or loss of the license to practice.

Express Terms in the Doctor-Patient Contract

Terms that are stated, orally or in writing, are called express terms. They usually include the service that is to be provided by the dentist, how long treatment will take, and the payment arrangement. A dentist and patient may include any terms in the contract for care that are not illegal, provided the patient is not subjected to terms that are the result of coercion because the patient is placed in an unfair bargaining position by having to accept unreasonable terms in order to receive needed treatment. For example, if a patient chooses a practitioner who is reputed to have special skills in providing implants but refuses to provide the service unless the patient agrees not to sue the dentist for malpractice, the courts may look upon the agreement as an "adhesion contract," and therefore unenforceable.

Implied Duties in the Doctor-Patient Contract

Implied duties are obligations that exist as a result of the doctor-patient relationship. These implied duties do not have to be explicitly stated or written to be legally effective.

The Dentist's Implied Duties. The dentist automatically gives certain warranties to the patient, including the following:

1. The dentist will use knowledge and skill with reasonable care in the provision of services as measured against customary (acceptable) standards of other practitioners of the same school of practice in the community. The court definition of the word "community" has undergone major changes. Previ-

ously, it was strictly defined as the "local community" in which the dentist practiced. As communication and travel became more accessible most states changed to a "similar community" definition. Some states further expanded the geographic community to include the entire state. Currently, there is a national trend to apply a national standard of care for judging specialists. In some jurisdictions a national standard has also been applied to generalists.

2. The dentist will be properly licensed and registered, and meet all other legal requirements to engage in the practice of dentistry.
3. The dentist will employ competent personnel and provide for their proper supervision.
4. The dentist will maintain a level of knowledge in keeping with current advances in the profession, e.g., participate in continuing dental education and subscribe to scientific journals.
5. The dentist will use methods that are acceptable to at least a "respectable minority" of reasonable practitioners in the community (see No. 1 above). Court decisions are made on a case-by-case basis. There is no set number that constitutes an "acceptable minority."
6. The dentist will not use experimental procedures or drugs without the patient's knowledge and written consent. There is no clear definition of what constitutes an experimental procedure or drug.
7. The dentist will obtain the informed consent of the patient before instituting any examination or treatment. (See the section on Consent and Informed Consent later in this chapter.)
8. The dentist will not abandon the patient.
9. The dentist will ensure that care is available in emergency situations.
10. The dentist will charge a reasonable fee for services based upon community standards. What is reasonable is determined by what other practitioners in the community charge. However, if a fee is stated, and the patient agrees, it is binding no matter what the amount.
11. The dentist will not permit any person acting under his or her supervision to engage in unlawful acts.
12. The dentist will keep the patient informed about his or her progress.
13. The dentist will not undertake any procedure for which the dentist is not qualified either by training, experience, or licensure.
14. The dentist will complete the care in a timely manner.
15. The dentist will keep accurate records of the examination and treatment of the patient.
16. The dentist will maintain confidentiality of information.
17. The dentist will inform the patient of any unusual occurrences during treatment.
18. The dentist will request consultations when appropriate and make referrals for care when indicated.
19. The dentist will comply with all laws regulating the practice of dentistry.
20. The dentist will practice in a manner consistent with codes of ethics of the profession.

The Patient's Implied Duties. The patient also gives certain warranties to the dentist, including the following:

1. The patient will keep appointments.
2. The patient will notify the dentist (office) in a timely manner if appointments cannot be kept.
3. The patient will provide honest answers to health questions and histories.
4. The patient will inform the dentist if changes in his or her health status occur.
5. The patient will cooperate with the dentist in his or her care (e.g., home hygiene, prescription medication schedule, diet and nutrition, alcohol, smoking and drug use).
6. The patient will pay reasonable fees in a timely manner.

All of the above and more may be included in the contract of care between the dentist and patient, thus becoming part of the express agreement.

Breach of Terms

In contract law, if one party breaches any of the terms, express or implied, the other party is relieved of duty to perform. The courts have modified the rules as it applies to health care. For example, in the provision of orthodontic care for a minor, if the parent does not pay the fee as agreed, the dentist may not remove the appliances and place the child's oral health at risk. The courts have declared that the dentist's remedy is in the courts and that the dentist cannot hold the minor's health as "hostage" to collect the fee from the delinquent parent. In the provision of health care in general, the courts have held that although the patient breaches a duty, the practitioner must not withhold treatment if that would adversely affect the patient's health. In addition, the patient must be given enough time to obtain a substitute care.

In other situations the courts treat breaches in contracts of health care as they do other contracts with the caveat that a breach by a patient does not justify a counter breach by the doctor at a time when the patient's health may be adversely affected. For example, if a dentist and patient agree to a treatment plan of ten individual crowns and the patient refuses to pay the agreed fee after two crown preparations are begun, the dentist must complete the treatment of those two crowns. At this point, however, the dentist is not obligated to treat the remaining eight "untouched" teeth.

Guarantees

An important risk management caveat is to never guarantee the outcome of care. To do so is foolish because a guarantee cannot be legitimately made in health care. In some states it is a violation of law for a health care provider to guarantee the outcome of care. In many cases it leads to expectations by the patient that, if not achieved, could lead to a law suit. Finally, if the patient should claim that the contract was breached by the dentist because the guaranteed result was not achieved, the suit may be subject to contract law, which places no burden on the patient to produce an expert witness rather than malpractice law, which requires the testimony of an expert.

CLINICAL TIP. The admonition to never guarantee results should be strictly observed by dentists performing cosmetic dentistry.

STANDARDS OF CARE

The traditional standard of care to which dentists are held is undergoing a rapid change as evidenced by some recent court decisions. The traditional view was that a dentist was held to a customary standard as practiced by reasonable practitioners in the same community. This is known as the strict locality rule. Over the years courts in many jurisdictions have substituted "a similar community" for the "same community." Another modification substitutes the word "acceptable" for "customary." With the substitution the courts recognized that what may be customary as practiced by the practitioners in a particular community may not be acceptable by any reasonable standard. The application of this legal concept is rare, but it has been used. The current trend is to apply a national standard of care to board certified specialists. States that have adopted, by court law, a national standard for board certified specialists include: Alaska, Arizona, Colorado, Connecticut, Georgia, Iowa, Kansas, Louisiana, Maine, Massachusetts, Michigan, Minnesota, Missouri, Nevada, New Jersey, New Mexico, Ohio, Pennsylvania, South Carolina, and Wisconsin. One appellate department in New York has been added to the list. The effect, as one court stated, is a two-tiered standard: one for board certified specialists and another for other practitioners of the profession.

Based on the court decisions, and in the absence of legislation, dentists practicing cosmetic dentistry are held to the modified local standard of care. Unless a specialty group is formed for these dentists, or courts apply a national standard for generalists, the current situation will prevail.

CONSENT AND INFORMED CONSENT
Consent

Examining or treating a patient without consent constitutes an unauthorized touching (trespass to the person), and makes the one who commits the act guilty of a battery and liable to the patient in a civil suit. The trend in most courts today is to treat allegations of faulty consent as professional negligence. To support the theory, the courts have stated that to sustain an allegation in battery it must be shown that intent to harm was present in the commission of the act. This essential element can rarely be shown in cases brought against health practitioners. However, some courts have stated that if there is no consent at all, an action in battery may be appropriate. In the latter situation, the defendant dentist is at a distinct legal disadvantage, may not be covered by his professional liability insurance policy, may be subject to criminal action, and may be assessed punitive damages.

The fact that the act on which the suit is brought may have been necessary and of benefit to the patient does not affect liability. Similarly, liability is not altered if the service is provided at no fee. Only if a true emergency exists at the time the service is provided can the practitioner proceed at no risk without the consent of the patient. Most jurisdictions state that an emergency exists when care must be rendered at once to protect the life or health of the patient. When these conditions are met, and time is of the essence, consent need not be obtained; it is implied by law. Most courts also apply two other tests: would consent have been given if the patient had been able to grant consent, and would a reasonable person in the same situation have granted consent?

Consent may also be implied by the actions of the patient. For example, a patient enters a dentist's office and after reporting a health complaint, asks to be examined. The patient is told by the doctor that radiographs of the teeth will be taken. The patient allows the radiographs to be taken without objection. Consent is thus implied by the action of the party. The key elements are: the patient was aware of the nature of the problem or the need for treatment and knew or should have known of the treatment (examination) being provided, and the patient made no objection when treatment was begun.

Informed Consent

Treating a patient without consent raises a different issue than treating a patient without *informed* consent. As stated above, treating a patient without consent constitutes a battery, and may subject the dentist to a criminal charge and punitive damages. Therefore, it is better to obtain consent that is faulty rather than no consent at all.

For consent to be valid it must be informed and it must be obtained from one who is competent to grant it. The person must be an adult of sound mind. It is questionable whether a patient under the influence of alcohol or other drugs has sufficient mental acuity to grant a valid consent. A patient under stress, as most patients are when faced with an immediate surgical procedure, presents similar problems. When consent is obtained and the patient appears to be under the influence of drugs or alcohol, treatment should be postponed. If the patient appears to be experiencing stress when faced with a surgical procedure, it is best to allow the patient to take the consent form, if one is used, home. If no form is used, allow the patient to delay the decision for a period of time, ideally overnight.

Except in special circumstances not directly related to dental care, consent obtained from a mentally retarded adult is invalid. In some jurisdictions the parent of a mentally incompetent adult cannot grant a valid consent on behalf of the patient unless appointed as guardian by the court. Other jurisdictions, such as New York, have ruled that, for health care, the mentally incompetent adult may be considered a minor, and the parent may grant consent for care without being legally appointed as guardian.

Generally, cosmetic dentistry qualifies as health care, and a marginally retarded adult may benefit in job placement following cosmetic dental treatment.

Only the parent of a minor can grant a valid consent for care of the minor. Siblings, grandparents, or other relatives may not grant consent. The parents, however, may authorize another party to grant consent, e.g., the administrators of a resident school or a neighbor during the parents' absence.

Either parent may grant a valid consent, even over the objection of the other parent. By common law, a minor is anyone who has not reached the 21st birthday. The age has been reduced by statute to 18. In most jurisdictions there are special statutes granting minors the right to consent to health care without the consent of the parent. In New York, as in most states, minors may grant consent to health care at 18, as set by statute. In Alabama, this age is 14.

By common law, minors may be emancipated and thus may consent to health care without the consent of the parent. Generally, a minor who is financially independent of parental support is emancipated. Many states, such as New York, have codified common law and may list the conditions under which a minor becomes emancipated. These usually include minors who are married, pregnant, or living outside the parental home.

In some cases the courts have stated that a minor may grant a valid consent if the minor understands the nature of the treatment and the risks. This is known as the "mature minor rule." The youngest age at which it has been applied is 14. In many jurisdictions a minor of any age may consent to care for the treatment of venereal diseases, for sex related advice and treatment, and for abortions without the consent of the parent. In many jurisdictions disclosure of this information to the parent places the practitioner at legal risk of criminal action by the state and of civil action by the child for breach of confidentiality.

Consent granted by a spouse is not valid. However, in emergency situations when the consent of the patient cannot be obtained, it is wise to obtain the assent of the spouse. Consent granted by an adult child for a parent or by one sibling for another also is not valid.

For consent to be valid, it must be freely granted. Courts have declared consent invalid because the patient, in order to secure needed care, was required to consent to conditions not in his or her best interest. These consents are known as adhesion contracts, and have been declared unenforceable by many courts. (See the section on Express Terms in the Doctor-Patient Contract earlier in this chapter.)

The courts also look with disfavor on consents that contain exculpatory language, that is, language that relieves the practitioner of liability for negligence. An example is a consent that contains the following provi-

sion: "I accept this treatment with the understanding that I will hold the doctor harmless for any negligence in the performance of the treatment." The courts have stated, in strong terms, that exculpatory language in consents to health care is void as against public policy.

The trend in the courts and the legislatures during the past 20 years has been to demand that the health care provider disclose more information to the patient, thus the concept of "informed consent" has been superimposed on the consent issue. Basic to the concept of informed consent is that the patient must be given, in understandable language, enough information about the proposed treatment to make an intelligent decision about whether to proceed with the proposed treatment, and the patient must have an opportunity to ask questions and have them answered.

Both the courts and the legislatures, in most jurisdictions, have provided specific guidelines as to the required elements of informed consent. In general, for the consent to be valid and effective:

1. It must be freely given.
2. The proposed treatment and its prognosis must be described.
3. The patient must be informed of the risks and benefits of the proposed treatment, including the prognosis if no treatment is provided.
4. Alternative treatment(s) to the one suggested, including their risks and benefits must be described.
5. The patient must be given an opportunity to ask questions and have them answered.
6. All communication with the patient must be in language the patient understands.
7. The consent must be obtained from a patient authorized to grant consent.

The element that causes problems for the courts and practitioners is, "How much detail of the risks should be told to the patient?" There are two different tests applied by the courts. One holds the provider to the standard of what other doctors in the community tell their patients in the same or similar circumstances (the professional community standard). The other standard requires the doctor to provide the patient with sufficient information for him or her to make an intelligent decision as to whether to proceed with the proposed treatment (the reasonable person standard). When the former standard is used by the court, experts from the community must appear for the plaintiff/patient. When the latter is used, no expert testimony is required. Also, in the latter, some courts apply the objective standard, that is: "Is the information provided sufficient for a reasonably intelligent person to make an intelligent choice?" Other courts apply the subjective standard, considering only what the patient was told. New York has adopted, by statute, the professional community standard for all health care providers, and requires expert testimony to establish the standard to which the defendant doctor is held.

In the reasonable person standard, the risks to be communicated to the patient are described as "material." In the professional community standard, they are described as "foreseeable."

It appears from the decisions of the courts that the more invasive the procedure, or the greater the risk attached to it, the more detail regarding the risk the provider is required to disclose to satisfy the "informed" standard.

CLINICAL TIP. Consent given over the telephone, when properly executed, is acceptable to the courts. It must, however, contain all the elements that constitute a valid consent. In addition, it should be properly documented. In the case of a minor, the parent or guardian should be contacted by phone, and told that a third party is listening on an extension. The parent should be told of the situation, and the need for treatment, including all the facts that would be required to meet a valid consent. After the consent is received, appropriate notes should be made in the patient's chart, signed by the person who obtained the consent and by the third party.

Consent need not be written to be valid, however, in some jurisdictions written consent is required for surgical procedures. New York requires written consent for some surgical procedures, e.g., donation of human organs, acupuncture, and abortion in minors.

An oral consent is subject to challenge as to content and whether consent was, in fact, obtained. The degree to which the doctor wishes to document that consent was obtained is a personal decision. In some situations a written signed consent is appropriate, while in others an oral consent might suffice.

It is advised that when the treatment is invasive or the risks are significant, the consent should be written, notwithstanding that local law does not require that consent be written.

Recent court decisions have addressed the issue of who should obtain the consent to care. Options include the operating surgeon (the treating dentist), an associate, a hygienist, an assistant, or a receptionist (secretary).

In a recent New York case, the court referred to a case decided in Pennsylvania, stating that it was the only case on record in which a court was called upon to decide whether the treating doctor or an office employee can obtain valid consent from a patient. In the Pennsylvania case, the dentist's wife, acting as his assistant, obtained the consent of a patient. The court stated that it is the scope of the information that the patient had been given, rather than the identity of the person making the communication that is important. In the opinion of the Pennsylvania court, the operating surgeon is not required to obtain consent.

In the New York case, the court, following the lead of the Pennsylvania court, stated, "a nurse trained in obtaining informed consent to a particular procedure could act as an agent for the treating physician."

Although the appellate courts of two states, Pennsylvania and New York, have ruled that an office worker may obtain the effective consent to care of a patient, there are certain caveats that a doctor should keep in mind before delegating this responsibility. First, the office worker should be trained in obtaining informed consent and, second, the degree of invasiveness and the risks attached to the procedure, should dictate who answers questions asked by the patient about the procedure. If the doctor delegates the responsibility to obtain consent to another, he or she should be available to answer questions asked by the patient.

Examples of consent forms appear in Appendix D.

RECORDS

When the facts regarding what took place in the treatment of the patient conflict, and the records support the dentist's position, an attorney consulted by a potential plaintiff, upon review of the dentist's record, often is likely to dissuade the client from suing.

CLINICAL TIP. Patient treatment records, properly maintained, are the best defense against a claim of negligence where there is no negligence. Plaintiff attorneys, juries, and judges can be positively influenced by records that are neat, legible, and appear to be accurate representations of the treatment the patient received.

In many states it is mandated by law, rule of the licensing agency, or by the state health department, that records of each patient must be kept. There also are rules regarding how long the practitioner is required to retain the records of the patient, and what the record must contain. For this information dentists are advised to contact a local attorney.

Financial information should not be kept on the treatment record. The treatment record should be reserved for treatment and patient reactions to treatment. Financial information should be kept on separate sheets and placed within the folder. The presence of financial information on the treatment record may affect the outcome of the case. For example, if a juror believes the fees to be excessive, this may influence the juror's decision on matters unrelated to fees. In addition, any financial information appearing on the treatment record cannot be kept from the jury.

The following rules should be followed regarding patient treatment records.

1. Entries should be legible, written in black ink or black ball point pen. (Pencil notes should be avoided.)
2. There should be no erasures on the record.
3. Erroneous entries should not be blocked out so that they cannot be read. Instead, a single line should be drawn through the entry, and a note made above it stating "error in entry, see correction below." The correction should be dated at the time it is made.
4. Entries should be uniformly spaced on the form. There should be no unusual or irregular blank spaces.
5. In offices where more than one person makes entries, the entries should be signed or initialed.

In addition to treatment information, the following items should be included in every patient record.

1. Document that consent to care was obtained before treatment was begun. Include all risks and benefits of the treatment presented to the patient and any remarks made by the patient during the discussion.
2. Record all cancellations, late arrivals, and changes of appointments.
3. Document all requests for consultations with other

health practitioners.

4. Document the failure of a patient to comply with a consultation or with a consultant's recommendations.
5. Carefully document all conversations with other health practitioners relating to any consultation or care of the patient.
6. Inform the patient of any adverse occurrences or untoward events that take place during the course of treatment, and document in the record that the patient was informed.
7. Note in the record if the patient has not complied with home care instructions.

Information obtained from the patient on the health history, during conversations, or during the course of treatment, is confidential and should be guarded carefully.

Subjective evaluations, such as an opinion about the patient's mental health, should not be included in the treatment record unless the practitioner is qualified and licensed to make such evaluations. In jurisdictions where the patient is entitled to a copy of the record such notes may be counterproductive to the dentist. Notes about the patient's mental state or other personal evaluations should be made on a separate sheet.

If the practice of dentistry is discontinued, the local law should be checked to determine the requirements on how, where, and in what form the records must be retained.

CLINICAL TIP. *Never surrender original records or radiographs to anyone, except by order of a court. This rule includes a specialist to whom you have referred a patient.*

In one court case, failure of the defendant to produce the original radiographs was interpreted as an attempt to conceal information and resulted in a decision against the doctor. In addition, retaining the original radiographs is required by law in some states.

CLINICAL TIP. *Never tamper with a record once there is an indication that legal action is contemplated by the patient. This is fraud, and may result in loss of the suit and severe punishment by the courts and the insurance company.*

The Health History

An oral history with no record that questions were asked of the patient and answers given, will not meet the test of responsible office practice. Only a written history will meet a reasonable standard of care in history taking.

Recent malpractice suits have centered around failures to obtain an accurate health history of the patient. Some of the problems resulted from the use of a self administered form that uses check marks or circles to indicate a "yes" or "no" answer to a health question. In a recent trial there was conflicting testimony regarding who made the check marks or circled the answers. Also, answers other than "yes" or "no" are possible to almost all questions. For example, "I do not understand the question," and "I am not certain of the answer" are possible answers. To avoid problems, the questionnaire should be designed with open ended questions in which the patient writes the response. An analysis of the handwriting leaves no doubt as to the author.

Errors most commonly associated with medical problems are:

1. Failure to discover a potential drug incompatibility.
2. Failure to learn of drug allergy or potential drug allergy.
3. Failure to discover a medical condition that may result in serious injury to the patient as a result of dental treatment.

Errors most commonly associated with dental problems are:

1. Failure to determine that the patient presented with a history of problems associated with temporomandibular dysfunction.
2. Failure to discover that the patient exhibited a reaction to the administration of a local anesthetic.
3. Failure to discover problems associated with periodontal disease.

Several other notable problems have surfaced in recent cases, such as: who completed the history form, who reviewed it, and who discussed it with the patient. To deal with these concerns, appropriate notes should be made on the history forms and in the treatment record.

Ideally, the treating dentist should take the history. However, if the responsibility of history taking is delegated, the rules are:

1. The person to whom the task is delegated should be specially trained in history taking.
2. The treating doctor should review the history with the patient.
3. Document that the history was reviewed with the patient by the doctor.

In multiple practitioner offices where more than one person may treat a patient, each provider should review the patient's health history before treatment is begun. The same is true as it relates to the consent to care. It is not sufficient to rely on the ability of others in the office, even another treating doctor or hygienist, to obtain an adequate health history or a valid consent. The rule is that the one who provides the care is responsible for ensuring that the care he or she is providing is compatible with the health of the patient and that consent was obtained.

All history forms should include the following:

1. The patient's name at the top (to avoid misfiling should the form become separated from the main record).
2. The patient's signature.
3. The signature of the party completing the form if it is not the patient.
4. The signature of a witness to the patient's signature.
5. The signature of the dentist who reviewed the form with the patient.

The form and all signatures should be completed in black ink or black ball point pen supplied by the office. Not all copiers are capable of reproducing colors other than black.

A sample health history form meeting all the requirements described above is shown in Appendix D.

History Updates

There is no law or fixed rule about how often the medical history should be updated; it is a professional judgment the dentist should make with each patient. For an apparently healthy teenager with uncomplicated dental problems, one may decide to update the health history at every recall visit. For a geriatric patient with a history of diabetes, one may decide to update the health history each month during an extended dental treatment process. Based on professional judgment, it may be sufficient to simply ask, "Has there been any change in your health since your last visit to the office?" If it is felt that this is sufficient, it should be documented in the patient's record that the question was asked and the answer given by the patient.

CLINICAL TIP. The patient's medical and dental condition should be monitored at intervals appropriate to the patient's age and medical and dental status.

When a formal update is required the patient should be given a copy of his or her most recently completed self-administered history form for review. If the patient states that there are no changes, it should be noted in the patient's record or on a form specially designed for that purpose. If the patient indicates that changes have occurred, it may be advisable to have the patient complete another history form and for the dentist to repeat the entire history taking process. Sample copies of this and all office forms are located in the Appendix D.

CLINICAL TIP. There is less health risk to the patient and less legal risk to the dentist when the error is on the side of needless effort than when the review process is shortened and information that is vital to the safe treatment of the patient is overlooked.

In the field of cosmetic dentistry it is essential to thoroughly evaluate the patient's attitude toward dental care. Suitable questions should be designed by the practitioner, either orally or in writing, to determine the mind set of the patient. The questions and responses should be accurately documented in the record. It may be important for the patient to demonstrate oral hygiene procedures. Questions designed to elicit the patient's attitude toward cosmetics in general, and cosmetic dentistry in particular, may be of interest to the cosmetic dentist. Forms alone are not enough for the dentist to properly and safely plan a treatment. A discussion and interview with the patient following the completion of the forms is essential.

Reviewing the completed forms, reading radiographs, evaluating consultant reports and test results, and reviewing the patient interview, completes the health history and prepares the dentist to discuss the treatment plan and alternatives with the patient.

THE STATUTE OF LIMITATIONS

The statute of limitations defines the time within which a law suit may be brought against an individual or any other form of legal entity. It is designed to prevent the threat of a suit from lasting forever. In addition, the statute takes into account fading memories and the unavailability of witnesses due to death or relocation. The statute prevents the execution of stale claims. If the statute has expired, the patient cannot maintain a suit.

Basic issues in limitations statutes are:

1. When does the clock begin to run?
2. What events or conditions toll (delay) the running of the statute?
3. How long does the statute run?

There is no nationwide consistency about the issues noted above. Therefore, if a dentist wishes to know the times related to the statute, he should consult a local attorney. What follows are some generalizations about the statute of limitations applied to malpractice suits against dentists.

Commencement of the Statute of Limitations

Usually, the statute of limitations begins when the act of negligence takes place, whether or not the patient is aware of it. States that follow this rule are called "occurrence states." However, some states consider that the statute of limitations starts when the patient discovers, or should have discovered, that an act of negligence caused injury. States that follow this rule are call "discovery states." Additional possibilities for the start of the statute of limitations include:

1. When the course of treatment in which the negligent act took place ends.
2. When the doctor-patient relationship ends.
3. Should the negligence relate to leaving a foreign object in the body that was not intended to remain in the body, the statute begins to run when the patient discovers, or should have discovered it.

All states have some combination of the above starting dates. For example, in New York the statute of limitations begins when the negligence takes place. However, there are exceptions for foreign objects and continuous treatment.

Tolling of the Statute of Limitations

The statute of limitations is tolled during infancy and generally does not begin to run until the minor reaches majority. However, during the malpractice crises of the 1970s and 1980s, states enacted tort reform legislation in an attempt to control the growing number of malpractice suits. Some changes modified the tolling of the statute of limitations for infancy and placed a maximum tolling years regardless of when the minor reaches adulthood.

Other factors that toll the statute of limitations are of little consequence to dentists, and include the imprisonment of the plaintiff, periods of mental incompetency, and the absence of the plaintiff from the jurisdiction of the court.

Expiration of the Statute of Limitations

Even if the statute of limitations has run, the patient may still enter suit against the dentist. It then becomes the dentist's burden, through his or her attorney, to answer the initial filing of the claim with an affirmative defense raising the running of the statute of limitations. Then the court will rule on whether the suit will continue.

The time in which suit may be brought is controlled by state law, and varies between 1 and 5 years, with most states in the 2 to 3 year category. The time in which the statute begins, and how long it runs, lend confusion and lack of uniformity to the issue. For example, in a state in which the statute does not begin to run until the patient discovers that a fractured root tip was left in the bone during an extraction, the statute may not begin to run until several years after treatment and continue for the time of the statute. In effect, the statute of limitations may be for an indefinite period. In another state in which the statute begins at the time of the incident, i.e., the breaking of the root tip, the statute begins to run without the knowledge of the patient and continues for the time set by local law.

FRAUDULENT CONCEALMENT

Courts take a dim view of a doctor withholding information from a patient about an act of negligence committed during the course of treatment. Many states have enacted legislation on this issue. In those states, the statute of limitations is tolled because of the fraudulent concealment committed by the practitioner; it does not begin to run until the patient discovers, or should have discovered, the fraud and then the statute of limitations for alleged fraud is applied, which may be considerably longer than that for malpractice. Therefore, even in an occurrence state with a fixed statutory time, if the dentist withholds a fact from the patient, such as about a broken root tip, the court may use fraudulent concealment to extend the period in which the patient may bring suit.

CLINICAL TIP. When things go awry during the course of treatment, inform the patient and document in the record the event and that the patient was informed. This fixes the time the statute can run, offers time-related protection to the dentist in discovery states, and avoids tolling of the statute of limitations due to fraudulent concealment in all states.

Knowing how long a patient may exercise the right to sue for an act of negligence, or an alleged act of negligence, may bring peace of mind to the practitioner. To obtain this information, consult a local attorney.

ASSOCIATES AND EMPLOYEES

The legal concept of vicarious liability is applied when an innocent party is held liable to a third party for the negligence of another. It occurs most often in associate practice. Respondeat Superior is a form of vicarious liability in which the parties are in an employer-employee relationship, such as a dentist held liable for the negligent act of an employee dentist, hygienist, or dental assistant. The innocent dentist may be held liable even if the act performed by the associate or employee was prohibited or unlawful.

CLINICAL TIP. In partnership practice each partner may be held liable for the negligent act of any partner under the vicarious liability doctrine. In professional corporations this may not be true; only the negligent dentist and the corporation are held liable, not other stockholders (dentists) in the corporation.

When the associate dentist is an independent contractor, the liability of the principal for the negligence of the independent contractor depends on the relationship between the two, the manner in which professional decisions are made, and the source of patients. Decisions by the courts as to liability are made on a case-by-case basis. However, the Internal Revenue Service has taken a firm position that although the parties may claim an independent contractor relationship, it may in fact be an employer-employee relationship for tax purposes. Before entering into any relationship with another dentist it is best to consult an attorney and an accountant.

CLINICAL TIP. It is recommended that the dentist select and monitor with extreme care those who may vicariously impart their negligence on others in the practice.

FORMS AND RELEASES

The increase in paper work in the modern dental office has become oppressive to many dentists, especially those who remember the "good old days." The practice of dentistry has become more complex due to the expansion of services provided by the profession. New techniques, such as orthognathic surgery, the increased use of implants, new diagnostic procedures, increased concern about temporomandibular joint problems, new awareness by the public about adult orthodontics, and the rapidly growing field of cosmetic dentistry, have added to the complexity of modern dentistry. Further complicating dental practice is the emergence of third party insurance programs and other forms of third party payment programs. The latest intrusion has been the need to build practice management defenses in the form of risk management to counter what is taking place in the legal arena. Complete and carefully designed record keeping systems are essential to a modern practice. Computers in the office are almost as common and necessary as x-ray machines.

A practice that is aware of risk management includes

a series of forms that enable the dentist to practice in a legal worry-free environment. The forms include:

1. **Release of information form.** To enable the dentist to obtain health information about the patient from other practitioners and health facilities, including hospitals.
2. **Waiver of confidentiality form.** To permit the dentist to release information about the patient to insurance carriers, third party payers, and other practitioners.
3. **Informed consent form.** To document that the patient has agreed to the treatment. This is essential when the treatment is invasive or the risks are great.
4. **Informed refusal form.** To document that the dentist has informed the patient of the consequences of not following the dentist's advice regarding recommended care, referrals, and specialty treatment. This form is particularly useful when periodontal consultation or treatment is recommended and refused by the patient.
5. **Permission to take photographs, slide, and videos.** To allow the taking, use, and publications of photographs, slide, or videos. This is especially important in cosmetic dentistry.
6. **Release of all claims form.** When a fee is returned to a patient, it is essential to have the patient sign this form. A dentist should never return a fee to a patient without having this form signed by the patient.

Sample copies of these and all office forms are located in Appendix D.

PROCEDURE WHEN A SUIT IS INSTITUTED

The shock of a malpractice suit may bring a variety of inappropriate responses. Among them are psychologic denial, in which the papers are ignored. Unfortunately, deadlines must be met. There may be a desire to telephone the patient or to contact his lawyer. This is improper because there is a clause in all professional liability insurance contracts that binds the dentist to cooperate with the insurance company and to refrain from any activity that may compromise the suit. Payments made by the dentist to or for the patient, except for first aid, usually are prohibited and should not be made without prior approval by the insurance carrier. Additional things *not* to do include:

1. Do not respond to questions about the case or the treatment of the patient with anyone not known to be a representative of the insurance company or your attorney.
2. Do not surrender your original records to anyone except your attorney or the insurance company and do get a receipt.
3. Do not speak to a dentist that you know treated the patient or wrote a report about the treatment you performed.
4. Do not alter, or add any notes to the patient's treatment record.

5. Do not lose any of the patient's records, radiographs, test results, or reports.
6. Do not agree to see the patient, regardless of the reason. Once the patient elects to file suit, the doctor-patient relationship ends and the adversarial relationship begins. Notify your attorney of the request.
7. Do not make any entries on the patient's record about the law suit or any other matter relating to the suit, such as receipt of the summons, demand for records, or communications with the insurance company or your attorney. These and similar notes related to the case should be recorded on a separate sheet and labeled "confidential."
8. Do not tell anyone that you are insured.
9. Do not speak to your colleagues about the case. All information about the case must remain confidential. Your attorney is in charge, and he or she should decide before any action is taken.
10. Do not tell anyone that you are being sued.

Some appropriate thing to *do* are:

1. Remain calm.
2. Record the manner in which you were served; not on the patient's record, but on a separate sheet headed "confidential."
3. Make a copy of all the papers that were included in the service.
4. Read your professional liability insurance policy to determine where the suit papers are to be sent. If the information is not present, call the carrier.
5. Notify your insurance carrier by certified mail, return receipt requested, as soon as possible. Send the original of all papers included in the service, including the envelope, if it was sent to you through the mail, after you have made copies for your record.
6. Contact all carriers if your carrier changed during the course of the patient's treatment. Include a copy of all papers included in the service to each, after you have made copies for your record.
7. Make a copy of all records and radiographs related to the care of the patient, and secure the originals in a safe place.
8. Write a detailed narrative description of all treatment provided to the patient using your records to refresh you memory. Title the sheet "confidential." Include all you recall about conversations held with the patient and statements made about the treatment. Date and sign the narrative. Send a copy to your insurance carrier. Lock the original in a safe place.
9. Inform your office staff about the suit and caution them about speaking with anyone about the case or the patient.
10. Contact your personal attorney, if you have one, to inform him about the suit. If you do not have a personal attorney, you may consider retaining one. If the amount of the suit exceeds the limits of your

RISK MANAGEMENT IN COSMETIC DENTISTRY

policy, you should retain an attorney to watch over your financial interests.

Patient dissatisfaction with the results of care increases the risk of suit. A poor result by the patient's standard is not always a poor result by the dentist's standard. Too often, patients fail to realize the limitations placed upon achieving a perfect outcome. This is particularly true when cosmetic results are important. Therefore, dentists who practice this art and science are at greater risk than those who practice nonelective and noncosmetic procedures. Although all dentists practice some form of cosmetic dentistry, those whose practice is primarily dedicated to cosmetic dentistry must meticulously adhere to risk management principles because of the increased risk of a suit.

Special precautions must be taken because subjective opinions about the outcome of care may determine whether the patient sues. Consent issues before care is begun become a major factor in determining the patient's expectations of the outcome. Patient expectations must be realistic to avoid problems when the care is completed. The nature and content of the consent may determine whether the patient initiates a suit. Predictable limitations in outcomes must be incorporated into the consent form. Documentation is essential.

CLINICAL TIP. Keeping the patient informed during each step that impacts on the cosmetic result and continuing the involvement of the patient as the treatment progresses may prevent a result which the patient will perceive as a poor one.

Behavioral science plays a greater role in cosmetic dentistry than in most other fields of dental practice. Failure is measured in litigation. When cosmetic dentists include in their treatment procedures the use of general anesthetics, intravenous sedatives, orthodontics, orthognathic surgery, or implants, they take on the added level of legal risk associated with those procedures.

Although risk management applied to cosmetic dentistry is no different from that applied to dental practice in general, more emphasis should be placed in the following areas to avoid legal difficulties following treatment.

1. Record keeping must be meticulous.
2. Consent forms must be carefully constructed and executed.
3. The patient must be involved in all stages when cosmetics is a consideration.
4. Documentation rules must be carefully observed.
5. False and unrealistic hopes should not be presented to the patient.
6. The patient must be kept informed.
7. Guarantees about outcome or patient satisfaction should be carefully avoided. The dentist and office personnel should not use words that imply a guarantee or patient satisfaction.

CONCLUSION

The past decade has seen a dramatic extension in services that fall within the dentist's scope of practice. Basic to many has been the improvement in restorative materials that has contributed to improved esthetics. Improved and expanded techniques have matched the new materials. The use of implants and advances in orthognathic surgery has added to the armamentarium of the profession. There is no doubt that the services available to patients, particularly in the field of cosmetic dentistry, have increased. Patients want more and dentists are able to provide more than ever before.

With the increase in what the modern dentist is able to provide to a demanding public, has come a concurrent increase in litigation. The present legal environment has demonstrated that good professional care is not enough. Good records are part of good care. The patient is entitled to decide what should be done to his or her own body, and before it is done, to have enough information to make an informed decision. Documentation is essential to defend a law suit. Communication with the patient to keep him or her informed about the care is essential. When cosmetics is part of the care, because of its elective nature and subjective evaluations, special care must be taken to ensure that all legal preventive measures are followed. And finally, good risk management is as important as good professional care. Without both dentistry becomes a high risk profession.

ESTHETICS AND ADVANCED TECHNOLOGY

Kenneth W. Aschheim, D.D.S.

29

Advances in electronic technology have influenced every aspect of our society, including dentistry. Each year, new technologies are introduced that will someday make current dental procedures obsolete. The incorporation of these advances into an esthetic dental practice will enable the practitioner to offer a wider range of services and provide additional treatment options.

TERMINOLOGY

The complex nature of the subject matter in this chapter necessitates the use of terminology with which the reader may not be familiar. In this section all italized words contained within a definition are also separately defined.

Annotation. The addition of explanatory text to an image.

Backwards compatibility. The ability of newer *computer* models or *software* to perform all the tasks of the older models they replace.

Byte. The unit of measurement for the amount of *memory* in a *computer*.

CCD. See *charged coupled device.*

Central processing unit (CPU). The brain of the *computer.* It is synonymous with *microprocessor.* Since more than just the CPU determines what a computer understands, computers from two different manufacturers utilizing the same CPU, may not always be able to run the same *programs.*

Character generator. A specialized device used to *annotate* (add text to) an image.

Charged coupled device (CCD). An electronic *sensor,* made up of hundreds of thousands of individual sensors, which "sees" the image. CCDs are often re-

ferred to as *solid state devices* in order to distinguish them from old style vacuum tubes.

CIS. See *computer imaging system* in the section on Equipment Categories later in this chapter.

Compatibility. The ability of different *computers* from different manufacturers to run the same *software.* For example, a *program* written for an IBM brand PC will run on any IBM-compatible computer (e.g., Compaq, NEC, or Dell PC). However, a *program* written for an IBM computer will not run on an Apple Macintosh. (See also *CPU compatibility* and *software.*)

Composite video signal. A single signal carrying all the video information from the *sensor* to the *video controller* (see also *RGB signal*).

Computer. A major *hardware* component that, unlike a microwave oven which is preset at the factory to perform a single task, can be instructed to do different tasks via *software* instructions called *programs.*

Computer imaging system (CIS). See *computer imaging system* in the section on Equipment Categories later in this chapter.

Computer resolution. The sharpness of the image on a *computer screen,* usually defined by the number of dots that make up the image. *Computer* systems do not adhere to the *NTSC* standard and usually follow a standard which is unique to each brand of computer. (see also high definition television, pixels, video board).

Computer screen. See *monitor.*

Computer-aided design and computer aided manufacturing (CAD/CAM). See *computer-aided design and computer aided manufacturing (CAD/CAM) systems* in the section on Equipment Categories later in this chapter.

Controller. See *video controller.*

CPU. See *Central processing unit.*

CPU compatibility. There are two major manufacturers of *CPUs* for personal *computers*, Intel and Motorola. Each manufactures a family or group of CPUs. Each CPU within a particular family is able to understand a similar set of instructions, which for the most part is unique to that "family." The Motorola 68000/68020/68030/68040 family of CPUs is used in Apple Macintosh, Atari ST, and Commodore Amiga computers. Intel's 8088/8086/80286/80386/80486 family is used by all IBM and IBM-compatible computers. CPU compatibility does not ensure *compatibility*. For example, a *program* written for an Apple Macintosh computer with a 68000 CPU will not run on an Atari ST computer with a 68000 CPU. (See also *compatibility* and *software*.)

Cursor. A small line, dot or arrow that appears on the *computer screen* and marks the current working position on the screen. The position of the cursor can be changed by the user.

Digitizer. A device capable of "reading" a photographic image and translating it into an electronic form that a *computer* can understand (see also *graphics tablet*).

Disk. A thin, flat, circular sheet upon which information is magnetically stored (see also *floppy diskette, hard disk*).

Double density. A type of floppy diskette (see also *floppy diskette*).

Floppy disk drive. A tape recorder-like device that is capable of retrieving (reading) and storing (writing) information onto a *floppy diskette* (see also *hard disk drive* and *optical disk drive*).

Floppy diskette or floppy disk. A round, flat, plastic *disk* encased in a protective soft cardboard or hard plastic shell. The disk, which is the thickness of a piece of paper, has an iron-oxide coating and is capable of magnetically storing information. Including the protective shell, disks usually measure either 3.5 or 5.25 in. and can be up to one-eighth of an inch thick. In addition to different sizes, disks also have different storage capacities. The terms *single, double, high* and *quad density* are used to describe the relative storage capacities of different types of diskettes (see also *floppy disk drive* and *optical disk drive*).

Full screen view. A graphic image that fills the entire viewing screen.

Graphical environment. A *program* that enables the user to direct the *computer* to perform desired functions. The user "points" to small *icons* on the screen with a *mouse* (see also *icons, nongraphical environment*).

Graphics tablet (digitizer). A device for inputting information or manipulating images on the screen. It consists of a solid plastic board, a *mouse*-like device or a pointing device called a *stylus*.

Hard copy. A printed page or photograph obtained from a *computer, VIS,* or *CIS*.

Hard disk. A metal coated *disk* encased in a *hard disk drive* that is capable of storing 20 to 1000 times more data than a *floppy disk* (see also *hard disk drive* and *optical disk drive*).

Hard disk drive (Winchester drive). A disk drive system containing the *hard disk*. Unlike a *floppy diskette*, a hard disk is permanently attached to its drive and cannot be removed from the *computer*. (See also *optical disk drive*.)

Hardware. The actual equipment: the *computer*, the video camera, the *monitor*, or any components that interact with these devices. Hardware establishes the capabilities of a system, whereas the *software* determines how these capabilities are utilized.

HDTV. See *high definition television*.

High definition television (HDTV). A proposed higher *resolution* standard to replace *NTSC* which would produce a more photograph-like image on a video screen. Proposed HDTV standards could increase the maximum number of horizontal lines (currently 525) to over one thousand (see also *computer resolution,* and *NTSC*).

High density. A type of *floppy diskette* (see also *floppy diskette*).

Icon. A small picture on a video screen that represents various functions the *computer* can perform.

Input. The information that is entered into a *computer*.

Interface. See *user interface*.

Keyboard. A typewriter-like device used to send *(input)* information to a *computer*.

Kilobyte. One thousand *bytes*.

Laser systems. See *laser systems* in the section on Equipment Categories later in this chapter.

LCD. See *liquid crystal displays*.

LED. See *light emitting diodes*.

Light emitting diodes (LED). Specialized light bulbs which draw very little power, usually red in color.

Liquid crystal displays (LCD). Very thin display panels that perform the same function as a computer *monitor*. Because of their light weight and low power consumption, they are ideal for use in battery operated portable *computers*. The most common LCDs are the displays found on digital watches.

Macro lens. A close-up lens capable of sharply focusing on and magnifying a small object at very close range.

Megabyte. One million *bytes*.

Memory. See *random access memory*.

Microprocessor. See *central processing unit (CPU)*.

Modem. An acronym for **mo**dulating and **dem**odulating device; used to transmit or receive *computer* information over a telephone line.

Monitor. A specialized television used to display *computer* text or graphics.

Mouse. A device attached by a wire to the *computer* that is used to manipulate images on a screen.

Mouse pen. A smaller pen-shaped *mouse* with a button on the side.

Multi-image view. The ability to place multiple images on the same screen.

Nongraphical environment. A *program* that requires the user to type commands from a *keyboard* in order to direct the *computer* to perform a desired function (see also *graphical environment*).

NTSC (National Television Standards Committee). The Federal Communications Commission and the electronics industry have defined standards regarding how a video image may be displayed. NTSC *resolution* is described by the number of lines that make up the image. NTSC sets the maximum number of horizontal lines at 525, although, for technical reasons, rarely are more than 450 of these lines displayed. The number of vertical lines varies among manufacturers, from 250 to 400, depending on the quality of the television. The resolution of video cameras and video recorders is defined in the same way as television (see also *high definition television, computer resolution, pixels*).

Optical disk drive. A very high capacity plastic disk drive system capable of storing 200 to 10,000 times more data than a *floppy disk*. Like a *hard disk*, most are permanently attached to and cannot be removed from the *computer*.

Output. The information that is obtained from a *computer*.

Picture elements. See *pixels*.

Pixels (picture elements). A definition of *resolution* in a *CIS* based on the number of dots that make up the image. Although this unit is analogous to the lines on a television, the two units are not the same and there is no easy way to compare lines to dots. In addition, a number of other factors, such as the number of colors available, can affect the perceived resolution of a system. Thus, the number of pixels alone cannot be the sole criteria for comparing the resolution of different systems (see also *computer resolution* and *video board*).

Processing unit. See *central processing unit*.

Program. See *software*.

Quad density. A type of *floppy diskette*.

Radiographic image processing system (RIPS). See *radiographic image processing systems* in the section on Equipment Categories later in this chapter.

Radiographic imaging systems (RIS). See *radiographic imaging systems* in the section on Equipment Categories later in this chapter.

RAM. See *random access memory*.

Random access memory (RAM). The electronic portion of the *computer* where currently used *programs* and data are placed. The size of the RAM is measured in *kilobytes* or *megabytes*. In general, the more RAM a computer has, the more powerful the programs it is able to run (see also *byte, kilobyte, megabyte*).

Resolution. The sharpness of a picture.

RGB signal. A signal divided into multiple frequencies of information. By separating the signal by color (usually Red, Green and Blue) a higher fidelity picture is obtained. This is analogous to the way audio signals are separated into low (bass), medium (midrange), and high (treble) frequencies in order to obtain high fidelity sound.

Sensor. An electronic device that "sees" an object.

Single density. A type of *floppy diskette* (see also *floppy diskette*).

Software. An electronic set of instructions, called a *program*, that tells the *hardware* exactly what to do and when to do it. Software is machine specific: a program written for an Apple Macintosh *computer* will not run on an IBM computer. The program is stored on a *floppy diskette* and is read (loaded) into the machine via the floppy or *hard disk* drive. Because it is time consuming to write programs, the software often costs as much or more than the hardware.

Software compatibility. See *compatibility*.

Solid state devices. See *charged coupled device (CCD)*.

Stylus. A pointing device attached to a *graphics tablet*.

User interface. The method by which options from a *program* are selected (see also *software*).

Video board. An electronic component that determines the maximum *resolution* of a particular *computer*. Resolution varies from between 320 × 200 *pixels* (low resolution) to 1024 × 768 pixels (high resolution). For dental imaging, a special video board is required to convert *NTSC* signals to a form the computer can understand. In general, computers are able to process much higher resolutions than those obtained from reasonably priced commercially available video cameras. Thus, the use of video boards capable of resolutions greater than the NTSC standard is of limited value in dental imaging.

Video controller. A specialized *computer* used to manipulate a video image.

Video head. The area of the handpiece where the *CCD* is placed.

Video imaging system (VIS). See *video imaging system* in the section on Equipment Categories later in this chapter.

Video transmission cable. The wire that transmits the image from the video handpiece to the *central processing unit*.

VIS. See *video imaging system* in the section on Equipment Categories later in this chapter.

Winchester drive. See *hard disk drive*.

EQUIPMENT CATEGORIES

Technologic trends in dentistry can be divided into seven major categories:

1. **Video imaging system (VIS).** VISs consist of specialized video cameras, controllers, and monitors designed to display on a screen, record, and print intraoral video images (Fig. 29–1).
2. **Computer imaging system (CIS).** CISs are extensions of VISs and allow for the modification of color, shape, and size of intraoral images (Fig. 29–2).
3. **Computer-aided design and computer-aided manufacturing (CAD/CAM) system.** CAD/CAM systems are extensions of CISs. They create a modified intraoral image, which is used as an "electronic die" to fabricate a restoration (Fig. 29–3).
4. **Radiographic imaging system (RIS).** RISs consist of specialized sensors capable of recording, storing, and enhancing radiographic images (Fig. 29–4).
5. **Radiographic image processing system (RIPS).** RIPSs are capable of "reading" the image from a radiographic film, calculating cephalometric measurements, and displaying the measurements on a monitor or a printout (Fig. 29–5).

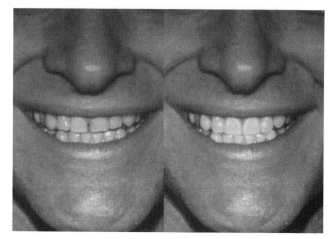

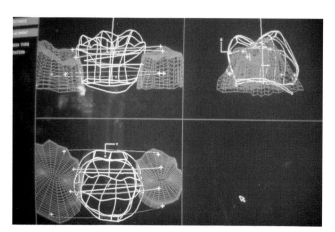

FIG. 29–1. A intraoral video image of a fractured first premolar.

FIG. 29–2. A computer imaging system allows for modification of the color, shape, and size of an intraoral image. (Courtesy of McAndrews-Northern Dental Laboratory).

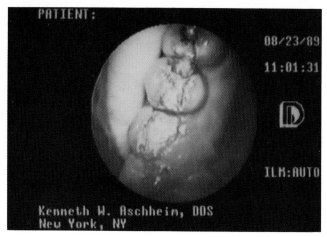

FIG. 29–3. A computer image of a CAD/CAM system calculating the shape of a crown restoration. (Duret system courtesy of Hennson International.)

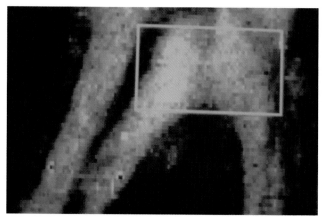

FIG. 29–4. A computer enhanced radiovisiographic image of a dental apex. (Courtesy of Trophy U.S.A., Inc.)

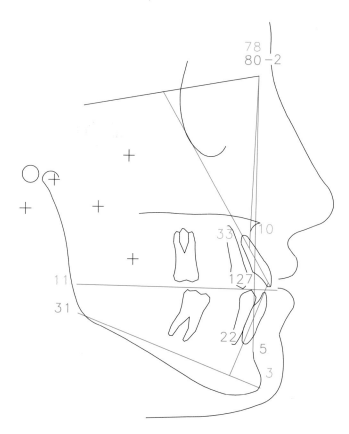

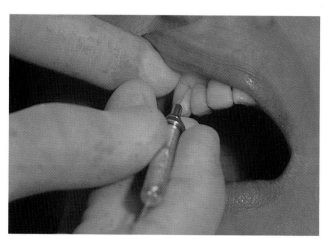

FIG. 29–6. A laser curettage treatment. (Courtesy of American Dental Laser.)

FIG. 29–5. A color plot of a cephalometric tracing. (Courtesy Dr. Daniel Buchbinder.)

6. **Laser systems.** Laser systems are capable of gingival recontouring, caries removal, and enamel etching (Fig. 29–6). (However, currently not all of these procedures are FDA-approved.)
7. **Other systems.** Other systems include those that use the computer to analyze oral non-image information, such as centric occlusion analyses or periodontal pocket measurements (Fig. 29–7).

Video Imaging Systems

Video imaging systems (VISs) were among the first electronic devices to be used in dentistry. Original VISs were modified gastroenterology endoscopes, however, newer models have been designed exclusively for dental use. VISs are primarily used to enhance clinical visualization by displaying intraoral images on a monitor. In addition, these systems can store, retrieve, and reproduce the images. They also are capable of limited image annotation.

Advantages

1. **Increased visibility.** VISs provide an unparalleled view of the oral cavity, allowing the clinician to view areas that are difficult, if not impossible, to see by any other method. Newer systems, equipped with special macro lenses, allow for visualization of endodontic canal systems and periodontal pockets.
2. **Patient education and marketing.** VISs allow patients to see their clinical situations on a monitor. This aids in the proper understanding of treatment options, which may lead to increased acceptance of proposed treatment plans.[1]
3. **Medicolegal documentation.** All VISs are capable of producing prints of images, which provide visual documentation for archival, legal, and educational purposes.
4. **Evaluation of treatment effectiveness.** VISs have the ability to create prints, which provide serial documentation of the effectiveness of long-term treatments. Results of periodontal therapy, bleaching techniques, or patient home care, for example, can be compared with previous images.

Disadvantages

1. **High cost.** The initial start-up costs of a VIS can range from 3,000 to over 30,000 dollars, depending on the options selected. Leasing may help to amortize the cost to a few hundred dollars each month.[1]
2. **Complexity.** All of these systems require an expenditure of considerable time to learn how to properly use them.
3. **Increased chair time.** These systems can increase the amount of time necessary to present simple cases. With experience, presentation time can be reduced. In addition, the initial viewing of a patient's oral condition can be delegated to an auxiliary employee.[1]
4. **Moderate resolution.** The resolution of most systems is limited by current television and video standards. With the future introduction of high definition television (HDTV), this problem should be rectified.

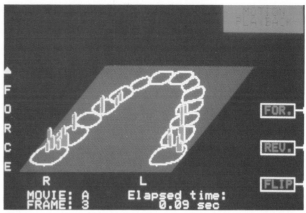

FIG. 29–7. A computerized occlusal analysis. (Courtesy of Tekscan, Inc.)

5. **Limited extraoral imaging.** Most video systems have extraoral imaging capability, however, since they have been optimized for macroscopic imagery, their extraoral video quality is inferior to a standard video camera or 35 mm single lens reflex camera. Many tend to produce a distorted "fish-eyed" appearance.
6. **Large size.** These systems require substantial operatory space. When the monitor is placed on an optional mobile cart, the system can exceed 5 feet in height and 2 feet in both width and depth.
7. **Removable hard storage.** VISs use different types of removable media (e.g., video cassette tape, floppy disk) for storage. As the number of images increases, retrieval may become time consuming and careful records must be kept regarding which disks or tapes hold older images.
8. **Evolving technology.** Current systems may quickly become obsolete due to rapid advances in microelectronics. Increases in resolution, graphics capability, and storage capability, as well as decreases in size and price, are inevitable.

Components

Although hardware varies from system to system, all have certain common elements (Figs. 29–8, 29–9).

1. **Video input device.** Most video input devices are small, free standing video cameras designed to mimic a dental handpiece, or are specially designed video cameras that attach to a dental mirror. Selection is usually based on individual preference. Newer units utilize higher resolution solid state imaging devices, which are smaller than older units and provide sharper images at lower light levels.
2. **Video transmission cable.** Video transmission cable is the "wire" that transmits the image from the video handpiece to the central processing unit. Some cables function as "two lane highways," also transmitting a very bright light from the processing unit to help illuminate the image. In these cases, the fiber optic cable may, if abused, degrade over time.
3. **Light source.** A xenon or quartz light source is built into each unit. Xenon bulbs are always located

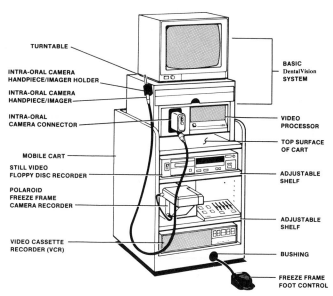

TURNTABLE

INTRA-ORAL CAMERA
HANDPIECE/IMAGER HOLDER

INTRA-ORAL CAMERA
HANDPIECE/IMAGER

INTRA-ORAL
CAMERA CONNECTOR

MOBILE CART

STILL VIDEO
FLOPPY DISC RECORDER

POLAROID
FREEZE FRAME
CAMERA RECORDER

VIDEO CASSETTE
RECORDER (VCR)

BASIC
DentalVision
SYSTEM

VIDEO
PROCESSOR

TOP SURFACE
OF CART

ADJUSTABLE
SHELF

ADJUSTABLE
SHELF

BUSHING

FREEZE FRAME
FOOT CONTROL

FIG. 29–8. A diagram of a typical video imaging system (VIS).

in the central processing unit, are stroboscopic (flash on and off at a set rate), and produce a very bright light. They also may produce an audible "clicking" when the unit is on. Although long-lasting, xenon bulbs can be expensive to replace. Other systems utilize a continuously illuminating quartz bulb, which can be located in either the video handpiece head or the central processing unit. Not as bright as a xenon bulb, the video heads in these systems are usually adjusted to overcome this problem. Units with bulbs located in the central processing unit often have a built-in cooling fan.

4. **Video display.** Different sizes of high resolution video displays are available. These are usually RGB type video monitors with a higher resolution than the more common composite video monitors, which have resolutions similar to those of NTSC televisions found in the home.

5. **Central processing unit.** The central processing unit processes the image. Processing includes image freeze, color adjustment, graphics input, and text annotation. The image is "frozen" with a foot pedal, and some units also include a detachable keyboard for annotating the image.

6. **Video storage unit.** Manufacturers offer a number of options for electronically storing the image. All storage media are removable, the two most common types being video cassette recorders (VCR) using standard video cassettes and floppy disk-based devices using special 2 in. hard-cased floppy diskettes. VCR devices are inexpensive and reliable but can store at only the lower NTSC resolution. Since images are stored sequentially, access may require fast-forwarding and rewinding the tape until the specific image is found. Floppy disk-based systems are expensive, but they allow instant access to an image on the disk. Utilizing a special floppy diskette, they are based upon a newer video still camera technology and can store an RGB image.

7. **Video output device.** Video output devices provide hard copy of the displayed image. The quality of the output is directly proportional to the cost of the output device. The least costly units usually utilize a Polaroid Freeze-Frame (Fig. 29–10), which is capable of producing 35 mm slides as well as instant color prints. The most expensive units use color graphics printers, which can produce high quality pictures.

Available Products

CLINICAL TIP. Products are continually being updated and revised. It is important to check with the manufacturer prior to purchase to determine which options are still available, what enhancements have been made to the unit, and if current limitations still exist. In addition, new products may have been introduced that make current products obsolete.

CLINICAL TIP. A great deal of time and effort is required to master the complexities of video imaging systems. It is important to locate a dealer who can provide ample instruction and maintenance support. If a "bargain system" does not include servicing, the full capability of the system may never be realized.

Dentalvision (Dentsply International, Inc.). This is a xenon-based system, which is connected by a fiber optic cable to a computer with a detachable keyboard. The video head is very small, resembling a handpiece. The image is frozen via an attached foot pedal. The computer is attached to an RGB monitor and can magnify an 8 mm central incisor to a size of 10 cm. The image produced is contained within a circle 15 cm in diameter.[1] No full screen view is available and "fish-eye" distortion occurs with extraoral images. Numerous output devices are available, the most common being the Polaroid Freeze-Frame. Images can be stored on either a VCR or floppy disk system. The unit uses a liquid defogging agent. This unit is being replaced by the Perspective Dental Imaging System (see below).

Fuji Dentacam EDC 2 (Patterson Dental Co.) (Fig. 29–11). This xenon-based imaging system uses a video head attached to an instrument that resembles a mouth mirror. The fiber optic cable also serves as a conduit for compressed air to prevent mirror fogging. The image is processed by the built-in computer and is displayed on a high resolution RGB monitor. The system can magnify an 8 mm central incisor to a size of 13 cm.[1] The image produced is contained within a circle 23 cm in diameter. No full screen view is available. Images can be stored on a VCR or floppy disk system and prints are made on a high resolution color printer, which can produce multiple images on a single page (Fig. 29–12). The detachable keyboard allows for annotation of the image. This system is easily integrated into Fuji's Vision Plus Computer Imaging System (see the section on Computer Imaging Systems, Available Products, later in this chapter).

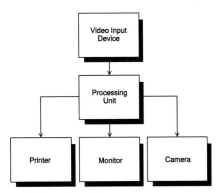

FIG. 29–9. A flow chart of a typical video imaging system (VIS).

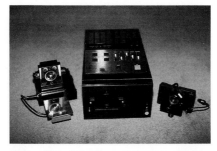

FIG. 29–10. The Polaroid Freeze-Frame system. (Courtesy of Polaroid, Inc.)

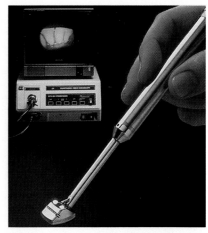

FIG. 29–11. The Fuji Dentacam EDC 2 system. (Courtesy of Patterson Dental Co.)

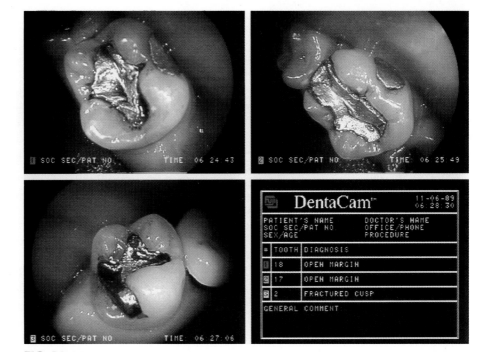

FIG. 29–12. A high resolution color printer permits multiple images to be printed on a single page and allows for the addition of text. (Courtesy of Patterson Dental Co.)

FIG. 29-12

Oral Scan Video Imaging System (Lester A. Dine, Inc.) (see Oral Scan Computer Imaging System, Fig. 29–27, later in this chapter).

Unlike many other systems, the Oral Scan produces a full screen rectangular image on an RGB screen, utilizing a large cylindrically shaped video head attached to a 30 mm mirror. Images are stored on a VCR and are printed on a Polaroid Freeze-Frame. The unit cannot annotate the image. Defogging can be accomplished by attaching compressed air.

Oral Video Scope (Video Dental Concepts). The

Oral Video Scope system utilizes a CCD video head at-

tached by a fiber optic cable to a quartz halogen light source. Magnification of up to 30 times normal is available using two detachable magnifying mirrors. Options include a VCR recorder, a video floppy disk recorder, and a color printer (Fig. 29–13).

KTD Dentvision (KTD, Inc.). Dentvision is a quartz-based system that uses a small hand-held camera similar to that of the Visioner system (see below). Unlike other systems, Dentvision is designed for both single operatory or multiple operatory environments. The VCR and video processing unit can remain in one operatory on a stationary rack with each satellite operatory equipped with a keyboard, camera, light source, and

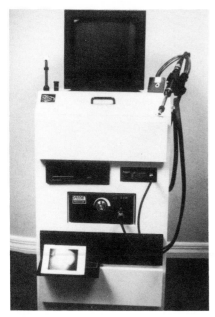

FIG. 29–13. *The Oral Video Scope system. (Courtesy of Video Dental Concepts.)*

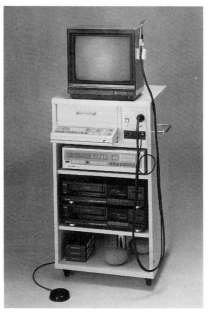

FIG. 29–14. *The KTD Dentvision. (KTD, Inc.)*

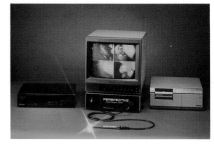

FIG. 29–15. *The Perspective Dental Imaging System. (Courtesy of Dentsply International, Inc.)*

monitor (Fig. 29–14). These satellite operatories must be wired to the central video processing unit. The system is capable of image annotation.

Perspective Dental Imaging System (Dentsply International, Inc.). The Perspective Dental Imaging System is smaller than the Dentalvision system and eliminates both the noise and stroboscopic effects of the xenon bulb. The system produces a full screen, rectangular image. The handpiece is similar in size to the conventional DentalVision handpiece. Magnification of up to 38 times normal is possible, and images are stored on a VCR, which also allows for the simultaneous audio dictation of clinical findings. Options include a multi-image display, an on-screen character generator for annotation, a floppy disk storage system, and a color video printer. (Fig. 29–15).

Ultra-Eye (Trojan Intra-Oral Camera Systems). The Ultra-Eye is a CCD-based camera attached by fiber optic cable to a quartz-halogen unit. Two separate beams of light provide for increased illumination. Two mirrors (0.75 in. and 1.25 in.) attach to the small video head to provide magnifications of up to 40 times normal. The image is viewed through a round window. Options include a VCR, video floppy disk recorder, a Polaroid Freeze-Frame, and a color printer. The system easily attaches to the company's Imagemaker Computer Imaging System. (See the section on Computer Imaging Systems, Available Products, later in this chapter.)

Visioner 21A (J. Morita USA, Inc.). The Visioner is a quartz-based system with a hand-held, solid state camera. It is unique in that the manufacturer claims that interchangeable lenses allow for viewing both sub-

gingivally and within the pulp chamber. The smallest lens is 0.69 mm in diameter. Images are stored on a video floppy disk system.

Clinical Procedure

Although the individual controls of all these systems vary greatly there are certain common elements:

Armamentarium

- Video imaging system

Clinical Technique. The technique for operating these systems are extremely simple. They include:

1. Adjust the operatory lights for optimum viewing according to the manufacturer's recommendation.

CLINICAL TIP. Most xenon-based video heads are designed specifically for use with a xenon light source. To obtain an optimum image, dim the overhead and room lights to prevent background light from interfering with color balancing.

2. Aim the video head at the desired image.
3. Freeze the image on the video screen by activating the foot pedal.
4. Store the image on the VCR or a floppy disk of a still video system (optional).
5. Print the image (optional).

CLINICAL TIP. It is prudent to bracket the image (take multiple images at different light intensities) when using a film-based output device. Although the Polaroid Freeze-Frame is capable of "image previewing" on a separate monitor, it is often of limited value since the video image does not faithfully duplicate the film colors.

FIG. 29–16. Patients are shown "what-if" scenarios. (Courtesy of McAndrews Northern Dental Laboratory.)

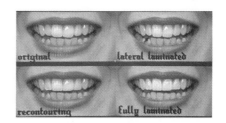

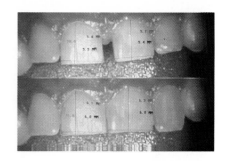

FIG. 29–17. Computer generated superimposed measurements predict the final dimensions of the teeth following proposed diastema closure.

Computer Imaging Systems

The computer imaging system (CIS) is slowly revolutionizing diagnosis and treatment planning. Intraoral and extraoral images can be manipulated, creating "what if" scenarios (Fig. 29–16). Patients see not only their current condition, but also the possible results of various treatment plans. Most CISs have the following capabilities:

1. **Magnify or shrink an image.** CISs can alter the size of the entire image or an individual section of the image.
2. **Crop an image.** CISs can crop (isolate) sections of the image and remove extraneous information. This aids the patient in focusing on problem areas.
3. **Move an image.** CISs can move a section of an image from one area to another. The possible results of proposed orthodontic treatment, for example, can be seen immediately.
4. **Copy an image.** CISs can duplicate images of individual teeth and move them to edentulous areas, enabling the patient to see the results of tooth replacement.
5. **Change shading.** The shade of any section of an image can be altered, allowing patients to see the possible results of bleaching, laminate veneer procedures, or other shade altering treatments.
6. **Change the shape of an image.** The shape of any section of an image can be altered to allow patients to see the possible results of porcelain laminate veneers, esthetic recontouring, or other reconstructive procedures.
7. **Store and retrieve image cutouts.** CISs have the ability to save small sections of an image, retrieve them instantly, and add them to the appropriate position on the display screen. This creates a "library" of prosthetic parts. The dentist can, for example, instantly show a patient the effects of placing a pontic or wrought wire clasp.
8. **Create a print of the altered image.** Once a treatment goal has been established, a print of the image can be conveyed to the laboratory in order to aid in the fabrication of the final prosthesis. Some systems allow for the immediate electronic telephone transmission of the image.
9. **Take measurements directly from the screen.** Most systems can take measurements of the image on the viewing screen. The measurement can be used when fabricating the restoration (Fig. 29–17).
10. **Models available for manipulation of entire facial features.** Many of the systems were first developed for plastic and cosmetic surgery and are also capable of predicting the possible results of orthognathic and other maxillofacial surgical procedures.

Advantages

CISs have the same advantages as VISs plus the following:

1. **Create "what if" scenarios.** By allowing manipulation of the images, different treatment alternatives can be explored.
2. **Decrease the chance of patient misunderstanding.** Because the patient sees predicted treatment results, there is less chance of miscommunication.
3. **Convey the desired treatment goals to the dental laboratory.** After the dentist and patient produce an acceptable treatment plan, the information can be conveyed to the dental laboratory. Some systems allow the immediate transmission of the image directly to the laboratory over a standard telephone line.
4. **Contain large capacity storage system.** Unlike most VISs, CISs have large capacity hard disks or optical disks that can store hundreds of images. This increases the ease and efficiency of information retrieval.
5. **Accept images from multiple sources.** All units can accept images obtained from a VIS.

Disadvantages

CISs have the same disadvantages as VISs plus the following:

1. **May inaccurately predict the final result.** The major drawback of these systems is the possibility that the optimal results predicted on a preoperative computer simulation will not be achieved clinically.

CLINICAL TIP. *The method by which images are manipulated is different from the way teeth are treated clinically. It is important to emphasize to the patient that a predictive simulation is therefore only an approximation.*

It is uncertain at this time if an inadequate clinical result following a favorable prediction by a computer simulation is a valid basis for litigation.

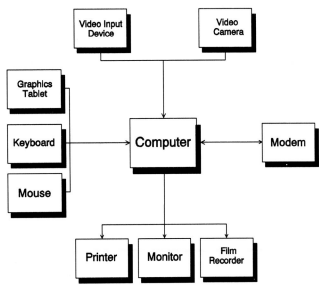

FIG. 29–18. A flow chart of a typical computer imaging system (CIS).

2. **May duplicate video imaging equipment.** Many of the components found in these systems may duplicate those found in video imaging equipment. However, although a CIS can function as a VIS it cannot function as well as a VIS. For example, a CIS can produce adequate images of anterior teeth but is limited in its ability to obtain intraoral images of the posterior regions of the mouth. Although most CISs can accept images obtained from a VIS, the cost of purchasing both systems may be prohibitive.

Hardware Components

All CISs are similar in terms of their hardware components. They all consist of the following (Fig. 29–18):

1. **Video input device.** Most systems utilize an extraoral RGB video camera (Fig. 29–19). All units can accept input from any VIS. However, since many of the intraoral VISs tend to distort extraoral images, an extraoral camera is also required.
2. **Light source.** All systems that use extraoral RGB video cameras require photographic studio lights in order to obtain good color balance (Fig. 29–20).
3. **Video display.** Most systems use a standard 19 in. RGB color monitor, although smaller monitors are available.
4. **Video board.** Most systems use either an Everex Video 16 or a TrueVision Raster Graphics Adapter 16 (Targa) video board. However, some companies (e.g., Fuji) have manufactured custom video boards for their own CISs.
5. **Central processing unit** (Fig. 29–21). All systems utilize IBM compatible computers with a minimum of between 512 kilobytes (512 K) and 2 megabytes (2 M or 2000 K) of random access memory (RAM), depending on the system. They require an Intel 80286, 80386SX, 80386, 80486SX, or 80486 central processing unit, and are capable of running MS-DOS and OS/2 software. The 80386 and 80486 based sys-

tems tend to run more quickly then the 80286 system. All systems can be controlled by a detachable keyboard.
6. **Alternate input devices.** In order to manipulate the image, all systems require either a mouse, a mouse pen, or a Summagraphics graphics tablet (Fig. 29–22).
7. **Video storage unit.** Unlike VISs, CISs are all equipped with large, internal storage devices. Large capacity hard disks store images magnetically. Very large capacity optical disks store the images "optically." Access to an image on either type of disk is immediate.
8. **Video output device.** These devices are identical to those discussed for VISs.

Software Components

A major difference among the different computer imaging systems is software. All use menu systems, but their implementation is different. Early systems were written under a graphical environment called Truevision Imaging Software (TIPS). This is a very powerful program which allows such extreme customization that it is virtually impossible to determine which systems utilize TIPS software and which use a different program. Other systems use a graphical environment called Freestyle or other proprietary operating system in order to obtain additional features.

The method by which the dentist selects various options available within a program is termed the user interface. Currently there are three types of user interfaces available on CISs.

1. **Icon.** The icon system utilizes little pictures (objects or icons) on a screen (Fig. 29–23). Each icon represents a different function that the computer can perform. The dentist selects the appropriate icon by moving a cursor over the object with the aid of a mouse. When the cursor is over the correct object, the dentist pushes (clicks) the button on the mouse. This system is similar to one used by the Apple Macintosh computer.
2. **Pull down menu.** In pull down menu systems the choices are contained in a word list (Fig. 29–24). After the cursor is used to select a given choice another set of suboptions is displayed ("pulled down") on the screen. The appropriate suboption is also selected with the cursor.
3. **Simple menu.** This system is similar to the pull-down menu except that the menu is confined to a small area of the screen, usually just the top one or two lines and is limited to one or two words per option. The goal is to eliminate "clutter" on the screen.

Individual preference seems to be the major determinant of which system is most efficient.

CLINICAL TIP. *Products are continually being updated and revised. It is important to check with the manufacturer prior to any purchase to determine whether current limitations still exist, which options are still available, and what enhancements have been made to the unit. In addition, new products may have been introduced that make current products obsolete.*

ESTHETIC DENTISTRY

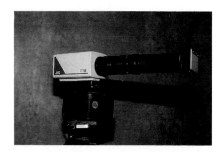

FIG. 29–19. An RGB video camera with slide adapter to allow for direct input of color slides. (Courtesy of Dr. Cary Ganz.)

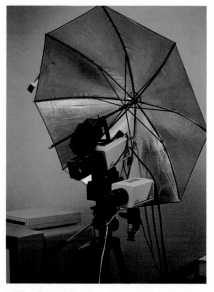

FIG. 29–20. A color corrected light source with umbrella reflector and video cameras. (Courtesy of McAndrews-Northern Dental Laboratory.)

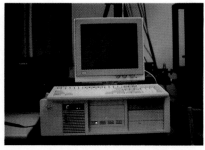

FIG. 29–21. A typical IBM-compatible computer with keyboard and video unit. (Courtesy of McAndrews-Northern Dental Laboratory.)

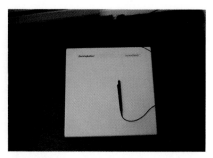

FIG. 29–22. A Summagraphics graphics tablet. (Courtesy of McAndrews-Northern Dental Laboratory.)

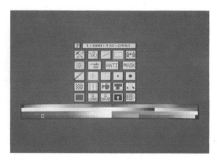

FIG. 29–23. An icon-based system displays small pictures (icons) on a screen. (Courtesy of McAndrews-Northern Dental Laboratory.)

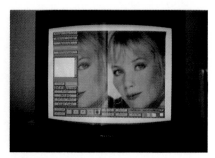

FIG. 29–24. A menu-based system utilizes a hierarchical menu system. (Courtesy of Dr. Cary Ganz.)

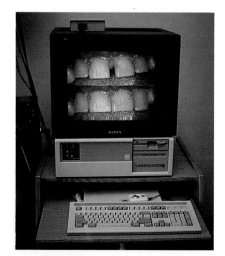

FIG. 29–25. The Dentavision^Plus system. (Courtesy of Envision Imaging Technologies.)

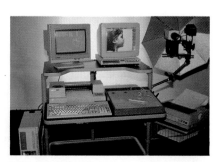

FIG. 29–26. The Imagemaker system. (Courtesy of Trojan Imaging Systems, Inc.)

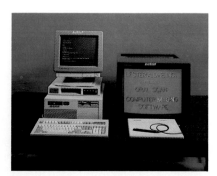

FIG. 29–27. The Oral Scan Computer Imaging System. (Courtesy of Lester A. Dine, Inc.)

CLINICAL TIP. A great deal of time and effort is required to master the complexities of computer imaging systems. It is important to locate a dealer who can provide ample instruction and maintenance support. If a "bargain system" does not include servicing, the full capability of the system may never be realized.

Available Products

CIS-2—(Cosmetic Imaging Systems). The CIS-2 is an IBM-compatible, 80286-based system utilizing an extraoral RGB camera, a high resolution image controller, and a graphics tablet with stylus. It has menu driven software which tends to use keyboard commands more than stylus input.

Dentavision^Plus (Envision Imaging Technologies, formerly Business Information Technologies, Inc.) (Fig. 29–25). This icon-based system consists of an RGB video camera, 80286 based IBM compatible computer, large screen RGB monitor, and a Polaroid Freeze-Frame output device. Optional accessories include a high speed modem, which allows the dentist to send the image over the telephone line to any laboratory which has the Dentavision^Plus system. Optional hardware includes a high capacity optical storage device.

Fuji Vision Plus—(Patterson Dental Co). Fuji has designed a CIS that uses a proprietary video board and custom software. The system is built around a 80386 CPU with the high resolution video camera and keyboard attached to the integrated cabinet. The software is menu driven, using a mouse pen to manipulate the image. The system is fully integrated with the Dentacam Video Imaging System. Output can be viewed on a 13 in. monitor or a high resolution color printer.

Imagemaker (Trojan Intra-Oral Camera Systems) (Fig. 29–26). The Trojan Imagemaker utilizes an Everex 80286 Computer as well as a video board (Everex Vision 16 High Speed Imaging Board). The image is recorded by a JVC RGB CCD camera and viewed on a 13 in. Sony RGB monitor. The Freestyle software is icon oriented. Input is controlled by a Summagraphics digitizing tablet, which accepts images from the Ultra-Eye Camera.

Oral Scan Computer Imaging System (Lester A. Dine, Inc.) (Fig. 29–27). Unlike some of the other systems, the Lester Dine system is an extension of the manufacturer's VIS. Utilizing the same camera and monitor, this system can be purchased as a unit or the video system can be upgraded to a complete CIS. The system is a simple menu system, operating under a proprietary graphical environment. (The program was not written under TIPS, but rather under a system specially designed and customized by Lester A. Dine, Inc.)

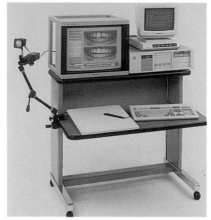

FIG. 29–28. The Preview system. (Courtesy of New Visions, Inc.)

Preview (New Visions, Inc., formerly McGhan InstruMed Corporation) (Fig. 29–28). The Preview system utilizes pull down menus, an RGB video camera, 80286-based IBM compatible computer, large screen RGB monitor, and a Polaroid Freeze-Frame output device. A high capacity hard disk drive is used for storage.

Retrospective Treatment Consultant—(Dentsply Co.). The Retrospective Treatment Consultant is an IBM-compatible, 80286-based system consisting of a high resolution image capturing board, a digitizing tablet with stylus and an extraoral RGB camera. A focal length chain is attached to the camera to facilitate subject placement and image standardization. The menu-driven software is easy to use but can take up half the screen, thus reducing the patient's image.

Clinical Procedure

Although system operation techniques vary greatly, the following are common to all:

Armamentarium

- Computer imaging system

Clinical Technique

Clinical techniques are extremely simple. Because of the flexible nature of the software, there are many ways to achieve the same result. Personal experience with the system is required in order to understand which method will have the greatest predictive value of the final outcome of a case.

1. Obtain a video image of the patient and duplicate the entire image on the video monitor according to the manufacturer's recommendations (Fig. 29–29).
2. After a discussion with the patient, determine a proposed final result.
3. Highlight the images you wish to duplicate (Fig. 29–30).
4. Select the correct orientation of the highlighted image (Fig. 29–31).

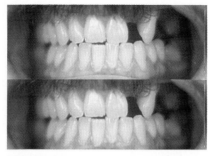

FIG. 29-29

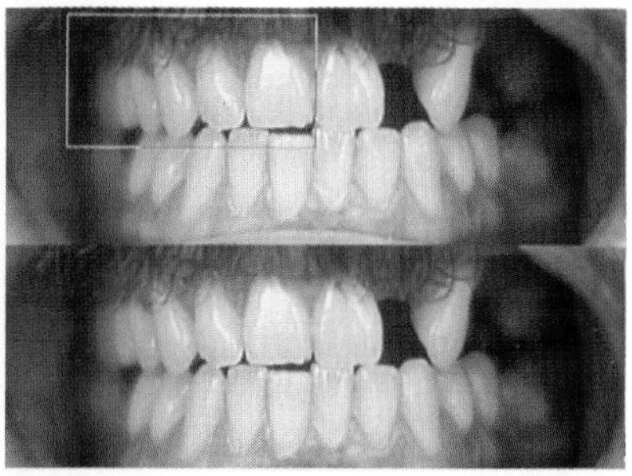

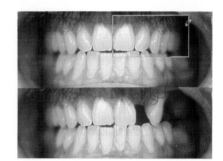

FIG. 29-30

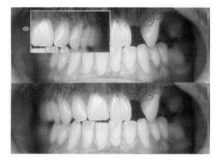

FIG. 29-31

FIG. 29-32

FIG. 29–29. A duplicated video image of the patient.

FIG. 29–30. The image segment to be duplicated is highlighted.

FIG. 29–31. The correct orientation of the highlighted image segment is selected.

FIG. 29–32. The image segment is moved to the proper position.

5. Move the image to the proper position (Fig. 29–32).
6. "Paste" the image into the new position.
7. Blend the colors as necessary.
8. Save the image.

The technique illustrated above was designed for simplicity; other methods would probably provide a more accurate prediction of the final esthetic results. In the example, the right arch (which was intact) was duplicated, inverted (a mirror image created), and superimposed on the left side where two teeth were missing. This does not take into account the relative position of any of the remaining teeth on the left side of the arch, which, fortunately in this case, were ideally positioned. If, however, there was migration or tipping of the teeth in the left arch, although the computer simulation would have produced a perfect result, the actual treatment plan would require preprosthetic orthodontics in order to properly position the proposed abutment teeth. The manner in which the images are manipulated (duplicating the right side and superimposing it on the left side) is not the same manner in which the teeth are manipulated (preparing the teeth in their current position or in their postorthodontic position and then fabricating a fixed prosthesis). Thus, it is important to attempt to simulate clinical technique as closely as possible (e.g., placing pontics in the edentulous areas of the left side, as with a conventional bridge, as opposed to merely duplicating the right side).

Computer-Aided Design and Computer Aided Manufacturing (CAD/CAM) Systems

These systems, still in their infancy, promise to revolutionize dentistry. All systems receive a video input, ma-

CLINICAL TIP. Although the computer simulation may yield a mutually agreeable final result, only the dentist can determine if a treatment plan exists that can obtain these results. Because most of the techniques used by the computer to "rehabilitate" an arch are different from those used by a dentist to fabricate a prosthesis, a less desirable final result sometimes must be accepted. CIS can be extremely valuable in these cases because the dentist can simulate these limitations. This prevents unrealistic patient expectations and documents the possibility of less than optimal results.

CLINICAL TIP. Because various proposed final results may be contemplated, it is important to clearly mark and save each result prior to manipulating a new image.

nipulate the image, and guide a computer controlled milling device, which fabricates a final restoration (Fig. 29–33).

Advantages

1. Eliminates impression making. Because some of these systems are video based, optical computer images replace impression making.
2. Dentist controls the manufacturing of the restoration. Some systems currently under development allow the milling device to be placed in the dental office, thus eliminating the need for a dental laboratory.
3. One-visit restoration. Those systems with in-office milling devices are usually able to fabricate the restoration in less than 1 hour.
4. Alternative materials. Because all CAD/CAM systems utilize milling machines, the dentist is not limited to castable materials.[2]

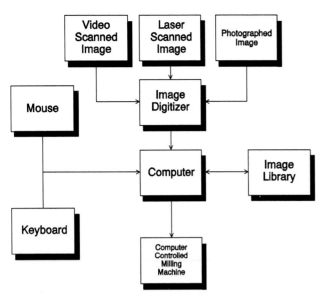

FIG. 29–33. A flow chart of a typical Computer Aided Design/Computer Aided Manufacturing (CAD/CAM) system.

Disadvantages

1. **Still in developmental or early introductory stage.** Widespread use of these systems is unlikely within the next 5 to 10 years.
2. **Limitations in the fabrication of multiple units.** Most systems currently in development can only fabricate single units, however, some systems claim to be able to fabricate fixed bridges of up to four units.[3]
3. **Inability to characterize shades.** Although some systems can fabricate porcelain-based restorations, they utilize monochromatic porcelain blocks available in only a few shades. None of the systems is capable of manipulating variations in shading, unless they are added by a laboratory technician.
4. **No long-term studies on the durability of the restorations.** The recent introduction of these systems precludes any long-term studies comparing these restorations to those fabricated in the dental laboratory.
5. **Inability to image in a wet environment.** No system is capable of obtaining an accurate image in the presence of excessive saliva, water, or blood.
6. **Incompatibility with other imaging systems.** Because of the unique nature of these systems, none are compatible with currently available VISs and CISs.
7. **Expense.** These systems are extremely expensive due to their limited availability. However, most are leased and the cost of the actual restorations can be competitive with laboratory fees.

Clinical Products

CLINICAL TIP. Currently, only one system (Cerec) is commercially available and only on a limited basis. It is unlikely that any system in development will resemble the eventual commercially released product except in principle. It is therefore crucial to verify the current status of these products with the manufacturer prior to purchase.

Celay System (Mikrona Technolgie). This system utilizes a small stylus attached to a digitizer (pantograph). A direct acrylic "inlay" is fabricated intraorally and then removed. The stylus is passed over the acrylic inlay and the shape is recorded and stored in a computer. This recording system is analogous to a key copying machine.[4] A computer controlled milling machine then fabricates an all-porcelain inlay. The milling device uses a flat disk and is therefore incapable of machining the occlusal anatomy.

The Cerec System (Siemens Corp.) (Fig. 29–34). This system, designed to fabricate porcelain inlays, onlays, and laminate veneers, was developed in Switzerland and first demonstrated in 1986.[5–7] First introduced commercially by Siemens in Europe, it is available in limited quantities in the United States. The system utilizes a noncontacting scan head containing an LED and a CCD. A white, glare-free powder containing titanium oxide (Cadvision, Svedia Dental Industry) is placed on the tooth. A visual light in the scan head aids in aiming the scanner while the infrared image is captured on the CCD sensor in less than .2 sec.[6] The system is capable of a resolution of 256×256 pixels.[8] A self-contained microprocessor displays the digitized image. The dentist then highlights the outline form of the inlay preparation. Preformed porcelain or Dicor (Dentsply International, Inc.) blocks are placed in a numerically controlled three-axis micromilling machine, which fabricates the prosthesis (Figs. 29–35, 29–36). Currently, the porcelain blocks are available in four Vita shades and the Dicor blocks are available in two shades. Milling time is less than 10 min. The occlusal surface is adjusted in the mouth, the material is finished, acid etched, silane activated, and cemented with a dual-cured composite resin luting agent. The system can fabricate a porcelain laminate veneer which must be custom stained with conventional porcelain stains and oven glazed (Figs. 29–37, 29–38) (see Appendix A—Custom Staining).

The DentiCAD System (DentiCAD USA). This system consists of a miniaturized robotic arm that can be used either intraorally or with an indirect model to digitize the preparation. Intraorally, the arm is attached with a mounting post and compound to adjacent teeth. Clinically, the probe inputs information by moving (like an explorer) over the prepared tooth, the opposing teeth, and the contact areas of the adjacent teeth, recording information.[4] The information is obtained in a manner similar to that used with a key copying machine. Once the image is obtained, the restoration is fabricated on a computer controlled milling machine. Currently, the system can only produce inlays, however the ability to fabricate full coverage and multiple unit restorations is planned. The system is capable of using machinable ceramics, most dental metals (including titanium), and composite resins.

The Duret System (Hennson International) (Fig. 29–39). This system, developed by Dr. Francois Duret,

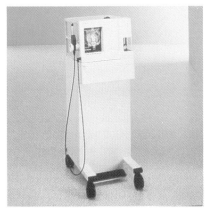

FIG. 29-34. The Cerec System (Siemens Corp.). (Courtesy of Drs. Karl Leinfelder and Barry Isenberg.)

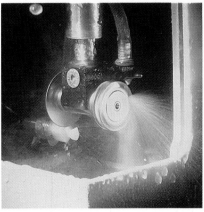

FIG. 29-35. A computer controlled milling machine fabricating a porcelain inlay. (Courtesy of Drs. Karl Leinfelder and Barry Isenberg.)

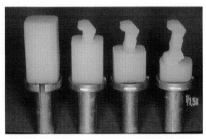

FIG. 29-36. The sequential steps in the fabrication of a porcelain inlay. (Courtesy of Drs. Karl Leinfelder and Barry Isenberg.)

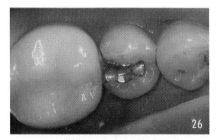

FIG. 29-37. A preoperative view of a second premolar that will receive a porcelain inlay. (Courtesy of Drs. Karl Leinfelder and Barry Isenberg.)

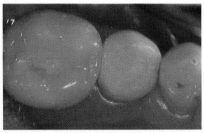

FIG. 29-38. A postoperative view of the patient in Figure 29-37 showing the CAD/CAM manufactured porcelain inlay. (Courtesy of Drs. Karl Leinfelder and Barry Isenberg.)

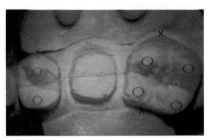

FIG. 29-39. A scanned image produced on the Duret system. (Courtesy of Hennson International.)

uses a laser scanner to produce images of the tooth (Fig. 29-39) and is capable of producing inlays, onlays, full crowns, fixed bridges of up to four units, and complete dentures from a solid block.[2] Following conventional dental preparations, the gingiva is retracted and the tooth is coated with a white nontoxic material. Five images (buccal, lingual, mesial, distal, and opposing occlusal surfaces) are made with the laser scanner, which resembles a dental handpiece.[9] A Euclid CAD/CAM system (Matra Datavison), running on a MicroVAX II computer (Digital Equipment Corp.), integrates the image. The dentist then highlights contact areas, cuspal heights, occlusal grooves, and cusp alignment of the opposing arch. A "library" of theoretic tooth forms aids in the design of the external anatomy (Fig. 29-40).[9] A numerically controlled micromilling machine fabricates the prosthesis from gold, composite resin, nonprecious metal, or ceramic.[10] Porcelain prostheses are custom stained in a conventional glazing oven (Fig. 29-41) (see Appendix A—Custom Staining).

The DUX (Titan) System (DCS Dental). This system consists of a contact digitizer (pantograph). The stylus is passed over a conventional die and the information is

transferred to a computer in a manner similar to that used by a key copying machine.[4] A milling machine is then used to fabricate a uniform thickness titanium coping onto which porcelain is added by a laboratory technician.

The Procera System (Nobelpharama, Inc.). This system requires a conventional impression and stone model. The shape of the restoration is "read" into a computer by running a stylus from a pantograph across the die in a manner similar to that used with a key copying machine. After the information is processed, an electric discharge machine "cuts" a titanium coping onto which porcelain is added by a laboartory technician.[4]

The Rekow System (Digital Dental Systems). Unlike other systems which record the image directly into electronic form, this system is photographically based. A standard 35 mm camera is modified with a 10 mm diameter single-rod laryngopharyngoscope (Fig. 29-42). Developers of this system claim that it is impossible for a computer to obtain resolutions higher than 512 × 512 pixels in real time (during a single scan

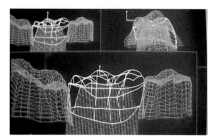

FIG. 29–40. A computer designed crown generated by the Duret system. (Courtesy of Hennson International.)

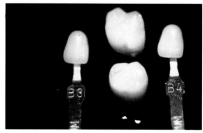

FIG. 29–41. A completed restoration from the Duret system. (Courtesy of Hennson International.)

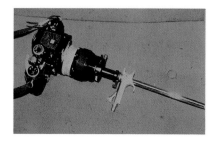

FIG. 29–42. A 35 mm camera is modified with a 10 mm diameter single-rod laryngopharyngoscope in the Rekow system. (Courtesy of Digital Dental Systems.)

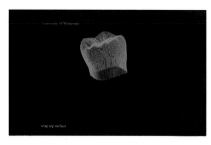

FIG. 29–43. A CAD/CAM system calculating tooth morphology on the Rekow system. (Courtsey of Digital Dental Systems.)

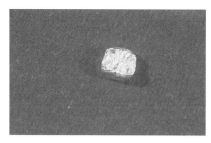

FIG. 29–44. A completed all-gold restoration from the Rekow system. (Courtesy of Digital Dental Systems.)

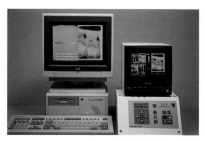

FIG. 29–45. A radiovisiography system. (Courtesy of Trophy U.S.A., Inc.)

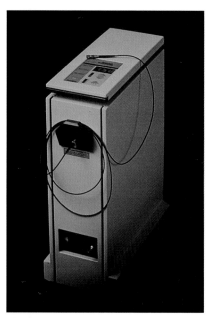

FIG. 29–46. A dental laser system. (Courtesy of American Dental Laser.)

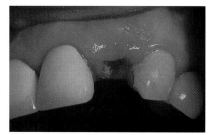

FIG. 29–47. A preoperative view of a tooth requiring a periodontal crown lengthening procedure. (Courtesy of American Dental Laser.)

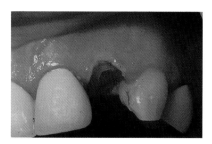

FIG. 29–48. An immediate postoperative view of the crown lengthening procedure performed with a dental laser. (Courtesy of American Dental Laser.)

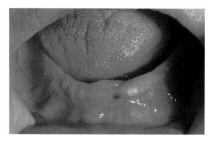

FIG. 29–49. A preoperative view of a healed edentulous ridge with implants in place. (Courtesy of American Dental Laser.)

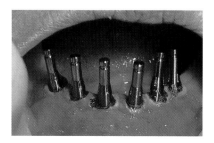

FIG. 29–50. An edentulous ridge following Stage II implant surgery using a dental laser. (Courtesy of American Dental Laser.)

of the tooth of less than 1 sec. duration). Therefore, a high resolution image is captured on film in order to allow the computer to scan the image more slowly.[11] A modified camera records a stereo image of the prepared tooth, proximal contacting teeth, and the opposing occlusal surface on Ektachrome ASA 400 film. The image is then sent to the dental laboratory and input via a digitizer into a minicomputer. A CAD/CAM system calculates the internal surface of the crown while a library of ideal tooth morphologies is used to determine the external surface (Fig. 29–43). The restoration is then milled on a five-axis milling machine. The system is capable of fabricating inlays, onlays, and full crowns (Fig. 29–44).

Radiographic Imaging Systems

Xeroradiography, originally developed by Xerox, Inc., is a method of producing radiographic images without using conventional x-ray film. After exposure to a conventional x-ray source, a sensor transfers the image onto specially treated glossy paper. A newer technology, radiovisiography (Trophy U.S.A., Inc.) also uses a conventional x-ray source, but the x-ray film is replaced with an intraoral CCD sensor (Fig. 29–45). The sensor is attached to an image processing computer that digitizes the image, which can then be displayed on a video screen, enhanced, and, if desired, colorized by the computer. The image can be output to a 35 mm camera, Polaroid Freeze-Frame, or high resolution thermal printer.

Radiographic Image Processing Systems

This broad category includes the hardware and software needed to process radiographic images. The most common use is to obtain cephalometric measurements from lateral and anterior facial films. There are many systems that can be used on most personal computers. Most systems require the dentist to place the film on a Summagraphics graphics tablet and mark the appropriate points. The computer can output both the appropriate measurement and a cephalometric tracing (see Figure 29–5).

Laser Systems

A laser (an acronym for **L**ight **A**ctivation by **S**timulated **E**mission of **R**adiation) is a device capable of producing an intense, highly focused monochromatic beam of light which, among other uses, can instantly vaporize living tissue. The use of lasers in dentistry has been considered for over 20 years.[12-14] Early findings concluded that the energy levels needed to remove dental caries would cause irreversible pulpal necrosis.[12-14] Extensive hard and soft tissue damage also occurred when early lasers were used on gingival and mucosal tissues.[12-14] In addition, most common laser delivery systems were too cumbersome for dental use.

Recent studies, however, have shown that pulpal necrosis and damage to hard and soft tissue can be minimized by the substitution of a carbon dioxide (CO_2) or neodymium yttrium-aluminum-garnet (Nd:YAG) laser for the previously used ruby laser.[15,16] Although these lasers produce higher energy levels, they can be pulsed (turned on and off) at rates of 10 to 30 times per second. Therefore, they are less likely to cause damaging heat build-up because the tissue is allowed to cool between pulses.[17] In addition, both the CO_2 and Nd:YAG laser beams can be delivered via a fiber optic cable to a dental handpiece, which allows for easy intraoral use.

Uses

CO_2 and Nd:YAG lasers have been used by physicians for a number of years. Currently, the FDA has only approved their use in dentistry for *soft* tissue procedures. Companies such as American Dental Laser (Nd:YAG-type)(Fig. 29–46), Laser Endo Technic (Nd:YAG-type), and Luxar Corporation (CO_2 type) have begun manufacturing devices specifically designed for dental use.

The types of soft tissue procedures that can be performed using dental lasers are similar to those that can be performed using an electrosurgical unit. These procedures include gingivoplasty, gingivectomy, crown lengthening (Figs. 29–47, 29–48), frenectomy, subgingival curettage, biopsy, gingival troughing for crown and bridge procedures, and esthetic recontouring of gingival tissue. In addition, lasers produce excellent hemostasis.[18] They have been used to uncover implants in Stage II surgery (Figs. 29–49, 29–50); however, further study is needed to determine if implants are affected by possible heat build-up.

Presently, clinical studies are evaluating hard tissue uses for dental lasers. These lasers are unable to penetrate enamel and no laser is currently approved for hard tissue use. They have, however, been shown to be effective for caries removal in dentin and are capable of inducing anesthesia.[19-22] Both lasers have been used for tooth desensitization, the removal of incipient decay in pits and fissures, the removal of extrinsic stains, and enamel etching.[19,20]

Controversy still exists regarding which type of laser is best suited for dental use. Laser penetration is a function of the wavelength of the laser used, as well as the absorption characteristics of the target tissue. In soft tissue, CO_2 lasers are readily absorbed by water (the predominant component of soft tissue) and thus little peripheral tissue damage results.[21,22] However, despite the greater penetration of a Nd:YAG laser, as compared with a CO_2 laser, the actual depth of a cut is less for the former.[21,22] In addition, the greater penetration ability of the Nd:YAG laser may make it more effective for the removal of vascular malformations than CO_2 lasers.[21,22] Further study is need to determine which type of laser is the most appropriate for each specific dental procedure.

Recent laboratory tests using a new type of pulsed laser, an erbium:YAG laser, have also been promising. This laser appears to be capable of vaporizing enamel with no detectable damage to the surrounding hard tissue.[23]

Other Systems

As electronic technology has evolved many other types of systems have become available. Some examples follow:

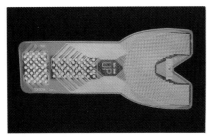

FIG. 29–51. A special mylar sensor is used to analyze occlusion. (Courtesy of Tekscan, Inc.)

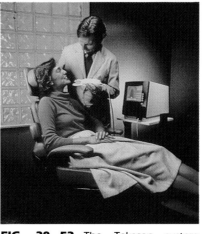

FIG. 29–52. The Tekscan system. (Courtesy of Tekscan, Inc.)

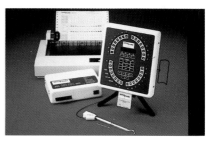

FIG. 29–53. The Interprobe system. (Courtesy of Bausch and Lomb Oral Care Division.)

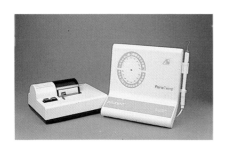

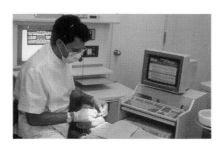

FIG. 29–54. The Periotemp system. (Abiodent, Inc.)

FIG. 29–55. The Simplesoft Voice Chart system. (Avanti Computer Associates.)

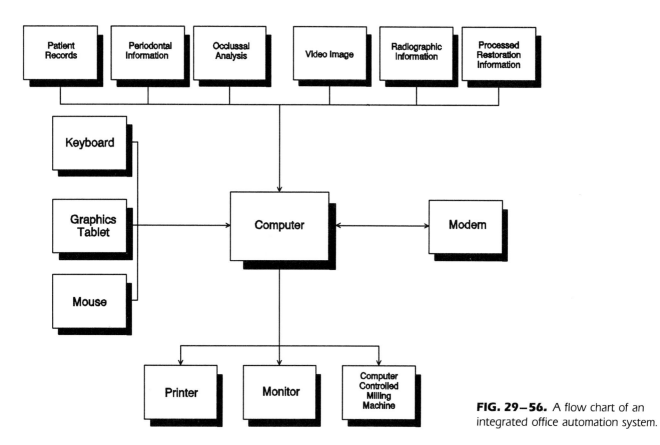

FIG. 29–56. A flow chart of an integrated office automation system.

Occlusal analysis systems. New computer systems are able to locate occlusal prematurities and provide analyses from the point of initial tooth contact to the point of maximum intercuspation. The T-Scan (Tek-scan, Inc.) utilizes a special mylar sensor (Fig. 29–51) and allows the dentist to analyze and record a patient's occlusion (Fig. 29–52). The dentist can subsequently verify that the appropriate occlusion has been duplicated in a prosthesis. The T-Scan is available as a free standing unit which can communicate with a computer or can be used as an addition to any IBM-compatible computer.

Periodontal analysis. Periodontal charting can be automatically recorded with the Interprobe system (Bausch & Lomb Oral Care Division) (Fig. 29–53). Another company (Abiodent, Inc.) manufactures a microtemperature probe (Periotemp) (Fig. 29–54) that records intrasulcular temperature postulated to correlate with the state of periodontal health.[24]

Automated Record Keeping. Many computer based office management systems now store patient charting information in a computer, allowing quick access to patient data. Newer systems (Simplesoft Voice Chart, Avanti Computer Associates) (Fig. 29–55) allow the system to "learn" the dentist's voice pattern for voice activated "hands free" data entry. In addition, these systems provide excellent charting, data analysis, and longitudinal comparison of a patient's periodontal condition.[25,26] In the future, automated record keeping systems will be able to link video, computer, and radiographic images, occlusal, restorative, and periodontal information and allow instant access to a patient's complete dental record (Fig. 29–56).

CONCLUSION

Electronic and computer technology are evolving at a rapid pace. The amount and types of diagnostic patient information are expanding rapidly. New technologies are replacing the photographic camera with a video camera, the x-ray film with a CCD sensor, and ultimately the high speed dental handpiece with a laser handpiece. Although these transformations are still incomplete, advances in technology are turning this vision into reality.

REFERENCES

1. Christensen, R.: Clinical Television, Intra- and Extraoral. Clin Res Assoc News, 13:1, 1989.
2. Rekow, D.: Prosthesis by computer. NY State Dent J 54:4, 1988.
3. Freeman, G.: Long-awaited robotics has come to the dental profession. Dent Today 8:8, 1989.
4. Rekow, D.: Dental CAD-CAM systems, J Am Dent Assoc, 122:43, 1991.
5. Brandestini, M., Moermann W., Lutz F., and Krejci I.: Computer machined ceramic inlays: in vitro marginal adaptation (Abstract). J Dent Res 64:208, 1985.
6. Moermann W., Brandestini M., Ferru A., et al.: Marginale adaptation von adhaesiven porzellaninlays in vitor. SSO: Schweiz Monatsschr Zahnmed, 95:118, 1985.
7. Moermann W., Jans H., Brandestini, M., et al.: Computer machined adhesive porcelain inlays: marginal adaptation after fatigue stress (Abstract). J Dent Res 65:762, 1986.
8. Moermann W., Brandestini, M.: Method and apparatus for the fabrication of custom-shaped implants. US Patent No. 4,575,805, March 11, 1986.
9. Duret F., Blouin, J.L., and Duret, B.: CAD-CAM in dentistry. J Am Dent Assoc 117:6, 1988.
10. Reed, O.: Addenda for Francois Workshop. Phoenix, AZ, Napoli International, 1986.
11. Rekow, D.: Computer-aided design and manufacturing in dentistry: a review of the state of the art. J Prosthet Dent 58:512, 1987.
12. Stern, R.H. and Sognnaes, R.F.: Laser beam effects on hard tissues. J Dent Res 43:873, 1964.
13. Sognnaes, R.F. and Stern, R.H.: Laser effects on resistance of human dental enamel to demineralization in vitro. J South Cal Dent Assoc 33:328, 1965.
14. Goldman, L., Gray, J., Goldman, J., et al.: Effects of laser beam impacts on teeth. J Am Dent Assoc 70:601, 1965.
15. Meyers, T.D. and Meyers, W.D.: The use of laser debridement of incipient caries. J Prosthet Dent 53:6, 1985.
16. Meyers, T.D. and Meyers, W.D.: A review of lasers in dentistry. IL Dentista Moderno, 7:1, 1989.
17. Meyers, T.D.: What laser can do for dentistry and you. Dent Man 29:26, 1989.
18. Meyers, T.D., Meyers, W.D., and Stone, R.M.: First soft tissue study utilizing a pulsed Nd:YAG dental laser. Northwest Dent, Mar-Apr, 1989.
19. Dunlap, J.: Is there a laser in your future? Dent Econ, Sept, 1988.
20. Case Study Procedures with an American Dental Laser, American Dental Laser Co, Inc.
21. Garber, D.: Dental laser—myths, magic, and miracles? Part 1. Introduction to lasers in dentistry. Compend Cont Educ Dent 12(7):448,
22. Garber, D.: Dental laser—myths, magic, and miracles? Part 2. Present and future uses. Compend Cont Educ Dent, 12(10):698,
23. Paghdiwala, A.F.: Does the laser work on hard dental tissue? J Am Dent Assoc 122:79, 1991.
24. Fedi, P.F. Jr. and Killoy, W.J.: Temperature differences at periodontal sites in health and disease. J Dent Res 69:273, 1990.
25. Christensen, R.: Computer Software, Charting and Diagnosis Clinical Research Associates Newsletter, 14:9, 1990.
26. Baumgarten, H.S.: A voice-input computerized dental examination system using high resolution graphics. Compend Contin Educ Dent 9(6):446, 1988.

Kenneth W. Aschheim, D.D.S.
Barry G. Dale, D.M.D.

CUSTOM STAINING

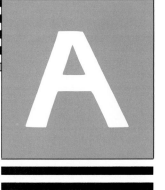

FUNDAMENTALS OF CUSTOM STAINING

A fundamental understanding of hue, value, chroma, complementary hue, and the color wheel is essential before attempting custom staining. (See Chapter 2, Fundamentals of Esthetics and Chapter 4, Color Modifiers and Opaquers.)

Dominant Hues

Hue is the name of the color. Chroma is the saturation or intensity of color (hue), therefore chroma can only be present when there is hue. Value is the relative whiteness or blackness of a color (hue). A light tooth has a high value; a dark tooth has a low value. (For detailed definitions, see Chapter 2, Fundamentals of Esthetics.)

The dominant hue is the principle color of the "body" porcelain. Prior to custom staining, the dominant hue of a restoration must be determined. Shades are then altered from this baseline. The dominant shade is only represented in the middle one-third of a tooth. The incisal edge is usually more translucent and the gingival one-third stained more heavily.

Known Shades. If a standard shade is selected, a simple reference table can be utilized (Tables A–1, A–2).

Unknown Shades. Unknown shades should be evaluated under three different lighting situations or in the lighting situation most appropriate for the individual. (See Chapter 2, Fundamentals of Esthetics.) Certain basic rules apply to dominant shade determination.

1. Avoid staring at a shade for a long period of time. The first glance is usually the most accurate.
2. The longer one stares at a shade, the grayer the shade appears to the eye.
3. Only focus on the middle one-third of the tooth.

CLINICAL TIP. To aid in determining a shade, mask the incisal and gingival thirds of a tooth with white adhesive tape.

Complementary Hues

The concept of complementary hues allows for certain clinically important modifications. Complementary hues are directly opposite one another on the color wheel. (See Chapter 2, Fundamentals of Esthetics.)

1. When placed side-by-side, complementary hues appear to intensify each other. A green stain applied to the incisal edge of a red-dominant shade (e.g., Bioform B–65), intensifies the approximating dominant red hue.
2. When blended in equal amounts, complementary hues produce a neutral gray. If a red-dominant shade (e.g., Bioform B–65) is gradually overlapped with its complementary hue (green stain) a neutral gray will eventually result. Other complementary pairs (violet-yellow and pink*-green) produce similar results.
3. When complementary hues are blended in unequal proportions, the dominant hue will be reduced both in value (look grayer) and chroma (look less intense). When a red-dominant shade (e.g., Bioform B–65) is overlaid with a green stain, both the value and chroma of the red shade are reduced.

Portions of this appendix were adapted from the Ceramco Stain System Technique Manual.

*In dental stains, a true red is difficult to achieve and seldom necessary, so pink is always substituted.

TABLE A-1. DOMINANT HUE RANGE OF SELECTED BIOFORM PORCELAIN SHADES

B-51	Red-brown range	B-59	Yellow range	B-69	Red-gray range	B-91	Gray range
B-52	Yellow range	B-62	Red-gray range	B-77	Yellow range	B-92	Red-gray range
B-53	Red-brown range	B-63	Red-brown range	B-81	Red-gray range	B-93	Red-gray range
B-54	Red-brown range	B-65	Red-brown range	B-83	Red-brown range	B-94	Gray range
B-55	Yellow range	B-66	Red-gray range	B-84	Red-brown range	B-95	Gray range
B-56	Yellow range	B-67	Yellow range	B-85	Red-brown range	B-96	Gray range

(Adapted from the Trubyte Bioform Color Ordered Shade Guide.)

TABLE A-2. DOMINANT HUE RANGE OF SELECTED VITA-LUMIN PORCELAIN SHADES

A-1	Orange range	B-1	Yellow range	C-1	Brown range	D-2	Orange range
A-2	Orange range	B-2	Yellow range	C-2	Brown range	D-3	Yellow range
A-3	Orange range	B-3	Yellow range	C-3	Brown range	D-4	Orange range
A-3.5	Orange range	B-4	Yellow range	C-4	Brown range		
A-4	Orange range						

CHAIRSIDE STAINING

Basic Principles

A few simple steps, meticulously adhered to, will produce optimal chairside staining results.

1. Apply chairside stains prior to glazing the ceramic.
2. Complete all anatomic and functional adjustment prior to applying stains.
3. Keep all brushes and instruments clean to avoid contamination.
4. Lay out the powders of the stains (the "feeder" supply) on the left side of a clean, dry, glazed porcelain palette.
5. Take care to avoid contaminating the "feeder" supply by accidentally mixing powders. Therefore, mix shades on the right side of the palette to avoid contamination.
6. Mix stains to a thick, toothpaste-like consistency. This can later be diluted to the desired consistency.
7. If a feeder supply dries out, reconstitute it by adding the liquid medium.

CLINICAL TIP. Chairside stains should never be applied intraorally because an absolutely dry field is necessary.

Applying Stains

Armamentarium

- Basic staining setup including:
    Stain kit (e.g., Ceramco Fine Grain Stain Kit, Ceramco, Inc.)
    Glazing oven or stain set (e.g. Ceramco Stain Set, Ceramco, Inc.)
    Porcelain cleaning agent (e.g., Spar-Cling, Spartan Ceramic Studio) (if necessary)
    Red sable brushes
    Locking pliers or curved hemostat
    Ceramic firing support
    Shade guide

Clinical Technique

1. Preheat the glazing oven to 1200°F (649°C).
2. Dilute the surface stains on the working side (right side) of the palette to a paint-like consistency to allow for easier transfer to the brush. The stain should neither drip nor run.
3. Wet a clean red sable brush with liquid medium, "flick" off the excess liquid, and draw the brush tip to a point.
4. Wash the crown with distilled water and thoroughly dry it with an oil-free air syringe or hair dryer.

CLINICAL TIP. If a restoration has been in the mouth for an extended period, bacteria may adhere to the porcelain surface. If bacteria are not completely removed they can cause the porcelain to crack when heated in the glazing oven. Soaking the restoration in a porcelain cleaning agent (e.g., Spar-Cling, Spartan Ceramic Studio) eliminates bacteria.

5. Hold the restoration securely with locking pliers or a curved hemostat.
6. Apply the stain in a series of light dapping motions.

CLINICAL TIP. Do not over-apply stain. You are looking for the effect of the stain, not the stain itself. Chroma can be controlled by avoiding excess powder in the mixture and controlling the dispersion of the stain particles with the tip of the brush.

7. If the stain is extended beyond the intended area, wipe the brush on a tissue until it is semi-dry and use the tip to absorb excess stain and medium.

CLINICAL TIP. Incorrect stains can be wiped off with a clean tissue and new stain can be applied.

CLINICAL TIP. Two or three test stainings may be necessary prior to obtaining an acceptable result.

CLINICAL TIP. If a glazing oven is not available in the office, an adhesive-type medium (e.g., Ceramco Stain Set) can be used in place of the conventional liquid medium. After the completion of staining, gently heat the restoration by holding it 1 in. above a bunsen burner flame. This causes the Stain Set to evaporate and an "onion skin" surface to form. The stained surface can now be handled without risk and can be sent to the laboratory for final firing. A two-minute application of a companion product (e.g., Ceramco Stain Wet) can restore the natural glaze appearance to the dried Stain Set restoration.

8. After the desired hue, value, and chroma have been obtained, place the restoration in front of the open door of the preheated glazing oven.
9. Leave the restoration in place until the liquid medium has evaporated and a powdery film covers the stained surface.
10. Place the restoration on a ceramic firing support.
11. Gradually move the restoration into the oven.
12. When the restoration is in place, close the oven door.
13. Gradually increase the furnace temperature from 1200°F (649°C) to between 1650°F and 1750°F (898°C to 940°C) at a rate of 90°F to 100°F (32°C to 38°C) per minute. No vacuum is needed.

CLINICAL TIP. If high-temperature firing is undesirable (e.g., to avoid thermal stress in a fixed bridge), a lower temperature glaze or stain can be used. No vacuum is needed.

14. Upon completion, slowly remove the restoration from the furnace and allow it to bench cool.
15. Evaluate the case intraorally.
16. Repeat the above steps, if necessary. If necessary, the surface stain can be removed by gently grinding the restoration with a green stone.

CLINICAL TIP. If a large, multiple-unit restoration must be modified, a shade tab or single unit of the prosthesis can be custom stained with Stain Set and the laboratory can duplicate the shade throughout the rest of the prosthesis.

ADJUSTING HUE, CHROMA, AND VALUE

Shades should always be adjusted from lighter to darker. The converse can only be accomplished by applying a more opaque stain over the shade to be lightened. This rarely produces an esthetically satisfactory result.

Adjusting Hue

In general, only minor adjustments to hue should be made with custom stains. Adjusting colors with complementary hues also decreases value. If major adjustments to hue are necessary, it is preferable to replace the porcelain with the proper shade.

Armamentarium

- Standard staining setup. (See the section on Applying Stains earlier in this chapter.)

Clinical Technique

1. Determine the dominant hue of the existing restoration (the "original" hue) (e.g., vita-Lumin D−2 = orange) and the dominant hue to be achieved (the "desired" hue) (e.g., Vita-Lumin D−3 = yellow).
2. Apply the *complementary* hue to the original hue (e.g., the complementary hue of Vita-Lumin D−2 is blue).
3. Incrementally add sufficient amounts of the complementary hue until the original hue is neutralized.
4. Apply the *dominant* hue of the desired hue (e.g., the dominant hue of Vita-Lumin D−3 is yellow) until the desired hue is obtained.

CLINICAL TIP. Steps 2 and 4 often can be combined into a single step. Since blue (step 2 above) and yellow (step 4 above) form green when mixed together, this procedure can be done in a single step if green stain is used.

CLINICAL TIP. If the original hue contains no dominant hue (e.g., Bioform B−91), simply apply the desired stain.

5. After the desired result is obtained, fire and glaze the restoration. (See the section on Applying Stains earlier in this chapter.)

Increasing Chroma
Armamentarium

- Standard staining setup (see the section on Applying Stain)

Clinical Technique

1. Determine the dominant hue of the existing restoration (the "original" hue) (e.g., Vita-Lumin A−1 = orange) and the dominant hue to be achieved (the "desired" hue) (e.g., Vita-Lumin A−4 = orange).
2. Apply the *dominant* hue to the original hue (e.g., the dominant hue of Vita-Lumin A−1 is orange).
3. Add a sufficient amount of the dominant hue until the desired hue is obtained.
4. After the desired result is obtained, fire and glaze the restoration. (See the section on Applying Stains earlier in this chapter.)

Decreasing Chroma
Armamentarium

- Standard staining setup. (See the section on Applying Stains earlier in this chapter.)

Clinical Technique

1. Determine the dominant hue of the existing restoration (the "original" hue) (e.g., Vita-Lumin A−4 = orange) and the dominant hue to be achieved (the "desired" hue) (e.g., Vita-Lumin A−3.5 = orange).
2. Apply a sufficient amount of the *complementary* hue to the original hue (e.g., the complementary hue of

Vita-Lumin A−4 is blue) until the desired hue is obtained.

CLINICAL TIP. Reducing chroma by applying the complementary hue also decreases value.

3. After the desired result is obtained, fire and glaze the restoration. (See the section on Applying Stains earlier in this chapter.)

Decreasing Value While Changing Hue

Armamentarium

- Standard staining setup. (See the section on Applying Stains earlier in this chapter.)

Clinical Technique

1. Determine the dominant hue of the existing restoration (the "original" hue) (e.g., Bioform B−65 = red-brown) and the dominant hue to be achieved. (the "desired" hue) (e.g., Bioform B−77 = yellow).
2. Apply the *complementary* hue to the original hue (e.g., the complementary hue of Bioform B−65 is green). This will yield a neutral hue, which also lowers the value.
3. Continue adding the complementary hue (green) until the value matches that of the desired hue.

CLINICAL TIP. If over-correction occurs, you may neutralize the complementary hue by adding a small amount of the original dominant hue. This will also reduce the value of the final restoration. However, it is usually better to remove all stain and start over.

4. Add the dominant hue (e.g., the dominant hue of Bioform B-77 is yellow) until the desired hue is obtained.
5. After the desired result is obtained, fire and glaze the restoration. (See the section on Applying Stains earlier in this chapter.)

Decreasing Value Without Changing Hue

Armamentarium

- Standard staining setup. (See the section on Applying Stains earlier in this chapter.)

Clinical Technique

1. Determine the dominant hue of the existing restoration (the "original" hue) (e.g., Bioform B−65 = red-brown).
2. Apply the *complementary* hue to the original hue (e.g., the complementary hue of Bioform B−65 is green).
3. Add a sufficient amount of the complementary hue until the original hue is neutralized or until the value is lowered appropriately.
4. Reapply the *dominant* hue of the original hue (e.g., the dominant hue of Bioform B−65 is red-brown), if necessary. Because this is being applied over the previously neutralized hue, the "added gray" will serve to reduce the value without changing the hue.
5. After the desired result is obtained, fire and glaze the restoration. (See the section on Applying Stains earlier in this chapter.)

ADJUSTING TRANSLUCENCY

Translucency is the ability of material to allow light transmission. The greater the amount of light transmitted, the greater the "real" translucency. In custom staining, an illusion of translucency can be created that is called "apparent" translucency.

Increasing Real Translucency

Because real translucency is a quality of the material used, it is impossible to increase real translucency with surface stains.

Decreasing Real Translucency

Decreasing real translucency is the same as increasing opacity. This is usually accomplished by applying a white stain. This opaque stain can be adjusted to more closely match the desired shade by applying other stains on top of this opaque layer.

Increasing Apparent Translucency

Adjustments in translucency are most often required at the incisal edge of the tooth. Changes in apparent translucency are accomplished by alterating the amount of blue stain in the incisal area.

CLINICAL TIP. Variants of blue, such as blue-violet or blue-green, often must be used to adjust translucency because they contain complementary hues that neutralize excess amounts of yellow or pink which may be visible in the incisal area.

Armamentarium

- Standard staining setup. (See the section on Applying Stains earlier in this chapter)

Clinical Technique

1. Examine the incisal area closely for excess pink, red, or yellow.
2. If pink or red is present, select a blue-green stain.
3. If yellow is present, select a blue-violet stain.
4. Apply the stain to the incisal area.
5. After the desired result is obtained, fire and glaze the restoration. (See the section on Applying Stains earlier in this chapter.)

CLINICAL TIP. Complementary colors, when placed side by side, intensify each other. To further increase the apparent translucency, "rim" the incisal edge with white or yellow/orange (the complement of violet or blue).

Decreasing Apparent Translucency

A decrease in apparent translucency is accomplished by decreasing the amount of blue by applying its complementary hue, orange. In theory this will also decrease value, but because the hues are so dilute, it is unlikely that any perceivable change in value will occur.

CLINICAL TIP. *Translucency alterations are subtle effects. Do not over-apply the stain. Begin with very dilute amounts of orange and light applications.*

Adjusting the Incisal-Gingival Blend

Often the shade and translucency of a tooth are correct but the proportion of body shade to incisal translucency is incorrect. The incisal area can be altered by changing the surface area of apparent translucency. If the incisal area must be lengthened, the appropriate amount of dominant body hue should be neutralized with the complementary hue. If the incisal area is too long, a stain should be blended to match the body shade.

CLINICAL TIP. *If the dominant hue of the tooth is yellow and the blue incisal area is pronounced, the resultant hue may have a greenish tint. If this is unesthetic, it can be neutralized with a small amount of violet stain.*

CHARACTERIZATION OF TEETH

Truly esthetic restorations often require the duplication of flaws that exist in adjacent teeth. As patients age, their dentition changes and they may wish to have these imperfections duplicated. Characterization is accomplished with the use of opaque white, brown-gray, and black stains. It is sometimes easier to use a sharp-edged instrument, a trimmed fine point brush, or a single bristle to apply these stains.

CLINICAL TIP. *Characterization should be visible, but not glaringly obvious. Some applications may be so subtle that one is barely aware of the effect.*

Although variations in tooth characterization are limitless, certain types are quite common.

Decalcification

Decalcified areas are common and are easy to reproduce.

Armamentarium

- Standard staining setup. (See the section on Applying Stains earlier in this chapter.)

Clinical Technique

1. Mix the white stain to a moderately thick consistency.
2. Place white stain with a brush or pointed instrument.

CLINICAL TIP. *Vary the opacity within the opaque area to create a more realistic decalcification effect.*

CLINICAL TIP. *If additional areas of decalcification are required on the same tooth, differ their shapes and depths of opacity.*

3. After the desired result is obtained, fire and glaze the restoration. (See the section on Applying Stains earlier in this chapter.)

Enamel Cracks and Checks

Enamel cracks are thin white lines that begin at the incisal edge and extend less than one-third the length of the tooth. They generally occur in younger patients. Over time these cracks discolor and then are termed enamel checks. They range in shade from orange to brown, sometimes with a grayish cast. Cracks and checks often cast a slight shadow along their length.

Armamentarium

- Standard staining setup (see the section on Applying Stains earlier in this chapter.)

Clinical Technique

1. To create a crack, mix a white stain to a moderately thick consistency. For a check, use orange, brown, or gray stain.
2. Press a wetted brush against the porcelain palette to form a flat, "chisel" edge.
3. After picking up the stain, run the "chisel" edge of the brush from a point one-third of the way up the tooth toward the incisal edge. This should be done in a single, fast, light stroke.

CLINICAL TIP. *A sharp edge, a single bristle, or pointed instrument may be used instead of a brush.*

4. If the line is too thick or uneven, clean and "point" the brush, wipe it semi-dry, and run the point along the side of the "line" to remove excess stain.
5. After a line with the proper thickness has been created, clean the brush, reform the "chisel edge" and create a shadow effect by running a faint black line along one side of the white "crack."
6. After the desired result is obtained, fire and glaze the restoration. (See the section on Applying Stains earlier in this chapter.)

Stained Composite Resin or Silicate Restorations

Old anterior restorations tend to be opaque and are usually discolored. In addition, they often exhibit marginal staining.

Armamentarium

- Standard staining setup. (See the section on Applying Stains earlier in this chapter.)

Clinical Technique

1. Determine the dominant hue of the restoration.
2. Mix a white stain to a moderately thick consistency to reduce the tendency of the material to run.
3. With a brush or instrument, create the simulated restoration with the white stain as a base and add gray, black, or other appropriate hues until the dominant hue of the restoration is approximated.
4. Use orange or brown stain to precisely outline the restoration.

CLINICAL TIP. In younger patients, with light translucent teeth, a hairline of black or gray stain may be used as an outline.

---

5. If discoloration is desired, use a brush to form an uneven halo of orange-brown-gray. The discoloration should not abut the outline, but should fade out in a narrow, uneven, feathery pattern.

CLINICAL TIP. Reflected undermining of teeth may be simulated by applying gray or brown stain, either individually or blended together in a semihalo effect on the incisal portion of the simulated restoration.

---

6. After the desired result is obtained, fire and glaze the restoration. (See the section on Applying Stains earlier in this chapter.)

Random Discolorations

One type of characterization consists of slight intensifications of chroma in random areas of the tooth surface. This is sometimes accompanied by a slight change of hue. By varying the amount of medium used to dilute the stains, different degrees of discoloration can be produced.

Fissures and Apertures

Characterization of fissures and apertures is usually restricted to older patients. It is accomplished by applying thin orange or brown lines to the fissures, grooves, sulci, and proximal apertures. It is also possible to replicate worn enamel edges of mandibular anterior teeth by utilizing an orange-brown or brown stain to mimic exposed dentin.

Barry G. Dale, D.M.D.

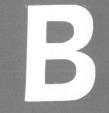

NINETY-SECOND RUBBER DAM PLACEMENT

It is highly unlikely that a dentist would be faulted for routinely using a rubber dam. Few procedures in dentistry are more universally accepted. Ironically, the infrequency of rubber dam usage demonstrates that few dental procedures are more universally rejected as well.[1]

This paradox is further complicated by the reasons given for the rejection of rubber dam placement as a routine part of the daily practice of dentistry. Those who shun the technique cite patient disapproval, inconvenience, lack of necessity, and additional time requirements as the rationale for rejection.[2] Advocates hold diametrically opposing views, indicating patient preference, work simplification and convenience, necessity, and an overall time savings.[1,3-5]

The dental student's early experiences with rubber dam application are often negative because of a typical and expected lack of manual dexterity. The virtually total avoidance of rubber dam usage, except during endodontic therapy, routinely begins immediately upon graduation.

A simplified technique, along with the naturally acquired manual adeptness of the average practitioner, allows placement of the rubber dam in ninety seconds or less to be a quickly attainable reality. With a minimum of practice, placement time can be decreased further. The average rubber dam application time (isolating an average of 4.6 teeth) of five private practitioners who routinely used rubber dam was 50.7 seconds.[5]

RUBBER DAM CLAMP SELECTION

Rubber dam clamp selection can be confusing because of the vast array of available clamp sizes and styles. The following basic assortment, however, will accommodate virtually every clinical situation (Table B-1).

Armamentarium

- 6 in. × 6 in. rubber dam, medium gauge (e.g., Dental Dam, The Hygenic Corp.; Rubber Dam, Miles, Inc. Dental Products)
- 5 in. × 5 in. metal U-shaped rubber dam frame
- Rubber dam hole punch
- Rubber dam hole placement template or rubber stamp (e.g., The Hygenic Corp.; Miles, Inc. Dental Products)
- Unwaxed regular dental floss (e.g., Johnson & Johnson)
- Rubber dam clamp assortment (see Table B-1)
- Rubber dam clamp forceps

Clinical Technique

The approximate time required to perform each step is indicated at the end of the description.

1. Punch a double hole in the rubber dam at the point corresponding to the tooth to be clamped. For a single occlusal restoration, clamp only the tooth to be restored, and skip to step 3. For a single multiple surface tooth restoration or when restoring more than one tooth, clamp one tooth distal to the tooth to be restored (if possible). **(3 seconds)**

CLINICAL TIP. *Punching a double-sized hole facilitates the placement of the rubber dam around the clamp (Fig. B-1).*

---

2. Punch single holes corresponding to the positions of the teeth to be isolated (Fig. B-1). A rubber dam stamp (Fig. B-2) or rubber dam template (Fig. B-3) is helpful for properly positioning the holes. **(7 seconds)**

TABLE B–1. RUBBER DAM CLAMPS

WINGED TYPE	WINGLESS TYPE	INDICATION
14A	W14A	Most adult molars
14	W14	Small adult molars; adult premolars, primary molars
8A	W8A	More aggressive clamp for adult molars
1	W1	Mandibular anterior teeth
211	212	Maxillary and mandibular anterior teeth (Class V restorations)

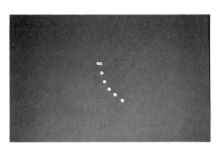

FIG. B–1. A double hole corresponding to the tooth to be clamped facilitates rubber dam clamp placement.

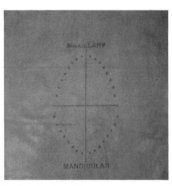

FIG. B–2. A rubber dam stamp aids in determining the proper position for the holes.

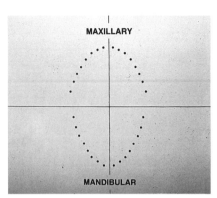

FIG. B–3. A rubber dam template aids in determining the proper position for the holes.

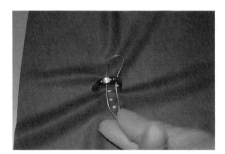

FIG. B–6. A loop of dental floss is placed under the bow of the rubber dam clamp.

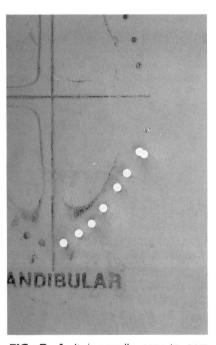

FIG. B–4. It is usually easy to pass floss and rubber dam material through the interproximal contact areas of the incisor teeth. Therefore, extending isolation to include one central incisor facilitates the placement of the rubber dam.

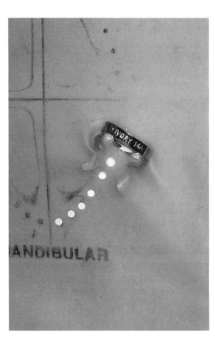

FIG. B–5. The rubber dam clamp is positioned in the rubber dam with the open end of the clamp facing mesially.

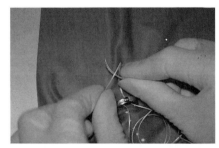

FIG. B–7. Both ends of the floss are brought over the bow of the rubber dam clamp and through the loop of floss.

CLINICAL TIP. When isolating several teeth always extend isolation to include one central incisor. This significantly increases the efficiency of rubber dam placement because the interproximal contact areas of the incisor teeth usually are not resistant to the passage of the rubber dam material (Fig. B–4).

3. Position the double hole in the rubber dam over the bow of the clamp. Push the bow through the hole (Fig. B–5). The open end of the clamp should face mesially. **(5 seconds)**
4. Tie dental floss to the bow of the rubber dam clamp. **(5 seconds)**

CLINICAL TIP. The following ligation is easily placed and is more easily removed than a square knot:
A. Place a loop of floss under the bow of the rubber dam clamp (Fig. B–6).
B. Bring both free ends of the floss over the bow of the rubber dam clamp and through the loop of floss (Fig. B–7).
C. Tighten the floss securely in the center of the bow (Fig. B–8).

CLINICAL TIP. Do not ligate the clamp through the holes that are often found on the wings of the clamp. Ligation in this area will complicate rubber dam placement.

5. Attach the rubber dam clamp to the rubber dam clamp forceps. Hold the forceps with the dominant hand (i.e., right hand for right-handed dentists) and gather the rubber dam material with the other hand so that the "teeth" of the rubber dam clamp are readily visible (Fig. B–9). **(5 seconds)**
6. Place the clamp on the appropriate tooth (Fig. B–10). **(5 seconds)**

CLINICAL TIP. Mandibular teeth: If lingual anesthesia has been achieved along with mandibular block anesthesia, position the "teeth" of the rubber dam clamp onto the *lingual* surface of the tooth. Then, gently slide the clamp onto the buccal surface. This sequence provides adequate control of clamp placement in the area of the unanesthetized buccal gingiva.

Maxillary teeth: If buccal anesthesia has been achieved, position the "teeth" of the rubber dam clamp onto the *buccal* surface of the tooth. Then, gently slide the clamp onto the palatal surface. This sequence provides adequate control of clamp placement in the area of the unanesthetized palatal gingiva.

7. For single tooth isolation, skip to step 8. For all other situations, position the most anterior three holes of the rubber dam over the corresponding anterior teeth. Attempt to slip the rubber dam through the interproximal contact areas of all three teeth in a single quick maneuver (Fig. B–11). Usually at least one of the anterior contact areas will permit easy passage of the dam material and often all three teeth can be isolated with one quick maneuver. Do not use dental floss at this time. **(5 seconds)**

CLINICAL TIP. The key to rapid rubber dam placement is the flexibility and tear resistance of modern rubber dam material. It can be stretched to the thinness of dental floss and used as such (Fig. B–12).

CLINICAL TIP. If a template or rubber dam stamp was not used, the holes may be properly spaced relative to one another, but the "arch" of holes may be improperly positioned within the square of rubber dam. Use a 5 in. × 5 in. frame and a 6 in. × 6 in. rubber dam sheet to compensate for this error.

8. Position the rubber dam frame (Fig. B–13). **(5 seconds)**

CLINICAL TIP. This placement sequence allows for the positioning of the rubber dam frame as soon as possible. Once the frame is in place, the efficiency and ease of rubber dam placement are significantly increased because unobstructed visibility is assured and both hands are freed.

9. Fold any excess rubber dam material that contacts the nose under the top of the rubber dam frame (Fig. B–14). If the material does not remain in place:
   A. Release the rubber dam material from the top right and left retaining pins (Fig. B–15).
   B. Momentarily stretch an additional amount of rubber dam material over the nose (Fig. B–16) and reattach the rubber dam to the frame (Fig. B–17).
   C. Fold the excess rubber dam material under the top of the frame. The additional bulk of rubber dam material will now remain in place (Fig. B–18). **(5 seconds)**
10. Slip the rubber dam over the teeth of the rubber dam clamp (Fig. B–19). **(2 seconds)**
11. Isolation for a single occlusal restoration is now complete. For all other restorations, attempt to position the remaining rubber dam material through all of the remaining contact areas in a single quick maneuver. Do not use dental floss at this time **(3 seconds)**
12. Forcefully attempt to pass the material through any individual resistant contact areas without using dental floss. Stretch the material until it is as thin as dental floss (Fig. B–20), and, using a sawing motion, "work" it through the interproximal contact area as if it were dental floss (Fig. B–21, B–22). **(10 seconds)**

CLINICAL TIP. Avoiding the use of dental floss at this time is an important time saving strategy.

13. Use dental floss to position any remaining rubber dam material that could not be negotiated through the corresponding contact areas (Fig. B–23). **(15 seconds)**

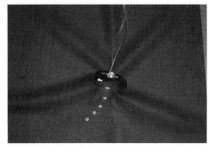

FIG. B–8. The floss is securely tightened in the center of the bow.

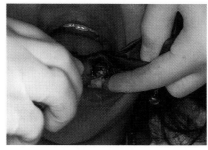

FIG. B–9. After attaching the rubber dam clamp to the rubber dam clamp forceps, the forceps are held with the dominant hand (i.e., right hand for right-handed dentists) and the rubber dam material is gathered with the other hand. The "teeth" of the rubber dam clamp will be readily visible.

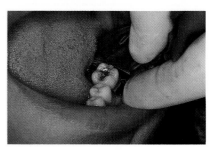

FIG. B–10. The rubber dam clamp is placed on the appropriate tooth.

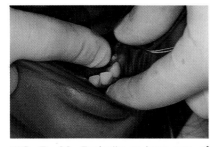

FIG. B–11. Typically at least one of the anterior incisor interproximal contact areas will readily allow the passage of rubber dam material without the necessity of using dental floss. Often all three anterior teeth can be isolated with one quick maneuver.

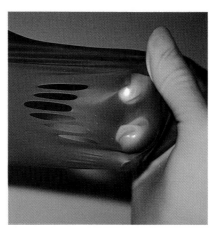

FIG. B–12. Modern rubber dam material can be stretched to the thinness of dental floss and still resist tearing while being "worked" through the interproximal contacts. This is the key to efficient rubber dam placement.

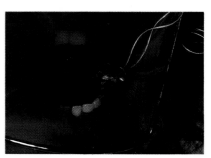

FIG. B–13. The rubber dam frame is positioned.

14. Use scissors to cut any rubber dam material (Fig. B–24) that could not be negotiated through the corresponding contact area (Fig. B–25). **(15 seconds)**

Total time: 90 seconds.

RUBBER DAM INVERSION

It is sometimes necessary to invert the rubber dam into the gingival sulcus to achieve better isolation and visibility (Fig. B–26). This is easily accomplished in the following manner:

1. Stretch the rubber dam buccally so that it does not contact the cervical areas of the teeth.
2. Dry the teeth with compressed air (Fig. B–27).
3. Slowly release the tension on the rubber dam until it contacts the teeth. The dam will usually "self-invert" (Fig. B–28).
4. Any areas that do not "self-invert" can be properly positioned with a flat-ended plastic instrument (Fig. B–29).

PATIENT REACTIONS TO RUBBER DAM USE

In a preliminary study, patients were asked to indicate their reactions to the use of a rubber dam during operative procedures, compared to similar procedures performed without a rubber dam.[5] More than 87% preferred or were neutral about the use of rubber dam. Rubber dam use may, therefore, be a practice builder, especially when presented favorably.

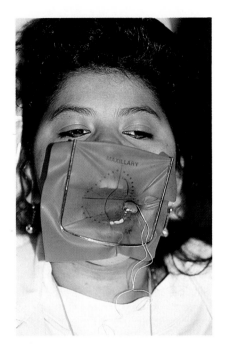

FIG. B–14. The rubber dam covers the patient's nose.

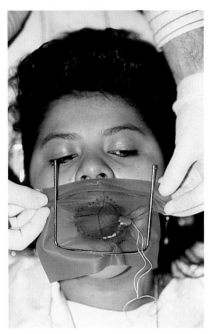

FIG. B–15. The rubber dam is released from the top retaining pins of the rubber dam frame.

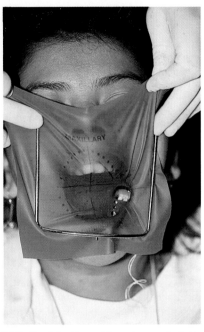

FIG. B–16. The rubber dam material is stretched over the nose.

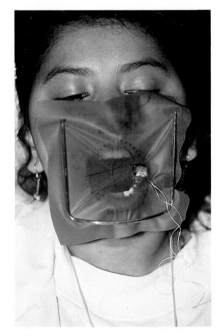

FIG. B–17. The rubber dam material is reattached to the rubber dam frame.

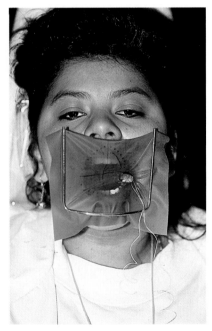

FIG. B–18. The rubber dam material is folded under the top of the frame. The additional bulk of rubber dam material will now remain in place.

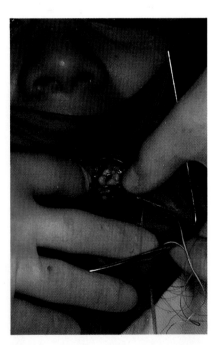

FIG. B–19. The rubber dam is slipped over the wings of the rubber dam clamp.

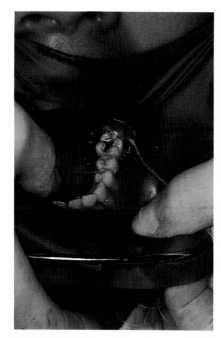

FIG. B–20. The rubber dam material is stretched to the thinness of dental floss and forcefully "worked," using a sawing motion, through the interproximal contact areas.

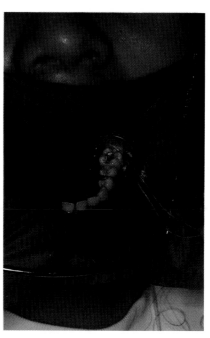

FIG. B–21. Most interproximal contact areas have been negotiated without the use of dental floss.

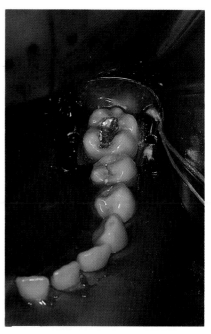

FIG. B–22. Placement through the contact area between the first and second premolars requires dental floss in this case.

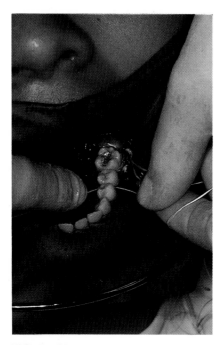

FIG. B–23. Dental floss is used to position the rubber dam material between the premolars.

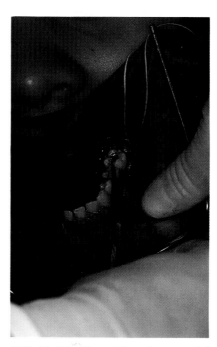

FIG. B–24. The rubber dam material corresponding to any impenetrable interproximal contact areas can be cut.

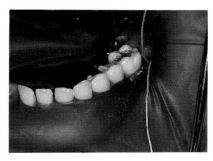

FIG. B–25. Cutting the rubber dam material usually does not result in a clinically significant loss of isolation.

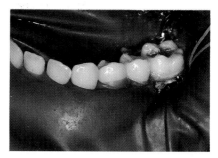

FIG. B–26. The rubber dam material is not properly inverted around the first and second premolars.

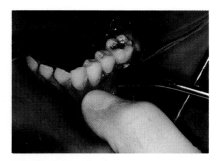

FIG. B–27. The rubber dam material is stretched away from the cervical area. A stream of air is directed at the cervical region of the first premolar until the area is dry.

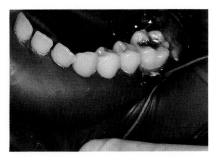

FIG. B–28. When the rubber dam material is slowly released, it "self-inverts" into the gingival sulcus.

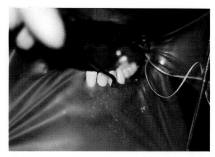

FIG. B–29. A plastic instrument is used to invert the rubber dam material if the above sequence is not successful.

The following introductory statements can further reinforce a positive patient response to rubber dam use:

1. The rubber dam prevents tooth structure, decay, debris, and restorative material from being swallowed.
2. The rubber dam prevents moisture contamination, which can adversely affect the properties and longevity of the medicaments and restorative materials.
3. The rubber dam, by virtue of its elasticity, reduces the muscle fatigue associated with maintaining an open mouth posture.
4. The rubber dam allows the patient to breathe through both the mouth and the nose. The rubber dam is only water-tight around the individual teeth.
5. The rubber dam merely "muffles" the patient's speech, as when a napkin is held to the mouth; however, verbal communication is still possible.

CLINICAL TIP. The napkin analogy is particularly useful because it relates the rubber dam to a common, helpful object.

6. The rubber dam clamp should be referred to as a "ring". The sensation caused by clamp placement should be termed "tight and secure."

REFERENCES

1. Going R. and Sawinski V.: Parameters related to use of rubber dam. J Am Dent Assoc 77:598, 1968.
2. Going R. and Sawinski V.: Frequency of use of the rubber dam: a survey. J Am Dent Assoc 75:158, 1967.
3. Stebner C.M.: Economy of sound fundamentals in operative dentistry. J Am Dent Assoc 49:294, 1954.
4. Ireland L.: The rubber dam, it's advantages and application. Texas Dent J 80:6, 1962.
5. Dale, B.G.: Unpublished data.

Barry G. Dale, D.M.D.
Kenneth W. Aschheim, D.D.S.

SMILE ANALYSIS

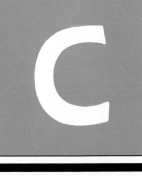

USING THE SMILE ANALYSIS

The smile analysis is an effective patient education and marketing aid. The analysis form can be filled out in the reception area or in the operatory before treatment, or it can be mailed to the patient along with an appointment reminder. A "yes" or "unsure" response on the form indicates an area that requires further evaluation for possible treatment. When completed, the smile analysis form becomes part of the patient's permanent record.

SMILE ANALYSIS

Patient Name: _____

Please look into a mirror and evaluate the following:

Number
How many teeth are visible in a full smile (circle correct number)? 2   4   6   8   10   12

Color

Are your teeth:

	yes	no	unsure		yes	no	unsure
too yellow?	☐	☐	☐	too brown?	☐	☐	☐
too dark?	☐	☐	☐	too uneven in color?	☐	☐	☐
too spotted?	☐	☐	☐	too discolored?	☐	☐	☐

Do your teeth have unattractive fillings or restorations? .... ☐   ☐   ☐

Position

	yes	no	unsure
Are your teeth too crowded?	☐	☐	☐
Do your teeth have spaces between them?	☐	☐	☐

If your tetth have spaces between them
how many spaces (circle correct number)? 1   2   3   4   5   6

Size

Are your teeth:

	yes	no	unsure		yes	no	unsure
too long?	☐	☐	☐	too short?	☐	☐	☐
too wide?	☐	☐	☐	too narrow?	☐	☐	☐
too large?	☐	☐	☐	too small?	☐	☐	☐

Are your two upper center front teeth the same length or shorter
than the two neighboring teeth? .... ☐   ☐   ☐

Shape

	yes	no	unsure
Are your teeth unattractively shaped?	☐	☐	☐

Are your teeth:

	yes	no	unsure		yes	no	unsure
too square?	☐	☐	☐	too rounded?	☐	☐	☐
too irregular in shape?	☐	☐	☐				

Gums

	yes	no	unsure
Do you show too much gum tissue (gummy smile)?	☐	☐	☐
Are your gums red and/or swollen?	☐	☐	☐
Does the shape of the gums surrounding the teeth appear unattractive?	☐	☐	☐

Please list anything else about your smile that you wish to discuss:

_____

_____

_____

Signature: _____   Date: _____

Copyright 1992 Barry G. Dale D.M.D. and Kenneth W. Aschheim D.D.S.

ESTHETIC DENTISTRY

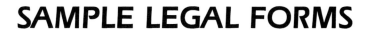

SAMPLE LEGAL FORMS

D

Forms are reproduced courtesy of ProSystems. They may be purchased from ProSystems, 118 Cain Drive, Brentwood, New York, 11717, 800-232-3366. Additional forms are available to complete a total dental office record keeping system.

MEDICAL–DENTAL HISTORY

Medical
Alert
Sticker

Patient's Name _____ DOB __/__/__ SSN _____

The following information is essential for this office to provide dental care in a manner that is compatible with your general health. Your cooperation in providing accurate information is necessary to meet your dental needs safely and efficiently. Incorrect information can be dangerous to your health.

MEDICAL HISTORY

* Write the answer to each question in the space provided.
* If the question is not understood, you are not certain of the answer, or have any question, indicate so in the space, and discuss the matter with the doctor.
* All questions must be answered.
* Use black ink or ball point pen.

Name of Physician _____ Phone _____

Address _____

Date of Last Visit _____ Reason For Last Visit _____

1. Are you currently under the care of a physician? If yes, for what reason or condition? _____

2. Are you currently taking any medication? If yes, what medication and for what reason or condition?

Have You Ever Had Or Been Treated For:
3. Rheumatic fever, rheumatic heart disease, heart murmur or congenital heart disease? _____

4. Heart trouble, heart attack, angina, heart surgery, a pacemaker, or irregular beats? _____

5. Stomach or intestinal disease? _____

6. Abnormal blood pressure, excessive bleeding, or anemia? _____

7. Breathing problems, asthma, tuberculosis, or hay fever? _____

8. Cancer, X-ray treatments, or chemotherapy? _____

9. Diabetes? _____

10. Hepatitis, jaundice, or liver disease? _____

11. Kidney problems or renal dialysis? _____

12. Venereal disease or AIDS? _____

© Budmor Enterprises Ltd. 1987
All Rights Reserved

13. A stroke, convulsions, or fainting spells? _____

_____

14. Tumors or growths? _____

_____

15. Arthritis or rheumatism? _____

_____

16. Allergic reactions to medications? _____

_____

17. Have you ever had a major operation? If yes, describe. _____

_____

18. Have you ever had a serious injury to your head or neck? If yes, describe. _____

_____

19. Are you on a special diet? If yes, for what reason and describe. _____

_____

20. Do you smoke? If yes, describe type and quantity. _____

_____

21. Have you consulted or been treated by a psychiatrist, psychologist or counsellor? If yes, describe. _____

_____

22. Are there any other problems about your health of which you are aware? _____

_____

23. For women: are you pregnant? _____

_____

DENTAL HISTORY

Date of your last visit to a dentist _____

Reason for your last visit (or series of visits) _____

Do you have any of your X-rays or dental records? _____

In respect to any previous dental treatment have you:

24. Ever fainted? _____

_____

25. Had an allergic reaction? _____

_____

26. Had abnormal bleeding? _____

_____

27. Any other complications during or following dental treatment? If yes, describe. _____

_____

28. Do your gums bleed on brushing or eating? _____

_____

29. Does food catch between your teeth? _____

_____

30. Have your teeth shifted, are there spaces between your teeth now where there were none, are your teeth flaring, or are some of your teeth becoming loose? _____

_____

31. Are any of your teeth sensitive to heat, cold, or pressure? _____

_____

32. Do you grind your teeth or clench your jaws? _____

_____

33. Do you have pain or clicking in the jaw joint around your ear? _____

_____

34. Have your jaw muscles ever been sore? If yes, describe. _____

_____

35. Are there any sores or growths in your mouth? _____

_____

36. Do any of your teeth ache? _____

_____

37. Do you have any other dental complaint? _____

_____

NOTE: A change in your health status should be reported to the office at the earliest possible time.

To the best of my knowledge, the foregoing questions have been accurately answered.

Permission To Release Health Information
  I grant the right to the dentist to release health information obtained from me, and information about my dental treatment to third party payors, and/or other health practitioners.

Person completing the form: Signature _____

Print Name: _____

If other than patient, indicate relationship: _____ Date _____/_____/_____

Dentist's History Review & Significant Findings

_____

_____

_____

_____

_____

_____

_____

_____

_____

_____

_____

_____

_____

_____

_____

_____

_____

_____

Signature Dr. _____ Date _____

Date: _____

I have reviewed the attached MEDICAL HISTORY. My general health status and medication has changed as follows (if no change, write "NO CHANGE"):

_____

_____

Person Completing The Update: Signature _____

Print Name _____

If other than the patient, indicate relationship: _____

Update reviewed by Dr. _____

- -

Date: _____

I have reviewed the attached MEDICAL HISTORY. My general health status and medication has changed as follows (if no change, write "NO CHANGE"):

_____

_____

Person Completing The Update: Signature _____

Print Name _____

If other than the patient, indicate relationship: _____

Update reviewed by Dr. _____

- -

Date: _____

I have reviewed the attached MEDICAL HISTORY. My general health status and medication has changed as follows (if no change, write "NO CHANGE"):

_____

_____

Person Completing The Update: Signature _____

Print Name _____

If other than the patient, indicate relationship: _____

Update reviewed by Dr. _____

- -

Date: _____

I have reviewed the attached MEDICAL HISTORY. My general health status and medication has changed as follows (if no change, write "NO CHANGE"):

_____

_____

Person Completing The Update: Signature _____

Print Name _____

If other than the patient, indicate relationship: _____

Update reviewed by Dr. _____

(c) Budmor Enterprises Ltd. 1987
All Rights Reserved

HISTORY UPDATES

REQUEST FOR RELEASE OF HEALTH INFORMATION

I, _____, hereby grant permission to
                    (Print Name)

_____
                 (Print Name of Doctor or Hospital)
to release information related to my health history, status, and treatment, and copies of my health
record, X-rays, and any test results to;

_____

At _____

_____

Signature _____ Date _____
          (If a minor, parent or guardian must sign)

© Budmor Enterprises Ltd. 1987
All Rights Reserved

I, (print name) _____ , hereby

authorize Dr. (print name) _____ to take photographs, slides, and/or videos of my face, jaws, and teeth.

I understand that the photographs, slides, and/or videos will be used as a record of my care, and may be used for educational purposes in lectures, demonstrations, and professional publications.

I further understand that if the photographs, slides, and/or videos are used in any publication, or as part of a demonstration, reasonable attempts will be made to conceal my identity.

_____
Patient's Signature

_____
If a Minor, Signature of Parent
or Guardian

_____
Witness Signature

_____
Doctor's Signature

_____
Date

FORM # 2013D

© Budmor Enterprises Ltd. 1989
All Rights Reserved

PERMISSION TO TAKE PHOTOGRAPHS, SLIDES, & VIDEOS

I, (print name) _____ have been

informed by Dr. (print name) _____, of the need to

undergo dental treatment as presented to me on _____.

I have been fully informed about the details of the recommended treatment and alternatives, and agree to accept the treatment as recommended by the doctor.

I understand that as the treatment proceeds there may be need to change the treatment plan. If this occurs I expect to be informed before any change is instituted.

I further understand that individual reactions to treatment cannot be predicted, and that if I experience any unanticipated reactions during or following any treatment, I agree to report them to the office as soon as possible.

I have been told that the success of the recommended treatment depends upon my cooperation in keeping scheduled appointments, following home care instruction, including oral hygiene and dietary instructions, and reporting to the office any change in my health status as soon as possible.

I have discussed all of the above with the doctor, and all my questions have been answered.

I acknowledge that no guarantees or assurances have been given by anyone as to the results that may be obtained.

Following the explanation, the discussion, and the answers to my questions, I authorize the doctor to complete the treatment as described.

_____	_____
Patient's Signature	If a Minor, Signature of Parent or Guardian
_____	_____
Witness Signature	Doctor's Signature
_____	
Date	

FORM # 2013F

© Budmor Enterprises Ltd. 1989
All Rights Reserved

CONSENT TO DENTAL TREATMENT

I, (print name) _____, hereby authorize

Dr. (print name) _____ to complete orthodontic treatment

for my child (print name) _____

The procedure used in the provision of care has been fully explained to me, and I understand it.

I have been told that the success of the treatment depends upon several factors under my and my child's control, such as: following recommended oral hygiene procedures, diet and nutrition, home care advice, cooperate with maintaining the appliances, and keeping office appointments.

I understand that regular dental examinations by our family dentist are essential to the success of the orthodontic treatment. In addition, referrals to other dental specialists may be required e.g., an oral surgeon, a periodontist, etc.

I further understand that despite all estimates of the success of the treatment, there are many personal biologic factors that cannot be predicted in advance that may affect its success.

I have been informed that one of the complications of orthodontic treatment may be problems associated with the temporomandibular joint. This is the joint located in front of each ear and connects the lower jaw to the skull. If there is any discomfort in the joint during treatment I am to report it to the dentist as soon as possible. I understand that if this occurs further consultation and treatment may be necessary.

I understand that following completion of treatment my child may be required to use retaining devices to maintain the position of the corrected bite.

I have been informed that some grinding and reshaping of the teeth may be necessary to adjust the bite and correct the occlusion.

I have discussed all of the above with the doctor, all my questions have been answered, and I fully understand why the orthodontic treatment is necessary, its limitations, estimates of success, and the effect on my child's dental health for refusing to accept the recommended care.

I agree to report any change in my child's health, and any problem that my child has with the treatment or the appliances to the office as soon as possible.

_____   _____
     Signature of Parent   Signature of Doctor
        or Guardian

_____   _____
     Witness Signature   Date

FORM # 2013K

© Budmor Enterprises Ltd. 1989
All Rights Reserved

CONSENT FOR OTHODONTIC TREATMENT

I, _____, hereby request and

authorize Dr. _____ to provide me with oral implants.

The procedure has been fully explained to me, and I understand, that success with implants depend on the cooperation of the patient, and on the individual body response that cannot be accurately determined prior to the placement of implants.

I have been made aware of the following possible complications: improper occlusion, prosthetic and/or material failure, loss of permanent teeth, loss of prosthesis and/or the implant should dental disease develop due to improper home care, loss of the implant and/or prosthesis should systemic disease develop, and wear or breakage of the implant component and or the prosthesis. Other complications may occur that cannot be predicted at this time. Should any of the complications occur, I understand that there may be a need to surgically remove the implant and the use of alternative forms of treatment.

Specific complications related to my care may include: _____

_____

_____

I have been made aware that smoking and the excessive use of alcohol and sugar will have an adverse effect on my body's response, and may therefore affect the success of the implant, as will my cooperation in performing prescribed home care.

I understand that should the implant fail for any of the above reasons, I may require corrective surgery, and/or the modification of the restoration.

Alternative treatment plans have been fully explained to me along with possible outcomes and risks.

I understand that I am to return to the dental office at regular intervals for the purpose of examining the status of the implant and my oral health, and that a reasonable fee will be charged for such visits.

I hereby authorize the taking of photographs of my mouth and implants during the course of treatment, and that they may be used for educational purposes, with the understanding that reasonable efforts will be taken to hide my identity.

I acknowledge that no guarantees or assurances have been made to me concerning the results intended from the use of the implants.

I have been given this form to be taken home on _____ for review.

I have had the opportunity to discuss all of the above on _____ with

Dr. _____, and have had all my questions answered.

I certify that I fully understand all matters as described in this AUTHORIZATION AND CONSENT FOR IMPLANTS.

_____   _____
             Doctor   Patient

Date _____   Time _____   _____
                                                         Witness

© Budmor Enterprises Ltd. 1989
All Rights Reserved

FORM # 2013B

AUTHORIZATION AND CONSENT FOR IMPLANTS

I, (print name) _____, parent of

(print name) _____, have been informed by

telephone on (date) _____, of the need to have the

following treatment performed on him/her:

_____

_____

_____

_____

_____

During the telephone conversation the service(s) were described, along with risks, benefits, and alternatives.

Following the receipt of the information on the telephone, and having all my questions answered, I authorized

Dr. (print name) _____ to perform the service(s) as listed above.

_____   _____
        Signature of Parent or Guardian   Date

FORM # 2013H

© Budmor Enterprises Ltd. 1989
All Rights Reserved

FOLLOW UP OF TELEPHONE CONSENT

RELEASE OF ALL CLAIMS

I, _____, as Releasor, being of lawful age,

for the sole consideration of _____ dollars

($ _____), paid to me, do hereby, and for my heirs, acquit and forever discharge

Dr. _____, as Releasee, and his or her agents, associates,

and employees from any and all claims, causes of actions, demands, damages, loss of services, expenses and

compensation whatsoever, which I now have, or which may hereafter accrue on account of, or in any way

may have been the result of treatment received now or in the past from the above named Releasee.

It is understood and agreed that this settlement is the compromise of a doubtful and disputed claim, and

that the payment made is not to be construed as an admission of liability on the part of the party or parties

hereby released, and that said Releasee denies liability therefor and intend merely to avoid litigation and buy

their peace.

_____   _____
(Signature of Patient)   (Print Name)

_____   _____
(Signature of Doctor)   (Print Name)

_____   _____
(Signature of Witness)   (Print Name)

                                       _____
                                                     (Date)

RELEASE OF ALL CLAIMS © Budmor Enterprises Ltd. 1989
All Rights Reserved

RELEASE FROM LIABILITY AGAINST DENTAL ADVICE

I, _____, the undersigned, being of lawful age,

hereby release from liability Dr. _____, and his or her

associates, employees, and agents from any injury I may currently, or in the future suffer as a result of my

refusal to have the following service(s) or consultation(s) performed:

_____

_____

_____

The need for the service(s) or consultation(s) has been fully explained to me, along with the consequences

of not having the service(s) or consultation(s) performed.

I have discussed the matter with the doctor, all my questions have been answered, and I fully understand

why the recommendation has been made, and the effects of my refusal.

_____   _____
(Signature of Patient)   (Print Name)

_____   _____
(Signature of Doctor)   (Print Name)

_____   _____
(Signature of Witness)   (Print Name)

                                        _____
                                                (Date)

FORM # 2016

© Budmor Enterprises Ltd. 1989
All Rights Reserved

RELEASE FROM LIABILITY AGAINST DENTAL ADVICE

LIST OF MANUFACTURERS

The list of manufacturers is compiled by Clinical Research Associates, 3707 N. Canyon Rd., Suite 6, Provo, UT, 84604. For more information, write or call 801-226-2121. The information in this list may not be current because of significant changes that occur annually.

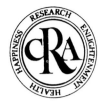

Clinical Research Associates

3707 North Canyon Road, Suite 6 ● Provo, UT 84604 ● (801) 226-2121

DENTAL COMPANY LIST (1/92)

A

1. **21st CENTURY HEALTH CARE PRODUCTS, INC.**
225 Madison Street
Jefferson City, MO 65101
(800) 325-0277
(314) 634-3575
FAX: (314) 634-8812

2. **3M DENTAL PRODUCTS DIV.**
Bldg. 225-4S-11
3M Center
St. Paul, MN 55144
(800) 634-2249
(612) 733-8524
FAX: (612) 733-2481

3. **7L CORP.**
25 East Poplar
Harrisburg, IL 62946
(800) 4-684-9274
(618) 253-4721
FAX: (618) 252-2846

4. **AALBA DENT INC.**
400 Watt Drive
Cordelia, CA 94585
(800) 227-1332
(707) 864-3334
FAX: (707) 864-2403

5. **ABIODENT, INC.**
33 Cherry Hill Drive
Danvers, MA 01923
(800) 648-1802
(508) 777-5386
FAX: (508) 774-4822

6. **ABRASIVE TECHNOLOGY**
8400 Green Meadows Drive
P.O. Box 6127
Westerville, OH 43081
(614) 548-4100
FAX: (614) 548-6249

7. **ACCARDI ENTERPRISES, INC.**
34 Lucille Lane
Dix Hills, NY 11746
(516) 427-6469
FAX: (718) 482-0601

8. **ACCOR, INC.**
P.O. Box 21020
Cleveland, OH 44121
(216) 381-2868

9. **ACCRA-LINE DENTAL TAB, INC.**
1002 Broad Street, Suite 301
P.O. Box 66
Augusta, GA 30903
(404) 724-0891
FAX: (404) 721-6210

10. **ACCU BITE DENTAL SUPPLY, INC.**
5001 West St. Joseph
P.O. Box 85707
Lansing, MI 48917
(800) 248-2746
(517) 351-0911
FAX: (517) 351-0908

11. **ACCU-DENT RESEARCH & DEVELOPMENT CO., INC.**
85 Industrial Way
Suite F
Buellton, CA 93427
(800) 344-5457
(805) 686-4672
FAX: (805) 688-7928

12. **ACCU-LINER SYSTEMS INC.**
13401 Bel-Red Road
Bellevue, WA 98005
(206) 746-0023

A (cont.)

13. **ACCUTRON, INC.**
8932 North Second Street
Phoenix, AZ 85020
(800) 531-2221
(602) 995-3145
FAX: (602) 861-2036

14. **ACKERMAN DENTAL MFG.**
(Mfr. name change. See Orange-Sol,
Inc., dba/Ackerman Dental Mfg.)

15. **ADAM DENTAL MFR. CORP.**
Schoolhouse Lane
Hurley, NY 12443
(800) 232-6810
(914) 339-4993

16. **ADCOA, INC.**
2142 North Killingsworth
Portland, OR 97217
(800) 876-8276
(503) 285-1534
FAX: (503) 285-8084

17. **A-DEC, INC.**
2601 Crestview Drive
P.O. Box 111
Newberg, OR 97132
(800) 547-1883
(503) 538-7478
FAX: (503) 538-0276

18. **A & D ENGINEERING, INC.**
1555 McCandless Drive
Milpitas, CA 95035
(800) 726-3364
(408) 263-5333
FAX: (408) 263-0119

19. **ADIUM DENTAL PRODUCTS, INC.**
3301 Olive Avenue
Long Beach, CA 90807
(800) 892-2150
(213) 595-5693
FAX: (213) 426-5509

20. **ADOLPH GASSER, INC.**
5733 Geary Boulevard
San Francisco, CA 94121
(415) 751-0145
FAX: (415) 387-6566

21. **ADVANCED CLINICAL TECH., INC.**
P.O. Box 2599
Westwood, MA 02090
(800) 922-9801
(617) 762-9801
FAX: (617) 762-1529

22. **ADVANCED DENTAL CO. OF CANADA**
Box 958
5079 Victoria Avenue
Niagra Falls, Ontario,
Canada L2E 6V8
(416) 356-0848
FAX: (416) 356-6330

23. **ADVANCED DENTAL CONCEPTS, INC.**
7 North Pinckney Street
Suite 305
Madison, WI 53703
(800) 369-3698
(608) 256-0344
FAX: (608) 256-1000

24. **ADVANCED DIAMOND INSTRUMENTS**
(See American Diamond Instruments)

25. **ADVANCED ORAL TECHNOLOGY, INC.**
307 Los Pinos Way
San Jose, CA 95119
(408) 629-6848
FAX: (408) 578-3384

A (cont.)

26. **ADVANTAGE DENTAL PRODUCTS, INC.**
P.O. Box 214767
Auburn Hills, MI 48321
(800) 388-6319
(313) 373-6319

27. **AD VICE ADVERTISING**
31921 Camino Capistrano
Suite 9238
San Juan Capistrano, CA 92675
(800) 634-7467
(714) 496-4874
FAX: (714) 661-8364

28. **AEI MUSIC NETWORK INC./NOVATONE**
900 East Pine Street
Seattle, WA 98122
(800) 426-1600
(206) 329-1400
FAX: (206) 329-9952

29. **AESTHETE LABORATORIES, INC.**
1000 East William Street
Suite 100
Carson City, NV 89701
(800) 544-4915
(702) 885-7435
FAX: (702) 883-4874

30. **AFFORDABLE DENTAL PRODUCTS**
855-C Conklin Street
Farmingdale, NY 11735
(800) 666-9008
(516) 249-4495

31. **AGUDA NORTH AMERICA, INC.**
(Mfr. name change. See J.L. Blosser,
Inc.)

32. **AIMES DISPOSABLES INC.**
1211 Rainbow Avenue
Pensacola, FL 32505
(904) 438-7317
FAX: (904) 438-4134

33. **AIR TECHNIQUES INC.**
70 Cantiague Rock Road
P.O. Box 870
Hicksville, NY 11801
(516) 433-7676
FAX: (516) 433-7684

34. **AIR & WATER DOCTOR, INC.**
931 East 4500 South
Salt Lake City, UT 84117
(801) 268-4941

35. **ALADAN CORP.**
630 Columbia Highway
P.O. Box 8308
Dothan, AL 36304
(205) 793-4509
FAX: (205) 792-2753

36. **ALCIDE CORP.**
One Willard Road
Norwalk, CT 06851
(800) 543-2133
(203) 847-2555
FAX: (203) 846-3331

37. **ALL-GEL CORP.**
1135 Northwest 51st Street
Seattle, WA 98107
(206) 789-9147
FAX: (206) 789-0819

38. **ALLIANCE SUPPLY CORP.**
2949 Bayview Drive
Fremont, CA 94538
(415) 659-1460
FAX: (415) 683-9653

A (cont.)

39. **ALLIED PHOTO PRODUCTS CO.**
5440-A Oakbrook Parkway
Norcross, GA 30093
(800) 262-9333
(404) 448-0250
FAX: (404) 448-0257

40. **ALLSEASONS ENVIRONMENTAL CONTROL., INC.**
51 Esna Park Drive
Unit 5
Markham, Ontario
Canada L3R 1C9
(416) 475-9795
FAX: (416) 475-6597

41. **ALMORE INT'L., INC.**
P.O. Box 25214
Portland, OR 97225
(800) 547-1511
(503) 643-6633
FAX: (503) 643-9748

42. **ALOE VERA OF AMERICA, INC.**
P.O. Box 801428
Dallas, TX 75380
(214) 343-5700
FAX: (214) 343-8322

43. **ALPHA PROTECH, INC.**
903 West Center St., Bldg. E
North Salt Lake, UT 84054
(800) 527-7689
(801) 298-3240
FAX: (801) 298-3250

44. **ALPINE AIR PRODUCTS**
9405 Brush Creek
Eagle, CO 81631
(303) 328-6543

45. **ALRICH/GIRARD CO.**
3627 North Andrews Avenue
Oakland Park, FL 33309
(800) 654-5705
(305) 561-8597
FAX: (305) 563-1124

46. **ALTO BOOKS/ADEPT INSTITUTE**
(Publishers of the ADEPT Report)
P.O. Box 5433
Santa Rosa, CA 95402
(707) 544-2586
FAX: (707) 575-4033

47. **ALVIN J. BERNARD**
7600 Dr. Phillips Boulevard
Suite 62
P.O. Box 690098
Orlando, FL 32819
(407) 351-5536

48. **ALZA CORP.**
950 Page Mill Road
P.O. Box 10950
Palo Alto, CA 94303
(415) 494-5000

49. **AMADENT/AMERICAN MEDICAL & DENTAL CORP.**
P.O. Box 733
Cherry Hill, NJ 08003
(800) 289-6367
(609) 429-8297
FAX: (609) 429-2953

50. **AMBU INC.**
611 North Hammond Ferry Road
Suite A
Linghicum, MD 21090
(800) 262-8462
(301) 636-1144
FAX: (301) 636-9964

51. **AMCO**
American Consolidated Mfg. Co.
2 Union Road
West Conshohocken, PA 19428
(800) 523-0740
(215) 825-2630
FAX: (215) 825-1958

52. **AMDRECOR**
5414 Antoine
Suite B
Houston, TX 77091
(800) 356-2938
(713) 681-4777

53. **AMERICAN DENTAL LASER**
2600 West Big Beaver
Troy, MI 48084
(800) 359-1959
(313) 649-0000
FAX: (313) 649-3252

54. **AMERICAN DENTAL SUPPLY INC.**
2600 William Penn Highway
Easton, PA 18042
(800) 558-5925
(215) 252-1464
FAX: (215) 252-2822

55. **AMERICAN DENTECH CORP.**
4910 Neptune Street
Corpus Christi, TX 78405
(800) 462-7990
(512) 882-2033
FAX: (512) 882-1726

56. **AMERICAN DIAMOND INSTRUMENTS**
869 McEllen Way
Lafayette, CA 94549
(800) 537-7474
(415) 284-3208
FAX: (415) 284-4129

57. **AMERICAN DIVERSIFIED DENTAL SYSTEMS**
Division of MDS Products, Inc.
1440 S. State College Blvd., Suite 3-H
Anaheim, CA 92806
(800) 637-2337
(714) 991-1371
FAX: (714) 991-9540

58. **AMERICAN MEDICAL ASSOC.**
P.O. Box 2964
Milwaukee, WI 53201
(800) 621-8335
(312) 464-5000
FAX: (312) 464-5600

59. **AMERICAN MEDICAL PUBLISHING CO., INC.**
P.O. Box 1087
Branford, CT 06405
(203) 488-0505

60. **AMERICAN ORTHODONTICS CORP.**
1714 Cambridge Avenue
P.O. Box 1048
Sheboygan, WI 53082
(800) 558-7687
(414) 457-5051
FAX: (414) 457-1485

61. **AMERICAN SHIELD CO.**
2390 South Orange Blossom Trail
Orlando, FL 32805
(407) 422-4000

62. **AMERICAN SOCIETY OF DENTISTRY FOR CHILDREN**
211 East Chicago Avenue
Suite 1430
Chicago, IL 60611
(800) 637-2732
(312) 943-1244
FAX: (312) 943-5341

63. **AMERICAN TOOTH INDUSTRIES**
Justi Division
1200 Stellar Drive
Oxnard, CA 93033
(800) 235-4639
(805) 487-9868
FAX: (805) 483-8482

64. **AMINODERM LABORATORIES, INC.**
4911 Van Nuys Boulevard
Suite 301
Sherman Oaks, CA 91403
(800) 426-1681
(818) 995-6751
FAX: (818) 995-1269

65. **AMSCO SCIENTIFIC**
Division of America Sterilizer Co.
1002 Lufkin Road
Apex, NC 27502
(800) 444-9009
(919) 362-0842
FAX: (919) 387-8335

66. **AMWAY CORP.**
7575 East Fulton Road
Ada, MI 49355
(616) 676-6000

67. **ANALGOTRONICS**
3049 Beacon Avenue South
Seattle, WA 98144
(206) 329-0500
FAX: (206) 329-0538

68. **ANALYTIC TECHNOLOGY CORP.**
15233 Northeast 90th Street
Redmond, WA 98052
(800) 428-2808
(206) 883-2445
FAX: (206) 882-3128

69. **ANCHOR CHEMICAL CO.**
777 Canterbury Road
Westlake, OH 44145
(216) 871-1660
FAX: (216) 871-0665

70. **A-NE ENTERPRISES**
6850 Klug Pines #31
Shreveport, LA 71129
(800) 256-1015
(318) 688-5600

71. **ANSELL INC.**
Cranberry Commons
446 Street Highway 35
Eatontown, NJ 07724
(800) 524-1377
(908) 542-9500
FAX: (908) 542-5569

72. **ANSON INT'L.**
P.O. Box 1902
Lynnwood, WA 98046
(800) 726-1628
(206) 745-3303
FAX: (206) 743-1145

73. **APM-STERNGOLD**
23 Frank Mossberg Drive
P.O. Box 839-A
Attleboro, MA 02703
(800) 243-9942
(508) 226-5660
FAX: (508) 226-5473

74. **APO HEALTH CO.**
13 Centre Street
Hempstead, NY 11550
(800) 365-2839
(516) 485-6700
FAX: (516) 485-6753

75. **APOLLO DENTAL PRODUCTS**
10427 Laramie Avenue
Chatsworth, CA 91311
(800) 233-4151
(818) 700-0380
FAX: (209) 442-4222

76. **ARDENT, INC.**
Box 666
Bromall, PA 19008
(215) 356-7997
(215) 544-8756

77. **ARGO INDUSTRIAL**
804 West 1700 South
Salt Lake City, UT 84104
(800) 827-1288
(801) 972-1482
FAX: (801) 973-0563

78. **ARTUS CORP.**
P.O. Box 511
201 South Dean Street
Englewood, NJ 07631
(800) 535-0086
(201) 568-1000
FAX: (201) 568-8865

79. **ASEPSIS INT'L., INC.**
943 Isles Road
Boynton Beach, FL 33435
(407) 738-6695
FAX: (716) 684-4692

80. **ASEPTICO, INC.**
P.O. Box 3209
Kirkland, WA 98083
(800) 426-5913 = USA
(800) 543-4470 = Canada
(206) 487-3157
FAX: (206) 487-2608

81. **ASH/DENTSPLY**
570 West College Avenue
P.O. Box 872
York, PA 17405
(800) 877-0020
(717) 845-7511
FAX: (717) 843-5951

82. **ASH TEMPLE**
31 Scardale Road
Don Mills, Ontario
Canada M3B 2R2
(416) 449-2300
FAX: (416) 449-5932

83. **A/S L. GOOF**
Usseroed Moelle
DK-2970 Hoersholm
Denmark
45-4286-2111
FAX: 45-4257-2726

84. **ASTRA PHARMACEUTICAL PROD.**
50 Otis Street
Wesboro, MA 01581
(800) 225-6333
(617) 366-1100
FAX: (508) 366-7406

85. **ASTRON DENTAL CORP.**
6250 Capitol Drive
Wheeling, IL 60090
(800) 323-4144
(708) 537-8787
FAX: (708) 537-8730

86. **ATHENA MFG., INC.**
(Mfr. name change. See AIMES Disposable Inc.)

87. **ATHENA TECHNOLOGY, INC.**
420 South Vernon Avenue
Glendora, CA 91740
(800) 253-1771
(818) 914-6632
FAX: (818) 852-0216

88. **ATTACHMENTS INT'L., INC.**
600 South Amphlett Boulevard
San Mateo, CA 94402
(800) 999-3003
(415) 340-0393
FAX: (415) 340-8423

89. **AUDRA, INC.**
21400 North Shore Drive
Sturgis, MI 49091
(800) 445-0170
(616) 651-9106
FAX: (616) 651-7611

90. **AUTHENTIC PRODUCTS, INC.**
4415 Piedras West
Suite 160
San Antonio, TX 78228
(800) 683-1025
(512) 735-1433

91. **AVANTI COMPUTER ASSOC.**
157 Valley Run Drive
Cherry Hill, NJ 08002
(800) 223-3672
(609) 354-8054
FAX: (609) 428-7348

92. **AVM CO., INC.**
P.O. 2274
Evansville, IN 47714
(812) 477-2555

93. **AVTEK**
P.O. Box 4406
Glendale, CA 91202
(800) 423-2868
(818) 240-1028
FAX: (818) 840-9239

94. **AXEL JOHNSON DENTAL AB**
(Mfr. name change. See AxTrade Dental AB)

95. **AXTRADE DENTAL AB**
P.O. Box 423
S-194 04 Upplands Vasby,
Sweden
46-760-99700
FAX: 46-760-898-93

B

96. **BALDOR ELECTRIC CO.**
2520 West Barberry Place
Denver, CO 80204
(800) 888-0360
(303) 623-0127
FAX: (303) 595-3772

97. **BALLARD MEDICAL PRODUCTS**
12050 Lone Peak Parkway
Draper, UT 84020
(801) 572-6800
FAX: (801) 572-6999

98. **BAND'AIDS SAFETY PROD., INC.**
2801 Boulevard, Suite D
Colonial Heights, VA 23834
(804) 526-8405

99. **BANDITT DENTAL INST. CO.**
P.O. Box 6841
Freehold, NJ 07728
(800) 222-0961
(908) 462-5457

100. **BANTEX CORP.**
P.O. Box 4098
Burlingame, CA 94011
(800) 633-4839
(415) 697-3545
FAX: (415) 697-3596

101. **BANYAN INT'L. CORP.**
P.O. Box 1779
Abilene, TX 79604
(800) 351-4530
(915) 677-1874
FAX: (915) 677-1372

102. **BARRIER CONCEPTS, INC.**
808-D Lady Street
Columbia, SC 29201
(800) 252-5262
(803) 252-3404
FAX: (803) 252-3533

103. **BARRIER PROTECTION CO., INC.**
3320 Industry Drive
Long Beach, CA 90806
(800) 367-5432
(800) 237-0097 (CA)
(213) 427-3223

104. **BARRIERS FOR DISEASES**
2724 7th Avenue South
Birmingham, AL 35233
(800) 233-1006
(205) 252-0075
FAX: (205) 252-0096

105. **BAUSCH & LOMB ORAL CARE DIV.**
5243 Royal Woods Parkway
Suite 100
Tucker, GA 30084
(800) 633-6363
(404) 934-1232
FAX: (404) 723-9522

106. **BA VIDEOGRAPHICS**
22187 Hibiscus Hill Drive
Woodland Hills, CA 91367
(818) 347-6238
FAX: (818) 592-0635

107. **BAXTER HEALTHCARE CORP.**
General Healthcare Division
One Parkway North, Suite 100
P.O. Box 851
Deerfield, IL 60015
(800) 423-2311
(708) 940-1990
FAX: (708) 940-1935

108. **BAXTER HEALTHCARE CORP.**
Medical Specialties Devices Group
Technology & Ventures Division
2132 Michelson Drive
Irvine, CA 92715
(714) 474-6400

109. **B.C. DECKER INC.**
(Mfr. name change. See Mosby-
Year Book)

110. **BEAVERS DENTAL/DIV. OF SYBRON
CANADA LTD.**
P.O. Bag 900
Morrisburg, Ontario
Canada K0C 1X0
(613) 543-3791
FAX: (613) 543-2525

111. **BECK, E.A. & CO.**
(See E.A. Beck & Co.)

112. **BECTON-DICKINSON, INC.**
1 Stally Street
East Rutherford, NJ 07073
(201) 460-2000
FAX: (201) 460-1104

113. **BELL INT'L.**
1313 North Carolan
Burlingame, CA 94010
(800) 523-6640
(415) 348-2055
FAX: (415) 348-3937

114. **BELLE DE ST. CLAIR, INC.**
20600 Plummer Street
Chatsworth, CA 91311
(800) 322-6666
(818) 718-7000
FAX: (818) 341-1142

115. **BENCHMARK ENTERPRISES**
5069 South 1000 East
Salt Lake City, UT 84117
(801) 972-5042

116. **BERNARD, ALVIN J.**
(See Alvin J. Bernard)

117. **BIG SKY DENTAL SUPPLY**
341 Springwood Lane
Idaho Falls, ID 83404
(208) 529-2228

118. **BILSOM INT'L., INC.**
109 Carpenter Drive
Sterling, VA 22170
(800) 733-1177
(703) 834-1070
FAX: (703) 834-1024

119. **BIO-CIDE INT'L., INC.**
P.O. Box 722170
Norman, OK 73070
(405) 329-5556
FAX: (405) 329-2681

120. **BIOLOGICAL RESCUE PROD., INC.**
566 High Street
Pottstown, PA 19464
(800) 882-0505
(215) 327-9449
FAX: (215) 327-9452

121. **BIOMEDICAL COMPOSITES LTD.**
9783 Halifax Street
Ventura, CA 93004
(805) 647-7035

122. **BIO-MEDICAL/DENTAL CORP.**
2143 Davcor Street Southeast
Salem, OR 97302
(800) 444-1765
(503) 399-1765
FAX: (503) 364-1934

123. **BIO-RESEARCH, INC.**
4113 North Port Washington Road
Milwaukee, WI 53212
(800) 251-2315
(414) 332-3003
FAX: (414) 332-5317

124. **BIOSAFETY SYSTEMS INC.**
8380 Camino Santa Fe
San Diego, CA 92121
(800) 421-6556
(619) 452-3500
FAX: (619) 452-3917

125. **BIOTECHNICA DIAGNOSTICS INC.**
(Mfr. name change. See Omnigene, Inc.)

126. **BIOTROL INT'L.**
P.O. Box 870199
2561 South 1560 West
Woods Cross, UT 84087
(800) 822-8550
(801) 298-0880
FAX: (801) 298-7339

127. **BISCO DENTAL PROD.**
1500 West Thorndale Avenue
Itasca, IL 60143
(800) 247-3368
(708) 773-6633
FAX: (708) 773-6949

128. **BLEACHMASTER, INC.**
2250 South Redwood Road
Suite 9
Salt Lake City, UT 84119
(800) 253-2246
(801) 972-3653
FAX: (801) 972-4002

129. **BLOCK DRUG CORP.**
Oral Health Care Division
105 Academy Street
Jersey City, NJ 07302
(800) 365-6500
(201) 434-3000
FAX: (201) 333-3117

130. **BLOSSER, J.L., INC.**
(See J.L. Blosser, Inc.)

131. **BLUE DOLPHIN PRODUCTS/
PRODUCTIVITY TRAINING CORP.**
6489 Camden Avenue
Suite 200
San Jose, CA 95120
(800) 448-8855
(408) 268-4355
FAX: (408) 268-6671

132. **BOECKELER INSTRUMENTS, INC.**
3280 East Hemisphere Loop #114
Tucson, AZ 85706
(800) 552-2262
(602) 573-7100
FAX: (602) 573-7101

133. **BONDAIRE, INC.**
198 Park Road
Pittsford, NY 14534
(800) 999-2473
(716) 383-0584
FAX: (716) 787-0314

134. **BOND POND**
East 12308 Broadway
Spokane, WA 99216
(800) 235-2663
(509) 928-5112

135. **BOSWORTH, HARRY J. CO.**
7227 North Hamlin Avenue
Skokie, IL 60076
(708) 679-3400
FAX: (708) 679-2080

136. **BOWEN LTD.**
811 South Grand
Santa Ana, CA 92705
(800) 821-1071
(714) 558-7501
FAX: (714) 835-7268

137. **BRADFORD, JAMES**
Portage Professional Bldg.
325 East Centre Street
Portage, MI 49002
(616) 323-1633

138. **BRAHLER PRODUCTS, INC.**
3200 Haskell, Suite 110
P.O. Box 4009
Lawrence, KS 66046
(913) 843-0932
FAX: (913) 832-1016

139. **BRANSON ULTRASONICS CORP.**
41 Eagle Road
Danbury, CT 06813
(203) 796-0400 ext. 532
FAX: (203) 796-2240

140. **BRASSELER U.S.A.**
800 King George Boulevard
Savannah, GA 31419
(800) 841-4522
(912) 925-8525
FAX: (912) 927-8671

141. **BREVET, INC.**
3630 Miraloma Avenue
Anaheim, CA 92806
(714) 630-5202
FAX: (714) 630-5527

142. **BRITE SMILE**
700 Sunhill Road
Suite 201
Birmingham, AL 35215
(800) 284-4656
(205) 856-7580
FAX: (205) 856-7585

143. **BROWN METALS CO.**
P.O. Box 3606
13249 Barton Circle
Santa Fe Springs, CA 90670
(800) 992-5015
(213) 946-4545
FAX: (213) 941-7822

144. **BRULIN CO., THE**
(See The Brulin Co.)

145. **BRUSHGUARD SYSTEMS INC.**
118 West Hazel Avenue
Inglewood, CA 90302
(213) 673-8616
FAX: (213) 673-9003

146. **BUFFALO DENTAL MFG. CO., INC.**
575 Underhill Boulevard
Syosset, NY 11791
(800) 828-0203
(516) 496-7200
FAX: (516) 496-7751

147. **BURRON MEDICAL, INC.**
824 12th Avenue
Bethlehem, PA 18018
(215) 691-5400
FAX: (215) 691-1785

148. **BUTLER, JOHN O. CO.**
4635 West Foster Avenue
Chicago, IL 60630
(800) 528-8537
(312) 777-4000
FAX: (312) 777-5101

C

149. **CADCO DENTAL PRODUCTS, INC.**
600 Hueneme Road
Oxnard, CA 93033
(800) 833-8267
(805) 488-1122
FAX: (800) 444-5170

150. **CALCITEK, INC.**
2320 Faraday Avenue
Carlsbad, CA 92008
(800) 854-7019
(619) 431-9515
FAX: (619) 431-9753

151. **CALGON VESTAL LABORATORIES**
P.O. Box 147
St. Louis, MO 63166
(800) 325-8005
(314) 535-1810
FAX: (800) 543-2680

152. **CALTECH INDUSTRIES, INC.**
P.O. Box 1139
Midland, MI 48641
(800) 234-7700
(517) 496-3110
FAX: (517) 496-0212

153. **CAMERON-MILLER, INC.**
3949 South Racine
Chicago, IL 60609
(800) 621-0142
(312) 523-6360
FAX: (312) 523-9495

154. **CAM VAC**
85 North Edison Way
Suite 10
Reno, NV 89502
(800) 327-4401
(702) 329-4401

155. **CAPCAD INC.**
P.O. Box 3092
Winnipeg, Manitoba,
Canada R3C 4E5
(204) 452-9469
FAX: (204) 284-2433

156. **CARMEL DENTAL CO.**
147 West Carmel Drive
Suite 105
Carmel, IN 46032
(317) 573-8505

157. **CAULK/DENTSPLY**
(See L.D. Caulk/Dentsply)

158. **C & C SYSTEMS, INC.**
P.O. Box 4244
Greenwich, CT 06830
(800) 836-3660
(914) 939-2393
FAX: (914) 939-9291

159. **CENTER FOR DENTAL TECHNOLOG
& BIOMATERIALS**
Karolinska Institute
Box 4064
S-14104 Huddinge, Sweden
011-46-8-7460200
FAX: 011-46-8-7793166

160. **CENTRA, INT'L.**
1100 East 80th Street
Minneapolis, MN 55420
(800) 328-5536
(612) 854-2881
FAX: (612) 854-8381

161. **CENTRIX INC.**
30 Stran Road
Milford, CT 06460
(800) 235-5862
(203) 878-7875
FAX: (203) 877-8017

162. **CERAMIC ENGINEERING ASSOC.**
3700 East Marion Street
Seattle, WA 98122
(206) 543-2032
FAX: (206) 543-3100

163. **CETYLITE INDUSTRIES, INC.**
9051 River Road
P.O. Box 90006
Pennsauken, NJ 08110
(800) 257-7740
(609) 665-6111
FAX: (609) 665-5408

164. CFI, INC.
P.O. Box 1454
Battleground, WA 98604
(800) 323-7922
(415) 924-4435

165. CHALLENGE PRODUCTS, INC.
Lake Road 54-22
P.O. Box 468
Osage Beach, MO 65065
(800) 322-9800
(314) 348-2227
FAX: (314) 348-2228

166. CHAMELEON DENTAL PROD., INC.
200 North 6th Street
Kansas City, KS 66101
(800) 366-0001
(913) 281-5552
FAX: (913) 621-7012

167. CHATSWORTH MEDICAL SUPPLY, INC.
21011 Itasca Street
Suite F
Chatsworth, CA 91311
(800) 752-6919
(818) 773-6680
FAX: (818) 773-8002

168. CHEM-MIX, INC.
625 Charlie Hicks Road
Jonesborough, TN 37659
(615) 926-4488
FAX: (615) 926-2087

169. CHESHEIM DENTAL ASSOC.
716 Bethlehem Pike
Philidelphia, PA 19118
(215) 233-0206

170. CHIGE, R., INC.
475 West Merrick Road
Valley Stream, NY 11580
(800) 645-2628
(516) 872-3530
FAX: (516) 872-2082

171. CHILD KEYPPERS INT'L.
P.O. Box 6456
Lake Worth, FL 33466
(407) 586-6695
FAX: (407) 585-4372

172. CHISWICK TRADING CO., INC.
33 Union Avenue
Sudbury, MA 01776
(800) 225-8708
FAX: (800) 638-9899

173. CINE FILM SYSTEMS, INC.
3511 Locke
Fort Worth, TX 76107
(800) 237-0740
(817) 738-7851
FAX: (817) 732-2463

174. CLARK DENTAL EQUIPMENT SYSTEMS
47 Hilltop Avenue
Hullbridge Hocky
Essex, England SS 56 BA
702-230-760
FAX: 702-231-587

175. CLEARCHEM CORP.
P.O. Box 446
2601 Adgate
Lima, OH 45802
(800) 962-2712
(419) 222-3275
FAX: (419) 222-4573

176. CLINICAL RESEARCH DENTAL SUPPLY
P.O. Box 1486
Dearborn, MI 48121
(800) 265-3444

177. CLINICOVERS- DIVISION OF
CLINETEX, INC.
1003 North Mesa Road
P.O. Box 1443
Montrose, CO 81402
(800) 336-1414
(303) 249-3733

178. CLIVE CRAIG CO.
600 Hueneme Road
Oxnard, CA 93033
(800) 833-8267
(805) 488-1122
FAX: (800) 444-5170

179. CLOROX, THE CO.
1221 Broadway
Oakland, CA 94612
(800) 292-2200
(415) 271-7000

180. CMP INDUSTRIES
413 North Pearl Street
Albany, NY 12207
(800) 833-2343
(518) 434-3147
FAX: (518) 434-1288

181. COAXCO, INC.
P.O. Box 489
12250 Southwest Myslony
Tualatin, OR 97062
(800) 637-0001
(503) 692-2900
FAX: (503) 692-3029

182. COE LABORATORIES, INC.
(Mfr. name change. See GC America,
Inc.)

183. COLGATE-HOYT LABORATORIES
One Colgate Way
Canton, MA 02021
(800) 225-3756
(617) 821-2880
FAX: (617) 821-2644

184. COLLA-TEC INC.
105 Morgan Lane
Plainsboro, NJ 08536
(609) 683-0900
FAX: (609) 799-3297

185. COLLIS CURVE INC.
313 West 48th Street
Minneapolis, MN 55409
(612) 822-2740
FAX: (612) 822-7209

186. COLORADO BIOMEDICAL, INC.
6851 Highway 73
Evergreen, CO 80439
(800) 962-2272
(303) 674-5447
FAX: (303) 674-1296

187. COLTENE AG
Feldwiesenstrasse 20
CH-9450
Altstatten, Switzerland
011-41-71-75-41-21
FAX: 011-41-71-75-1695

188. COLTENE/WHALEDENT
236 Fifth Avenue
New York, NY 10001
(800) 221-3046
(212) 696-8000
FAX: (212) 532-1644

189. COLUMBIA DENTOFORM CORP.
22-19 41st Avenue
Long Island City, NY 11101
(718) 482-1569
FAX: (718) 482-1585

190. COLUMBIA WORLD CORP.
1314 Jadwin
Richland, WA 99352
(800) 225-3881
(509) 946-3993
FAX: (509) 946-5353

191. COLUMBUS DENTAL
(Mfr. name change. See Miles, Inc.)

192. COLWELL SYSTEMS, INC.
201 Kenyon Road
Champaign, IL 61820
(800) 225-1448
(217) 351-5400
FAX: (217) 351-5413

193. COMLITE SYSTEMS, INC.
2570 Northeast Expressway
Atlanta, GA 30345
(800) 438-3406

194. COM-PAC INT'L.
800 Industrial Park Road
P.O. Box 2707
Carbondale, IL 62902
(800) 824-0817
(618) 529-2421
FAX: (618) 529-2234

195. CONFI-DENTAL PRODUCTS CO.
385 South Pierce Avenue
Louisville, CO 80027
(800) 383-5158
(303) 665-7535
FAX: (303) 666-4320

196. CONSERVE-A-DENT, INC.
809 West 26th Street
Erie, PA 16508
(814) 455-9949
FAX: (814) 453-5246

197. CONTINENTAL CARBIDE CORP.
5659 West 63rd Avenue
Arvada, CO 80003
(303) 422-2775

198. CONTINUING EDUCATION UPDATE
65 Prospect Street
Stamford, CT 06901
(203) 348-4646

199. COOKE & ASSOC., INC.
P.O. Box 34626
7602 Old Galveston Road
Houston, TX 77234
(800) 231-3058
(713) 941-8455
FAX: (713) 943-8797

200. CORE-VENT CORP.
15821 Ventura Boulevard
Suite 410
Encino, CA 91436
(800) 551-3838
(818) 783-0681
FAX: (818) 783-0788

201. CORNERSTONE IMAGING SYST. CO.
20291 Paseo Del Prado
P.O. Box 1373
Walnut, CA 91788
(714) 594-2766
FAX: (714) 598-9325

202. COSMEDENT, INC.
5419 North Sheridan Road
Chicago, IL 60640
(800) 621-6729
(312) 989-6844
FAX: (312) 989-1826

203. COSMETIC IMAGING SYSTEMS
309 Santa Monica Boulevard,
Suite 315
Santa Monica, CA 90401
(800) 258-2218
(213) 393-3993
FAX: (213) 395-3516

204. COTTRELL, LTD.
7399 South Tucson Way
Englewood, CO 80112
(800) 843-3343
(303) 799-9401
FAX: (303) 799-9408

205. COURTNEY DENTAL
723 Parkhurst Lane
Lexington, SC 29072
(803) 359-5539

206. COX STERILE PRODUCTS, INC.
5115 McKinney
Suite C
Dallas, TX 75205
(800) 247-6493
(214) 528-8900
FAX: (214) 528-0467

207. CREATION NORTH AMERICA, INC.
12720 West North Avenue
Brookfield, WI 53005
(800) 872-1588
(414) 789-0909
FAX: (414) 789-0916

208. CRESCENT DENTAL MFG. CO.
7750 West 47th Street
Lyons, IL 60534
(800) 323-8952
(708) 447-8050
FAX: (708) 447-8190

209. CREST ULTRASONICS CORP.
Scotch Road
P.O. Box 7266
Trenton, NJ 08628
(800) 441-9675
(609) 883-4000
FAX: (609) 883-6452

210. CROSSTEX
Cross Country Paper Products
P.O. Box 13188
10 Ranick Road
Hauppauge, NY 11788
(800) 223-2497
(516) 582-6777
FAX: (516) 582-1726

211. C.R. TRADING, INC.
(Mfr. name change. See Columbia
World Corp.)

212. CURA PHARMACEUTICAL, INC.
2000 Corporate Square #4
Jacksonville, FL 32216
(800) 326-5690
(904) 725-8447
FAX: (904) 720-0059

D

213. DANVILLE ENGINEERING
115-A Railroad Avenue
Danville, CA 94526
(800) 827-7940
(415) 838-7940
FAX: (415) 838-0944

214. DARBY DENTAL SUPPLY CO.
100 Banks Avenue
Rockville Centre, NY 11570
(800) 545-5916 ext. 2101
(516) 683-1800 ext. 2101
FAX: (516) 832-8771

215. DAVID'S DENTAL LABORATORY
3918 Seneca Street
West Seneca, NY 14224
(800) 628-3384
(716) 674-2770

216. DAVIS, F.A. CO/PUBLISHER
1915 Arch Street
Philadelphia, PA 19103
(800) 523-4049
(215) 568-2270
FAX: (215) 568-5065

217. DC DENTAL SPECIALTIES
2007 Wilshire Boulevard
Suite 813-815
Los Angeles, CA 90057
(800) 347-3096
(213) 413-3636
FAX: (213) 413-3599

218. DECKER, B.C., INC.
(Mfr. name change. See Mosby-
Year Book)

219. DEDECO INT'L., INC.
Route 97
Long Eddy, NY 12760
(800) 431-3022
(914) 887-4840
FAX: (914) 887-5281

220. **DEGUSSA CORP.**
Dental Department
3950 South Clinton Ave., Bldg. B
South Plainfield, NJ 07060
(800) 221-0168
(908) 754-6300
FAX: (908) 668-1174

221. **DELAR CORP.**
P.O. Box 226
Lake Oswego, OR 97034
(800) 669-7499
(503) 635-6820
FAX: (503) 635-2978

222. **DELDENT LTD.**
19 Keren Kayemet Street
49372 Petach Tikva
Israel
011-972-3-923-1649
FAX: 011-972-3-575-3346

223. **DEL-TUBE**
13901 Main Street
Menomonee Falls, WI 53051
(800) 558-8934
(414) 251-1077
FAX: (414) 251-1786

224. **DEMETRON RESEARCH CORP.**
5 Ye Olde Road
Danbury, CT 06810
(203) 748-0030
(212) 265-8680 (NY)
FAX: (203) 791-8284

225. **DENAR CORP.**
901 East Cerritos Avenue
Anaheim, CA 92805
(800) 854-9316
(714) 776-9000
FAX: (714) 776-9044

226. **DENBUR, INC.**
P.O. Box 3473
Oak Brook, IL 60522
(800) 992-1399
(708) 986-9667
FAX: (708) 986-9688

227. **DENDEV LABORATORIES, INC.**
4525 South Wasatch Boulevard
Suite 320
Salt Lake City, UT 84124
(800) 331-4437
(801) 273-0112

228. **DENERICA DENTAL CORP.**
550 Frontage Road
Northfield, IL 60093
(800) 336-7422
(708) 441-7070
FAX: (708) 441-7096

229. **DENIRO**
1118 East Adams Avenue
Suite B
Orange, CA 92667
(714) 538-5998

230. **DEN-MAT CORP.**
P.O. Box 1729
Santa Maria, CA 93456
(800) 433-6628
(805) 922-8491
FAX: (805) 922-6933

231. **DEN-MED SUPPLY CO.**
2616 Harmony Road
Louisville, KY 40299
(502) 267-4432

232. **DENOVO**
140 East Santa Clara Street
Suite 12
Arcadia, CA 91006
(800) 854-7949
(818) 446-5757
FAX: (818) 446-5871

233. **DENTACO PRODUCTS**
73 East Merrick Road
Freeport, NY 11520
(800) 645-2866
(516) 868-8649
FAX: (516) 868-1309

234. **DENTAL AIRE INC.**
5142 Blazer Memorial Parkway
Dublin, OH 43017
(617) 792-1906

235. **DENTAL ARTS LABORATORY, INC.**
241 North East Perry
Peoria, IL 61651
(800) 322-2213
(309) 674-8191
FAX: (309) 674-8174

236. **DENTAL COMPONENTS, INC.**
P.O. Box 228
Newburg, OR 97132
(800) 624-2793
(503) 538-8343
FAX: (503) 538-9302

237. **DENTAL CONCEPTS INC.**
9 North Goodwin Avenue
Elmsford, NY 10523
(914) 592-1860
FAX: (914) 592-4922

238. **DEN-TAL-EZ INC.**
(Star Dental/Custom Vacuum/
Columbia Dentoform/Den-Tal-Ez)
P.O. Box 896
Valley Forge Corporate Center
Valley Forge, PA 19482
(215) 666-9050
FAX: (215) 666-9062

239. **DENTAL HEALTH PRODUCTS, INC.**
4011 Creek Road
P.O. Box 355
Youngstown, NY 14174
(800) 828-6868
(716) 745-9933
FAX: (716) 754-4352

240. **DENTAL INVISIONS, INC.**
425-A Southeast 5th Avenue
Boynton Beach, FL 33435
(800) 322-7207
(407) 734-7207
FAX: (407) 734-7223

241. **DENTAL KINETICS**
1955 East Yalcrest Avenue
Salt Lake City, UT 84108
(801) 583-3169

242. **DENTAL MATERIALS GROUP, LTD.**
175 Commerce Drive
P.O. Box 12084
Hauppauge, NY 11788
(516) 434-7760/7810
FAX: (516) 434-7750

243. **DENTAL & MEDICAL INT'L.**
P.O. Box 2853
Scottsdale, AZ 85252
(602) 957-9052

244. **DENTAL NETWORK OF AMERICA, INC.**
Two TransAm Plaza Drive
Suite 500
Oakbrook Terrace, IL 60181
(800) 323-6840
(708) 691-1133 ext. 238
FAX: (708) 495-0575

245. **DENTAL OPTICS MFG., INC.**
203 Long Beach Road
Island Park, NY 11558
(800) 423-7688
(516) 889-5857
FAX: (516) 889-5874

246. **DENTAL RESOURCES, INC.**
530 River Street South
Delano, MN 55328
(800) 328-1276
(612) 972-3801
FAX: (612) 972-3807

247. **DENTAL SPECIALTY MFG. CO.**
3013 Mangum Dairy Road
Monroe, NC 28112
(704) 764-3424

248. **DENTAL SYSTEMS & COMPONENTS**
10850 Slater Avenue Northeast
P.O. Box 3447
Kirkland, WA 98083
(800) 654-4601
(206) 827-3885

249. **DENTAL TECHNICAL PUBLICATIONS**
3455 Northeast 12 Terrace
P.O. Box 23620
Oakland Park, FL 33307
(305) 565-9852
FAX: (305) 783-0097

250. **DENTAL TECHNOLOGIES, INC.**
1465 Post Road East
P.O. Box 901
Westport, CT 06881
(203) 255-2778

251. **DENTAL VENTURES OF AMERICA**
100 Chaparral Court, Unit #100
Anaheim Hills, CA 92808
(800) 228-6696
(714) 974-6280
FAX: (714) 283-2723

252. **DENTAMERICA**
Division of Royal Industries
P.O. Box 3200
Industry, CA 91744
(818) 912-1388
FAX: (818) 912-7554

253. **DENTA-SLEEVE**
Box 534
15870 Franklin Trail
Prior Lake, MN 55372
(800) 535-4370
(612) 440-1212

254. **DENTAURUM, INC.**
2 Pheasant Run
Newtown, PA 18940
(800) 523-3946
(215) 968-2858
FAX: (215) 968-0809

255. **DENTECHNICA**
12204 Green Lane
Montreal, Quebec
Canada H4K 2C3
(514) 336-4680
FAX: (514) 336-4072

256. **DENTEK, INC.**
155 Great Arrow Avenue
Buffalo, NY 14207
(716) 875-1770
FAX: (716) 875-1770

257. **DENTELLIGENT CORP.**
18751 Beach Boulevard
Huntington Beach, CA 92648
(800) 535-3955
(714) 375-2424
FAX: (714) 375-2433

258. **DENTICATOR**
11330 Sunrise Park Drive
Suite A
Rancho Cordova, CA 95742
(800) 227-3321
(916) 638-9303
FAX: (916) 638-0319

259. **DENTIFAX/DI-EQUI**
17 Old Route 9
Wappingers Falls, NY 12590
(914) 297-1014 = Dentifax
(914) 297-4387 = Di-Equi
FAX: (914) 297-1626

260. **DENTIQUE, LTD.**
34586 Lakeshore Bouldevard
Eastlake, OH 44094
(216) 946-7878

261. **DENT-MED CO.**
P.O. Box 4081
East Lansing, MI 48823
(517) 349-3212

262. **DENTO-PROFILE SCALE CO.**
P.O. Box 1107
Fond Du Lac, WI 54936
(414) 922-5446
FAX: (414) 921-3052

263. **DENTRADE INT'L.**
Div. of Bausch Articulating Papers
P.O. Box 15-B
San Francisco, CA 94115
(415) 929-1774
FAX: (415) 391-5475

264. **DENTRAN, INC.**
461 Manitou Drive
Kitchener, Ontario
Canada N2C 1L5
(519) 748-6846
FAX: (519) 748-9221

265. **DENTREX INC.**
7114 State Road
P.O. Box 17643
Philadelphia, PA 19135
(800) 344-2223
(215) 331-1242
FAX: (800) 446-9512

266. **DENTRONIX, INC.**
101 Steamwhistle Drive
Ivyland, PA 18974
(800) 523-5944
(215) 322-4220
FAX: (215) 364-8607

267. **DENTSPLY INT'L., INC.**
570 West College Avenue
P.O. Box 872
York, PA 17405
(800) 877-0020
(717) 845-7511
FAX: (717) 854-2343 ext. 565

268. **DENTURE LAB, INC., THE**
(Mfr. name change. See Lab One)

269. **DENT-X**
250 Clearbrook Road
Elmsford, NY 10523
(800) 225-1702
(914) 592-6665
FAX: (914) 592-6148

270. **DENT-ZAR CO.**
6362 Hollywood Boulevard
Suite 214
Los Angeles, CA 90028
(213) 465-3621

271. **DEPLAQUE INC.**
P.O. Box 255
Victor, NY 14564
(716) 924-3190

272. **DEPROCO, INC.**
(See Septodont)

273. **DESIGNS FOR VISION, INC.**
760 Koehler Avenue
Ronkonkoma, NY 11779
(800) 345-4009
(516) 585-3300
FAX: (516) 585-3404

274. **DEXIDE INC.**
7509 Flagstone Drive
Ft. Worth, TX 76118
(800) 645-3378
(817) 589-1454
FAX: (817) 595-3300

275. **DIAL CORP., THE**
(See The Dial Corp.)

276. **DIAMOND ROTARY & CARBIDE INT'L.**
P.O. Box 3092
Winnipeg, Manitoba
Canada, R3C 4E5
(204) 452-9469
FAX: (204) 284-2433

277. **DIAMOND TECHNOLOGIES CO.**
Suite 455
The Mall Office Center
400 Sherburn Lane
Louisville, KY 40207
(502) 893-2503
FAX: (502) 894-8940

D (cont.)

278. DICK PRIVAT DENTAL EQUIP.
23924 Walling Road
Geyserville, CA 95441
(707) 857-3726
FAX: (707) 857-3174

279. DIFFINDERFER SERVICES
6170 Woodside Drive
Rocklin, CA 95677
(916) 784-3537

280. DINE, LESTER A., INC.
Oral Scan Imaging Systems
PGA Commerce Park
351 Hiatt Drive
Palm Beach Gardens, FL 33418
(800) 237-7226
(407) 624-9100
FAX: (407) 624-9103

281. DIOPTICS
51 Zaca Lane
San Luis Obispo, CA 93401
(800) 422-9096
(805) 541-0554
FAX: (805) 541-0812

282. DISPOMED, INC.
118 Hillside Drive
Lewisville, TX 75057
(800) 873-4776
(214) 434-1154
FAX: (214) 221-9299

283. D & M MARKETING
1380 U.S. Highway 37
Libby, MT 59923
(406) 293-6289
FAX: (406) 293-4235

284. DMV CORP.
1024 Military Road
P.O. Box 2829
Zanesville, OH 43702
(800) 522-9465
(614) 452-4787
FAX: (614) 452-4501

285. DOLAN-JENNER IND., INC.
Blueberry Hill Industrial Park
P.O. Box 1020
Woburn, MA 01801
(800) 833-4237
(617) 935-7444
FAX: (617) 938-7219

286. D-O SCIENTIFIC PRODUCTS, INC.
1711 Pine Street
Philadelphia, PA 19103
(215) 545-4570
(215) 735-9469

287. D.R.A.C.
(See Diamond Rotary & Carbide Int'l.)

288. D & R MINER DENTAL
14 Lavina Court
Orinda, CA 94563
(415) 376-5802

289. DREXAM LABORATORIES, INC.
4521 East Virginia Avenue
Denver, CO 80222
(800) 237-3926
(303) 388-1736

290. DR. HOPF GmbH & CO. KG
BayernstraBe 9
D-3012 Langenhagen
Germany
(0511) 78 9924
FAX: 0511-74-1130

291. DUFFIN, DR. STEVEN, DDS, MBA
219-B Madrona Southeast
Salem, OR 97302
(800) 424-2835
(503) 585-8205
FAX: (503) 585-8269

292. DU-MORE, INC.
1751 South 1st
P.O. Box 1167
Rogers, AR 72757
(800) 643-3447
(501) 631-1088
FAX: (501) 631-1934

D (cont.)

293. DUNHALL PHARMACEUTICALS
(Mfr. name change. See Omnii Int'l.)

294. DW TECHNOLOGY
4055 South Spencer Street, #238
Las Vegas, NV 89119
(800) 448-4417
(702) 369-2800
FAX: (702) 734-0755

295. DYNA DENT
151 East Columbine Avenue
Santa Ana, CA 92707
(800) 228-4298 (CA)
(800) 448-8882
(714) 546-4891
FAX: (714) 546-1109

296. DYNA FLEX LTD.
10246 Bach Boulevard
St. Louis, MO 63132
(800) 444-0495
(314) 426-4020
FAX: (314) 429-7575

297. DYNAMIC MKTG. & SERVICES CO.
6010 West Cheyenne
Suite 958
Las Vegas, NV 89108
(800) 677-6789

298. DYNATRONICS RESEARCH CORP.
470 West Lawndale Drive, Bldg. D
Salt Lake City, UT 84115
(800) 874-6251
(801) 485-4739
FAX: (801) 467-5637

E

299. E.A. BECK & CO.
P.O. Box 10859
657 West 19th Street
Costa Mesa, CA 92627
(800) 854-0153
(714) 645-4072
FAX: (714) 645-4085

300. EASTMAN KODAK CO.
HSD/Dental Products
343 State Street
Rochester, NY 14650
(800) 242-2424
(716) 724-4000
FAX: (716) 724-5797

301. ECONO SYSTEMS
P.O. Box 1591
Vienna, VA 22180
(800) 527-2076

302. E & D DENTAL PRODUCTS, INC.
560 Springfield Avenue
Suite 1B
Westfield, NJ 07090
(800) 526-4911
(908) 233-5001
FAX: (908) 233-7811

303. ED-UCATION SYSTEMS
305 West 12th Avenue
P.O. Box 188
Columbus, OH 43210
(614) 292-3830
FAX: (614) 292-7619

304. EFOS, INC.
190 Lawrence Bell Drive
Suite 100
Williamsville, NY 14421
(800) 826-8701
(716) 634-5601
FAX: (716) 634-5698

305. ELECTRO MEDICAL SYSTEMS SA
GH Piquet 17
CH 1347
Le Sentier, Switzerland
41-21-845-4771
FAX: 41-21-845-6963

E (cont.)

306. ELECTRONIC WAVEFORM LAB, INC.
15683 Chemical Lane
Huntington Beach, CA 92649
(800) 874-9283
(213) 598-8513
FAX: (714) 894-3920

307. ELLMAN INT'L. MFG. CO.
1135 Railroad Avenue
Hewlett, NY 11557
(800) 835-5355
(516) 569-1482
FAX: (516) 569-0054

308. EMERY DENTAL
(Mfr. name change. See McCleay
Dental Inc.)

309. EMF CORP.
701 Spencer Road
Ithaca, NY 14850
(800) 456-7070
(607) 272-3320
FAX: (800) 456-3227

310. ENDO TECHNIC CORP.
3002 Dow Avenue
Suite #114
Tustin, CA 92680
(800) 323-3913 (CA)
(800) 323-3917
(714) 838-6499
FAX: (714) 838-0317

311. ENGELHARD CORP./BAKER DENTAL
700 Blair Road
Carteret, NJ 07008
(800) 631-5599
(908) 205-5800
FAX: (908) 205-7453

312. ENGLER ENGINEERING CORP.
1099 East 47th Street
Hialeah, FL 33013
(800) 445-8581
(305) 688-8581
FAX: (305) 685-7671

313. ENVIRO-AMERICAN, INC.
22 Northeast 46th
Oklahoma City, OK 73105
(800) 729-2048
(405) 528-0414
FAX: (405) 528-0416

314. ENVIRONMENTAL AUTOMOTIVE SYST.
13497 Gracie Road
Nevada City, CA 95959
(916) 265-2486
FAX: (916) 265-2486

315. ENVISION IMAGING TECH., INC.
One College Park
8910 Purdue Road
Suite 690
Indianapolis, IN 46268
(800) 432-2442
(317) 879-8700
FAX: (317) 897-4090

316. EPI PRODUCTS
2525 Ocean Park Boulevard
Santa Monica, CA 90405
(800) 444-5347
(213) 399-2525
FAX: (213) 836-7578

317. EQUIMED CORP.
3650 Annapolis Lane
Plymouth, MN 55447
(800) 451-7470
(612) 557-6810
FAX: (612) 557-6814

318. ERA CORP.
2750 Niagra Lane North
Minneapolis, MN 55447
(800) 325-0932
(612) 550-1000
FAX: (612) 550-1237

319. ESMA CHEMICALS, INC.
2689 Waukegan
Highland Pk., IL 60035
(708) 433-6116

E (cont.)

320. ESPE GmbH & CO., KG—U.S. OFFICE
(Mfr. name change. See H.A. Opotow
Consulting Corp.)

321. ESPE-PREMIER SALES CORP.
P.O. Box 111
1710 Romano Drive
Norristown, PA 19404
(800) 344-8235
(215) 277-3800
FAX: (215) 277-4270

322. ESSENCE PERFUME, INC.
321 Lawndale Drive
Salt Lake City, UT 84115
(800) 888-7948
(801) 466-1375
FAX: (801) 467-5969

323. ESSENTIAL DENTAL SYSTEMS, INC.
89 Leuning Street
S. Hackensack, NJ 07606
(800) 223-5394
(201) 487-9090
FAX: (212) 487-5120

324. EURO-CON PLUS INC.
217 East 85th Street
Suite 189
New York, NY 10028
(800) 338-9909
(212) 288-2228
FAX: (212) 734-1881

325. EVAPORATED METAL FILMS
(Mfr. name change. See EMF Corp.)

326. EVELYN CO., INC., THE
(See The Evelyn Company, Inc.)

327. EVIDENT DENTAL CO. LTD.
110 Gloucester Avenue
Primrose Hill
London, England NWI 8HX
071-722-0072
FAX: 071-722-0976

328. EXPENDABLES PLUS/BENCHMARK
20574 Strawn Drive
Redding, CA 96003
(800) 332-4274
(916) 221-1147
FAX: (916) 222-6945

329. EXTRACTION SYSTEMS INC.
P.O. Box 1329
32 Mechanic Avenue
Woonsocket, RI 02895
(401) 769-1113
FAX: (401) 769-1118

330. E-Z FLOSS
P.O. Box 2292
Palm Springs, CA 92263
(800) 458-6872
(800) 227-0208 (CA)
(619) 325-1888
FAX: (619) 325-0290

331. EZ SPECIALTIES INC.
77 Second Avenue
Paterson, NJ 07514
Accept collect calls
(201) 345-0029
FAX: (201) 345-9085

F

332. FAIRFAX DENTAL INC.
2601 South Bayshore Drive
Suite 875
Miami, FL 33133
(800) 233-2305
(305) 859-7233
FAX: (305) 859-7433

333. FEINSTEIN, SAM
15 Franklin Street
Bridgeton, NJ 08302
(609) 455-1382

334. **FILHOL DENTAL**
2 Church Green
Witney
Oxon OX8 6AW
England
44-993-706222
FAX: 44-993-706646

335. **FISHER-SCIENTIFIC**
2170 Martin Avenue
Santa Clara, CA 95050
(800) 766-7000
FAX: (408) 727-4905

336. **FLORIDA PROBE CORP.**
1820 Northeast 23rd Avenue
Gainesville, FL 32609
(800) 443-2756
(904) 372-1142
FAX: (904) 372-0257

337. **FLOSSIE SENAIR-MOT INC.**
(Mfr. name change. See DeNiro)

338. **FLOW X-RAY**
420 Hempstead
West Hempstead, NY 11552
(800) 356-9729
(516) 485-7000
FAX: (516) 485-7012

339. **FLUID ENERGY INC.**
P.O. Box 7207
11616 Wilmar Boulevard
Charlotte, NC 28241
(704) 588-0854
FAX: (704) 588-4949

340. **FOREMOST DENTAL MFG., INC.**
242 South Dean
Englewood, NJ 07631
(201) 894-5500
FAX: (201) 894-0213

341. **FOREST MEDICAL PRODUCTS, INC.**
P.O. Box 989
Hillsboro, OR 97123
(800) 423-3555
(503) 640-3012
FAX: (503) 640-4008

342. **FUJI OPTICAL SYSTEMS, INC.**
170 Knowles Drive
Los Gatos, CA 95030
(800) 634-6244
(408) 866-5466
FAX: (408) 866-5038

G

343. **GAYSO BRIDGE-TECH**
3355 Poplar Avenue, #135 G
Memphis, TN 38111
(800) 662-2033
(901) 324-1901

344. **GC AMERICA INC.**
3737 West 127th Street
Chicago, IL 60658
(800) 323-7063
(708) 597-0900
FAX: (708) 371-5103

345. **GC INTERNATIONAL CORP.**
(Mfr. name change. See GC America Inc.)

346. **GC INT'L. CORP. (JAPAN)**
76-1, Hasunuma-cho
Itabashi-Ku
Tokyo 174, Japan
03-3-558-5181
FAX: 03-3-966-1470

347. **GEBAUER CO.**
9410 Saint Catherine Avenue
Cleveland, OH 44104
(800) 321-9348
(216) 271-5252
FAX: (216) 271-5335

348. **GEL-KAM CORP.**
P.O. Box 800009
Dallas, TX 75380
(800) 527-0222
(214) 233-2800
FAX: (214) 239-6859

349. **GENDEX CORP.**
Box 21004
Milwaukee, WI 53221
(800) 558-2900
(414) 769-2888
FAX: (414) 769-2868

350. **GENERAL DENTAL PRODUCTS, INC.**
2281 East Devon Avenue
Elk Grove Village, IL 60007
(708) 595-3930
FAX: (708) 595-2115

351. **GENERAL REFINERIES, INC.**
7227 North Hamlin Avenue
Skokie, IL 60076
(800) 323-4352
(708) 679-3400
FAX: (708) 679-2080

352. **GENT-L-KLEEN PRODUCTS, INC.**
3445 Board Road
York, PA 17402
(800) 233-9382
(717) 767-6881
FAX: (717) 767-6888

353. **GERI, INC.**
P.O. Box 9086
North St. Paul, MN 55109
(612) 681-9388
FAX: (612) 681-9388

354. **G. HARTZELL & SON**
2372 Stanwell Circle
P.O. Box 5988
Concord, CA 94520
(415) 798-2206
FAX: (415) 798-2053

355. **G.H. PORT DENTAL LABS**
150A Liverpool Street
Sidney, Australia 2010
011-61-2-360-6605

356. **GILCOM TECHNOLOGY, INC.**
10115 East Mill Plain
Vancouver, WA 98664
(800) 872-6444
(206) 892-5400
FAX: (206) 892-5533

357. **GILKERSON, DR. ROBERT**
3259 East Sunshine
Springfield, MO 65804
(417) 881-5115

358. **GILL MECHANICAL CO.**
P.O. Box 7247
Eugene, OR 97401
(503) 686-1606
FAX: (503) 342-1193

359. **GINGI-PAK**
P O. Box 240
4825 Calle Alto
Camarillo, CA 93011
(800) 437-1514
(805) 484-1051
FAX: (805) 484-5076

360. **GIRRBACH DENTAL GmbH**
P.O. Box 140120
Duerrenweg 40
D-7530 Pforzheim 14
Germany
(800) 638-6041 (USA)
07231-5804-0 (Germany)
FAX: (707) 539-8900 (USA)

361. **GLENROE TECHNOLOGIES**
2060 Whitfield Park Avenue
Sarasota, FL 34243
(800) 237-4060
(813) 753-8925
FAX: (813) 753-8926

362. **GLIDEWELL LABORATORIES**
303 West Palm
Orange, CA 92666
(800) 854-7256
(714) 633-3104
FAX: (714) 633-5249

363. **GLOBAL DENTAL PROD. CO., INC.**
2465 Jerusalem Avenue
P.O. Box 537
North Bellmore, NY 11710
(516) 221-8844
FAX: (516) 785-7885

364. **GNATHOS DENTAL PROD., INC.**
P.O. Box 655
Weston, MA 02193
(800) 325-0285
(617) 237-6029
FAX: (617) 237-1168

365. **GOFF, DR. CLIFF**
450 39th Street
Ogden, UT 84403
(801) 621-4422

366. **GO-JO INDUSTRIES**
P.O. Box 991
Akron, OH 44309
(800) 321-9647
(216) 920-8100
FAX: (216) 920-8119

367. **GOLDSMITH & REVERE**
242 South Dean Street
Englewood, NJ 07631
(201) 894-5500
FAX: (201) 894-0213

368. **GORE, W.L. & ASSOC., INC**
(See W.L. Gore & Associates, Inc.)

369. **GORLECHEN, DR. NORMAN S.**
21 Huckleberry Lane
Oyster Bay, NY 11771
(516) 922-3831

370. **G.P. DENTAL PRODUCTS, INC.**
6011-S 27th Street
Greenfield, WI 53221
(800) 236-7677 ext. 282
(414) 282-6440

371. **GREAT LAKES ORTHODONTIC PROD.**
199 Fire Tower Drive
Tonawanda, NY 14150
(800) 828-7626
(716) 695-6251
FAX: (716) 695-0810

372. **GREEN, WARREN H., INC**
8356 Olive Boulevard
St. Louis, MO 63132
(800) 537-0655
(314) 991-1335
FAX: (314) 997-1788

373. **GRESCO PRODUCTS INC.**
12603 Executive Drive
Suite 814
Stafford, TX 77477
(800) 527-3250
(713) 240-1811
FAX: (713) 240-2371

374. **GUARD AID**
271 Reservation Road
Suite #101
Marina, CA 93933
(408) 384-8020

H

375. **HALKYARD, DR. DOUGLAS**
110 East Jackson Street
Morris, IL 60450
(815) 942-0832

376. **HALL SURGICAL**
P.O. Box 730
1170 Mark Avenue
Carpinteria, CA 93013
(800) 544-3844
(805) 684-0356
FAX: (805) 684-3185

377. **H.A.L. PRODUCTS**
Dental Products Division
1457 Eastwind Circle
Westlake Village, CA 91361
(800) 962-7056
(818) 991-2081

378. **HAMILL, DR. MAURICE R., JR.**
Martin Building
1127 Norwood Street
Suite 201
Radford, VA 24141
(703) 639-0111
FAX: (703) 639-6111

379. **HAMLIN ASSOC., LTD.**
P.O. Box 932
Newtown, PA 18940
(215) 741-3559

380. **HAMPTON RESEARCH & ENG., INC.**
2670 West Interstate 40
Oklahoma City, OK 73108
(405) 232-5103
FAX: (405) 232-5104

381. **HANDLER MFR. CO., INC.**
P.O. Box 520
612 North Avenue, East
Westfield, NJ 07090
(800) 274-2635
(908) 233-7796
FAX: (908) 233-7340

382. **H.A. OPOTOW CONSULTING CORP.**
200 Lake Avenue #205
Lake Worth, FL 33460
(407) 586-7500
FAX: (407) 586-0315

383. **HARMONY-O-PRESS**
c/o Dr. Gary C. Hunt
85 Braemar Drive
Hillsborough, CA 94010
(415) 343-7010

384. **HARTZELL & SON, G.**
(See G. Hartzell & Son)

385. **HASCOM, INC.**
(Health & Safety Communications)
15110 Southwest Lower Boonsferry
Lake Oswego, OR 97035
(800) 348-7747
(503) 697-3881
FAX: (503) 697-7144

386. **HEALTH CAREER LEARNING SYST.**
37557 Schoolcraft
Livonia, MI 48150
(800) 899-4257
(313) 462-0550
FAX: (313) 462-2055

387. **HEALTHCO INT'L., INC.**
25 Stuart Street
Boston, MA 02116
(800) 225-2360
(617) 423-6045
FAX: (617) 423-6220

388. **HEALTHFIRST CORP.**
P.O. Box 279
Edmonds, WA 98020
(800) 331-1984
(206) 771-5733
FAX: (206) 775-2374

389. **HEALTHPAK, INC.**
607 West Jefferson Street
Shorewood, IL 60436
(800) 777-4725
(815) 744-4725
FAX: (815) 744-4734

390. **HEALTH SONICS CORP.**
1056 Serpentine Lane
Pleasanton, CA 94566
(800) 342-3096
(510) 462-4610
FAX: (510) 462-8024

391. **HERAEUS KULZER GmbH**
IM Dammwald 21
Postfach 1320
D-6382 Friedrichsdorf 1
Germany
06172/732-0
FAX: 011-49-6172-74689

392. **HERAEUS KULZER, INC. USA**
10005 Muirlands Boulevard, Unit G
Irvine, CA 92718
(800) 854-4003
(714) 770-0219
FAX: (714) 770-5019

393. **HERITAGE COMMUNICATIONS**
11469 Lippelman Road
Cincinnati, OH 45246
(513) 771-2230

394. **HERRCO ENTERPRISES, INC.**
1219-B Greenwood Road
Baltimore, MD 21208
(800) 522-3678
(301) 486-7274
FAX: (301) 486-9091

395. **HIGA MFG. LTD.**
P.O. Box 91160
West Vancouver, B.C.
Canada V7V 3N6
(604) 922-5261
FAX: (604) 922-5261

396. **HIT INC.**
1700 Pine Avenue
Niagara Falls, NY 14301
(416) 356-0848
FAX: (416) 356-6330

397. **HOBON**
P.O. Box 8243
Naples, FL 33941
(800) 521-7722
(813) 643-4636

398. **HO DENTAL CO.**
966 Embarcadero del Mar
Goleta, CA 93117
(800) 635-0555
(805) 968-8620
FAX: (805) 685-2125

399. **HOLMES DENTAL CO.**
P.O. Box 243
Hatboro, PA 19040
(800) 322-5577
(215) 675-2877
FAX: (215) 675-7147

400. **HOOKER SALES CO.**
707 West Givens Street
Box 295
Tavares, FL 32778
(800) 359-5180
(904) 343-5171
FAX: (904) 343-4700

401. **HTI SIME DARBY**
(Mfr. name change. See Sime Health
Limited)

402. **HU-FRIEDY CO.**
3232 North Rockwell Street
Chicago, IL 60618
(312) 975-6100
FAX: (312) 975-1683

403. **HUGHES, DR. THOMAS E., DDS**
5312 Comercio Lane
Woodland Hills, CA 91364
(818) 340-0416

404. **HUKUBA DENTAL CORP.**
914-1 Nazukari
Nagareyama-City, Chiba
270-01, Japan
0471-45-3516
FAX: 0471-45-3546

405. **HUNTINGTON LABORATORIES**
970 East Tipton Street
Huntington, IN 46750
(800) 537-5724
(219) 356-8100
FAX: (219) 356-6485

406. **HURD DENTAL LABORATORY INC.**
413½ North 20th Avenue
Yakima, WA 98902
(509) 452-8229

407. **H.W. ANDERSON PRODUCTS, INC.**
Health Science Park
Box 1050
Chapel Hill, NC 27514
(919) 376-3000
FAX: (919) 376-8153

408. **HYDRO FLOSS, INC.**
404 Business Center Drive
Birmingham, AL 35244
(800) 322-7955
(205) 733-1352
FAX: (205) 733-1353

409. **HYGENIC, THE CORP.**
(See The Hygenic Corp.)

410. **ICHTHYS ENTERPRISES**
P.O. Box 9424
Mobile, AL 36691
(800) 288-8765
(205) 443-9626

411. **ICN PHARMACEUTICALS, INC.**
3300 Hyland Avenue
Costa Mesa, CA 92626
(800) 548-5100
(714) 545-0100
FAX: (714) 556-0131

412. **I.C. PUBLICATIONS**
1150 East Nicholls Road
Fruit Heights, UT 84037
(801) 544-2146
FAX: (801) 544-2146

413. **I.D.E. INTERSTATE**
1500 New Horizon Boulevard
Amityville, NY 11701
(800) 666-8100
(516) 957-8300
FAX: (516) 957-1678

414. **IDENTALLOY COUNCIL**
205 Nassau Street
Princeton, NJ 08540
(908) 921-7740
FAX: (908) 651-8491

415. **IDENT CORP. OF AMERICA**
11709 Old Ballas Road, Suite 203
Creve Coeur, MO 63141
(314) 569-2635

416. **IDENTOFLEX A.G.**
Postfach 440
CH-9470 BUCHS
Switzerland
4185-6-63-67
FAX: 4185-6-13-32

417. **I.E.A. (ISHIYAKU EURO/AMERICA,
INC., PUB.)**
716 Hanley Industrial Court
St. Louis, MO 63144
(800) 633-1921
(314) 644-4322
FAX: (314) 644-9532

418. **IMAGES INT'L.**
150 East 400 North
Salem, UT 84653
(801) 423-2800
FAX: (801) 423-2350

419. **IMPLANT INNOVATIONS INC.**
1897 Palm Beach Lakes Boulevard
Suite 117
West Palm Beach, FL 33409
(800) 443-8166
(407) 683-9028
FAX: (407) 683-3515

420. **IMPLANT SUPPORT SYSTEMS**
4790 Irvine Boulevard
#105-137
Irvine, CA 92720
(800) 338-5620
(714) 259-8221
FAX: (714) 259-8288

421. **INDISPERSE INDUSTRIES INC.**
4080 E.C. Row, Unit 25
Windsor, Ontario
Canada N9A 6J3
(519) 948-8556
FAX: (519) 973-1108

422. **INDUSTRIAL SPECIALTIES, INC.**
2741 West Oxford, Unit #6
Englewood, CO 80110
(303) 781-8486
FAX: (303) 761-7939

423. **INFECTION CONTROL SERVICES INC.**
115 Tillicum Street
Renton, WA 98055
(206) 271-5394

424. **INFECTION CONTROL SYSTEMS, INC.**
3095 Kerner Boulevard
San Rafael, CA 94901
(800) 835-3003
(415) 459-0367
FAX: (415) 459-0553

425. **INLAND DENTAL DISTRIBUTORS**
10569 111th Street
Edmonton, Alberta
Canada T5H 3E8
(403) 420-6901
FAX: (403) 425-2241

426. **INNOVATIVE DENTAL DESIGNS**
4411 Bee Ridge Road
Suite 405
Sarasota, FL 34233
(800) 735-1264
(813) 925-1264

427. **INNOVATORS, INC.**
2721 Industrial Drive
Jefferson City, MO 65109
(800) 347-0985
(314) 893-4888
FAX: (314) 893-5244

428. **INTECARE INC.**
1303 Clear Springs Trace
Suite 210
Louisville, KY 40223
(800) 548-9089
(502) 426-6323
FAX: (502) 429-5208

429. **INTERNATIONAL SPECIALTY
DISCOUNT DENTAL SUPPLY**
2435 South West Timberline Drive
Portland, OR 97225
(800) 232-7345
(503) 228-1499
FAX: (503) 297-5936

430. **INTERPORE INT'L.**
P.O. Box 19369
Irvine, CA 92714
(800) 722-4489
(714) 261-3100
FAX: (714) 261-9409

431. **INTERSTATE DENTAL EQUIPMENT
& SUPPLY INC.**
(See Patterson Dental)

432. **ISLAND POLY**
514 Grand Boulevard
Westbury, NY 11590
(800) 338-4433
(516) 338-4433
FAX: (516) 338-4405

433. **IVIE TAILORING**
P.O. Box 538
Gunnison, UT 84634
(801) 528-7097

434. **IVOCLAR NORTH AMERICA**
(Williams-Ivoclar-Vivadent)
175 Pineview Drive
Amherst, NY 14228
(800) 533-6825
(716) 691-0010
FAX: (716) 691-2285

435. **IVOCLAR-VIVADENT CANADA**
23 Hannover Drive
Saint Katherines, Ontario
Canada L2W 1A3
(416) 988-5400
FAX: (416) 244-8286

436. **JAMES MARTIN CORP.**
P.O. Box #993
Edmonds, WA 98020
(206) 778-8350

437. **JAVA CROWN, INC.**
6111 FM 1960 West
Suite 215
Houston, TX 77069
(800) 322-5282
(713) 583-9373

438. **JAYTEC, INC.**
520 West 9th
Winfield, KS 67156
(800) 336-4737
(316) 221-2460

439. **J.B. DENTAL SUPPLY CO.**
7301 Southwest Kable Lane #100
Portland, OR 97224
(800) 777-0577
(503) 624-0603
FAX: (503) 639-7177

440. **JELENKO, J.F. & CO.**
99 Business Park Drive
Armonk, NY 10504
(800) 431-1785
(914) 273-8600
FAX: (914) 273-9379

441. **JENERIC/PENTRON INC.**
53 North Plains Industrial Road
P.O. Box 724
Wallingford, CT 06492
(800) 243-3969
(203) 265-7397
FAX: (203) 284-3310

442. **JENNIFER de ST. GEORGES & ASSOC.,
INC.**
P.O. Box 35640
Monte Sereno, CA 95030
(800) 366-7004
(408) 354-4144
FAX: (408) 354-1931

443. **JENSEN INDUSTRIES, INC.**
50 Stillman Road
North Haven, CT 06473
(800) 243-2000
(203) 239-2090
FAX: (203) 234-7176

444. **J.L. BLOSSER, INC.**
22 North Main Street
Liberty, MO 64068
(800) 445-9528
(816) 781-3206
FAX: (816) 781-0164

445. **J.M. NEY CO.**
Ney Industrial Park
Bloomfield, CT 06002
(800) 243-1942
(203) 242-2281
FAX: (203) 242-5688

446. **J. MORITA**
(See Morita, J. USA Inc.)

447. **JOHNSON & JOHNSON CONSUMER
PRODUCTS**
Professional Dental Division
199 Grandview Road
Skillman, NJ 08558
(800) 526-3967
(908) 874-1000
FAX: (908) 874-2545

J (cont.)

448. JOHNSON & JOHNSON MEDICAL, INC.
(For Johnson & Johnson asepsis prod.)
P.O. Box 130
Arlington, TX 76004
(800) 433-5170
(817) 465-3141
FAX: (817) 784-5468

449. JONES, TED
14065 Victoria Trail
Suite 206
Edmonton, Alberta
Canada T5Y 2B6
(403) 476-3358

450. J.S. DENTAL MFG., INC.
P.O. Box 904
Ridgefield, CT 06877
(800) 284-3368
(203) 438-8832
FAX: (203) 431-8485

451. JUMAR CORP.
P.O. Box 5252
Carefree, AZ 85377
(602) 488-0881
FAX: (602) 488-0940

K

452. KAYCOR INT'L. LTD.
3611 Commercial
Northbrook, IL 60062
(800) 323-4612
(708) 564-4334
FAX: (708) 564-9040

453. KEELER INSTRUMENTS INC.
456 Parkway
Broomall, PA 19008
(800) 523-5620
(215) 353-4350
FAX: (215) 353-7814

454. KEITH ILLUMINATION CORP.
61963 West Road
P.O. Box 908
La Grande, OR 97850
(800) 433-9698
(503) 963-3616
FAX: (503) 963-9406

455. KELLER LABORATORIES INC.
10966 Gravois Industrial Court
St. Louis, MO 63128
(800) 325-3056
(312) 842-4320

456. KEM PUBLISHING
4318 South Eastern Avenue
P.O. Box 28734
Las Vegas, NV 89126
(702) 735-0612

457. KENT DENTAL INC.
25 Commerce Drive
Aston, PA 19014
(800) 345-8202
(215) 485-7400
FAX: (215) 485-0723

458. KERR MFG. CO.
P.O. Box 455
28200 Wick Road
Romulus, MI 48174
(800) 537-7123
(313) 946-7800
FAX: (313) 946-8316

459. KERSTEN MFG./R & D
2767 Quail Valley Road
Solvang, CA 93463
(805) 688-9786
FAX: (805) 688-9786

460. KILGORE INT'L., INC.
P.O. Box 98
Coldwater, MI 49036
(800) 892-9999
(517) 279-9000
FAX: (517) 278-2956

K (cont.)

461. KINETIC INSTRUMENTS INC.
Berkshire Boulevard
Bethel, CT 06801
(800) 233-2346
(203) 743-0080
FAX: (203) 790-1227

462. KINGSWOOD LABORATORIES, INC.
10375 Hague Road
Indianapolis, IN 46256
(317) 849-9513
FAX: (317) 849-9514

463. KINKHORST & ASSOC.
4540 Persimmon Road
Reno, NV 89502
(702) 829-8652

464. KISCO
232 North Seneca
Wichita, KS 67203
(800) 325-8649
(316) 262-1456

465. KLH MEDICAL, INC.
5400 Mitchelldale Street
Suite B-5
Houston, TX 77092
(800) 328-8884
(713) 682-1111
FAX: (713) 682-8884

466. KORAL, DR. STEPHEN M.
2006 Broadway
Boulder, CO 80302
(303) 443-4984

467. KOWA AMERICAN CORP.
1140 Avenue of the Americas
New York, NY 10036
(800) 221-2076
(212) 869-0990
FAX: (212) 869-4457

468. KROMOPAN USA, INC.
1267 Rand Road
Des Plaines, IL 60016
(708) 298-1259
FAX: (708) 803-6229

469. KULZER, INC., USA
(Mfr. name change. See Heraeus
Kulzer, Inc. USA)

470. KURARAY CO. LTD.
Dental Material Department
1-12-39 Shin-Hankyu Building
Umeda, Kita-Ku
Osaka 530, Japan
011-81-6-348-2604
FAX: 011-81-6-348-2552

471. KYOCERA AMERICA, INC.
8611 Balboa Avenue
San Diego, CA 92123
(800) 421-5735
(619) 576-2683
FAX: (619) 694-0157

L

472. LAB ONE
1003 Norfolk Square
Suite 6
Norfolk, VA 23502
(804) 455-8686

473. LAB SAFETY SUPPLY
P.O. Box 1368
Janesville, WI 53547
(800) 356-0783
(608) 754-2345
FAX: (800) 543-9910

474. LACLEDE RESEARCH LABS
15011 Staff Court
Gardena, CA 90248
(800) 922-5856
(213) 770-0463
FAX: (213) 515-1154

475. LACTONA/UNIVERSAL
201 Commerce Drive
Montgomeryville, PA 18936
(800) 523-2559
(215) 368-2000
FAX: (215) 368-1659

L (cont.)

476. LA-MAN CORP.
P.O. Box 487
100 Homestead Drive
Hamilton, IN 46742
(800) 348-2463
(219) 488-3511
FAX: (219) 488-3409

477. LA MAR INDUSTRIES
645-2 Woodside Sierra
Sacramento, CA 95825
(916) 971-1712

478. LANCER ORTHODONTICS, INC.
6050 Avenida Encinas
P.O. Box 819
Carlsbad, CA 92008
(800) 854-2896
(619) 438-4112
FAX: (619) 438-3637

479. LANG DENTAL MFG. CO., INC.
P.O. Box 969
175 Messner Drive
Wheeling, IL 60090
(800) 222-5264
(708) 215-6622
FAX: (708) 215-6680

480. LARES RESEARCH
295 Lockheed Avenue
Chico, CA 95926
(800) 347-3289
(916) 345-1767
FAX: (415) 345-1870

481. LAWHORN INNOVATIONS
218 East Front Street
Suite 302
Missoula, MT 59802
(406) 543-3777

482. L.D. CAULK/DENTSPLY
Lakeview & Clarke Avenues
P.O. Box 359
Milford, DE 19963
(800) 532-2855
(302) 422-4511
FAX: (800) 788-4110

483. LEARNING RESOURCES SERVICES
VA Medical Center
Washington, D.C. 20054
(202) 745-8458
FAX: (202) 745-8274

484. LEE PHARMACEUTICALS
1444 Santa Anita Avenue
P.O. Box 3836
South El Monte, CA 91733
(800) 423-4173
(818) 442-3141
FAX: (818) 578-8607

485. LEHN & FINK
(See L & F Products Inc.)

486. L & F PRODUCTS INC.
225 Summit Avenue
Montvale, NJ 07645
(800) 526-0321
(201) 573-5700
FAX: (201) 573-6046

**487. LIFECORE BIOMEDICAL, INC./
ORTHOMATRIX DIVISION**
3515 Lyman Boulevard
Chaska, MN 55318
(800) 752-2663
(612) 368-4300
FAX: (612) 368-3411

488. LIFE-TECH, INC.
10920 Kinghurst
P.O. Box 36221
Houston, TX 77236
(800) 231-9841
(713) 495-9411
FAX: (713) 495-7960

489. LINK ERGONOMICS DIV.
3149 California Boulevard, Suite C
P.O. Box 2877
Napa, CA 94558
(800) 424-5465
(707) 255-4822
FAX: (707) 255-7191

L (cont.)

490. L & L DENTAL
1480 Wharton Way
Concord, CA 94521
(415) 689-2900

491. LORVIC CORP.
8810 Frost Avenue
St. Louis, MO 63134
(314) 524-7444
FAX: (314) 524-7446

492. LOUDON AMALGAM VACUUM TRAPS
(Mfr. name change. See Professional
Technology Inc.)

493. L & R MFG. CO.
577 Elm Street
Kearny, NJ 07032
(800) 572-5326
(201) 991-5330
FAX: (201) 991-5870

494. LUCKMAN CORP.
1930 Old York Road
Abington, PA 19001
(215) 659-1664
FAX: (215) 659-5506

495. LUSTGARTEN MULTI-TECH INT'L.
73 Dalton Road
Suite 8-B
Holliston, MA 01746
(508) 429-7225
FAX: (508) 429-7306

496. LUXAR CORP.
11816 North Creek Parkway, North
Suite 102
Bothell, WA 98011
(206) 483-4142
FAX: (206) 483-6844

497. LYNCH, JOSEPH A.
51 East First Avenue
Hialeah, FL 33010
(305) 888-2756

M

498. MACAN ENGINEERING & MFG. CO.
1564 North Damen
Chicago, IL 60622
(312) 772-2000
FAX: (312) 772-2003

499. MACK BLEVINS ENTERPRISES
819 Southeast Madison Boulevard
Bartlesville, OK 74006
(800) 654-7311
(918) 335-1455
FAX: (918) 335-1789

500. MACROCHEM CORP.
9 Linnell Circle
Billerica, MA 01821
(800) 622-3685
(508) 670-5800
FAX: (508) 670-5824

501. MADA EQUIPMENT CO., INC.
60 Commerce Road
Carlstadt, NJ 07072
(800) 332-6232
(201) 460-0454
FAX: (201) 460-3509

502. MADAUS MEDTEC INC.
901 Bethlehem Pike
Spring House, PA 19477
(215) 641-0544
FAX: (215) 641-0756

503. MAJESTIC DRUG CO., INC.
711 East 134th Street
Bronx, NY 10454
(800) 238-0220
(212) 292-1310
FAX: (212) 292-2835

504. MARION MERRELL DOW
Consumer Products Division
10123 Alliance Road
Cincinnati, OH 45242
(513) 948-9111
FAX: (513) 948-7311

505. **MARKLINE BUSINESS PROD. CO.**
P.O. Box 171
Belmont, MA 02178
(800) 343-8572
(617) 891-8954
FAX: (617) 899-9833

506. **MARTIN FOX CO.**
Custom Aluminum Bur Blocks
10320 Bilston
St. Louis, MO 63141
(314) 567-1833

507. **MASEL INC.**
2701 Bartram Road
Bristol, PA 19007
(800) 423-8227
(215) 785-1600
FAX: (215) 785-1680

508. **MASTERS SERIES VIDEO STUDY CLUB**
3553 Wheeler Road
Agusta, GA 30909
(800) 521-8913
(404) 738-8070

509. **MASTERSONICS, INC.**
12877 Industrial Drive
Granger, IN 46530
(219) 277-0210
FAX: (219) 277-0210

510. **MATECH, INC.**
13038 San Fernando Road
Sylmar, CA 91342
(800) 292-6620
(818) 367-1745

511. **MAY PELL CHEMICAL DEV. CO.**
211 South Street
Davison, MI 48423
(313) 653-1830

512. **McBINN LTD., INC.**
1948 East Kenwood Drive
St. Paul, MN 55117
(612) 771-3148
FAX: (612) 778-9610

513. **McCLEAY DENTAL INC.**
422 Lancaster Northeast
Salem, OR 97301
(800) 367-1993
(503) 378-0523

514. **McHENRY LABORATORIES, INC.**
118 North Wells
Edna, TX 77957
(512) 782-7617
FAX: (512) 782-5438

515. **M-DEC**
16604 Southeast 17th Place
Bellevue, WA 98008
(800) 321-6332
(206) 747-5424
FAX: (206) 746-6332

516. **M & D INT'L. ENTERPRISES**
P.O. Box 1294
517 Maple Avenue
Carpinteria, CA 93013
(805) 684-4528
FAX: (805) 684-5207

517. **M.D. PRODUCTS, INC.**
4720 Southeast Fort King Street
Ocala, FL 32671
(800) 255-5493
(904) 694-5776
FAX: (904) 694-7330

518. **MDS PRODUCTS, INC.**
American Diversified Dental Systems
1440 South State College Boulevard
Suite 3H
Anaheim, CA 92806
(800) 637-2337
(714) 991-1371
FAX: (714) 991-9540

519. **MDT CORP.**
19645 Rancho Way
Rancho Dominiquez, CA 90220
(800) 347-4638
(213) (608)-2290
FAX: (213) 618-9105

520. **MEDICAL I.D. SYSTEMS, INC.**
3954 44th Street Southeast
Grand Rapids, MI 49512
(800) 262-2399
(616) 698-0535
FAX: (616) 698-0603

521. **MEDICAL LETTER, INC., THE**
(See The Medical Letter, Inc.)

522. **MEDICAL SYSTEMS RESEARCH INC.**
130 South Redwood Road
Building "G"
North Salt Lake, UT 84054
We accept collect calls
(801) 292-5353

523. **MEDIDENTA INT'L., INC.**
39-23 62nd Street
P.O. Box 409
Woodside, NY 11377
(800) 221-0750
(718) 672-4670
FAX: (718) 565-6208

524. **MEDIMARK**
2651 East Chapman Avenue
Suite 101
Fullerton, CA 92631
(800) 548-9389
(714) 526-5168
FAX: (714) 526-5669

525. **MED-INDEX**
5225 Wiley Post Way
Suite #500
Salt Lake City, UT 84116
(801) 536-1000
FAX: (801) 536-1009

526. **MEDITOX, INC.**
1239 East Newport Center Drive
Suite 114
Deerfield, Beach, FL 33442
(305) 429-1004
FAX: (305) 429-1008

527. **MEISINGER**
c/o F. Scherer & Co.
6831 Aura Avenue
Reseda, CA 91335
(818) 609-9605
FAX: (818) 609-9615

528. **MELALEUCA, INC.**
560 Broadway
Idaho Falls, ID 83402
(800) 522-3156
(208) 522-0700
FAX: (208) 524-7413

529. **MELTON, JOHN C.**
120 West Chestnut
Las Cruces, NM 88005
(505) 524-2001

530. **MERCK, SHARP & DOHME**
P.O. Box 4
West Point, PA 19486
(800) 637-2579
(215) 661-5000

531. **MERLIN DENTAL PRODUCTS**
131 Chesterfield Road
Box 573
Bogart, GA 30622
(800) 828-6521

532. **METREX RESEARCH CORP.**
P.O. Box 646
Parker, CO 80134
(800) 841-1428
(303) 841-5842
FAX: (303) 841-5915

533. **METTLER ELECTRONICS CORP.**
1333 South Claudina Street
Anaheim, CA 92805
(800) 854-9305
(714) 533-2221
FAX: (714) 635-7539

534. **MICROBEX ASEPTICS INC.**
680 Denison Street
Markham, Ontario
Canada, L3R 1C1
(416) 477-5442
FAX: (416) 477-0740

535. **MICROCOPY**
3120 Moon Station Road
P.O. Box 2017
Kennesaw, GA 30144
(800) 235-1863
(404) 425-5715
FAX: (404) 423-4996

536. **MICROCOR, INC.**
424 East 500 South, Suite 109
Salt Lake City, UT 84111
(801) 596-2300
FAX: (801) 596-1999

537. **MICRODONTICS**
100 Northfield Avenue
West Orange, NJ 07052
(201) 731-4800
FAX: (201) 731-1153

538. **MICRON SPECIALISTS, INC.**
5948 East Corrine Drive
Scottsdale, AZ 85254
(602) 991-4801

539. **MICR-O-REG**
40-49 74th Street
Jackson Heights, NY 11373
(718) 429-7555

540. **MICRO-VAC INC.**
4132 East Speedway Boulevard
Tucson, AZ 85712
(800) 729-1020
(602) 325-2968
FAX: (602) 327-6659

541. **MICRO-VIBE CO.**
P.O. Box 8547
South Main Street
Penacook, NH 03303
(603) 763-5892

542. **MIDWEST DENTAL PRODUCTS CORP.**
901 West Oakton Street
Des Plaines, IL 60018
(708) 640-4800
FAX: (708) 640-6165

543. **MILES INC. DENTAL PROD.**
4315 South Lafayette Boulevard
South Bend, IN 46614
(800) 343-5336
(219) 291-0661
FAX: (219) 291-0720

544. **MILLSTEIN, DR. PHILIP L.**
15 Langdon Street
Cambridge, MA 02138
(617) 864-3446

545. **MILTEX INSTRUMENT CO., INC.**
6 Ohio Drive
Lake Success, NY 11042
(800) 645-8000
(516) 775-7100
FAX: (516) 775-7185

546. **MINIATURE SPECIALISTS, INC.**
(Mfr. name change. See Micron
Specialists, Inc.)

547. **MINNTECH CORP.**
14605 28th Avenue North
Minneapolis, MN 55447
(800) 328-3340
(612) 553-3300
FAX: (612) 553-3387

548. **MIRAGE DENTAL SYSTEM**
(Mfr. name change. See Chameleon
Dental Prod., Inc.)

549. **MISSION DENTAL, INC.**
2301 Leeds Avenue, Suite 405
Charleston, SC 29405
(800) 323-5087
(803) 745-1690
FAX: (803) 745-1692

550. **MITER, INC.**
P.O. Box 1133
Warsaw, IN 46581
(800) 325-8566
(219) 267-6662
FAX: (219) 267-6157

551. **MIZZY, INC.**
616 Hollywood Avenue
Cherry Hill, NJ 08002
(800) 333-3131
(609) 663-4700
FAX: (609) 663-0381

552. **M & M INNOVATIONS INC.**
4 Carteret Road
Brunswick, GA 31520
(800) 668-3384
(912) 265-7110

553. **M & M PHARMACEUTICALS**
153 Lakeview Circle
Brunswick, GA 31520
(800) 473-2759
(912) 262-9080

554. **MOLLOPLAST REGNERI GmbH &
CO., KG.**
RoonstraBe 23 a
P.O. Box 2106
D-7500 Karlsruhe
Germany
3407000 0
(0721) 8202-0
FAX: 0721-820250

555. **MOLULYCHE HEALTH CARE AB**
S-435 81
Molnlycke, Sweden
46-31-98-50-00
FAX: 46-31-88-32-15

556. **MONARCH LEARNING SYSTEMS**
P.O. Box D.E. (Dental Education)
Pacific Grove, CA 93950
(408) 649-1055
FAX: (408) 649-0567

557. **MOORE, DR. C.E.**
420 Magazine Street
Tupelo, MS 38801
(601) 842-1036

558. **MOORE, E.C. CO., INC.**
13325 Leonard Street
Dearborn, MI 48121
(800) 331-3548
(313) 581-7878
FAX: (313) 581-8348

559. **MORACK, INC.**
9132 Windsor Drive
Palos Hills, IL 60465
(800) 837-9696
(708) 598-0580
FAX: (708) 598-9203

560. **MORITA, J. USA INC.**
14712 Bentley Circle
Tustin, CA 92680
(800) 752-9729
(714) 544-2854
FAX: (714) 730-0783

561. **MOSBY-YEAR BOOK, INC.**
11830 Westline Industrial Drive
St. Louis, MO 63146
(800) 426-4545
(314) 872-8370
FAX: (314) 432-1380

562. **MOTLOID CO., THE**
(See The Motloid Co.)

563. **MOYCO INDUSTRIES, INC.**
S.E. Corner 21st & Clearfield Streets
Philadelphia, PA 19132
(800) 523-3676
(215) 229-0470
FAX: (215) 229-3291

564. **M-R SULLIVAN MFR. CO.**
6115 South Kyrene
Suite 103
Tempe, AZ 85283
(800) 456-2014
(602) 345-2014
FAX: (602) 897-8777

565. MTI PRECISION PRODUCTS
P.O. Box 221
175 Oberlin North Avenue
Lakewood, NJ 08701
(800) 367-9290
(908) 905-7440
FAX: (908) 905-7445

566. MULTIPIX
441 North Water Streets
Silverton, OR 97381
(503) 873-8735

**567. MURDOCK PHARMACEUTICALS, INC./
NUTRITION PROFESSIONALS, INC.**
1400 Mountain Springs Park
Springville, UT 84663
(800) 962-8873
(801) 489-3631
FAX: (801) 489-3639

568. MYDENT RESEARCH CORP.
175 Commerce Drive, Suite M
P.O. Box 12094
Hauppauge, NY 11788
(516) 434-3190
FAX: (516) 434-7750

569. MYO-TRONICS RESEARCH, INC.
720 Olive Way #800
Seattle, WA 98101
(800) 426-0316
(206) 622-2121
FAX: (206) 625-9933

N

570. NAPCOR
9852 Crescent Center Drive
Unit 801
Rancho Cucamonga, CA 91730
(714) 989-1641
FAX: (714) 944-3427

571. NATIONAL DENTAL PRODUCTS
17 Phyllis Drive
East Northport, NY 11731
(516) 499-6279

572. NATIONAL KEYSTONE PRODUCTS CO.
616 Hollywood Avenue
Cherry Hill, NJ 08002
(800) 333-3131
(609) 663-4700
FAX: (609) 663-0381

573. NATIONAL LABORATORIES
225 Summit Avenue
Montvale, NJ 07645
(800) 753-4855
(201) 573-5280
FAX: (201) 573-5275

574. NATIONAL PATIENT MEDICAL
P.O. Box 419 Lake Road
Dayville, CT 06241
(800) 243-1172
(203) 774-8541
FAX: (203) 774-1507

575. NATIONAL SALES COORDINATOR
P.O. Box 30162
Pensacola, FL 32504
(904) 438-4154

576. NATURAL WHITE, INC.
One Argonaut, Suite 200
Aliso Viejo, CA 92656
(800) 544-4915
(714) 454-9008
FAX: (702) 883-4874

577. NATURE'S WAY PRODUCTS, INC.
1375 North Mountain Springs Parkway
Box 4000
Springville, UT 84663
(800) 866-4404
(801) 489-3631
FAX: (801) 489-3639

578. ND LABS INC.
3379 Shore Parkway
Brooklyn, NY 11235
(718) 646-7998
FAX: (718) 646-3028

579. NEOLOY PRODUCTS CO.
14807 South McKinley Avenue
Posen, IL 60469
(800) 628-7336
(708) 371-8880/8881
FAX: (708) 371-8217

580. NETWORK INT'L.
1720 East Garry Avenue
Suite 109
Santa Ana, CA 92705
(714) 863-7133
FAX: (714) 863-7135

581. NEVIN LABORATORIES, INC.
5000 South Halsted Street
Chicago, IL 60609
(800) 544-5337
(312) 624-4330
FAX: (312) 624-7337

582. NEW HORIZONS
Route 3
Box 67
Somerville, AL 35670
(800) 445-0523

583. NEW IMAGE INDUSTRIES INC.
21218 Vanowen Street
Canoga Park, CA 91303
(800) 634-7349
(818) 702-0285
FAX: (818) 702-8868

584. NEW WORLD PROJECTS, INC.
2915 Waters Road
Suite 100
Eagan, MN 55121
(800) 766-2002
(612) 452-3648
FAX: (612) 452-3877

585. NEY, J.M. CO.
(See J.M. Ney Co.)

586. NOBELPHARMA USA, INC.
5101 South Keeler Avenue
Chicago, IL 60632
(800) 621-0176
(312) 735-0600
FAX: (312) 735-1833

587. NOBELPHARMA USA, INC.
Western Division
2425 Colorado Avenue, Suite 212
Santa Monica, CA 90404
(800) 637-3220
(310) 470-7584
FAX: (310) 453-5306

588. NOBILIUM
935 Broadway
P.O. Box 488
Albany, NY 12201
(800) 833-2343
(518) 434-3147
FAX: (518) 434-1288

589. NOIR MEDICAL TECHNOLOGIES
P.O. Box 159
6155 Pontiac Trail
South Lyon, MI 48178
(800) 521-9746
(313) 769-5565
FAX: (313) 769-1708

590. NORDENT MFG., INC.
1374 Jarvis Avenue
Elk Grove Village, IL 60007
(708) 437-4780
FAX: (708) 437-4786

591. NORTHERN ELECTRIC CO.
(Mfr. name change. See Sunbeam
Home Comfort)

592. NORTHWEST DENTAL, INC.
175 Southeast 2nd
Hillsboro, OR 97123
(800) 346-5709
(503) 640-0911/1007
FAX: (503) 693-1431

593. NORTHWEST DENTAL LABORATORY
600 South Federal Highway
Deerfield Beach, FL 33441
(800) 872-1525
(305) 426-4666
FAX: (305) 426-8535

594. NOVOCOL PHARMACEUTICAL, INC.
(See Septodont)

595. NOXLOX, INC.
P.O. Box 701021
West Valley City, UT 84170
(800) 766-9569
(801) 573-4979

596. NUCLEAR ASSOC.
(Division of VICTOREEN)
100 Voice Road
Carle Place, NY 11514
(516) 741-2166
FAX: (516) 741-5414

597. NUDANSU INC.
(Mfr. name change. See Nu-Dent, Inc.)

598. NU-DENT, INC.
145 East 49th Street
8th Floor
New York, NY 10017
(800) 645-4333
(212) 888-4746
FAX: (212) 888-6021

599. NUPERCO, INC.
P.O. Box 689
799 Franklin Avenue
Franklin Lakes, NJ 07417
(800) 672-3368
(201) 891-7027
FAX: (201) 891-0705

O

**600. OFFICE OF OCCUPATIONAL SAFETY
& HEALTH**
D.C. Dept. of Employment Serv.
950 Upshur Street, Northwest
Washington, D.C. 20011
(202) 576-6339

601. OHLENDORF CO.
2840 Clark Avenue
St. Louis, MO 63103
(800) 325-8921
(314) 533-3440
FAX: (314) 533-7331

602. OLSON LABORATORIES, INC.
P.O. Box 171
Port Washington, WI 53074
(414) 284-9755
FAX: (414) 284-7448

603. O.M.I.
P.O. Box 940
Tillamook, OR 97141
(800) 845-8798
(503) 842-4538

604. OMNIA-DENT USA
8895 Lawrence Welk Drive
Escondido, CA 92026
(800) 328-8895
(619) 749-7500

605. OMNIGENE, INC.
85 Bolton Street
Cambridge, MA 02140
(800) 433-0364
(800) 342-6556 (MA)
(617) 576-1966
FAX: (617) 547-9256

606. OMNII INT'L.
P.O. Box 100
Highway 59 North
Gravette, AR 72736
(800) 643-3639
(501) 787-5232
FAX: (501) 787-6507

607. OMNII PRODUCTS INT'L.
1153 East 250 South
Bountiful, UT 84010
(800) 777-2972
(801) 298-7663
FAX: (801) 298-2984

608. OMNITEC MEDICAL CORP.
(Mfr. name change. See Cottrell Ltd.)

609. OP-D-OP INC.
198 Cirby Way
Suite 120
Roseville, CA 95678
FAX: (916) 783-5765

610. ORACHEM PHARMACEUTICALS
9990 Global Road
Philadelphia, PA 19115
(800) 523-0191
(215) 677-5200
FAX: (215) 677-7736

611. ORAL-B LABORATORIES
1 Lagoon Drive
Redwood City, CA 94065
(800) 446-7252
(415) 598-5000
FAX: (415) 592-4059

**612. ORAL CARE/DIVISION OF
PFIZER, INC.**
205 East 42 Street
9th Floor
New York, NY 10017
(212) 573-1400

613. ORAL DYNAMICS, INC.
Division of Anson Int'l.
2209 North 56th
Seattle, WA 98103
(800) 726-1628
(206) 545-7971
FAX: (206) 743-1145

614. ORAL HEALTH U.S.A., INC.
255 Old New Brunswick Road, S-30
Piscataway, NJ 08854
(800) 533-5069
(201) 981-9440
FAX: (201) 981-9443

615. ORAL RESEARCH LABS., INC.
205 42nd Street, 9th Floor
New York, NY 10017
(212) 573-1400
FAX: (212) 573-3894

**616. ORANGE-SOL, INC. DBA/
ACKERMAN DENTAL MFG.**
P.O. Box 306
Chandler, AZ 85224
(800) 877-7771
(602) 497-8822
FAX: (602) 497-0444

617. ORATEC CORP.
485 Spring Park Place
Suite 600
Herdon, VA 22070
(800) 368-3529
(703) 471-0377
FAX: (703) 471-1632

618. ORTEC, INC.
904 Sumneytown Pike
Springhouse, PA 19477
(215) 628-2828

619. ORTHOMATRIX INC.
(Mfr. name change. See Lifecore
Biomedical, Inc./Orthomatrix Div.)

620. ORTHOTRONICS, INC.
29 North Main Street
Gloversville, NY 12078
(800) 800-1410
(518) 725-2455
FAX: (518) 725-9522

621. O'RYAN INDUSTRIES, INC.
12711 Northeast 95th Street
Vancouver, WA 98682
(800) 426-4311
(206) 892-0447
FAX: (206) 892-6742

622. OSADA ELECTRIC CO., INC.
8242 West Third Street
Suite 150
Los Angeles, CA 90048
(800) 426-7232
(213) 651-0711
FAX: (213) 651-4691

623. OSC INNOVATIVE PRODUCTS INC.
Harris Pond Office Park
32 Daniels Webster Highway
Suite 21
Merrimack, NH 03054
(603) 886-0540

624. OSHA
(See Office of Occupational Safety &
Health Association)

625. OSMED INC.
(Mfr. name change. See THM Biomedical Inc./Osmed)

626. O-SO ® ATTACHMENT SYSTEMS/
SCODENCO
P.O. Box 2426
1818 South Cincinnati Avenue
Tulsa, OK 74101
(800) 274-1050
(918) 587-6786

627. OWEN, DR. ALBERT H.
3624 North Hills Drive, #B101
Austin, TX 78731
(512) 345-0311

628. OXYFRESH USA, INC.
P.O. Box 3723
East 12928 Indiana
Spokane, WA 99220
(800) 333-7374
(509) 924-4999
FAX: (509) 924-5285

P

629. PAC-AID CORP.
P.O. Box 404
West Boylston, MA 01583
(508) 835-4111

630. PACIFIC RIM DENTAL INNOVATIONS
2780 Millstream Road
Victoria, British Columbia
Canada, V9B 3S6
(604) 478-4114

631. PAIN PREVENTION, INC.
P.O. Box 301
Vernon Hills, IL 60061
(800) 648-0999

632. PAIN RESOURCE CENTER, INC.
P.O. Box 2836
Durham, NC 27705
(800) 542-7246
(919) 286-9180
FAX: (919) 286-4506

633. PALCO DENTAL/PALMERO SALES
CO., INC.
120 Goodwin Place
Stratford, CT 06497
(800) 344-6424
(203) 377-6424
FAX: (203) 377-8988

634. PALODENT, THE CO.
75 Bear Gulch Drive
Portola Valley, CA 94028
(415) 851-0267

635. PARAMED TECHNOLOGY, INC.
510 Logue Avenue
Mountain View, CA 94043
(800) 421-3257
(415) 961-2545
FAX: (415) 965-1153

636. PARKELL
155 Schmitt Boulevard, Box 376
Farmingdale, NY 11735
(800) 243-7446
(800) 323-6349 (NY)
(516) 249-1134
FAX: (516) 249-1242

637. PARKER, CARL ASSOC., INC.
175 Commerce Drive
P.O. Box 12084
Hauppauge, NY 11788
(516) 434-7760/7810
FAX: (516) 434-7750

638. PASCAL CO., INC.
P.O. Box 1478
Bellevue, WA 98009
(800) 426-8051
(206) 827-4694
FAX: (206) 827-6893

639. PASS-IT CO., THE
(See The Pass-It Co.)

640. PATIENT VIEW SYSTEMS
523 Remington Street
Fort Collins, CO 80524
(800) 283-7843
(303) 482-6891

641. PATTERSON DENTAL CO.
(We deal with Centra)
1100 East 80th Street
Minneapolis, MN 55420
(800) 328-5536
(612) 854-2881
FAX: (612) 854-8381

642. PAULI, DR. RICHARD
3500 LaTouche
Suite #210
Anchorage, AK 99508
(907) 563-3046

643. PEARCE-TURK DENTAL LAB
P.O. Box 760
201 North Emporia
Wichita, KS 67202
(800) 835-2776
(800) 362-2204 (KS)
(316) 263-0284
FAX: (316) 263-5869

644. PEERLESS INT'L., INC.
A & A Industrial Park
228 Tosca Drive
P.O. Box 430
Stoughton, MA 02072
(800) 527-2025
(617) 344-6587
FAX: (617) 344-6040

645. PELTON & CRANE
A Siemens Company
P.O. Box 241147
Charlotte, NC 28224
(800) 659-6560
(704) 523-3212
FAX: (704) 529-5523

646. PERIO-MONITOR SYSTEMS
c/o Dr. Lawrence Snow
372 Central Park West
New York, NY 10025
(212) 663-2269

647. PERLINK USA INC.
290 Stuyvesant Avenue
Rye, NY 10580
(800) 874-0120
(914) 967-7663
FAX: (914) 967-6176

648. PERTUSSIN LABORATORIES
425 Fillmore Avenue
Tonawanda, NY 14150
(800) 828-7669
(716) 694-7100
FAX: (716) 694-0462

649. PETROLEUM PRODUCTS OF AMERICA
8787 East Mt. View #1031
Scottsdale, AZ 85258
(602) 991-6780

650. PFINGST & COMPANY, INC.
P.O. Box 377
105 Snyder Road
South Plainfield, NJ 07080
(800) 221-1268
(201) 561-6400
FAX: (201) 561-3213

651. PFIZER, INC.
(Mfr. name change. See Oral Care,
Division of Pfizer, Inc.)

652. PINNACLE PRODUCTS, INC.
624 South Smith
St. Paul, MN 55107
(612) 222-3042
FAX: (612) 222-3904

653. P.J. MAXWELL CO., INC.
1817 18th Avenue
Rockford, IL 61104
(815) 399-1180
FAX: (815) 398-1047

654. P.J. SPECIALTY CO., INC.
151 South Pfingsten
Unit E
Deerfield, IL 60015
(708) 564-8680
FAX: (708) 564-5033

655. PLAK SMACKER TOOTHBRUSH, INC.
2941 McAllister Avenue
Riverside, CA 92503
(800) 228-9021
(714) 359-3434
FAX: (714) 359-3008

656. PLANMECA, INC.
935 Dillon
Wood Dale, IL 60191
(708) 595-7077
FAX: (708) 595-7135

657. PLASTEK CO.
P.O. Box H
Sturgis, MI 49091
(616) 651-9136
FAX: (616) 651-7810

658. POPE, BRYAN M.
(Mfr. name change. See 21st Century
Health Care Products, Inc.)

659. PORCEMETRIC SYSTEMS, INC.
(Mfr. name change. See PSI Dental
Materials)

660. PORTER INSTRUMENT CO., INC.
Township Line Road
P.O. Box 326
Hatfield, PA 19440
(215) 723-4000
(215) 723-2199

661. POWDERHORN TEXTILES
(Mfr. name change. See CliniCovers—
Division of ClinTex, Inc.)

662. PRACTICE MADE PERFECT, INC.
21800 Devonshire Street
Chatsworth, CA 91311
(818) 341-3642

663. PRACTICE PERSONNEL SYSTEMS
21622 Marguerite Parkway, Suite 535
Mission Viejo, CA 92692
(714) 859-9479
FAX: (714) 859-6951

664. PRACTICON, INC.
4 Doctors Park
Greenville, NC 27834
(800) 334-0956
(919) 752-5183
FAX: (919) 752-2439

665. PREAT CORP.
1120 7th Avenue
San Mateo, CA 94402
(800) 232-7732
(415) 342-5700
FAX: (415) 342-5233

666. PREMIER DENTAL PRODUCTS CO.
1710 Romano Drive
P.O. Box 111
Norristown, PA 19404
(800) 344-8235
(215) 277-3800
FAX: (215) 277-4270

667. PREMIUM LATEX PRODUCTS, INC.
8439 Warner Drive
Culver, CA 90232
(800) 755-4588
(213) 287-0380
FAX: (213) 287-0384

668. PREVENTATIVE SYSTEMS, LTD.
P.O. Box 2664
Fair Oaks, CA 95628
(916) 338-0468

669. PREVENTIVE DENTAL ENTERPRISES
107 Monmouth Street
P.O. Box 8817
Red Bank, NJ 07701
(800) 448-5089
(908) 842-7605
FAX: (908) 842-3633

670. PREVEST, INC.
23420 Lakeland Boulevard
Cleveland, OH 44132
(800) 526-1725
(216) 731-6800
FAX: (216) 731-7390

671. PROCTER & GAMBLE
1 Procter & Gamble Plaza
Cincinnati, OH 45202
(800) 447-4865
(513) 983-1100
FAX: (513) 983-5593

672. PRO-DEN SYSTEMS, INC.
7814 North Interstate
Portland, OR 97217
(800) 252-5863
(503) 285-0733
FAX: (503) 285-5567

673. PRO-DENTEC
P.O. Box 4129
Batesville, AK 72503
(800) 228-5595
(501) 698-2300
FAX: (501) 793-5554

674. PRODUCTIVITY TRAINING CORP.
15900 Concord Circle
Unit 1
Morgan Hill, CA 95037
(800) 448-8855
(408) 776-0433
FAX: (408) 776-0145

675. PROFESSIONAL DENTAL SUPPLIES
PTY. LTD.
4B Bell Street
Yarra Glen, Vic. 3775
Australia
011-61-3-730-1073
FAX: 011-61-3-730-1073

676. PROFESSIONAL LAB SERVICES
125 Walnut Street
Watertown, MA 02172
(800) 634-3480
(617) 923-9616

677. PROFESSIONAL RESULTS, INC.
(Makers of the Tooth Slooth)
29 Merano
Laguna Niguel, CA 92677
(800) 350-3705
(714) 249-3705
FAX: (714) 495-5642

678. PROFESSIONAL TECHNOLOGY INC.
645 Valley Mall Parkway
East Wenatchee, WA 98802
(509) 884-0399
FAX: (509) 884-5599

679. PRO FLOW INC.
1500 New Horizons Boulevard
Amityville, NY 11701
(800) 645-7171
(516) 957-8300
FAX: (516) 957-1678

680. PRO PULSE, INC.
(Mfr. name change. See Vipont
Pharmaceutical)

681. PRO-SAFE PROFESSIONAL LINENS,
INC.
304 West Main Street
Grand Junction, CO 81501
(303) 245-7870
FAX: (303) 241-0771

682. **PRO TECH, INC.**
Dental Products Division
12 Lynhaven Place
Centereach, NY 11720
(800) 872-8898
(516) 732-1144
FAX: (516) 732-1025

683. **PRO TECH INDUSTRIES OF IL, INC.**
P.O. Box 99
Vernon Hills, IL 60061
(800) 477-4776
FAX: (708) 680-4390

684. **PSI DENTAL MATERIALS**
P.O. Box 88988
Atlanta, GA 30356
(800) 443-5459
(404) 395-9422
FAX: (404) 393-2069

685. **PULPDENT CORP.**
80 Oakland Street
P.O. Box 780
Watertown, MA 02272
(800) 343-4342
(617) 926-6666
FAX: (617) 926-6262

686. **PYMAH CORP.**
89 Route 206
P.O. Box 1114
Somerville, NJ 08876
(800) 526-3538
(908) 526-1222
FAX: (908) 526-9358

687. **PYRAMID INC.**
522 North Ninth Avenue East
Newton, IA 50208
(515) 792-2405
FAX: (515) 792-2478

Q

688. **QUALIDENT MFR. CO.**
2910 Weber Drive
Spirit Lake, IA 51360
(712) 336-3037

689. **QUALITY LATEX PRODUCTS, INC.**
P.O. Box 3273
Terre Haute, IN 47803
(800) 292-3273
(812) 235-2122

690. **QUANTUM LABS INC.**
422 5th Avenue
Suite 310
Madison, MN 56256
(800) 328-8213
(612) 545-1984

691. **QUICK INT'L., INC.**
4380 Southeast 57th Lane
Ocala, FL 32671
(904) 867-7034

692. **QUINTESSENCE PUBLISHING CO., INC.**
551 North Kimberly Drive
Carol Stream, IL 60188
(800) 621-0387
(708) 682-3223
FAX: (708) 682-3288

R

693. **RAMVAC CORP.**
120 East Michigan Street
P.O. Box 640
Spearfish, SD 57783
(605) 642-4614
FAX: (605) 642-3776

694. **RECIGNO LABORATORIES INC.**
519 Davisville Road
Willow Grove, PA 19090
(800) 523-2304
(215) 659-7755
FAX: (215) 657-1505

695. **RECSEI LABORATORIES**
330 South Kellogg, Building M
Goleta, CA 93117
(805) 964-2912

696. **REDDI-PRODUCTS CO.**
One Ocean Avenue
Massapequa, NY 11758
(516) 799-1183
FAX: (516) 799-1197

697. **REDWOOD DENTAL SUPPLY**
(Mfr. name change. See Dick Privat
Dental Equip.)

698. **REED & CARNRICK PHARMACEUTICAL**
c/o Block Drug
257 Cornelison Avenue
Jersey City, NJ 07302
(800) 545-5423
(201) 434-3000 ext. 1426
FAX: (201) 434-0842

699. **REGENCY DIAMOND CO.**
11999 Katy Freeway
Suite 388
Houston, TX 77079
(800) 669-3353
(713) 493-3353

700. **REGENT LABS, INC.**
600 South Federal Highway
Deerfield Beach, FL 33441
(800) 872-1525
(305) 426-4403
FAX: (305) 426-8535

701. **RELAX, INC.**
P.O. Box 15815
New Orleans, LA 70175
(504) 895-1137

702. **RELIANCE ORTHODONTIC PRODUCTS**
P.O. Box 678
Itasca, IL 60143
(800) 323-4348
(708) 773-4009
FAX: (708) 250-7704

703. **RESEARCH INFORMATION SERVICES**
One Raleigh Road
Marshfield, MA 02050
(800) 235-6646 ext. 615
(617) 834-6199

704. **RESTORATIVE TECHNICS DIV.**
73 Dalton Road
Suite B
Holliston, MA 01746
(800) 274-2230
(508) 429-7225
FAX: (508) 429-7306

705. **RHELCO INC.**
P.O. Box 325
Easton, CT 06612
(203) 222-9666

706. **RIBBOND INC.**
1003 Cobb Medical Center
Seattle, WA 98101
(800) 624-4554
(206) 624-8500

707. **RICHMOND DENTAL CO.**
P.O. Box 34276
Charlotte, NC 28234
(800) 438-0342
(704) 376-0380
FAX: (704) 342-1892

708. **RIDGELY PRODUCTS, INC.**
18 Gwynns Mills Court
Owings Mills, MD 21117
(301) 581-8860
FAX: (301) 581-8864

709. **RINN CORP.**
1212 Abbott Drive
Elgin, IL 60123
(800) 323-0970
(708) 742-1115
FAX: (800) 544-0787

710. **R.J. LABORATORIES INC.**
3901 MacArthur Boulevard
Suite 200
Newport Beach, CA 92660
(800) 825-8532
(714) 222-5700
FAX: (714) 642-1215

711. **ROBELL RESEARCH**
635 Madison Avenue
New York, NY 10022
(212) 751-3263
FAX: (212) 308-5182

712. **ROCKY MOUNTAIN ORTHODONTICS**
P.O. Box 17085
Denver, CO 80217
(800) 525-6375

713. **RODE, CHAS. W., INC.**
P.O. Box 1238
San Clemente, CA 92674
(714) 492-3524

714. **ROEKO U.S.A. INC.**
75 Union Avenue
Sudbury, MA 01776
(800) 626-7729
(508) 443-7729
FAX: (508) 443-7730

715. **RONVIG DENTAL & KIRURGI**
Gl. Vejlevej 57
DK-8721 Daugaard
Denmark
0-11-45-75-89-57-11
FAX: 0-11-45-75-89-57-44

716. **ROSCO LABS**
36 Bush Avenue
Port Chester, NY 10573
(800) 767-2669
(914) 937-1300
FAX: (914) 937-5984

717. **ROTH INT'L. LTD.**
669 West Ohio Street
Chicago, IL 60610
(800) 445-0572
(312) 733-1478
FAX: (312) 733-7398

718. **ROWLAND CO., THE**
(See The Rowland Co.)

719. **ROYDENT DENTAL PRODUCTS INC.**
6964 Crooks Road, Suite 4
Troy, MI 48098
(800) 992-7767
(313) 828-1019
FAX: (313) 828-1633

720. **RUBIN, DR. ROBERT M.**
302 East Little Creek Road
Norfolk, VA 23505
(804) 583-2333
FAX: (804) 480-2555

721. **RUTHAL INDUSTRIES LTD.**
6059 Jericho Turnpike
Commack, NY 11725
(800) 445-6640
(516) 493-0200
FAX: (516) 543-0777

722. **RX HONING MACHINE CORP.**
1301 East Fifth Street
Mishawaka, IN 46544
(800) 346-6464
(219) 259-1606
FAX: (219) 259-9163

S

723. **SABRA - THE DENTAL PROD. GROUP**
7642 North Kolmar
Skokie, IL 60076
(800) 537-2272
FAX: (708) 675-8722

724. **SAFCO DENTAL SUPPLY CO.**
527 South Jefferson Street
Chicago, IL 60607
(800) 621-2178
(312) 922-8118
FAX: (312) 922-5577

725. **SAFESKIN CORP.**
12520 High Bluff Drive
Suite #290
San Diego, CA 92130
(800) 456-8379
(619) 792-1414
FAX: (619) 792-1433

726. **SAFE T FACE CORP.**
279 South Beverly Drive
Suite 1090
Beverly Hills, CA 90212
(800) 669-3366
(213) 858-6765
FAX: (916) 421-3358

727. **SAFEWARE SUPPLIES**
Division of Safeware, Inc.
200 Inman Terrace
Willow Grove, PA 19090
(215) 659-0408
FAX: (215) 659-2629

728. **SAFE-WAVE PRODUCTS, INC.**
320 Dungate Drive
St. Louis, MO 63017
(314) 569-0808
FAX: (314) 434-2704

729. **SALVIN DENTAL SPECIALTIES**
6723 Colony Road
Charlotte, NC 28226
(800) 535-6566
(704) 542-1700
FAX: (704) 541-0097

730. **SANTA BARBARA MEDCO**
6483 Calle Real
Suite B
Goleta, CA 93117
(800) 346-3326
(805) 683-1486

731. **SAVAGE LABORATORIES**
60 Baylis Road
Melville, NY 11747
(800) 231-0206
(516) 454-9071
FAX: (516) 420-1572

732. **SCHEIN, HENRY INC.**
5 Harbor Park Drive
Port Washington, NY 11050
(800) 772-4346
(516) 621-4300
FAX: (516) 621-4300 ext. 4350

733. **SCHUSTER, DR. MICHAEL**
Center for Professional Development
7272 East Indian School Road
Suite #100
Scottsdale, AZ 85251
(800) 288-9393
(602) 941-9393
FAX: (602) 970-2494

734. **SCHUTZ-DENTAL GmbH**
Homburger Straße 64
D-6365 Rossbach I
Germany
(06003) 814-0
FAX: (06003) 321-7

735. **SCHWED, CHARLES B. CO., INC.**
138 Audley Street
Kew Gardens, NY 11418
(800) 847-4073
(718) 441-0526
FAX: (718) 441-4507

736. **SCICAN**
260 Yorkland Boulevard
Toronto, Ontario
Canada M2J 1R7
(800) 667-7733
(416) 491-5000
FAX: (416) 491-5040

737. **SCIENTIFIC PHARMACEUTICALS**
3221 Producer Way
Pamona, CA 91768
(800) 634-3047
(714) 595-9922
FAX: (714) 595-0331

738. **SCIENTIFIC SERVICES**
P.O. Box 698
Chester, SC 29706
(803) 385-2135
FAX: (803) 385-2137

739. **SCM MEDICAL**
P.O. Box 3855
Cherry Hill, NJ 08034
(800) 338-2707
(609) 427-0808
FAX: (609) 795-7157

740. **SCOTT ALL-SPORTS, INC.**
120 Professional Drive
West Monroe, LA 71291
(318) 322-1500
FAX: (318) 322-9714

741. **S.D.I. GROUP, INC.**
742 Central Avenue
Deerfield, IL 60015
(800) 227-8507
(708) 405-0030
FAX: (708) 405-0199

742. **SELECT CARE PRODUCTS**
P.O. Box 251
Woodland Hills, CA 91365
(800) 541-3347
(818) 716-1757
FAX: (818) 718-2974

743. **SEMANTODONTICS, INC.**
(Mfr. name change. See Smart Practice)

744. **SEPTODONT**
245-C Quigley Boulevard
New Castle, DE 19720
(800) 872-8305
(302) 328-1102
FAX: (302) 328-5653

745. **SHAKLEE CORP.**
444 Market Street
San Francisco, CA 94111
(415) 954-3000
FAX: (415) 986-0808

746. **SHERWOOD MEDICAL**
1915 Olive Street
St. Louis, MO 63103
(800) 325-7472
(314) 621-7788
FAX: (314) 241-3127

747. **SHOFU DENTAL CORP.**
4025 Bohannon Drive
Menlo Park, CA 94025
(800) 827-4638
(415) 324-0085
FAX: (415) 323-3180

748. **SHORNEYS OPTICAL**
1849 Yonge Street
Toronto, Ontario
Canada M4S 1Y2
(416) 488-1127

749. **SHYWAR MANAGEMENT CORP.**
2095 Kingston Road
Scarborough, Ontario
Canada, M1M 1P1
(416) 265-1400
FAX: (416) 785-7301

750. **SILVERMAN'S DENTAL SUP., INC.**
420 Feheley Drive
King of Prussia, PA 19406
(800) 448-3384
(215) 272-3500
FAX: (215) 272-8770

751. **SIME HEALTH LTD.**
1200 Sixth Avenue South
Seattle, WA 98134
(800) 726-8205
(206) 622-9596
FAX: (206) 622-9872

752. **SIMPLEX EQUIPMENT CORP.**
13535 Southeast Beech
Milwaukie, OR 97267
(800) 462-4823
(503) 654-0466

753. **SIMPLIFIED SYSTEMS, INC.**
4014 Chase Avenue, Suite PH
Miami Beach, FL 33140
(800) 888-0900
(305) 672-7676
FAX: (305) 531-5339

754. **SMART MOUTH, THE**
(See The Smart Mouth)

755. **SMART PRACTICE**
P.O. Box 29222
Phoenix, AZ 85038
(800) 522-0800
(602) 225-9090
FAX: (800) 522-8329

756. **SMITHKLINE BEECHAM**
1500 Spring Garden Street
Philidelphia, PA 19101
(800) 366-8900
(215) 751-5644
FAX: (215) 751-3400

757. **SMITH & NEPHEW, MPL**
Division of Smith & Nephew, Inc.
9400 King Street
Franklin Park, IL 60131
(800) 621-6421
(708) 678-7555
FAX: (708) 678-7585

758. **SMITH & NEPHEW PERRY**
1875 Harsh Avenue Southeast
Massilion, OH 44646
(800) 321-9752
(216) 833-2811
FAX: (216) 833-5991

759. **SOLID STATE INNOVATION, INC.**
1007 Rockford Street
Mt. Airy, NC 27030
(800) 346-4112
(919) 789-5767

760. **SONIX IV**
17622 Metzler Lane
Huntington Beach, CA 92647
(800) 878-2769
(714) 842-7622
FAX: (714) 843-1867

761. **SOUTHERN DENTAL ASSOC.**
P.O. Box 36972
Birmingham, AL 35236
(205) 985-9488
FAX: (205) 733-1006

762. **SOUTHERN DENTAL IND. LTD**
5-9 Brundson Street, Bayswater
P.O. Box 314
Victoria, Australia 3153
(800) 228-5166 (USA only)
011-61-3-729-9088
FAX: 0-11-61-3-720-2435

763. **SOUTH WADSWORTH DENTAL LAB**
1360 South Wadsworth
Lakewood, CO 80226
(303) 989-0337

764. **SPARTAN CHEMICAL CO., INC.**
110 North Westwood Avenue
P.O. Box 3495
Toledo, OH 43607
(800) 537-8990
(419) 531-5551

765. **SPARTAN U.S.A., INC.**
1725 Larkin Williams Road
Fenton, MO 63026
(800) 325-9027
(314) 343-8300
FAX: (314) 343-5794

766. **SPECIAL PRODUCTS, INC.**
102 Western Court
Santa Cruz, CA 95060
(800) 538-6836
(408) 425-0240
FAX: (408) 425-8565

767. **SPORICIDIN INT'L.**
5901 Montrose Road
Rockville, MD 20852
(800) 424-3733
(301) 231-7700
FAX: (301) 231-8165

768. **SPRING HEALTH PRODUCTS**
501 South Main Street
Spring City, PA 19475
(800) 800-1680
(215) 948-8141
FAX: (215) 948-8151

769. **SPRING WHITE CO.**
(Mfr. name change. See Spring Health Products)

770. **S.S. WHITE BURS, INC.**
1145 Towbin Avenue
Lakewood, NJ 08701
(800) 535-2877
(908) 905-1100
FAX: (908) 905-0987

771. **STAHMER, WESTON & CO., INC.**
602 Park Point Drive
Golden, CO 80401
(800) 423-7188
(303) 526-5520
FAX: (303) 526-1143

772. **STAR DENTAL**
(See Den-Tal-EZ Inc.)

773. **STARDENT LABORATORIES**
6510 South Cottonwood Street
Murray, UT 84107
(800) 678-1162
(801) 264-8952
FAX: (801) 261-3171

774. **STAR X-RAY**
63 Ranick Drive
Amityville, NY 11701
(516) 842-3010
FAX: (516) 842-5901

775. **STEINMAN SERVICES INC.**
237 North Main Street
Edwardsville, IL 62025
(618) 692-0818
FAX: (618) 656-8856

776. **STEPPING STONES TO SUCCESS**
1311-A Jerry Murphy Road
Pueblo, CO 81001
(800) 548-2164
(719) 545-0511

777. **STERI-DENT CORP.**
1330-13 Lincoln Avenue
Lincoln Towers
Holbrook, NY 11741
(516) 737-4646
FAX: (516) 737-0036

778. **STERI-DERM CORP.**
1723 Cypress Point Glen
Escondido, CA 92026
(619) 746-5017
FAX: (619) 738-6904

779. **STERI-OSS INC.**
901 East Cerritos Avenue
Anaheim, CA 92805
(800) 854-9316
(714) 776-9000
FAX: (714) 776-9044

780. **STERI-SAFE INC.**
P.O. Box 3059
New Haven, CT 06515
(203) 776-7233

781. **STERI-SHIELD PRODUCTS, INC.**
122 Industrial Drive
Ivyland, PA 18974
(800) 446-0041
FAX: (215) 355-5360

782. **STERLING-WINTHROP**
90 Allstate Parkway
Markham, Ontario
Canada L3R 6H3
(800) 668-7406 (Canada)
(416) 513-4444
FAX: (416) 513-6137

783. **STER-O-LIZER MFG. CORP.**
2109 West 2300 South
Salt Lake City, UT 84119
(801) 973-6400
FAX: (801) 973-6463

784. **STICK BRICK**
1524 Trafalgar Road
Ft. Worth, TX 76116

785. **STIRN INDUSTRIES**
Forsgate Technical Center
1095 Cranbury South River Road
P.O. Box 407
Dayton, NJ 08810
(609) 655-7500
FAX: (609) 655-4499

786. **STOUT, DR. KENNETH**
(Mfr. name change. See Chesheim Dental Associates)

787. **STRATFORD-COOKSON CO.**
904 Orlando Avenue
West Hempstead, NY 11552
(800) 241-5984
(516) 794-4920
FAX: (516) 683-0006

788. **STRAUMANN CO., THE**
(See The Straumann Co.)

789. **STRONG DENTAL PRODUCTS**
P.O. Box 2755
Saratoga, CA 95070
(800) 648-9729
(408) 376-0614
FAX: (408) 866-7034

790. **STRYKER DENTAL IMPLANTS**
420 Alcott Street
Kalamazoo, MI 49001
(800) 666-8603
(616) 381-3811
FAX: (800) 999-3811

791. **STUART PHARMACEUTICALS**
(See Coe Laboratories)

792. **SULCABRUSH INC.**
Canadian Head Office
45 Brisbane Road #10
Downsview, Ontario
Canada M3J 2K1
(800) 387-8777
(416) 665-0716
FAX: (416) 665-0893

793. **SULCABRUSH INC.**
U.S. address
908 Niagara Falls Boulevard
North Tonawanda, NY 14120

794. **SULTAN CHEMISTS, INC.**
85 West Forest Avenue
Englewood, NJ 07631
(800) 637-8582
(201) 871-1232
FAX: (201) 871-0321

795. **SUNBEAM HOME COMFORT**
P.O. Box 70
Highway 49 North
Hattilesburg, MS 39401
(601) 268-2880
FAX: (601) 268-2880

796. **SUPERPHARM CORP.**
1769 5th Avenue
Bayshore, NY 11706
(516) 434-4800
FAX: (516) 434-3188

797. **SUPER TOOTH PRODUCTS, INC.**
2629 Louisiana Avenue South
Minneapolis, MN 55426
(800) 522-7883
(612) 926-5324
FAX: (612) 926-6331

798. **SUTER DENTAL MFG. CO., INC.**
632 Cedar Street
Chico, CA 95928
(916) 893-8376
FAX: (916) 893-0473

799. **SYNAPSE DENTAL INFO. SYST.**
P.O. Box 882
Perrysburg, OH 43551
(419) 874-5419

T

800. **TACO DENTAL, INC.**
71 Northwest Drive
P.O. Box 338
Plainville, CT 06062
(203) 747-5597
FAX: (203) 747-5596

801. **TAKEDA MEDICAL**
(See A & D Engineering)

802. **TAK SYSTEMS**
P.O. Box 648
East Wareham, MA 02538
(800) 333-9631
(508) 295-9630
FAX: (508) 291-3240

803. **TALLADIUM, INC.**
25031 Anza Drive
Valencia, CA 91355
(800) 221-6449
(805) 295-0900
FAX: (805) 295-0895

804. **TANAKA DENTAL**
5135 Golf Road
Skokie, IL 60077
(800) 325-5266
(708) 679-1610
FAX: (708) 674-5761

805. **TARA CROWN, INC.**
80 Boylston Street
Suite 905
Boston, MA 02116
(800) 523-8272
(617) 423-4713
FAX: (800) 523-8272

806. **TAUB, GEORGE PRODUCTS**
277 New York Avenue
Jersey City, NJ 07307
(201) 798-5353
FAX: (201) 659-7186

807. **TAYLOR, DR. DONALD E.**
7509 Cantrell Road, Suite 208
Little Rock, AR 72207
(501) 664-3279

808. **TECH CHEM INC.**
Route 2 Box 209
West Highway 32
Stockton, MO 65785
(800) 852-5641
(417) 276-5154
FAX: (417) 276-5742

809. **TECHNICRAFT INDUSTRIES, INC.**
Plaza Terrace Office Building
445 East 2nd South, Suite 308
Salt Lake City, UT 84111
(801) 363-8537
FAX: (801) 521-5494

810. **TECHNOLOGY UNLIMITED, INC.**
146 South Bever Street
P.O. Box 723
Wooster, OH 44691
(216) 262-3600
FAX: (216) 264-5464

811. **TECNOL, INC.**
7201 Industrial Park Boulevard
Fort Worth, TX 76180
(800) 832-6651
(817) 581-6424
FAX: (817) 581-9354

812. **TEKSCAN INC.**
451 "D" Street
Boston, MA 02210
(800) 248-3669
(617) 737-8734
FAX: (617) 737-2763

813. **TELEDYNE GETZ**
1550 Greenleaf Avenue
Elk Grove Village, IL 60007
(800) 323-6650
(708) 593-3334
FAX: (708) 593-0569

814. **TELEDYNE HANAU**
80 Sonwil Drive
Buffalo, NY 14225
(800) 457-1700
(716) 684-0110
FAX: (716) 684-5155

815. **TELEDYNE/WATER PIK**
1730 East Prospect Street
Fort Collins, CO 80525
(800) 525-2020
(303) 484-1352
FAX: (303) 221-8715

816. **TEMKET, INC.**
5000 South East End Avenue
Chicago, IL 60615
(800) 932-0038
(312) 493-7976
FAX: (312) 288-5700

817. **TEMREX**
112 Albany Avenue
P.O. Box 182
Freeport, NY 11520
(800) 645-1226
(516) 868-6221
FAX: (516) 868-5700

818. **TENSOR LIGHTING CO.**
100 Justin Drive
Chelsea, MA 02150
(800) 872-5267
(617) 884-7744
FAX: (617) 889-2785

819. **TETRAHEDRON, INC.**
P.O. Box 402
Rockport, MA 01966
(800) 336-9266
(508) 546-6586
FAX: (508) 546-9226

820. **TEXELL PRODUCTS CO.**
3 Asbury Place
Houston, TX 77007
(713) 861-8121

821. **THE BRULIN CORP.**
2920 Dr. Andrew J. Brown Avenue
P.O. Box 270
Indianapolis, IN 46206
(800) 776-7149
(317) 923-3211
FAX: (317) 925-4596

822. **THE DIAL CORP.**
Headquarters Office
1850 North Central
Phoenix, AZ 85077
(800) 528-0849
(602) 207-4000

823. **THE DIAL CORP.**
Research Facility
15101 North Scottsdale Road
Scottsdale, AZ 85254
(800) 660-2018
(602) 991-3000
FAX: (602) 998-6336

824. **THE EVELYN COMPANY, INC.**
P.O. Box 35265
Tulsa, OK 74153
(800) 221-0518
(918) 250-5664

825. **THE HYGENIC CORP.**
1245 Home Avenue
Akron, OH 44310
(800) 321-2135
(216) 633-8460
FAX: (800) 633-7331

826. **THE MEDICAL LETTER, INC.**
1000 Main Street
New Rochelle, NY 10801
(914) 235-0500
FAX: (914) 576-3377

827. **THE MOTLOID CO.**
730 West Lake Street
Chicago, IL 60661
(800) 662-5021
(312) 648-2240
FAX: (312) 648-0319

828. **THE PASS-IT CO.**
P.O. Box 5892
Beaverton, OR 97006
(800) 346-8522
(503) 646-8522

829. **THERMAFIL**
5001 East 68th
Suite 500
Tulsa, OK 74136
(800) 662-1202
(918) 493-6598
FAX: (918) 493-6599

830. **THE ROWLAND CO.**
1675 Broadway
New York, NY 10019
(212) 527-8870
FAX: (212) 527-8989

831. **THE SMART MOUTH**
A Division of Nuperco, Inc.
P.O. Box 689
799 Franklin Avenue
Franklin Lakes, NJ 07417
(800) 672-3368
(201) 891-7027
FAX: (201) 891-0705

832. **THE STRAUMANN CO.**
One Alewife Center
Cambridge, MA 02140
(800) 448-8168
(617) 868-3800
FAX: (617) 868-9111

833. **THE WILKINSON CO.**
31011 Agoura Road Box 4558
Westlake Village, CA 91359
(800) 822-4653
(818) 889-0050
FAX: (818) 889-3810

834. **THE ZOO**
Route 2 Box 2086
Melrose, FL 32666
(904) 475-3357
FAX: (904) 378-6604

835. **THIERMAN PRODUCTS, INC.**
P.O. Box 435
Washougal, WA 98671
(503) 286-1158

836. **THM BIOMEDICAL INC./OSMED**
325 South Lake Avenue
Suite 608
Duluth, MN 55802
(800) 327-6895
(218) 720-3628
FAX: (218) 720-3715

837. **THOMPSON DENTAL MFG. CO.**
1201 South 6th West
P.O. Box 2902
Missoula, MT 59806
(800) 622-4222
(406) 728-0000
(406) 728-4885

838. **TIDI PRODUCTS, INC.**
P.O. Box 2150
360 South Lilac
Rialta, CA 92376
(800) 225-8434
(714) 421-0600
FAX: (714) 421-0808

839. **TIGER DENTAL MFG.**
Louisiana State Univ. Med. Ctr.
1100 Florida Avenue
New Orleans, LA 70119
(504) 948-8543

840. **TILLOTSON RUBBER CO./HPI INC.**
360 Route 101
Bedford, NH 03110
(800) 445-6830
(603) 472-6600
FAX: (603) 472-5151

841. **TIME DENTAL PRODUCTS**
1020 Timbertrail Road
Towson, MD 21204
(800) 441-5107
(301) 321-1363

842. **T K ENTERPRISES, INC.**
P.O. Box 7554
Menlo Park, CA 94026
(415) 854-9276
FAX: (415) 854-8011

843. **TOOTH SLOOTH**
(see Professional Results, Inc./
Tooth Slooth)

844. **TP ORTHODONTICS, INC.**
100 Center Plaza
P.O. Box 73
La Porte, IN 46350
(800) 348-8856
(219) 785-2591
FAX: (219) 324-3029

845. **TRIDENT DENTAL, INC.**
116 Lakeview Drive
Summerville, SC 29485
(803) 875-1500
FAX: (803) 875-9230

846. **TRI-DYNAMICS DENTAL CO., INC.**
616 Hollywood Avenue
Cherry Hill, NJ 08002
(800) 333-3131
(609) 663-4700
FAX: (609) 663-0381

847. **TRI HAWK CORP.**
849 South Broadway #811
Los Angeles, CA 90014
(800) 874-4295
(213) 622-0143
FAX: (213) 622-6962

848. **TROJAN RESEARCH & DEV.**
15500 Erwin Street
Suite 1021
Van Nuys, CA 91411
(800) 777-8102
(818) 908-5301
FAX: (818) 908-5341

849. **TROLLPLAST INC.**
P.O. Box 1703
New Milford, CT 06776
(800) 537-8765
(203) 775-4342
FAX: (203) 775-8385

850. **TSUMURA MEDICAL**
1000 Valley Park Drive
Shakopee, MN 55379
(800) 345-8084
(612) 448-4181
FAX: (612) 496-4747

851. **TULSA DENTAL PRODUCTS**
(Mfr. name change. See Thermafil)

852. **TURBINE INDUSTRIES, INC.**
10217 Buena Vista Avenue
Suite A
Santee, CA 92071
(800) 443-4812
(619) 258-4060
FAX: (619) 449-4346

853. **TUTTNAUER CO. LTD.**
1 Comac Loop
Ronkonkoma, NY 11779
(800) 624-5836
(516) 737-4850/4851
FAX: (516) 737-0720

U

854. **ULTRADENT PRODUCTS, INC.**
1345 East 3900 South
Salt Lake City, UT 84124
(800) 552-5512
(801) 277-3203
FAX: (801) 272-6716

855. **ULTRA LITE, INC.**
P.O. Box 2655
Orange Park, FL 32067
(800) 234-1557
(904) 272-1588

856. **UNION BROACH CORP.**
1212 Ave. of the Americas, 24th Floor
New York, NY 10036
(800) 221-1344
(212) 398-0700
FAX: (212) 398-0884

857. **UNITED SERVICE DENTAL CHAIR UPHOLSTERERS, INC.**
5669 147th Street North
Hugo, MN 55038
(800) 328-9689
(612) 429-8660

858. **UNITEK CORP./3M**
2724 South Peck Road
Monrovia, CA 91016
(800) 423-4588
(818) 445-7960
FAX: (818) 574-4500

859. **UNIVERSAL DENTAL ARTS**
2460 West 26th Avenue
Suite 40C
Denver, CO 80211
(303) 477-0003

860. **UNIVERSAL DENTAL IMPLEMENTS**
Oak Tree Business Center
906-B Oak Tree Road
South Plainfield, NJ 07080
(908) 754-8882

861. **UNIVERSAL MODEL-TRIMMER SHIELD**
45 Lottie Bennett Lane #5
San Francisco, CA 94115
(415) 346-9534

862. **UNIVERSITY OF PENNSYLVANIA SDM**
4001 Spruce Street
Philidelphia, PA 19104
(215) 898-5155
FAX: (215) 898-5243

863. **UPJOHN CO.**
7000 Portage Road
Kalamazoo, MI 49001
(800) 253-8600
(616) 323-4000
FAX: (616) 323-4077

864. **UP-RAD CORP.**
P.O. Box 163
Chewsville, MD 21721
(800) 327-8879
(301) 739-4556
FAX: (301) 739-4557

865. **USA DENTAL PRODUCTS, INC.**
11860 Magnolia #R
P.O. Box 201
Riverside, CA 92503
(800) 527-0393
(714) 359-3434
FAX: (714) 359-3008

866. **U.S. PHARMACOPEIA**
12601 Twinbrook Parkway
Rockville, MD 20852
(800) 227-8772
(301) 881-0666
FAX: (301) 816-8148

867. **U.S. SHIZAI CORP.**
2719 Wilshire Boulevard
Suite 201
Santa Monica, CA 90404
(800) 421-8501
(213) 820-7710
FAX: (213) 453-8049

V

868. **VANGUARD-HANDGUARD, INC.**
P.O. Box 652
Sterling Heights, MI 48311
(313) 977-0300

869. **VAN R DENTAL PRODUCTS INC.**
600 Hueneme Road
Oxnard, CA 93033
(800) 833-8267
(805) 488-1122
FAX: (800) 444-5170

870. **VERATEX CORP.**
1304 East Maple Road
P.O. Box 4031
Troy, MI 48083
(800) 521-2640
(313) 588-2970
FAX: (313) 588-1779

871. **VERMONT DIAMOND INSTRUMENTS, INC.**
River Road
P.O. Box 147
Bridge Corners, VT 05035
(800) 762-7689
(802) 672-3120
FAX: (802) 672-3127

872. **VIADENT, INC.**
1625 Sharp Point Drive
Fort Collins, CO 80525
(800) 842-3368
(303) 482-3126
FAX: (303) 482-0328

873. **VICON FIBER OPTICS CORP.**
90 Secor Lane
Pelham Manor, NY 10803
(914) 738-5006
FAX: (914) 738-6920

874. **VIC POLLARD DENTAL PROD., INC.**
755 Lakefield Road
Unit K
WestLake Village, CA 91361
(800) 235-1849
(800) 521-6939 (CA)
(805) 495-5222
FAX: (805) 379-3273

875. **VIDENT**
5130 Commerce Drive
Baldwin Park, CA 91706
(800) 828-3839
(818) 960-7531
FAX: (818) 962-4220

876. **VIKING ENGINEERING CO.**
P.O. Box 68
111 East Fayett
Pittsfield, IL 62363
(217) 285-4021

877. **VIPONT PHARMACEUTICAL, INC.**
1625 Sharp Point Drive
Fort Collins, CO 80525
(800) 962-2345
(303) 482-3126
FAX: (303) 482-0328

878. **V.I.R. ENGINEERING, INC.**
5580 Calle Real
Santa Barbara, CA 93111
(805) 964-0553
FAX: (805) 964-9588

879. **VISUAL HORIZONS**
180 Metro Park
Rochester, NY 14623
(716) 424-5300
FAX: (716) 424-5313

880. **VOCO GmbH**
Baudirektor-Hahn-StraBe 4
D-2190 Cuxhaven
Germany POB 767
49-4721/21045
FAX: 49-4721/61932

W

881. **WALDMANN LIGHTING CO.**
9 West Century Drive
Wheeling, IL 60090
(800) 634-0007
(708) 520-1060
FAX: (708) 520-1730

882. **WALKER ENTERPRISES**
2600 East Southern B1
Tempe, AZ 85282
(602) 839-4550

883. **WALL STREET CAMERA**
82 Wall Street
New York, NY 10005
(800) 221-4090
(212) 344-0011
FAX: (212) 425-5999

884. **WARNER-LAMBERT CO.**
201 Tabor Road
Morris Plains, NJ 07950
(800) 336-0567
(201) 540-6749
FAX: (201) 540-4400

885. **WASHINGTON SCIENTIFIC CAMERA CO., INC.**
615 Wood Avenue
Sumner, WA 98390
(206) 863-2854

886. **WEISSMAN TECH. INT'L., INC.**
192 Lexington Ave., Suite 901
New York, NY 10016
(800) 323-3136
(212) 481-1010
FAX: (212) 532-9026

887. **WESTERMAN, DR. ROBERT D.**
7931 Jefferson Highway
Baton Rouge, LA 70809
(504) 927-3442

888. **WESTERN M/D INC.**
1320 Marsten Road
Burlingame, CA 94010
(415) 343-1816
FAX: (415) 343-1816

889. **WESTNOFA USA, INC.**
7040 North Austin Avenue
Niles, IL 60648
(708) 647-7415
FAX: (708) 647-7715

890. **WESTONE LABORATORIES, INC.**
P.O. Box 15100
Colorado Springs, CO 80935
(800) 525-5071
(719) 634-8817
FAX: (719) 634-0563

891. **WESTPORT PHARMACEUTICALS INC.**
(Mfr. name change. See Gebauer Co.)

892. **WEST TEC INDUSTRIES, INC.**
224 West Plymouth Avenue #3
Salt Lake City, UT 84115
(801) 261-5421

893. **WHIP MIX CORP.**
361 Farmington Avenue
P.O. Box 17183
Louisville, KY 40217
(800) 626-5651
(502) 637-1451
FAX: (502) 634-4512

894. **WHITCOMB, DR. KENNETH R.**
4333 Palm Avenue, Suite C
La Mesa, CA 91941
(619) 461-6166

895. **WHITE GAPS**
3424 North First Street
#4500
Abilene, TX 79603
(800) 456-2272
(915) 672-8537
FAX: (915) 672-8532

896. **WHITELEY CHEMCIAL AUSTRALIA PTY. LTD.**
Medical Products Division
82-84 Ivy Street
Chippendale, New South Whales
Australia 2008
011-61-008-257352
011-61-2-699-1811
FAX: 011-61-2-698-2369

897. **WHITE, S.S. BURS, INC.**
(See S.S. White Burs, Inc.)

898. **WILKINSON CO., THE**
(See The Wilkinson Co.)

899. **WILLIAMS**
(A Division of Ivoclar North America)
175 Pineview Drive
Amherst, NY 14228
(800) 533-6825
(716) 691-0010
FAX: (716) 691-2285

900. **WINTHROP PHARMACEUTICALS**
90 Park Avenue
New York, NY 10016
(800) 446-6287
(212) 907-2000

901. **WISCONSIN DENTAL ASSOC.,**
633 West Wisconsin Avenue
Suite 507
Milwaukee, WI 53203
(800) 243-4675
(414) 276-4520
FAX: (414) 276-8431

902. **W.L. GORE & ASSOC., INC.**
3773 Kaspar Avenue
P.O. Box 2500
Flagstaff, AZ 86003
(800) 528-1866
(602) 526-3030
FAX: (602) 526-3878

903. **WOLFE PUBLISHING LTD.**
Brook House
2-16 Torrington Place
London WC1E 7LT
England
071-636-4622
FAX: 071-637-3021

904. **WORLDWIDE DENTAL, INC.**
3734-131 Avenue North
Suite 15
Clearwater, FL 34622
(800) 328-2335
(813) 541-3496
FAX: (813) 541-3496

905. **WYETH AYERST**
31 Morehall Road
Frazer, PA 19355
(215) 644-8000

906. **WYKLE RESEARCH, INC.**
2222 Hot Springs Road
Carson City, NV 89706
(800) 854-6641
(702) 887-7500
FAX: (702) 882-7952

907. **WYNMAN, WILBUR E.**
284 South Temelec Circle
Sanoma, CA 95476
(707) 996-4881

X

908. **X-RAY VISION, INC.**
5151 South Federal Boulevard
Littleton, CO 80123
(303) 795-1107

909. **X-RITE, INC.**
3100 44th Street, Southwest
Grandville, MI 49418
(616) 534-7663
FAX: (616) 534-9212

910. **XTTRIUM LABORATORIES**
415 West Pershing Road
Chicago, IL 60609
(312) 268-5800
FAX: (312) 924-6002

Y

911. **YARTER-TEK CORP.**
Dental Products Division
P.O. Box 38001
Denver, CO 80238
(303) 320-4500
FAX: (303) 399-6558

912. **YATES & BIRD**
730 West Lake Street
Chicago, IL 60661
(800) 662-5021
(312) 648-2150
FAX: (312) 648-0319

913. **YOUNG DENTAL**
13705 Shoreline Court East
Earth City, MO 63045
(800) 325-1881
(314) 344-0010
FAX: (314) 344-0021

914. **YOUNGER OPTICS**
3788 South Broadway Place
P.O. Box 77932
Los Angeles, CA 90007
(800) 421-2920
(213) 232-2345
FAX: (213) 232-2136

Z

915. **ZAHNARZT**
Tegernseer Landstrasse 62
8000 Muchen 90
Germany
011-49-697-3545
FAX: 011-49-651-7692

916. **ZEISS, CARL, INC.**
One Zeiss Drive
Thornwood, NY 10594
(800) 522-5204
(914) 747-1800
FAX: (914) 681-7409

917. **ZENITH DENTAL**
242 South Dean
Englewood, NJ 07631
(201) 894-5500
FAX: (201) 894-0213

918. **ZEST ANCHORS, INC.**
2061 Wineridge Place
Suite 100
Escondido, CA 92029
(619) 743-7744
FAX: (619) 743-7975

919. **ZEZA, INC.**
5400 South University Drive
Suite 103
Davie, FL 33328
(800) 527-8937
(305) 680-2566
FAX: (305) 680-9275

920. **ZILA® PHARMACEUTICALS**
5227 North 7th Street
Phoenix, AZ 85014
(602) 266-6700
FAX: (602) 234-2264

921. **ZIMMERMAN ENTERPRISES**
11416 Slater Avenue Northeast
Suite 101
Kirkland, WA 98034
(206) 822-8248

922. **ZINMAN, DR. EDWIN J.**
220 Bush Street
Suite 1600
San Francisco, CA 94104
(415) 391-5353
FAX: (415) 391-0768

923. **ZIRC CO.**
14420 21st Avenue North
Minneapolis, MN 55447
(800) 328-3899
(612) 475-2334
FAX: (612) 475-0401

924. **ZOO, THE**
(See The Zoo)

INDEX

Wire bending instrument, 334
Work authorization, ceramometal restoration and, 96
Working time, glass ionomer cement and, 70
Wrinkling
    collagen implant for, 382-383
    perioral, 396, 397, 405

XP-Primer, 17

Yashica cameras, 248-250
Yellow, 27
Yellow Pages advertising, 414
Yellow-brown, 27

20568